Bread and Its Fortification

Nutrition and Health Benefits

Food Biology Series

Bread and Its Fortification
Nutrition and Health Benefits

Editors

Cristina M. Rosell
Food Science Department
Institute of Agrochemistry and Food Technology
Avda Agustín Escardino
Paterna, Valencia
Spain

Joanna Bajerska
Department of Human Nutrition and Hygiene
Poznan University of Life Sciences
Poznań
Poland

Aly F. El Sheikha
Department of Biology
Al-Baha University
Al-Baha
Saudi Arabia

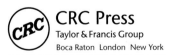

CRC Press
Taylor & Francis Group
Boca Raton London New York

CRC Press is an imprint of the
Taylor & Francis Group, an **informa** business

A SCIENCE PUBLISHERS BOOK

CRC Press
Taylor & Francis Group
6000 Broken Sound Parkway NW, Suite 300
Boca Raton, FL 33487-2742

First issued in paperback 2021

ISBN-13: 978-1-4987-0156-3 (hbk)
ISBN-13: 978-1-03-217963-6 (pbk)
DOI: 10.1201/b18918

Publisher's Note

The publisher has gone to great lengths to ensure the quality of this reprint but points out that some imperfections in the original copies may be apparent.

Visit the Taylor & Francis Web site at
http://www.taylorandfrancis.com

and the CRC Press Web site at
http://www.crcpress.com

Preface to the Series

Food is the essential source of nutrients (such as carbohydrates, proteins, fats, vitamins, and minerals) for all living organisms to sustain life. A large part of daily human efforts is concentrated on food production, processing, packaging and marketing, product development, preservation, storage, and ensuring food safety and quality. It is obvious therefore, our food supply chain can contain microorganisms that interact with the food, thereby interfering in the ecology of food substrates. The microbe-food interaction can be mostly beneficial (as in the case of many fermented foods such as cheese, butter, sausage, etc.) or in some cases, it is detrimental (spoilage of food, mycotoxin, etc.). The *Food Biology* series aims at bringing all these aspects of microbe-food interactions in form of topical volumes, covering food microbiology, food mycology, biochemistry, microbial ecology, food biotechnology and bio-processing, new food product developments with microbial interventions, food nutrification with nutraceuticals, food authenticity, food origin traceability, and food science and technology. Special emphasis is laid on new molecular techniques relevant to food biology research or to monitoring and assessing food safety and quality, multiple hurdle food preservation techniques, as well as new interventions in biotechnological applications in food processing and development.

The series is broadly broken up into food fermentation, food safety and hygiene, food authenticity and traceability, microbial interventions in food bio-processing and food additive development, sensory science, molecular diagnostic methods in detecting food borne pathogens and food policy, etc. Leading international authorities with background in academia, research, industry and government have been drawn into the series either as authors or as editors. The series will be a useful reference resource base in food microbiology, biochemistry, biotechnology, food science and technology for researchers, teachers, students and food science and technology practitioners.

Ramesh C. Ray
Series Editor

Preface

There is evidence that unleavened bread existed 9,000 years ago. Later (around 3,500 BC) the ancient Egyptians made the bread. From that time the heritage of bread, its economical, political and religious importance has persisted worldwide. Bread has changed in many ways since our ancestors, going from grainy flat bread to an aerated texture. Bread is the product of fermenting and baking a mixture of whole meal or refined flour, water, salt, and yeast or baking powder, as the basic ingredients. Bread provides over half of the caloric intake of the world's population including a high proportion of the intake of carbohydrates, proteins, minerals and vitamins. It is one of the largest consumed foodstuff, with an average consumption ranging from 41–303 kg/year per capita, which becomes an essential part of the human diet, enjoyed at various times of the day. Nevertheless, the term "bread" is a wide concept owing to the variety of products that can be obtained using different flours, additional ingredients and processes.

Besides the intrinsic nutritional benefits of bread owing its composition, bread can have a major role as nutrients carrier to ensure the supply and adequate intakes of nutrients as well as a healthy food. *Bread and its fortification for nutrition and health benefits* compiles the alternatives that food technologist have available for making healthy and nutritious breads understanding the role of the ingredients and processes.

After assessing the role of bread in human nutrition, the book presents the different alternatives for modulating and improving its nutritional and healthy benefits. Starting from raw commodities to the alternative ingredients currently in the market, besides the physical and chemical processes available for improving the nutritional value of bread, it discusses the raw materials and ingredients, fortification strategies, as well as safety considerations regarding bread storage and its shelf life, and health related aspects of breads like gluten in breads. In this book, innovative aspects and emerging fields have been identified, which are good examples of the driving forces in the bread market considering the nutrition and health concerns of consumers.

This book is intended to cover all aspect that could have an impact in the nutritional and health benefits of bread. We feel, the book is essential for research scientists, regulatory authorities, food chemists and technologists, dieticians, industrial bakers, academics and to the general public interested in nutrition.

Editors would like to thank all contributors for their excellent and critical revision to show the state of the art of the nutrition and health benefits of bread. Editors would like also to thank Dr. Ramesh C. Ray, the Series Editor, for inviting the editors for editing this book within CRC-FOOD BIOLOGY series.

February 2015

Cristina M. Rosell
Joanna Bajerska
Aly F. El Sheikha

Contents

1

Bread: Between the Heritage of Past and the Technology of Present

Aly F. El Sheikha[a,b]

1. Introduction

Around 7000 BC humans (probably the Egyptians) somehow learned to grind grains in water and heat the mix on hot stoves to make unleavened bread. Later (around 3500 BC) the ancient Egyptians made the bread. They made bread and beer from the two major cereals cultivated in Dynastic Egypt, emmer wheat (*Triticum dicoccum*) and six-row barley (*Hordeum vulgare* subsp. *Hexastichum*) (Bouthyette 2008). Bread was made from flour ground on grinding stones and mixed with water that was then kneaded and left to rise. The dough could be shaped in a flat loaf or baked in ceramic molds. Potsherds from bread molds are often found in the remains of ancient settlements. Figure 1, as the first photo, shows kitchen workers baking bread on a fairly large scale. The man with the large staff, while two of them standing behind him are doing two steps in the process of grinding grain. Other two bakers are work kneading the dough, and the crouching figure is reaching towards a beehive-shaped oven.[1]

"Is the bread-making technology makes forward progress?" Bakery engineers and the vendors supplying wholesale baking equipment can be justly proud of current bread-making technology. It reliably outputs loaf after loaf of consistent-quality bread at speeds that can exceed 180 pieces per minute. With the addition of automation and computer controls, such proven technology fits the needs for low-labor input and the low-margin, high-output products that populate the bread aisle. Yet the rising popularity

[a] Minufiya University, Faculty of Agriculture, Department of Food Science and Technology, 32511 Shibin El Kom, Minufiya Government, Egypt.
[b] Al-Baha University, Faculty of Sciences, Department of Biology, P.O. Box 1988, Al-Baha, Saudi Arabia.
  Email: elsheikha_aly@yahoo.com
[1] http://astromic.blogspot.com/2012/01/food-in-ancient-egypt.html

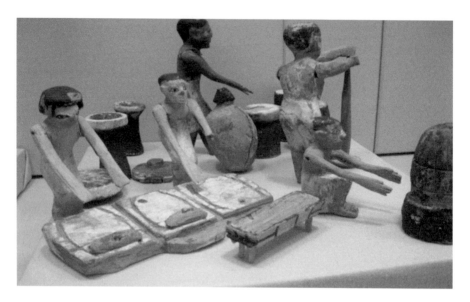

Figure 1. Kitchen workers baking bread on a fairly large scale.

of thins in sandwich bun and bagel formats, plus coiled-dough swirl breads and the attractive margins for artisan-style specialty loaves prompt the question, "Is it time to rethink bread-making technology?" The consensus of baking technology experts recently consulted by Baking & Snack was, "Yes," although they acknowledged that considerable institutional challenges exist. The opportunities are out there, particularly for high-margin and value-added products.[2]

More recently, the habit of eating bread in the form of sandwiches using European style white bread has taken hold, in particular among children. Cheese, processed, tinned or cooked meats, fried potatoes, pickled aubergines, eggs, and even bananas are some of the fillings that are used. For those who can afford them, the hamburger, pizza or the generously garnished composite modern sandwich are becoming popular (Wassef 2004).

The chapter highlights the heritage of bread and political importance. Today, bread supplies over half of the caloric intake of the world's population including a high proportion of the intake of Vitamins B and E. Bread therefore is a major food of the world. It then describes the traditional and modern technologies for bread making.

2. The history behind a loaf of bread

The bread-making process originated in ancient times. The basis of the operation is to mix flour with other ingredients, for example, water, fat, salt and some source of aeration followed by baking. The practice was to use a little old dough, or leaven, to "start" the new dough. These two doughs were mixed together and allowed to ferment

---

[2] http://www.bakingbusiness.com/News/News%20Home/Features/2011/5/Breadmaking%20
technology%20makes%20forward%20progress.aspx?cck=1

(rise) for some hours before baking. They made an astonishing 50 varieties of bread, paid wages with bread, and painted bread-making scenes in their tombs. A variety of methods have since been developed in making leaven. The Baker's Patent required the fermentation of hops and scalded malt for at least 2–3 d. In the early 1900's it was discovered that traditional long fermentation times could be reduced from 18 to 3–4 hr by the use of very small amounts of certain chemicals, called oxidants, in bread or flour. Oxidants, when added to dough, not only speed up the process but also produce a superior loaf.[3]

2.1 History of bread-making in Egypt

The Egyptians were curious why the effect of the bread 'rose' and attempted to isolate the yeast, to introduce directly into their bread. They also found that they could take a piece of dough from one batch and save it for the next day's batch of dough. This was how the origin of sour-dough came about and is a process still used today. Records also show that the Egyptians were baking bread as far back as 2500 yr ago and sometimes paid their officials with good bread.

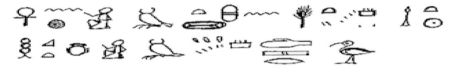

The Egyptian hieroglyphics above read: "let me live upon bread and barley of white my ale made of grain red".

Travelers took bread making techniques and moved out from the Egyptian lands; the art began spreading to all parts of Europe. As bread was valuable it was offered to the Gods such as Isis and Osiris, the protectors of grain and givers of bread. As milling processes were refined it was possible to bake whiter bread—which at that time was seen as the most valuable bread of them all. In old testament times, the evidence points to the fact that preparing the grain, making the bread and baking it, was the women's work. The bread was allowed to rise (leavened) into the shape of our familiar loaf. As the story goes, when the Israelites left Egypt in a hurry, described in the Book of Exodus in the Bible, they were prevented from allowing their bread to rise (leaven) as usual; the Jews today commemorate this event by eating unleavened bread on special occasions. The loaf of bread is 4000 yr old (approximately). The triangular loaf was one of many objects found under the foundation of Mentuhotep II's mortuary temple at Deir el Bahari in Western Thebes. Mentuhotep II reigned from c.2008 to 1957 BC. The Egyptians believed the temple was a miniature representation of the universe. The objects placed in the foundation deposits were intended to symbolically stabilize and protect the corners and the boundary walls of the temple. They believed they would be rewarded with a stable universe where there was an abundance of food such as bread.[4]

---

[3] http://www.bakeinfo.co.nz/Facts/Bread-making/
[4] http://www.dovesfarm.co.uk/about/the-history-of-bread/

2.2 The history continues with the romans

Baking flourished in the Roman Empire from as early as 300 BC but it wasn't until 168 BC that the first Bakers Guild was formed; within 150 yr there were more than three hundred specialist pastry chefs in Rome. The whole craft was incorporated in a guild of bakers—Collegium Pistorum—and was of so high repute in the affairs of the state that one of its representatives had a seat in the Senate. The ruins of Pompeii and other buried cities have revealed the kind of bakeries that existed in those historic times. The Romans enjoyed several kinds of bread, with interesting names. Lentaculum, made originally flat, round loaves made of emmer (a cereal grain closely related to wheat flour) with a bit of salt were eaten. There was also oyster bread (to be eaten with oysters); 'artolaganus' or cakebread; 'speusticus' or 'hurry bread', tin bread, Parthian bread and the Roman Style Slipper Loaf. Breads were made richer by adding milk, eggs and butter, but only the wealthy and privileged could afford these. The Egyptian grammarian and philosopher Athenaeus, who lived in the 3rd century AD, has handed down to us considerable knowledge about bread and baking in those days. He wrote: "the best bakers were from Phoenicia or Lydia, and the best bread-makers from Cappadocia". He also gave us a list of the sorts of bread common in his time; leavened loaves, unleavened loaves; loaves made from the best wheat flour; loaves made from groats, or rye, and some from acorns and millet. There were lovely crusty loaves too, loaves baked on a hearth and bread mixed with cheese, but the favorite bread of the rich was always white bread made from wheat.[4]

2.3 Bread in the Industrial Revolution

The Industrial Revolution really moved the process of bread making forwards. The first commercially successful engine did not appear until 1712 but it wasn't until the invention of the Boulton & Watt steam engine in 1786 which drove the Albion Flour mill in Battersea that the process was advanced and refined. For most of the 19th century millers continued using windmills and watermills, depending on their locations, to turn the machinery. It wasn't until 1874 that a Swiss engineer invented a new type of mill. Abandoning the use of the stone mill-wheels, he designed rollers made of steel which operated one above the other. It was called the reduction roller-milling system, and these machines soon became accepted all over Europe and in Britain.

At the time of the Industrial Revolution, the North American prairies which were ideally suited to grow wheat provided ample grain for the fast-growing population of Great Britain. This, together with the invention of the roller-milling system, meant that for the first time in history, whiter flour (and therefore bread) could be produced at a price which brought it within the reach of everyone—not just the rich.[4]

2.4 The Chorleywood bread process

In 1961 the Chorleywood Bread Process was developed, and revolutionized the way bread was made and produced. Now used to produce 80 percent of the bread in the UK it made an important impact on the domestic population.

The Chorleywood process is able to use lower protein wheat to produce bread; this development has enabled more bread to be produced in the UK where our wheat doesn't normally have high protein content (Cauvain 2007).

The process uses intensive high speed mixers to combine the flour, improvers, vegetable fat, yeast and water to make the dough. The whole process from flour to a ready loaf can be done in about 3½ hr. This is able to happen because introducing a number of high speed mixes the fermentation period quickens it up, making each loaf much faster. It is also important that the solid fats are used; this is because it's used to provide structure to the loaf during baking otherwise it would collapse.

This process can't be done in a normal kitchen because of the equipment required. The dough then needs to be shaken violently for around three minutes. This requires a lot of energy and the heat given off helps the dough to rise. The air pressure in the mixer headspace is maintained at a partial vacuum to prevent the gas bubbles in the dough from getting too large and creating an unwanted "open" structure in the finished crumb.

Once finished the dough is sliced and left to 'recover' for about eight minutes. After being placed in its tins it sits for about an hour. At this time it's very important to regulate the humidity and temperature of its local environment. After the time is up the bread is baked for around 20 minutes at 400 °F and then moved to cool down. After about two hours it's ready to be sliced, packaged and sent out.

Bread consumption has declined by half per person since 1960. If this were merely a consequence of affluence and the broadening of the national diet, there would be no problem. But for those who replace bread with foods high in saturated fats and refined sugars, the consequence may be seen in the ongoing epidemics of obesity, diabetes and coronary heart disease. Nutritional advice is that cereals, especially whole grains, should be a key component of a balanced diet (Cauvain 2007).

3. International experiences in bread industry

3.1 African (Egyptian) experience

The loaf of bread is considered one of the main diet components on the table of the Egyptian family whatever their level of living, where 90 percent of Egyptian households consume subsidized "Balady" bread. Egyptians eat food with bread, and not bread with food. Food other than bread is colloquially referred to as "ghomous" (literally, a dip): a piece of bread is broken off and dipped in the "ghomous". Food eaten with bread can be as simple as salt or a mixture of salt, cumin and sesame seeds, an onion, white radish leaves, some aged white cheese, or the more complete meal of cooked vegetables or legumes. In Egypt bread is called as "Aish", which is derived from the word of life and living, and perhaps the choice of the Egyptian people for the bread to be the first slogans during revolution of 25 January 2011 is a confirmation of the importance of bread to Egyptians across all centuries. "Balady" bread characterized that contains starch and significant content of mineral and protein in the daily diet of Egyptian citizen, as it provides the consumer about 70 percent of his food needs of carbohydrates and protein, and 52 percent of the calories, as well minerals such as iron and zinc. "Balady" bread is the only food commodity subsidized and available to all consumers without restriction, which will benefit all segments of society, especially low-income families, and its price is affected by the rise in the other commodities prices (IDSC 2010).

According to IDSC (2010), the subsidizing of bread rose by 179.3 percent during the period 2003/2004 to 2008/2009, as about 16.2 billion pounds of bread subsidies was allocated in 2008/2009 compared to 5.8 billion pounds in 2003/2004. Despite the rise in subsidizing for bread, the bread industry in Egypt is facing many difficulties and problems that escalated with the beginning of 2008, and these problems can be summarized as follow:

- Pre-production problems including provision of wheat and wheat milling process.
- Production problems including quality of bread, modern mechanization in production and auxiliary industries.
- Post-production problems including geographic distribution, consumption rates, wastage, profitability and economics of the bread industry.

There are many proposals and solutions to the problems of bread in Egypt, which are:

- Development of the production process including expansion to create bakeries, tighten the control process, the development of methods of production, using other sources of flour like maize, improving the quality of flour and improving the nutritional value of the bread.
- Development of the sales and marketing process including separating the production from distribution and determining the price on the basis of quality which called the price discrimination policy.
- Improving the quality, focusing in to improve the quality of a loaf of bread through its technical specifications.

3.2 European experience

Bread market is considered one of the largest segments of the food industry in the United Kingdom, where it is to produce 12 million loaves of bread per day (IDSC 2010). There are three basic segments of the baking industry in the United Kingdom:

- *Large plant bakers*: it is the largest sector of the production of bread, which produces 80 percent of the total amount of bread in the market.
- *In-store bakeries*: this sector produces about 17 percent of the total amount of bread in the market.
- *Craft bakeries*: produce the remaining three percent of the total amount of bread in the market.

What about the bread industry in Western Europe? In Western Europe, it is produced nearly 25 million tons of bread per year, Plant bakeries where contributes about 8 million tons. Germany and United Kingdom are considered the main producers for about 60 percent of the production of the "Plant bakeries". But for France, Netherlands and Spain produce 20 percent divided between these countries (IDSC 2010).

3.3 Asian experience

3.3.1 Malaysian experience

Bread industry in Malaysia faced many changes over the past decade; it started as a small-scale industry, then began to expand to become a medium-scale industry, and then expanded to the new direction called "boutique bakery". It is a kind of innovative marketing and relies on the concept of transparency between the producer and the consumer, as it allows the consumer to see the product during its preparation. Bread industry flourishes significantly in Malaysia and fast, to become bread products from more products that are gaining in popularity, in addition to being the best alternative for rice. Bakery products have recorded nearly two billion Malaysian ringgit in 2003, an increase of 65 million Malaysian ringgit from the previous year (IDSC 2010).

3.3.2 Yemeni experience

In Yemen, bread industry depends mainly on wheat. Yemen imports huge quantities of wheat annually for bread production, which is a negative indicator that the bread has become a net importer, where the rate of self-sufficiency in wheat is only 7.5 percent, according to data in 2002. The per capita arrived daily from bread to 245.7 g in 2002. It should be noted that the amount of bread covered by the daily per capita in developing countries has ranged from 137 g to 411 g. Based on the data of the Central Bureau of Statistics, the number of ovens increased by six percent per year, and can be classified by type into (IDSC 2010):

- *Popular ovens*: those used in the production of bread from kneading stage to baking stage. These ovens constitute 67 percent of the total number of ovens operating in Yemen.
- *Conventional ovens*: those in which some of the equipment in the production process, including kneading machines and the fermentation process, operate in the courtyard of the bakery. These ovens are made of stone and heated by diesel or gas. These ovens are 26 percent of the total number of operated ovens.
- *Semi-automatic bakeries*: these manufacturing machines are used in the production process, including kneading, shaping and fermentation (rooms where temperature and humidity can be controlled) with an automatic oven (which can adjust the temperature and baking time). These ovens are seven percent of the total number of operated ovens.

The output of the most bread ovens (popular and conventional) is of low quality as compared to the output of some semi-automatic bread bakeries. On the health side, the popular ovens and the most conventional ovens suffer from deteriorating situation (unclean production halls and manual handling of materials and the dough). However, most of semi-automatic bakeries are characterized by satisfactory health status. The storage places of production inputs (flour, yeast, improvers) are kept in the rooms that do not meet the conditions for the storage of these sensitive materials, especially in those areas with distinct climate, hot and humid in the summer (IDSC 2010).

3.4 Australian experience

Baking consists in Australia from three sectors, namely: bread, biscuits, and cake and pastry, with estimated total sales for the industry about $ 5.1 billion during the year 2001/2002. The sector of bread industry is the major one to contribute to the sales of the baked goods industry. It accounted for about 44 percent of total sales in this industry (IDSC 2010). There are four basic types of bread industry in Australia:

- *Corporate plant bakeries*: These produce bread and sell it wholesale, as well as to export part of its production abroad and thus is considered the largest producers of bread in Australia.
- *Traditional hot bread shops*: The second largest producers of bread in Australia, these are engaged in the manufacture and sale of bread directly through their stores.
- *Franchised hot bread shops*: These bakers also manufacture and directly sell bread in stores.
- *Supermarket in-store bakeries*: Establish the bakery shops within supermarkets, so as to encourage consumers to easily buy bread from them, as well as to compete with shops getting franchise bread.

3.5 North and South American experiences

In 1492, legend has it, Christopher Columbus brought a small crock of sourdough starter to the New World. Unleavened breads made from cornmeal, however, are believed to be the first breads embraced by European settlers in the Americas.

Due to the mechanization of yeast production, the industrialization of bread also became possible. Industrial bakers, particularly in the United States, were always on the lookout for quicker and cheaper production methods. Kneading times, proofing times and baking times were reduced to the absolute minimum. At the same time it became more and more difficult to find qualified personnel. As a result the bread lacked body and flavor.

In the United States the baking industry was built on marketing methods used during feudal times and production techniques developed by the Romans. Some makers of snacks such as potato chips or crisps have produced baked versions of their snack items as an alternative to the usual cooking method of deep-frying in an attempt to reduce the calorie or fat content of their snack products. Baking has opened up doors to businesses such as cake making factories and private cake shops where the baking process is done with larger amounts in bigger and open furnaces (Whitten 1990). Although Americans consumed more bread than any other single food well into the 21st century, the massive commodification and industrialization of bread has received almost no attention in scholarly work on the history and cultural politics of food in the U.S. and even less within the larger social historiography of early 21st century America. Discourses on hygiene, health, and food purity permeated in early

21st century American life and played a pivotal role in the making of modern bread (Bobrow-Strain 2005).

Certain South American countries are known for their breads made with cheese, eggs, and manioc flour (also known as yuca flour, cassava flour, or tapioca starch). In Brazil, there is the famous pão de quiejo. Colombians have pandebono and almojabanas. Paraguayans enjoy similar bread called chipa.

The unifying ingredient in these breads (except for almojabanas) is the yuca (cassava, tapioca) starch, which gives them their special texture (and makes them gluten-free). Some of that sour flavor is good in these recipes, but too much can be overwhelming.

Chipa and pandebono have both tapioca flour and corn meal (pão de queijo does not typically have corn meal). Chipa are made with a very finely ground corn meal. Processing US style corn meal for a few seconds in a food processor works well as a substitute. The corn meal used in Colombian pandebono is called masarepa, which is a precooked corn meal normally used to make arepas.

The cheese is another specialty ingredient. All three of these breads are made with a local salted version of fresh cow's milk cheese. In Brazil, pão de queijo is made with queijo minas cheese, from the Minas Gerais region. Substituting half feta and half farmer's cheese works well in all three of these recipes. Be sure to taste the dough for salt—some farmer's cheeses are saltier than others.[5]

4. Types of bread in the world

There are countless varieties of bread throughout the world, made from many different grains and flours (Hamelman 2004).

Around the world bread is found in many kinds, shapes and sizes, including baguettes, bagels, tortillas, rolls, crackers, popovers, pancakes, pretzels, pita, matzo, and many more. Making bread would be a great way to "rise" to the occasion as you explore grains and breads around the world.[6] There may be hundreds of variations of bread, but they fall into three main types.

4.1 Yeast breads

Yeast breads are leavened breads made with yeast, a microscopic, one-celled organism in the fungus family.

Yeast breads are eaten by most people in the United States, Canada, and many European nations. White bread is the most popular variety, but other yeast breads are gaining favor as world breads become growing enterprises. Yeast breads make up about 99 percent of the bread baked in the United States. Hamburger and hot dog buns, other rolls, croissants, Danish pastries, English muffins and crumpets (England), Kugelhopf (Austria and France), brioche (French buns), challah (Jewish braided bread), and loaves such as whole wheat, cracked wheat, pumpernickel, rye, and rolled oats are examples of yeast breads.

---

[5] http://southamericanfood.about.com/od/breads/a/cheesebread.htm
[6] http://www.americasheartland.org/education/teachers/003_breads_around_the_world.pdf

4.2 Quick breads

Quick breads are loaves that require no kneading or rising. They are descendants of hearth cakes of long ago. Some credit England's King Alfred with inventing "quick cakes" by accident. He forgot to watch the pot of porridge as he sat in his hut; he finally discovered that it had cooked into bread. The American Indians taught the early colonists to bake cornmeal over a fire into hot cakes.

Most quick breads contain baking soda and/or baking powder, other ways to leaven breads or make them rise. They can be made quickly and only require simple steps. Quick breads became popular in the United States in the last half of the 19th century when baking powder became readily available. Today's quick breads include quick loaves such as corn bread or banana bread, muffins, biscuits, coffee cakes, scones, pancakes and waffles.

4.3 Flat breads

Flat breads are more common in many parts of the world than in the United States. Most flat breads are unleavened. They are made from either batters or kneaded dough. They are easy to mix and quick to cook. Flat breads include tortillas (Mexico); Jewish matzah; crepes and crepelike chickpea flour bread (France); dosas, chapatis and parathas (India); Mandarin pancakes and scallion bread (China); okonomiyaki (Japan); pita bread and Lebanese wrapper bread (Middle East); and various crackers from around the world. Pita and Lebanese wrapper breads are made from yeasted dough and flattened to rise before baking. Crackers are rolled thinly and baked quickly; they all end up flat, including the ones which use leavening (Fig. 2).

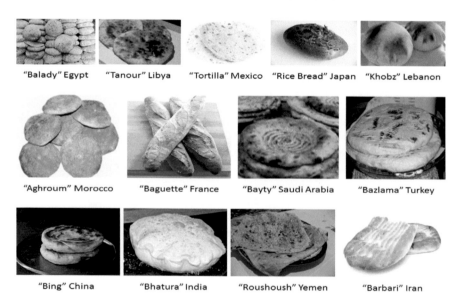

"Balady" Egypt   "Tanour" Libya   "Tortilla" Mexico   "Rice Bread" Japan   "Khobz" Lebanon

"Aghroum" Morocco   "Baguette" France   "Bayty" Saudi Arabia   "Bazlama" Turkey

"Bing" China   "Bhatura" India   "Roushoush" Yemen   "Barbari" Iran

Figure 2. Some of the bread types all over the world.

5. Science of bread-making

Dough is usually baked, but in some cuisines breads are steamed (e.g., mantou), fried (e.g., puri), or baked on an unoiled frying pan (e.g., tortillas). It may be leavened or unleavened (e.g., matzo). Salt, fat and leavening agents such as yeast and baking soda are common ingredients, though bread may contain other ingredients, such as milk, egg, sugar, spice, fruit (such as raisins), vegetables (such as onion), nuts (such as walnuts) or seeds (such as poppy). Referred to colloquially as the "staff of life", bread has been prepared for at least 30,000 years. The development of leavened bread can probably also be traced to prehistoric times. Sometimes, the word bread refers to a sweetened loaf cake, often containing appealing ingredients like dried fruit, chocolate chips, nuts or spices, such as pumpkin bread, banana bread or ginger bread.

The soft, inner part of bread is known to bakers and other culinary professionals as the crumb, which is not to be confused with small bits of bread that often fall off, called crumbs. The outer hard portion of bread is called the crust (Cauvain 2007).

Professional baker recipes are stated using a notation called baker's percentage. The amount of flour is denoted to be 100 percent, and the amounts of the other ingredients are expressed as a percentage of that amount by weight. Measurement by weight is more accurate and consistent than measurement by volume, particularly for dry ingredients.

The proportion of water to flour is the most important measurement in a bread recipe, as it affects texture and crumb the most. Hard US wheat flours absorb about 62 percent water, while softer wheat flours absorb about 56 percent (Cauvain and Young 2007). Common table breads made from these doughs result in a finely textured, light bread. Most artisan bread formulas contain anywhere from 60 to 75 percent water. In yeast breads, the higher water percentages result in more CO_2 bubbles and a coarser bread crumb. One pound (450 g) of flour will yield a standard loaf of bread or two French loaves.

5.1 Ingredients for bread-making

The basic ingredients in bread-making are flour, water, salt and yeasts. In modern bread-making, however, a large number of other components and additives are used. Knowledge of the baking process has grown. These components depend on the type of bread and on the practice and regulations operating in a country. They include "yeast food", sugar, milk, egg, shortening (fat), emulsifiers, anti-fungal agents, anti-oxidants, enzymes, flavoring and enriching ingredients (Okafor 2004). Based on the above, the ingredients of bread-making fall into four main categories:

5.1.1 Principal ingredients

Flour: Flour is a product made from grain that has been ground to a powdery consistency. Flour provides the primary structure to the final baked bread. While wheat flour is most commonly used for breads, flours made from rye, barley, maize, and other grains are also commonly available. Each of these grains provides the starch and protein needed to form bread. Several third world countries have encouraged the setting up of programs to study the feasibility of alternate locally available flours as a substitute for wheat flour. In Egypt, the local production of wheat is insufficient, and the Egyptian Government spends a lot to import wheat flour for bread and other baked food items. So, the substantial quantities for this cereal must be improved. Abdel-Kader (2000) suggested that the legumes may be used as wheat flour supplement in bread making to save the wheat flour and to improve the nutritional value at the same time. He reported that the replacement of wheat flour with up to 10 percent decorticated cracked broadbeans flour (*Vicia faba* L.) produced acceptable Egyptian "Balady" bread. The nutritional value of wheat flour (WF), decorticated cracked broadbeans flour (DCBF), wheat bread and DCBF-fortified breads are shown in Tables 1, 2 and 3. Table 2 concludes that the blending of the legume protein (DCBF) with the cereal protein (WF) should improve the protein quality of the bread, since the higher content of lysine in DCBF complements the lower content of lysine in WF, while the higher contents of sulfur-containing amino acids (methionine and cystine) in WF complement the lower contents in DCBF.

Table 1. Chemical composition of wheat flour (WF), decorticated cracked broadbeans flour (DCBF), wheat bread and DCBF-fortified breads (g/100 g dry matter).

Flours and breads	Moisture	Protein[a]	Fat[b]	Ash	Fiber	Carbohydrates[c]
Flour						
WF	12.91	12.52	1.25	0.61	0.55	85.07
DCBF	11.90	26.11	1.77	3.34	4.78	64.00
Bread						
Wheat bread	32.41	11.66	1.61	2.72	1.20	82.81
Fortified bread						
10% DCBF	32.49	14.13	1.76	3.12	1.55	79.44

[a] Protein was calculated (N × 6.25) except wheat flour samples (N × 5.70)
[b] Fat = ether extract
[c] Carbohydrates were calculated by difference
Source: Abdel-Kader (2001)

Table 3 shows that the DCBF contained greater amounts of all minerals analyzed than WF, because the ash content of DCBF was higher than its content in WF.

But it is still the quality bread-making related to the quality of flour which depends on the quality and quantity of its proteins. So, uniquely the wheat flour and some few cereal seeds flour contain type of proteins that have the ability to transform a gruel of flour and water into a glutinous mass (Cauvain 2007). Many consider gluten as the password of bread and bakery products for that the wheat was classified to types: "Hard" wheat with a high content of protein (over 12 percent) is best for making bread because the high content of glutenins enables a firm skeleton for holding the gases released during fermentation. "Soft" wheat with low protein contents (9–11 percent) is best for making cakes. Gluten is a protein complex found in wheat (including kamut and spelt), barley, rye and triticale which has the unique property of forming an elastic structure when moistened with water (Okafor 2004).

Table 2. Amino acid composition (g/16 g N) of WF, DCBF, wheat bread, DCBF-fortified breads and reference protein.

Amino acid	Flour		Wheat bread	Fortified bread	Reference protein[a]
	WF	DCBF		10%	
Essential					
Lysine	2.64	7.49	2.73	4.62	7.0
Histidine	2.02	3.31	2.47	3.49	2.4
Threonine	2.92	4.05	3.78	4.05	5.1
Valine	4.12	4.56	4.90	5.02	6.8
Methionine	1.61	1.17	2.05	2.19	3.4
Isoleucine	3.76	4.18	4.61	4.81	6.3
Leucine	6.51	7.78	7.42	8.52	8.8
Phenylalanine	4.49	4.04	6.94	7.14	5.7
No-essential					
Arginine	4.13	5.93	4.78	5.14	6.1
Aspartic acid	4.32	10.28	3.23	3.40	9.6
Serine	5.34	4.76	4.51	4.73	7.6
Glutamic acid	28.45	11.87	23.70	17.52	12.7
Proline	11.01	6.72	9.36	8.45	4.2
Glycine	3.02	2.95	2.98	3.27	3.3
Alanine	2.96	3.64	2.76	2.92	5.9
Tyrosine	3.39	4.01	3.11	3.40	4.2
Cystine	2.05	0.66	2.92	2.64	2.4

[a] Whole egg protein (FAO 1970)
Source: Abdel-Kader (2001)

Table 3. Mineral content (mg/100 g dry matter) of WF, DCBF, wheat bread and DCBF-fortified breads.

Minerals	Flour		Wheat bread	Fortified bread
	WF	DCBF		10%
Calcium	31.0	189	43.3	75.1
Magnesium	17.1	249	32.0	48.5
Sodium	2.2	38.5	380	502
Potassium	114	809	88	154
Phosphorus	121	505	138	178
Iron	1.19	10.22	1.78	2.15
Zinc	0.72	4.96	0.69	0.99
Copper	0.38	0.98	1.25	1.76
Manganese	0.90	28.09	0.28	0.38

Source: Abdel-Kader (2001)

Gluten-Free Bread…What and Why? Gluten-free bread is made with ground flours from a variety of materials such as almonds, rice (rice bread), sorghum (sorghum bread), corn (corn bread), or legumes such as beans (bean bread), but since these flours lack gluten it can be difficult for them to retain their shape as they rise and they may be less "fluffy". Additives such as xanthum gum, hydroxypropyl methylcellulose (HPMC), corn starch, or eggs are used to compensate for the lack of gluten (Schober and Bean 2008). Generally, a gluten-free diet is the only medically accepted treatment for celiac disease (Hischenhuber et al. 2006). Being gluten intolerant can often mean a person may also be wheat intolerant as well as suffer from the related inflammatory skin condition dermatitis herpetiformis. There are a smaller minority of people who suffer from wheat intolerance alone and are tolerant to gluten. Despite unknown benefits for non-celiacs and evidence to suggest adverse effects, a significant demand has developed for gluten-free food in the United States (Gaesser and Angadi 2012).

Water: After the flour, the next most important ingredient used in bread-making is water. It would be impossible to produce a loaf of bread without water in some form. There are several types of water. Hard water produces better quality bread than any type of water. Soft water weakens the gluten during mixing and fermentation. This can be corrected to some degree by increasing the percentage of salt in the formula slightly and by using mineral yeast food in the formula. Alkaline water is the most harmful, because it doesn't only weaken the gluten, but retards fermentation. Yeast likes a slightly acid medium to perform at its best. The weakening of the gluten and retarding effect on yeast can be corrected by using an acid ingredient such as vinegar (acetic acid) or lactic acid. Special types of mineral yeast food have been developed to correct this problem (Okafor 2004).

Yeasts: The yeasts used for baking are strains of *Saccharomyces cerevisiae*. The ideal properties of yeasts used in modern bakeries are as follows (Okafor 2004):

- ability to grow rapidly at room temperature of about 20–25°C;
- easy dispersibility in water;
- ability to produce large amounts of CO_2 rather than alcohol in flour dough;
- good keeping quality, i.e., ability to resist autolysis when stored at 20°C;
- ability to adapt rapidly to changing substrates such as are available to the yeasts during dough making;
- high invertase and other enzymes activity to hydrolyze to higher glucofructans rapidly;
- ability to grow and synthesize enzymes and coenzymes under anaerobic conditions of the dough;
- ability to resist the osmotic effect of salts and sugars in the dough; and
- high competitiveness, i.e., high yielding in terms of dry weight per unit of substrate used.

Salt: It is another essential ingredient in quality bread production. About two percent sodium chloride is usually added to bread. It has several functions as follows:

- it improves taste;
- it stabilizes yeast fermentation;

- has a toughening effect on gluten;
- helps retard proteolytic activity, which may be related to its effect on gluten; and
- it participates in the lipid binding of dough.

Because of the retarding effect on fermentation, salt is preferably added towards the end of mixing. For this reason flake-salt which has enhanced solubility is used and is added towards the end of the mixing. Fat-coated salt may also be used; the salt becomes available only at the latter stages of dough or at the early stages of baking (Okafor 2004).

5.1.2 Enriching ingredients

Sugar: Okafor (2004) reported that sugar is added:

- to provide carbon nourishment for the yeasts additional to the amount available in flour sugar;
- to sweeten the bread; and
- to afford more rapid browning (through sugar caramelization) of the crust and hence greater moisture retention within the bread. Sugar is supplied by the use of sucrose, glucose corn syrup (regular and high fructose), depending on availability.

Shortening: Animal and vegetable fats are added as shortenings in bread-making at about three percent (w/w) of flour to yield:

- increased loaf size;
- a more tender crumb; and
- enhanced slicing properties.

Butter is used only in the most expensive breads; lard (fat from pork) may be used, but vegetable fats especially soy bean oil, because of its most assured supply, is now common (Cauvain 2007).

Milk: Several years ago nonfat dry milk was the type of milk generally used in bread baking. Because of the rising cost of milk, skim milk and blends made from various components including whey, buttermilk solids, sodium or potassium caseinate, soy flour and/or corn flour are used. The milk substitutes are added in the ratio of 1–2 parts/100 parts of flour. Functions of milk are many. Milk is added to make the bread more nutritious. It has a stabilizing effect on fermentation, preventing wild fermentation. It improves crust color because of the lactose sugar and its buffering value. The lactose sugar is not fermentable by baker's yeast. It also improves texture, crumb color, flavor and taste, and keeping quality of the baked loaf. If nonfat dry milk is used in bread it must be heated to a high enough temperature during the drying process to destroy bacteria which weakens the gluten in the dough. Milk dried by the vacuum drying process must be properly heat treated prior to being dried otherwise considerable difficulty can be expected during mixing and fermentation of the dough (Okafor 2004).

5.1.3 Improving ingredients

Bleaching Agents: Flour bleaching agents are added to flour to make it appear whiter (freshly milled flour is yellowish), to oxidize the surfaces of the flour grains, and help with developing of gluten. Usual bleaching agents are nitrogen dioxide, azodicarbonamide "ADA", etc. (Hui and Cork 2006).

Oxidizing Agents: Originally flour was naturally aged through exposure to the atmosphere. The oxidizing agent strengthens gluten by its reaction with the proteins' sulphydryl group to provide cross-links between protein molecules and thus enhances its ability to hold gases released during dough formation. They may or may not also act as bleaching agents. The addition of these agents to flour will create stronger dough. Oxidizing agents which have been used include iodates, bromates and peroxide (Hui and Cork 2006).

Reducing Agents: It helps to weaken the flour by breaking the protein network. This will help with various aspects of handling strong dough. The benefits of adding these agents are reduced mixing time, reduced dough elasticity, reduced proofing time, and improved machinability (Hui and Cork 2006). Common reducing agents are fumaric acid, sodium bisulfate, non-leavened yeast and ascorbic acid.

Enzymes: These are also used to improve processing characteristics. Yeast naturally produces both amylases and proteinases, but additional quantities may be added to produce faster and more complete reactions. Amylases break down the starch in flours into simple sugars, thereby letting yeast ferment quickly. Malt is a natural source of amylase. Since most flours are deficient in α-amylase, flour is supplemented during the milling of the wheat with malted barley to provide this enzyme. Enzyme technology, especially aided by biotechnology, is a rapidly developing field. Scientists can now tailor enzymes with greatly improved functionality; for example, amylases that stop working at a specific point in bread baking, or proteases that can precisely control the strength of dough (Tenbergen 2000).

Emulsifiers (Surfactants): These are complex molecules that have both water- and fat-soluble regions. With one "end" of the molecule effectively dissolved in water and the other dissolved in fat, they are able to help form emulsions, which are stable mixtures of fats and water or water-containing fluids. Although several theories exist to explain how emulsifiers function in bread dough, their effects are well-known. Emulsifiers such as diacetyltartaric acid esters of mono-glycerides (DATEM) and stearoyl lactylates (SSL) effectively strengthen the dough and make it more extensible. This results in trapping more gas in smaller bubbles, reducing proofing time, giving softer, more even-textured bread. The added "stretch" also makes the dough more tolerant to over- or under-mixing. Emulsifiers are added as 0.5 percent flour weight (Tenbergen 2000; Okafor 2004).

Mold-Inhibitors (Antimycotics): The spoilage of bread is caused mainly by the fungi *Rhizopus*, *Mucor*, *Aspergillus* and *Penicillium*. Spoilage by *Bacillus mesenteroides* (ropes) rarely occurs. The main anti-mycotic agent added to bread is calcium propionate. Others used to a much less extent are sodium diacetate, vinegar, mono-calcium phosphate and lactic acid (Okafor 2004).

5.1.4 Optional ingredients

Flavoring Agents: It results in uniformity of products and efficiency of operations, assist in increasing the tolerances of doughs due to production variables, and help to satisfy the demand for variety in the flavor and taste of breads. The common flavoring agents added to bread types are rye flavoring, poppy seeds and sesame seeds (Okafor 2004).

Vitamins and Minerals: Bread is often enriched with various vitamins and minerals including thiamin, riboflavin, niacin and iron (Okafor 2004).

5.2 Leavening ... What?, How? and Why?

Leavening is the process of adding gas to dough before or during baking to produce lighter, more easily chewed bread. Optimally mixed dough is subjected to fermentation for a suitable length of time to obtain light aerated porous structure of fermented product. Fermentation is achieved by yeast (*Saccharomyces cerevisiae*) (Cauvain and Young 2007).

A simple technique for leavening bread is the use of gas-producing chemicals. There are two common methods. The first is to use baking powder or a self-rising flour that includes baking powder. The second is to include an acidic ingredient such as buttermilk and add baking soda; the reaction of the acid with the soda produces gas. Chemically leavened breads are called quick breads and soda breads. This method is commonly used to make muffins, pancakes, American-style biscuits, and quick breads such as banana bread (Okafor 2004).

5.2.1 Role of yeast in leavening process

The primary role of yeasts in bread-making is leavening. Leavening is the increase in size of the dough induced by gases by the metabolism of yeasts. During bread-making yeasts ferment hexose sugars mainly into alcohol, carbon dioxide and smaller amounts of glycerol and trace compounds of various other alcohols, esters, aldehydes and organic acids. The CO_2 dissolves continuously in the dough, until the latter becomes saturated. Subsequently the excess CO_2 in the gaseous state begins to form bubbles in the dough. It is this formation of bubbles which causes the dough to rise or to leaven. The total time taken for the yeast to act upon the dough varies from 2 to 6 hr or longer depending on the method of baking used (Williams and Pullen 2007).

Okafor (2004) concluded that the factors which effect the leavening action of yeasts are:

a) The nature of the sugar available.
b) Osmotic pressure.
c) Effect of nitrogen and other nutrients.
d) Effect on fungal inhibitors (anti-mycotic agents).
e) Yeast concentration.

5.2.2 What is the updating in bread fermentation?

Update in bread fermentation by lactic acid bacteria (LAB) is one of the recent updating in bread fermentation. Although sourdough bread is one of the oldest biotechnological processes but there are new developments on the biochemistry and physiology of LAB in the sourdough ecosystem, particularly in emphasis on anti-microbial compounds synthesis and decrease of certain allergen products derived from gluten which is present in wheat, barley and rye baked foods and is involved in celiac disease (Rollán et al. 2010; Thorigné et al. 2012).

Sourdough: Sourdough is an intermediate product between dough and traditional bread preparation, containing flour, water and metabolically active microorganisms, mainly lactic acid bacteria and yeast. During the fermentation of the dough, the metabolic products of LAB improve the organoleptic and technological properties of bread as well as their shelf life, nutritional value (Hammes and Gänzle 1998) and healthy aspect (De Angelis et al. 2010).

Types of Sourdoughs: On the basis of applied technology, sourdoughs have been grouped into three types: type I (sourdough which is restarted using a part of the previous fermentation), type II (generally used as dough-souring supplements in semi-fluid preparations) and type III (dried preparations) (Decock and Cappelle 2005). Unlike type I sourdoughs, type II and III doughs require the addition of baker's yeast (*S. cerevisiae*) as leavening agent (Corsetti and Settani 2007).

Impact of LAB in Sourdough Fermentation: The application of sourdough has a long tradition in the production of wheat and rye breads. Sourdough plays a crucial role in the development of the sensorial, nutritional and safety quality of fermented products. The metabolic activity of LAB during sourdough fermentation may contribute to the improvement of cereal products in different ways, such as improving the texture and palatability of whole grain, fiber-rich, or gluten-free products, stabilizing/increasing levels of bioactive compounds and enhancing mineral bioavailability (Arendt et al. 2007). Figure 3 illustrates the effects of sourdough on the nutritional quality of bread.

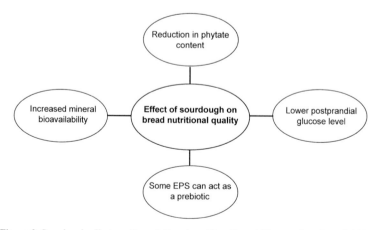

Figure 3. Sourdough effects on the nutritional quality of bread (Source: Arendt et al. 2007).

5.3 Staling and mould infection: reasons and novel strategies of control

Fresh bread is prized for its taste, aroma, quality, appearance and texture. Retaining its freshness is important to keep it appetizing. Bread that has stiffened or dried past its prime is said to be stale. Modern bread is sometimes wrapped in paper or plastic film or stored in a container such as a breadbox to reduce drying. Bread that is kept in warm, moist environments is prone to the growth of mold. Bread kept at low temperatures, in a refrigerator for example, will develop mold growth more slowly than bread kept at room temperature, but will turn stale quickly due to retrogradation (Cauvain 2007).

There are three ways in which bread stale. They are: starch retrogradation, infection by fungi, and infection by rope.

Although it has been studied for more than a century and a half, bread staling has not been eliminated and remains responsible for huge economic losses to both the baking industry and the consumer. Bechtel et al. (1953) defined staling as "a term which indicates decreasing consumer acceptance of bread caused by changes in crumb other than those resulting from the action of spoilages organisms".

Gray and Bemiller (2003) mentioned that the main changes which occur in bread as a result of staling are:

- Increase of crumb firmness.
- Increase in crumbliness of the crumb.
- Deterioration in flavor and aroma.
- Loss of crust crispiness.

Various methods and techniques have been used to measure staling in bread:

- Measurement of crumb firmness.
- Taste panel evaluations.
- Changes in the physical and chemical properties of the starch such as (decrease in soluble starch, decrease in enzyme susceptibility of the starch, increase in starch crystallinity, and changes in X-ray diffraction patterns).

5.3.1 Mechanism of staling

Bread staling is a complex phenomenon, certainly involving multiple factors. Much has been learned about bread staling, and application of this knowledge has led to considerable improvements in shelf life. However, without knowledge of the precise mechanism, addressing the problem of bread staling remains a process of formulating and testing more and more hypotheses. It is difficult to determine cause-and-effect relationships because involvement of a constituent may be indirect and additives, other changes in formulation, and process changes may alter more than one property and the effects may cancel each other.

Bread staling falls into two categories: crust staling and crumb staling. Crust staling is generally caused by moisture transfer from the crumb to the crust, resulting in a soft, leathery texture and is generally less objectionable than the crumb staling. Crumb staling is more complex, more important and less understood. The firmness of bread varies with position within a loaf, with maximum firmness occurring in the central portion of the crumb (Lin and Lineback 1990).

Schoch and French (1947) proposed a model that describes the heat-reversible aggregation of amylopectin as the principal cause of bread staling (Fig. 4). As illustrated in the Schoch and French model, amylose quickly associates in bread soon after baking, affecting initial firmness, but plays no further role in crumb firming. This firming is attributed to changes in the physical orientation of the branched amylopectin molecules of starch within the swollen granule. In fresh bread, the branched chains of amylopectin are unfolded and spread out within the limits of available water. These chains of the amylopectin polymer gradually aggregate, aligning with one another by various types of intra-molecular bonding. This effect results in increasing rigidity of the internal structure of the swollen starch granules causing crumb hardening (Pateras 2007).

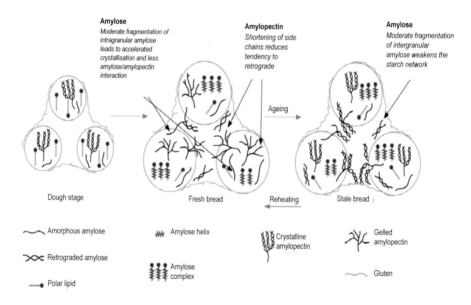

Figure 4. Mechanism of bread staling (Source: Schoch and French 1947).

5.3.2 Anti-staling

To avoid the losses and problems which result from bread staling, Pateras (2007) referred to certain groups of ingredients or processes which retard the staling process or minimize its effect such as enzymes, emulsifiers, pentosans, alcohol, sugars, freezing of bread and mold inhibitors.

5.3.3 Mold infection

Mold spoilage of bread is due to post-processing contamination. Bread becomes contaminated after baking from the mold spores present in the atmosphere surrounding loaves during cooling, slicing, packaging and storage. Mold growth is the most frequent cause of spoilage in bakery products mainly due to *Aspergillus, Fusarium* and *Penicillium* genera. Statistics show that Argentinean small factories register losses in packaged bread as high as 20–40 percent, mainly due to the lack of good manufacture practices in addition to the warm climate in the country (Gerez et al. 2009). The environment inside a bakery is not sterile because dry ingredients, especially flour, contain mold spores, and flour dust spreads easily through the air. It has been estimated that 1 g of flour contains as many as 8000 mold spores. In addition to the great economic losses derived from the presence of mold, another concern is the potential mycotoxin production that may cause public health problems (Legan 1993).

5.3.4 Novel strategies to mold control

Consumer demands for more natural foods have stimulated the research on biological (i.e., vegetal and microbial) preservation systems. In this aspect, LAB strains are organisms of interest for bio-preservation since they have been used for centuries in various fermented food, either by its natural presence in raw materials (spontaneous fermentation) or its addition as pure starter cultures. Recently, LAB have received scientific attention because of their antifungal potential since LAB strains from cereals with antifungal activity have been reported (Rouse et al. 2008). However, the application of these antifungal LAB cultures in baked food is still limited despite the advances on the characterization of antifungal metabolites (i.e., peptides, organic acids) regarding molecular weight, heat-resistance, spectrum of action and effectiveness. These novel strategies put into evidence the suitability of selected LAB strains to be used as natural food-grade bio-control agents for reducing mold spoilage in bakery products and assuring their safety and quality (Rollán et al. 2010).

6. Modern breads

6.1 Burger

Burger, or hamburger, is the name given to a grilled beef patty that is served in a bun, along with condiments like ketchup, mustard, mayonnaise, lettuce, tomato, onion, cheese, etc. A burger is usually accompanied with lots of French fries. With time, other ingredients, like potato, vegetables, fish and chicken, have started replacing the beef in the patty. Burger is a very popular fast-food among almost all the kids as well as college-goers. However, very few have ever thought about the history and origin of the delicious patty.[7]

History of burger

The origin of hamburger is a bit hazy and unclear. This is because there is no proper documentation to give us an idea about how the fast food came into being. Still, many

---

[7] http://lifestyle.iloveindia.com/lounge/history-of-burger-1702.html

people have claimed that the hamburger 'patty' was first noticed in the medieval times. Tartars (a band of Mongolian and Turkish warriors) used to place pieces of beef under their saddles. Under the weight of the rider and the saddle, the pieces used to turn tender enough to be eaten raw. Thus was born the initial beef 'patty'. A food item resembling the present-day burger, to some an extent, reached America around the 19th century. The dish, called Hamburg style beef, was brought to Hamburg (Germany) from Russia in the 14th century and when the German immigrants arrived in America, they brought it along with them. With time, the raw, chopped piece of beef evolved into the 'patty sandwiched in a bun'. Thus, it can be said that America had a major role in giving the world the hamburger, as we know of it today.[7]

6.2 Pizza

The term 'pizza' first appeared "in a Latin text from the southern Italian town of Gaeta in 997 AD, which claims that a tenant of certain property is to give the bishop of Gaeta 'duodecim pizze' ['twelve pizzas'] every Christmas Day, and another twelve every Easter Sunday" (Maiden 2012).

Pizza is an oven-baked, flat, round bread typically topped with a tomato sauce, cheese and various toppings. The modern pizza was invented in Naples, Italy, and the dish has since become popular in many parts of the world (Hanna 2006). An establishment that makes and sells pizzas is called a "pizzeria". Many varieties of pizza exist worldwide, along with several dish variants based upon pizza. Pizza is cooked in various types of ovens, and a diverse variety of ingredients and toppings are utilized. In 2009, upon Italy's request, Neapolitan pizza was safeguarded in the European Union as a Traditional Specialty Guaranteed dish.

Healthy benefits

Some studies have linked consumption of the antioxidant lycopene, which exists in tomato products that are often used on pizza, as having a beneficial health effect. European nutrition research on the eating habits of people with cancer of the mouth, oesophagus, throat or colon showed those who ate pizza at least once a week had less chance of developing cancer. Dr. Silvano Gallus, of the Mario Negri Institute for Pharmaceutical Research in Milan, attributed it to lycopene, an antioxidant chemical in tomatoes, which is thought to offer some protection against cancer.[8] Carlo La Vecchia, a Milan-based epidemiologist said, "Pizza could simply be indicative of a lifestyle and food habits, in other words the Italian version of a Mediterranean diet." A traditional Mediterranean diet is rich in olive oil, fiber, vegetables, fruit, flour, and freshly cooked food. In contrast to the traditional Italian pizza used in the research, popular pizza varieties in many parts of the world are often loaded with high fat cheeses and fatty meats, a high intake of which can contribute to obesity, itself a risk factor for cancer.

The innovation that led to flat bread pizza was the use of tomato as a topping. For some time after the tomato was brought to Europe from the Americas in the 16th

---

[8] http://www.marionegri.it/mn/en/index.html

century, it was believed by many Europeans to be poisonous (as are some other fruits of the nightshade family). However, by the late 18th century, it was common for the poor of the area around Naples to add tomato to their yeast-based flat bread, and so the pizza began.[9] The dish gained in popularity, and soon pizza became a tourist attraction as visitors to Naples ventured into the poorer areas of the city to try the local specialty.

7. Conclusions and future perspectives

As a foodstuff of great historical and contemporary importance, in many cultures in the West, Near and Middle East, bread has a significance beyond mere nutrition. Bread has ancient roots, and is a staple of many diets throughout the world, from thriving metropolises to developing nations. Bread comes in all shapes, flavors and forms, and is typically made from accessible and affordable ingredients. These ingredients are important because they help fill nutritional gaps in the diet as well as help you feel full and satisfied. The nearly ubiquitous consumption of bread all over the world gives bread an important position in international nutrition. In addition to their high starch contents as energy sources, bread also provides dietary fiber, protein (high in proline and glutamine, but low in lysine) and functional lipids rich in essential fatty acids. Important micronutrients present in bread include vitamins, especially many B vitamins, minerals, antioxidants and phytochemicals. In general, bread provides significant amounts of most nutrients. Because the awareness of a healthy lifestyle is increasing, breads containing whole grain, multi-grain or other functional ingredients will become more important in the bakery industry and the market. New ingredients or processing steps may therefore be necessary to develop breads with textures and appearances that can compete with the popularity of white breads. Research on the influences of those processes and ingredient innovations on the nutritional value of the finished bread is recommended. More work should be carried out to find out new and cheap substitutes of wheat flour for many reasons (the local production of wheat is insufficient in many developing countries and also to improve the nutritional value of wheat flour, e.g., lysine fortification). Also further researches should be focused on the production of dietetic breads of which gluten-free and sodium-reduced bread are the most important. Gluten-free breads have been produced from a large number of flours and starches (rice, corn, cassava, soybean, millet and sorghum) to satisfy the requirements of those suffering from coeliac disease (gluten intolerance).

Keywords: Anti-staling, Baking systems, Bread history, Bread ingredients, Bread types, Healthy bread, Modern bread, Mould control, Staling, Substitutes of wheat flour, Updating of bread fermentation

---

[9] http://www.pizzatoday.com/magazine/deep-dish-pizza#.Ulkb_1OUfSN

References

Abdel-Kader, Z.M. 2000. Enrichment of Egyptian 'Balady' bread. Part 1. Baking studies, physical and sensory evaluation of enrichment with decorticated cracked broadbeans flour (*Vicia faba* L.). Nahrung, 44: 418–421.

Arendt, E.K., L.A.M. Ryan and F. Dal Bello. 2007. Impact of sourdough on the texture of bread. Food Microbiology, 24: 165–174.

Bechtel, W.G., D.F. Meisner and W.B. Bradley. 1953. The effect of the crust on the staling of bread. Cereal Chemistry, 39: 160–168.

Bobrow-Strain, A. 2005. Since Sliced Bread: Purity, Hygiene, and the Making of Modern Bread. Proceedings of the Annual Meeting of the American Association of Geographers, USA. Available online: http://cgirs.ucsc.edu/conferences/whitefood/foodx/papers/bobrowstrain1.pdf.

Bouthyette, P.-Y. 2008. Introduction to fermentation and fermented foods. pp. 16–17. Fermentation Throughout the Ages. Available online: www.chemistrywithdrb.com/files/Fermentation.pdf.

Cauvain, S.P. 2007. Bread—the product. pp. 1–18. *In*: S.P. Cauvain and L.S. Young (eds.). Technology of Breadmaking. Springer, New York.

Cauvain, S.P. and L.S. Young. 2007. Technology of Breadmaking. Springer, New York.

Corsetti, A. and L. Settani. 2007. *Lactobacilli* in sourdough fermentation. Food Research International, 40: 539–558.

De Angelis, M., A. Cassone, C.G. Rizzello, F. Gagliardi, F. Minervini, M. Calasso, R. Di Cagno, R. Francavilla and M. Gobbetti. 2010. Mechanism of degradation of immunogenic gluten epitopes from *Triticum turgidum* L. *var durum* by sourdough *lactobacilli* and fungal proteases. Applied and Environmental Microbiology, 76: 508–518.

Decock, P. and S. Cappelle. 2005. Bread technology and sourdough technology. Trends in Food Science and Technology, 16: 113–120.

Gaesser, G.A. and S.S. Angadi. 2012. Gluten-free diet: Imprudent dietary advice for general population? Journal of the Academy of Nutrition and Dietetics, 112: 1314–1317.

Gerez, C.L., M.I. Torino, G. Rollan and G. Font de Valdez. 2009. Prevention of bread mould spoilage by using lactic acid bacteria with antifungal properties. Food Control, 20: 144–148.

Gray, J.A. and J.N. Bemiller. 2003. Bread staling: Molecular basis and control. Comprehensive Reviews in Food Science and Food Safety, 2: 1–21.

Hamelman, J. 2004. Bread: A Baker's Book of Techniques and Recipes. John Wiley & Sons. Inc., Hoboken, New Jersey.

Hammes, W.P. and M.G. Gänzle. 1998. Sourdough breads and related products. pp. 199–216. *In*: B.J.B. Woods (ed.). Microbiology of Fermented Foods, Vol. 1. Blackie Academic/Professional, London.

Hanna, M. 2006. American Pie. American Heritage Magazine 57. Available online: http://www.americanheritage.com/content/american-pie.

Hischenhuber, C., R. Crevel, B. Jarry, M. Mäki, D. Moneret-Vautrin, A. Romano, R. Troncone and R. Ward. 2006. Review article: safe amounts of gluten for patients with wheat allergy or coeliac disease. Alimentary Pharmacology and Therapeutics, 23: 559–575.

Hui, Y. and H. Cork. 2006. Bakery Products: Science and Technology. Blackwell Publishing. Iowa.

IDSC 2010. Information and Decision Support Center. Subsidized bread in Egypt—Facts and Figures. IDSC Monthly Reports in Food Security—Policies and Social Services, Egyptian Cabinet, Information and Decision Support Center, Cairo, 42: 11 pp.

Legan, J.D. 1993. Mould spoilage of bread: The problem and some solutions. International Biodeterioration and Biodegradation, 32: 33–53.

Lin, W. and D.R. Lineback. 1990. Change in carbohydrate fractions in enzyme-supplemented bread and potential relationship to staling. Starch/Statrke, 42: 385.

Maiden, M. 2012. Linguistic Wonders Series: Pizza is a German Word. Available online: http://www.yourdictionary.com/pizza.

Okafor, N. 2004. Fermented Foods and Their Processing. Encyclopaedia of Life Supporting Sciences, United Nations Educational Scientific & Cultural Organization, Paris.

Pateras, I.M.C. 2007. Bread spoilage and staling. pp. 275–298. *In*: S.P. Cauvain and L.S. Young (eds.). Technology of Breadmaking. Springer, New York.

Rollán, G., C.L. Gerez, A.M. Dallagnol, M.I. Torino and G. Font. 2010. Update in bread fermentation by lactic acid bacteria. Current Research, Technology and Education Topics in Applied Microbiology and Microbial Biotechnology, 2: 1168–1174.

Rouse, S., D. Harnett, A. Vaughan and D. Van Sinderen. 2008. Lactic acid bacteria with potential to eliminate fungal spoilage in foods. Journal of Applied Microbiology, 104: 915–923.

Schober, T.J. and S.R. Bean. 2008. Sorghum and maize. pp. 101–118. *In*: E.K. Arendt and F.D. Bello (eds.). Gluten-Free Cereal Products and Beverages. Academic Press, Massachusetts.

Schoch, T.J. and D. French. 1947. Studies on bread staling. 1. Role of starch. Cereal Chem., 24: 231–249.

Tenbergen, K. 2000. Dough and bread conditioners. Food Product Design Magazine. Available online: http://www.foodingredientsonline.com/doc/Dough-and-Bread-Conditioners-0001?VNETCOOKIE=NO.

Thorigné, A., L.G. Bermudez-Humaran, E. Chabrier, C. Cartier, F. Chain, S. Blugeon, J.J. Gratadoux, J. Rouillé, X. Dousset, P. Langella and B. Onno. 2012. Evaluation of probiotic strains among lactic acid bacteria isolated from cereals for food applications. Proceedings of a Symposium on Sourdough. Finland.

Wassef, H.H. 2004. Food habits of the Egyptians: newly emerging trends. Eastern Mediterranean Health Journal, 10: 898–915.

Whitten, D.O. 1990. Handbook of American Business History: Manufacturing. Greenwood Publishing Group, Connecticut.

Williams, T. and G. Pullen. 2007. Functional ingredients. pp. 51–89. *In*: S.P. Cauvain and L.S. Young (eds.). Technology of Breadmaking. Springer, New York.

2

Role of Bread on Nutrition and Health Worldwide

Concha Collar

1. Introduction

Cereals are basic, popular and healthy raw materials, providing excellent vectors for nutrition, health, diversity and innovation. Bread, made basically from wheat but also from other grains, is a staple food widely consumed all over the world since ancient times (10,000 BC) providing approximately half of consumed carbohydrates. The nearly ubiquitous consumption of bread places it in a position of global importance in international nutrition. Bread was initially baked in the home using simple home-ground wholemeal flours, and styles of bread, and the methods used to make them evolved to satisfy local tastes and eating habits. Flour milling and subsequent bread-making on a commercial scale emerged as vital components of local societies, and flour-based foods evolved into the current diversity (Fig. 1).

Bread baking is based on mixing flour and other ingredients with water to make dough, leavening with yeast which produces carbon dioxide, and baking to stabilize the solid protein foam formed, resulting in an elastic porous network. Bread is an excellent carrier of macro, micronutrients and bioactive components, that fulfills an increasing number of nutritional and health claims. Over the last and current decades, bread is being revisited as a key cereal-based baked good addressed to specific targeted groups of population (low caloric density for obesity prevention and control, gluten-free for

Cereals and Cereal-Based Products, Food Science Department, Instituto de Agroquímica y Tecnología de Alimentos (IATA), Consejo Superior de Investigaciones Científicas (CSIC). Avda. Catedrático Agustín Escardino, 7. 46980 Paterna. Spain.
Email: ccollar@iata.csic.es

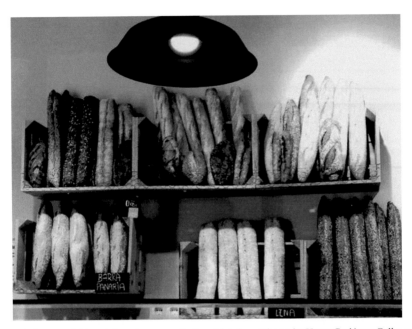

Figure 1. Commercial breads in a showcase of a Spanish bakery. Picture by Henar Gutiérrez-Collar, with permission.

coeliac patients, high-fiber goods to alleviate the low current intake of dietary fiber, low glycaemic index for diabetics and metabolic syndrome patients), and a wide array of tailored made breads is increasingly available.

The production and consumption of bread types across the world are presented and the traditional and innovative trends are highlighted. The role of wheat- and non wheat-breads in nutrition and health is emphasized and updated, and the value-added breads addressed to targeted groups of population are described.

2. Bread production and consumption worldwide: traditional and innovative trends

According to the Federation of Bakers (http://www.bakersfederation.org.uk/), a study for the European Commission in 2010 found that the European bread market was around 32 million tonnes in the EU 27 countries. Across the whole of the European countries the market share of the industrial bakers *vs.* the craft bakers was approximately 50/50, but there were great differences in different countries. One area of continued growth throughout Europe is the market for frozen dough and part-baked products which has transformed the market so that co-operatives and industrial baking companies are flourishing at the expense of the craft sector. In-store bakeries continue to be a growing sector. Bread production is relatively stable in most countries but there are some countries which are still showing a long term trend of a slow decline, 1–2%

per year, including the United Kingdom and Germany. The market structure varies throughout Europe, in the UK the industrial sector representing 80% of production, it is 40% in Germany, 35% in France, about 81% in the Netherlands and 19% in Spain. Bread consumption patterns differ widely within the EU but most countries have an average consumption of 50 kg of bread per person per year, mainly white bread. The Germans and Austrians eat the most bread at around 80 kg while the UK, Spain and Ireland are at the bottom of the list with annual consumption of less than 50 kg. As of 2000, the country with the largest per capita consumption of bread was Turkey with 200 kg per person. Turkish people eat more than three times their own body weight in bread annually. Turkey is followed in bread consumption by Serbia and Montenegro with 135 kg, and Bulgaria with 133 kg. In the UK and in Southern Europe, whole grain bread has a low market share (< 3%) while in countries with traditions of whole grain products, like Germany, the share is stable at 10% (Folloni and Ranieri 2013). Even in the Nordic countries, where whole grain breads have a larger share of the market, white bread is dominant and whole grain intake is still below recommended levels (Kyrø et al. 2011). In the Netherlands, whole grain, brown (50% whole grain) and white bread have about 25% of the market each, with white bread dominating the luxury and small bread market, followed by multigrain breads (Folloni and Ranieri 2013). There continues to be increased demand for greater variety of bread than ever with ethnic breads becoming more popular in Europe and greater varieties of wholemeal breads with oats, bran, seeds, etc. There is also a growing trend for increased production of sliced and wrapped bread in many countries across Europe including Germany and France. There will be continued growth in morning goods and specialty breads with many opportunities for innovation (Federation of bakers, http://www.bakersfederation.org.uk/). With respect to product innovation and development, health trends will continue with wholegrain, fiber and omega 3 all being important contributors. Whole grain launches across southern European food sectors continue to grow (Folloni and Ranieri 2013). In the Mediterranean area including France, Italy, Spain, Portugal, and Greece, new launches with whole grain claims have increased by 92% over 2005–2012, being the top four categories in 2011: bakery (52%), breakfast cereals (31%), side dishes (15%), and snacks (2%).

In North America, according to the Economic Research Service, USDA (2011, 2014), per capita grain availability, adjusted for losses, increased from 43.2 to 61.7 kg/year between 1970 and 2009, which corresponds to an increase in energy availability from 432 to 619 kcal/day during this interval. Per capita availability of flour and cereal products varied from 199.5 to 194.7 kg/year between 2000 and 2010. Breakdown of products between 2000 and 2012 was: wheat flour (146.3 to 134.4 kg), rye flour (0.5 to 0.5 kg), rice (19.2 to 20.4 kg in 2010), corn products (28.4 to 33.9 kg), oat products (4.4 to 5.2 kg), and barley products (0.7 to 0.6 kg). Consumers are interested in natural, convenience and indulgence and growing out of home consumption meaning less time spent on home food preparation and consumption. Bread is a staple food in the diets of many American consumers, as confirmed by NPD's National Eating Trends survey (International Markets Bureau 2012) which found that 68% of consumers reported eating bread in a two-week period, a frequency more than six times higher than the reported eatings of bagels, buns or crackers. Annual per capita consumption of bread at home or carried from home by Americans was 77 eatings in 2010. This is down slightly from the 80 eatings reported in 2006, but up from the low of 73 eatings per person, per year in 2009. Total retail sales of bread in the United States (U.S.) were US$21.4 million in 2010, according to Euromonitor (2011), with a compound annual growth rate (CAGR) of 1.6% since 2006. Sales are expected to reach US$23.6 million (CAGR of 1.2%). American consumers continue to embrace packaged/industrial bread, which accounts for about 66% of retail sales. Sales of packaged white and specialty breads have shown weakness over the 2006–2011 period, while sales of packaged whole wheat bread have grown. In fact, in 2010, sales of whole wheat bread surpassed sales of white bread for the first time. Euromonitor has attributed this shift to a number of factors, including more sophisticated consumer tastes and their desire for heartier or healthier and more nutritious food. Changes made by manufacturers have also influenced this shift, such as the removal of high-fructose corn syrup, lowering sodium, and experimenting with more exotic or ethnic varieties and new formats, like thinner slices. Despite increasing consumer interest, national brands have yet to respond to the gluten-free trend, which is currently a niche market. For consumers who currently report high consumption rates, price, longer-shelf life, less product waste is desired in the current economic climate (Collar and Rosell 2013). Easy-to-use formats, as well as improved nutritional attributes in line with the greater health interest and awareness of older consumers, are important considerations. In recent years, loaf bread has lost market share, mainly to alternatives such as rolls/buns, bagels, English muffins, tortillas (for wraps) and croissants. Much of this shift away from loaf bread and toward other types of bread-products has taken place to meet the taste demands of younger eaters (children and young adults), and of more affluent traditional or dual-income families without children. The challenge for manufacturers is to regain these consumer segments. This may mean increasing their nutritional profile and promoting healthier attributes which could include whole/ancient grains, flax seeds, chia seeds with high omega-3 content, gluten-free, all natural ingredients, high in protein, lower in sodium, fortified with vitamins/minerals, etc. (International Markets Bureau 2012).

South America wheat bread consumption is high only in Chile and Argentina (Cuniberti and Seghezzo 2009). In other South American countries the staples are maize and rice. In Argentina, wheat is the major source of calories and the second source of proteins after beef. Products derived from wheat supply 31% of the average Argentine's daily energy intake of some 12,000 kJ. Per capita bread consumption is 96 kg/year in Chile, 74 kg/year in Argentina (70 kg for craft bread and 4 kg for industrial bread), 28 kg/year in Peru, 27 kg/year in Brazil and 24 kg/year in Colombia. After Germany, Chile is the country with the highest per capita bread consumption of the world, currently.

3. Breads worldwide

Indigenous cereal-based foods from different cultures and civilizations define a wide variety of worldwide grain-related ethnic eating habits and foods disseminated in a globalized world with strong immigration movements. The assessment of the current and future impact of ethnic cereal-based foods on global eating patterns is a topic of transnational interest. Traditional and innovative approaches in ethnic goods are brought together, and significantly influence the grain market, convenience foods, and good nutrition (Collar 2009; Taylor and Cracknell 2009). Ethnic cereal-based foods are generally defined as products that are unique to a particular geographic region, or products that are produced from grains that are indigenous to a particular region. Western ethnic foods are defined as those wheat flour-based foods that initially became staples in Western Europe, and with European colonization, were transported around the world (Cracknell and Watts 2010) (Fig. 2).

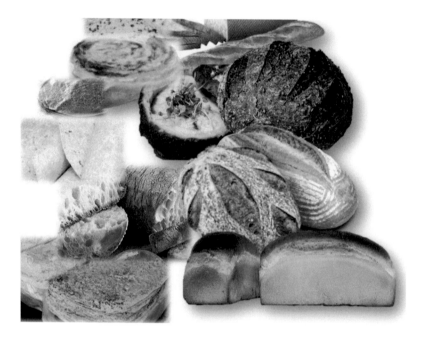

Figure 2. Assorted Western-style and flat ethnic breads.

3.1 Western ethnic breads

Cracknell and Watts (2010) reviewed in depth Western ethnic breads, of which a summary regarding bread types and breadmaking methods used follow. Pita is the oldest of known bread types with a range of potential countries of origin surrounding the Mediterranean Sea. Pita bread is a slightly leavened wheat bread, which is rolled flat and is either round or oval in shape and variable in size. It is commonly used as a wrap for a variety of filled pocket or rolled sandwiches and has spread throughout the world as a popular convenience food. *Sourdough* is a term used to describe bread produced where the leavening agent is a naturally occurring wild yeast or bacterium. The bread has a characteristic "sour" flavor and is as old as the history of leavened bread itself. Natural leavens or "starter" cultures consist of wild/natural yeast and lactobacilli maintained over time and used repeatedly, and produce breads with unique flavor, texture and keeping qualities. Hearth bread is the term used to describe the traditional baking method where a fermented doughpiece is baked on the floor of an often wood-fired oven. It is still widely used in small bakeries around the world, with an almost limitless range of local shapes and styles of bread. Hearth bread should have a distinctive appearance, taste and aroma with an open and coarse texture. Baguette (French bread and Vienna bread) is a hard crusty style of loaf associated with France, but developed in Vienna in the mid-19th century. Baguette is whiter, lighter and sweeter than the traditional sourdough breads. The golden-brown baguette, with crisp crust, sweet taste, characteristic external appearance with surface cuts, and white crumb with large irregular holes, is one of the most famous of all of the world's bread styles. Many regional adaptations of the baguette have developed across the world with the Pandesal of the Philippines, and the popular hearth type bread produced widely in Vietnam as examples. Pan bread is the term used to describe bread produced in a baking pan. It is a relatively recent innovation (18th century) that originates in England and Holland, which are the only European countries that routinely produce bread on a large scale in pans.

The regular shape, size and weight of the finished loaf led to the development of the sliced and wrapped loaf. Pan bread is produced by a range of methods, varying in mixing intensity, the use of rapid-acting maturing agents, and the length of bulk fermentation. The straight dough method is the traditional method of bread making with a bulk fermentation stage widely used in small bakeries in many parts of the world. The rapid dough method relies on full dough development during mixing, with no need for normal bulk fermentation as in the straight dough process. Doughs are divided, moulded and deposited direct into baking pans for proofing and baking. Bread is produced in two hours from start to finish, using medium strength, and medium protein flour. This is the popular method of bread manufacture in Australia, and it has spread to other countries which use Australian wheat (Cracknell and Watts 2010). The sponge and dough baking method is popular in the USA and successful marketing programs have seen it gain popularity in many Asian countries. The finished baked product has fine, even texture and excellent flavor which has contributed greatly to its popularity. The first stage or "sponge" is made by mixing a portion of the total flour and water together with the yeast and improver. The sponge is allowed to ferment up to four hours before the balance of the flour and other ingredients are added (including salt which if added sooner would inhibit fermentation) and remixed to form the complete dough. The dough is then allowed to relax, then divided, moulded and baked in a conventional manner to produce bread of high specific volume. The basic recipe of Focacciais thought to have originated from the Etruscans or ancient Greeks. It is likely to be the early precursor of the Pizza and whilst popular in Italy has spread all over the world. It comprises yeasted bread dough, often mixed or spread with oil, herbs, onion, garlic, sage, rosemary or oregano and cooked quickly. A bagel is a bread product, traditionally shaped by hand into the form of a ring from yeasted wheat dough, which is initially boiled for a short time in water then baked. The result is a dense, chewy, doughy interior with a browned and sometimes crisp exterior. Bagels are often topped with seeds baked on the outer crust, with the traditional ones being poppy or sesame seeds. Some may have salt sprinkled on their surface, and there are also a number of different dough types such as whole-grain or rye.

3.2 Ethnic breads

The first breads produced were probably cooked versions of a grain-paste, made from ground cereal grains and water. Descendants of these early breads are still commonly made from various grains worldwide, including the lavashs (Iran and Turkey), sangak (Iran), tortilla (Mexico), chapatti and roti (India) and pita (Middle East). Flatbreads are a simple form of bread made from flattened dough (Fig. 2). They may be leavened or unleavened, and they are still a very important stable or staple food among the people of the Middle East and India. Their use is spreading throughout the Western world due to their versatility (Koksel et al. 2009). Flatbreads are staples in Northeast Africa (Ethiopia, Eritrea and Sudan). They are made from a variety of different cereals, especially sorghum, finger millet and teff and resemble pancakes (Taylor and Taylor 2009). Unlike pancakes served in the West, many of these products have a leavened texture and an acidic flavor. These characteristics are a result of a mixed lactic acid bacteria and yeast fermentation. Probably the two most well-known flatbreads are injera and kisra. Injera is a large (some 50 cm in diameter), spongy textured pancake about 5 mm thick from Ethiopia and Eritrea. Its surface has a honeycomb-like appearance, very similar to a natural sponge, which is created by the escaping carbon dioxide during the steaming process. Teff is the preferred cereal for making injera in Ethiopia. This is due to the superior keeping qualities of teff injera when compared to injera made from other cereals such as sorghum. Kisra from Sudan is much thinner (1–1.5 mm thick) and smaller (approximately 30 cm in diameter) than injera. It is more like a flexible thin wafer. These flatbreads remain almost exclusively home-made products despite the fact that there are flourishing commercial bakeries in countries such as Ethiopia and the Sudan. In Kenya wheat flour chapattis are a very popular home-baked food in all communities. It is probable that this type of flatbread was introduced by Indians who settled in the country in the late 19th and early 20th century.

Steamed breads and buns are consumed throughout South East Asia but mostly in China, Japan, and Korea (Solah 2009). The characteristics of steamed breads and buns vary from country to country and region to region. Steamed buns can be filled (bao) or not filled (mantou). Mantou which is unfilled is the only product called steamed bread. Char siewbao, steamed buns with barbecue pork filling has white skin and splits open on steaming. This splitting is a positive quality characteristic. Char siewbao is very soft and cake-like and the highest quality is high in sugar (up to 30%) although low in fat. Low sugar char siewbao with a low-fat filling could contribute to a healthy diet. Hong Kong style char siewbao is made with low protein soft wheat and is usually sold fresh. The buns are usually chemically leavened with ammonia hydroxide which is released on baking. Singapore style char siewbao are firmer than Hong Kong style and use higher protein flour.

4. Nutritional value of bread: recommended intake and nutritional claims

Grains are sophisticated reservoirs of macronutrients, cell wall polysaccharides (dietary fiber) and many biologically active minor constituents. As 30–70% of daily energy according to the country income is derived from cereal-based foods, their role in nutrition is important. Cereal-based foods are an important source of carbohydrates, protein, dietary fiber, especially B vitamins and minerals. The starchy endosperm gathered most of the scientific and technological interest for food processing until the end of the previous century. The recognition of the importance of the outer grain layers for health maintenance created the interest to reveal the types, amounts and potential physiological significance of various vitamins, minerals and phytochemicals in the whole grain and food made thereof. It also has been recognized that food structure at different levels, to a large extent modified in food processing, is important in controlling the rate and extent of digestion of nutrients and the bioavailability of phytochemicals (Poutanen 2012). In the European Prospective Investigation into Cancer and Nutrition (EPIC) study populations, 27% of total carbohydrate intake was from bread. The majority of bread, as well as other baked goods, is made of refined white wheat flour, free of the outer grain layers rich in cell wall material and associated phenolic compounds, minerals and vitamins. Epidemiological studies constantly show that intake of whole grain and cereal dietary fiber protect against the rapidly increasing chronic diseases related to a sedentary lifestyle, such as cardiovascular disease and type 2 diabetes (Collar 2008).

4.1 Energy and macronutrients

With an energy content of around 2.2 kcal (9.2 kJ)/g, bread is considered a 'medium' calorie food from an energy density perspective (Rolls 2005). Most of the energy in bread comes from starch; therefore, bread is generally classified as a 'starchy food'. A medium slice of white bread typically provides 86 kcal (361 kJ). Continental breads (such as focaccia) contain oils (usually olive oil; rich in monounsaturated fatty acids) that increase the calorie content, with a 50 g serving of focaccia containing, on average, 180 kcal (756 kJ). An average slice of ciabatta (around 45 g) contains, on average, 116 kcal (487 kJ). Wholemeal (2.2 g/100 g) and brown flours (2 g/100 g) therefore contain slightly more fat than white flour (1.2 g/100 g) (O'Connor, 2012). Although white and brown flour provide a similar profile of saturated (e.g., palmitic acid), monounsaturated (e.g., oleic acid) and polyunsaturated fatty acids (e.g., linoleic acid), the specific flours differ in their fatty acid concentration, with wholemeal flour providing the greatest proportion of fatty acids. The amount of fat/100 g bread is small. However, the addition of fat during the bread-making process or in meal preparation can increase the fat content. Bread also contains considerable amounts of protein and carbohydrate.

The amount of fiber in the bread depends on the flour used to make it. A slice of 40 g of white wheat bread will deliver about 1 g of dietary fiber, and a similar slice of whole meal bread would deliver 3–4.5 g. During the day, the choice of bread has a large effect on intake of dietary fiber, and six portions of whole meal bread would provide close to the recommended intake of dietary fiber of 25–35 g per day (WHO 2003). A range of minerals, vitamins and phytochemicals have been detected to be concentrated in the same grain parts as most of the dietary fiber polymers (Table 1), and there is increasing evidence about their biological activity and possible interference with various disease pathologies.

Table 1. Vitamins and minerals of wheat and rye breads. Source: www.nutritiondata.com.

per 100 g bread	Wheat					Rye				
	Unit	Brown		Wholegrain		Unit	Refined		Whole	
			%RDA		%RDA			%RDA		%RDA
Vitamins										
Vitamin K	µg	7.8	6%	2.2	3%	µg	3.1	4%	1.2	1%
Thiamine	mg	0.4	25%	0.4	27%		0.5	30%	0.4	29%
Riboflavin	mg	0.2	18%	0.3	20%		0.3	19%	0.3	20%
Niacin	mg	4.7	26%	4.4	22%		4.4	22%	3.8	19%
Vitamin B6	mg	0.2	6%	0.3	17%		0.1	4%	0.1	4%
Folate	µg	50.0	21%	118	29%		111	28%	110	27%
PantothenicAcid	mg	0.7	8%	0.5	5%		0.2	2%	0.4	4%
Cholin	mg	23.9		~			14.6		~	
Betain	mg	180		~			102		~	
Minerals										
Ca	mg	107	14%	91.0	9%		151	15%	73.0	7%
Fe	mg	2.4	19%	3.5	19%		3.7	21%	2.8	16%
Mg	mg	82.0	12%	53.0	13%		23.0	6%	40.0	10%
P	mg	202	15%	176	18%		99.0	10%	125	12%
K	mg	248	5%	204	6%		100	3%	166	5%
Na	mg	472	22%	487	20%		681	28%	660	27%
Zn	mg	1.8	8%	1.3	8%		0.7	5%	1.1	8%
Cu	mg	0.4	8%	0.3	13%		0.3	13%	0.2	9%
Mn	mg	2.1	56%	1.5	74%		0.5	24%	0.8	41%
Se	µg	40.3	41%	29.5	42%		17.3	25%	30.9	44%

RDA: Recommended Dietary Allowances (percent daily values for adults or children aged 4 or older, and based on a 2,000 calorie reference diet) of different breads. Source: U.S. Department of Agriculture, Agricultural Research Service. 2012. USDA National Nutrient Database for Standard Reference, Release 25. Nutrient Data Laboratory Home Page, http://www.ars.usda.gov; Dietary Reference Intakes (DRIs): Recommended Dietary Allowances and Adequate Intakes. Elements. Food and Nutrition Board. Institute of Medicine. National Academies. http://www.nap.edu

4.2 Micronutrients

Bread provides various micronutrients, including calcium, iron, zinc, copper, magnesium, manganese, selenium and some B-vitamins, including folate (Table 1). Any food that provides 15% or 30% of the recommended daily allowance (RDA) for a specific vitamin or mineral, per 100 g, is considered a 'source of' or 'high in', respectively, in the named vitamin or mineral (European Commission 2006). As Table 1 outlines, bread can be considered a 'source of' and/or 'high in' many micronutrients. Brown and wholegrain wheat and rye breads are considered sources of Fe, P, Na, thiamine, riboflavin, niacin, vitamin B6 (wholegrain), and folate. Wholegrain breads are high in Mn and Se, while refined wheat and rye breads are source of Ca. In the wheat grain-refining process outer layers are removed, resulting in the loss of vitamins, minerals, and other health-related compounds (Collar 2008). According to the USDA Nutrient Database (2004), essential nutrients decrease to the following levels with respect to the levels occurring in wholewheat after refining: vitamin E (7%), vitamin B6 (13%), vitamin K (16%), Mg (16%), Mn (18%), riboflavin, niacin (20%), Zn (24%), K (26%), thiamin (27%), Fe (30%), P (31%), Cu (38%), Na (40%), pantothenic acid (43%), Ca (44%), Se (48%), and folate (59%).

The predominant vitamins in bread are the B-vitamins, specifically thiamine, niacin and folate (Table 1). Bread contains some vitamin B6 and vitamin E, in smaller amounts. Data from the National Diet and Nutrition Survey (NDNS) carried out in 2000/2001 in UK adults (O'Connor 2012) showed that cereal and cereal products were the main source of dietary thiamine, providing one-third of the mean daily intake (Henderson et al. 2003). Two medium slices of bread (72 g) provide around 0.19 g of thiamine. According to the criteria in the EU Nutrition and Health Claims Regulation (2006), white, brown, wholemeal and granary bread are a 'source of' thiamine and wheat germ bread is 'high' in thiamine. According to the Department of Health (1991), two medium slices of bread provide, on an average, almost 20% of the DRV for men and 24% of the DRV for women (O'Connor 2012), showing that bread can make a valuable contribution to meeting daily thiamine requirements. Concerning niacin, two medium slices of bread provide, on an average, 16% of the DRV for women, which is 13 mg/day, and 12% of the DRV for men, which is 17 mg/day (Department of Health 1991). Regarding folate, two medium slices of bread provide, on an average, 47 mg/day, which is 17% of the DRV for adults (200 mg/day). Thus, bread can make an important contribution to meet daily folate requirements.

Bread contains a variety of minerals, at varying concentrations, depending on the type of bread (Table 1). According to the 2000/2001 NDNS, bread provided more than 10% of the adult dietary intake of iron, zinc, copper, magnesium; about one-fifth of calcium; and more than one-quarter of manganese (Henderson et al. 2003; O'Connor 2012). Currently, bread is likely to have reduced its contribution to these nutrients according to the decreased bread intake over the past decade. White bread contributes 13% to the mean intake of calcium overall (Henderson et al. 2003), so that bread can make a considerable contribution to calcium intake. Two medium slices of bread provide, on an average, 18% of the DRV for adults, which is 700 mg/day according to (Department of Health 1991). Phytic acid can reduce calcium absorption from foods by forming an insoluble salt in the gut, calcium phytate. Phytates are present in wholegrain cereals, including wholemeal bread, suggesting that calcium from white bread may be more easily absorbed than the calcium from wholegrain versions. It has been demonstrated that calcium absorption from calcium-fortified white and whole wheat bread compared favourably with absorption from milk (Martin et al. 2002). Concerning Fe, two medium slices of bread provide, on an average, 11% of the DRV for women, which is 14.8 mg/day, and almost one-fifth of the DRV for men, which is 8.7 mg/day (Department of Health 1991). White bread alone contributes 6% of the total Zn intake in UK (Henderson et al. 2003) with two medium slices of bread containing 1.02 mg providing, on an average, 14% of the DRV for women, which is 7 mg/day and, on average, 11% of the DRV for men, which is 9.5 mg/day. On Mg, two medium slices of white bread provide, on an average, 13% of the DRV for women, which is 270 mg/day and, on average, 11% of the DRV for men, which is 300 mg/day (Department of Health 1991).

4.3 Phytochemicals

The highest amounts of phytochemicals are found in the outer layers of grains and include phenolic compounds, phytosterols and tocols (tocopherols and tocotrienols) (Mattila et al. 2005). These plant substances have been substantiated to have antioxidant properties *in vivo*. A study examining the total antioxidant capacity of various foodstuffs, including cereals (such as wheat) and 18 cereal products, found that wholemeal buckwheat and wheat bran had the greatest total antioxidant capacity value, while white flour showed the lowest total antioxidant capacity value, indicating that flour containing the outer layers of the wheat grain and germ has a greater potential antioxidant activity than white flour (Pellegrini et al. 2006). In a recent study the polyphenol qualitative and quantitative profile and antiradical properties of enzyme-digested extracts mimicking human gastrointestinal conditions, from single oat, rye, buckwheat and wheat and multigrain quaternary breads at different levels of wheat flour replacement, has been investigated, and the relationships between total and individual polyphenols and kinetics of reduction of the free radical 2,2-diphenyl-1-picrylhydrazyl (DPPH) have been established (Angioloni and Collar 2011a). The total phenol content amongst the single bread extracts were significantly higher in buckwheat (808 mg gallic acid equivalents (GAE)/kg) and decreased in the following order: buckwheat > wheat > oat > rye. Mixed breads exhibited increased polyphenol content (up to 1135 mg GAE/kg) and higher polyphenol bioaccessibility (from 55% to 80%) with increasing degree of wheat replacement. Similar trends were found for antioxidant power. DPPH reduction followed two-step kinetics in all cases, where a considerable amount of phenolic acids and flavonoids correspond to high antiradical activity and to slow-kinetic rates (protocatechuic acid, ferulic acid), particularly for mixed grain bread extracts.

5. Bread and health claims: matching a naturally healthy food

Accumulated epidemiological studies during the past 15 years have shown the protective role of whole grain foods against chronic diseases, such as cardiovascular disease, type 2 diabetes and colon cancer. Although it has been calculated that consuming up to 50% of all grain foods as refined grain foods, when they do not contain high levels of added fat, sugar, or sodium, is not associated with increased disease risk. Whole grain foods are considered to be protective for health. Cereal dietary fiber is considered to be the main contributor to the health protective effects of whole grain foods. In addition, the potential role of phenolic and other minor grain constituents in health maintenance has been emphasized (Poutanen et al. 2014).

Following reports of epidemiological studies showing the importance of whole grain as compiled by the Whole Grains Council (http://wholegrainscouncil.org/), numerous actions have been taken to promote the use of cereal foods containing whole grain and dietary fiber, as recently reported by Poutanen (2012) and Poutanen et al. (2014). In 2003, the WHO/FAO expert consultation recommended that whole grain cereals, fruits and vegetables are the preferred sources of non-starch polysaccharides, the intake of which should be 20 g/day. Dietary recommendations in the US (www. mypyramid.gov) are to consume at least half of cereal foods as whole grain, and the Nordic dietary recommendations also recommend eating cereal foods as whole grain products (http://www.norden.org/fi/julkaisut/julkaisut/nord-2013–009). In Australia, according to The Australian Guide To Healthy Eating (http://www.eatforhealth.gov. au/), the recommended number of daily cereal servings for adults aged 19 to 60 years is four to nine for women and six to 12 for men. A serving equates to two slices of bread. The Canada's Food Guide (http://www.hc-sc.gc.ca/fn-an/food-guide-aliment/ index-eng.php) recommends at least three servings a day of whole grain breads, oatmeal or whole wheat pasta for all Canadians aged 9 and up. (2007). In Denmark, whole grain foods have been promoted by a campaign and logo (http://www.fuldkorn. dk/english/) with the aim of reaching the recommended daily intake of 75 g whole grain, and in the US, by a stamp and communication by Whole Grains Council (http:// wholegrainscouncil.org/whole-grain-stamp) helping consumers to reach a daily intake of whole grain of at least 48 g. In Spain, the Spanish Society for Communitary Nutrition (SENC 2004) recommends a daily intake of 4–6 servings of cereal-based goods, half of them made of wholegrain. The German Nutrition Society (http://www. dge.de/) indicates similar recommendations.

In 1999, the US Food and Drug Administration (www.fda.gov) accepted a health claim for whole grain foods: "Diets rich in whole grain foods and other plant foods and low in total fat, saturated fat, and cholesterol may reduce the risk of heart disease and some cancers". The European Food Safety Authority (http://www.efsa.europa. eu/) has not accepted a health claim concerning whole grain foods, but some health claims can be used in connection with cereal ingredients, such as wheat and oat bran, rye fiber and oat ß-glucan. Some examples follow. Rye fiber contributes to normal bowel function for food which fulfils the high fiber claim with this fiber. Barley grain fiber, oat grain fiber and wheat bran fiber contribute to an increase in faecal bulk for food which fulfils the high fiber claim with every fiber. Wheat bran fiber contributes to an acceleration of intestinal transit for food which fulfils the high fiber claim with this fiber with a daily intake of ≥ 10 g of wheat bran. Consumption of arabinoxylan (AX) from wheat endosperm as part of a meal contributes to a reduction of the blood glucose rise after that meal for food which contains at least 8 g AX-rich fiber per 100 g of available carbohydrates in a quantified portion. Consumption of ß-glucans from oat or barley as part of a meal contributes to the reduction of the blood glucose rise after the meal for food which contains ≥ 4 g of ß-glucans from oats or barley for each 30 g of available carbohydrates in a quantified portion. ß-glucans contribute to the maintenance of normal blood cholesterol levels for food which contains ≥ 1 g of beta-glucans from oats, oat bran, barley, barley bran, or from their mixtures per quantified portion, 3 g needed per day. Replacing digestible starches with resistant starch in a meal contributes to a reduction of postprandial glucose when the final content of resistant starch is at least 14% of total starch.

In Europe, Regulation (EC) Nr. 1924/2006 of The European Parliament and of the Council of 20 December 2006 (European Commission 2006) on nutrition and health claims made on food provides a list of allowed nutrition claims (http://ec.europa.eu/food/food/labellingnutrition/claims/community_register/nutrition_claims_en.htm), many of which also are relevant to cereal foods, such as "source of fiber" for products containing at least 3 g DF/100 g product, and "rich in fiber" for those containing 6 g DF/100 g product. Also, a claim that a food is "energy-reduced, light or lite", and any claim likely to have the same meaning for the consumer, may only be made where the energy value is reduced by at least 30%, with an indication of the characteristic(s) which make(s) the food reduced in its total energy value. Some commercial and experimental breads (Table 2) fulfill these nutrition claims, and can be labeled either as "source of fiber" or "rich in fiber", and/or "light" (Fig. 3).

Protein, vitamins and omega-3 and polyunsaturated fatty acids also are among those food components where nutrition claims may be used to show a high content

Table 2. Nutritional composition of refined wheat flour breads with added dietary fiber.

Nutrition facts, per 100 g bread	Sandwich bread		White pan bread		Pan bread		
	Reference	Low calorie high-fiber bread[1]	Reference	High-fiber bread[2]	Reference	High-fiber light bread[3]	High-fiber white bread[4]
Moisture, g					36.1	43.3	35.3
Energy, kcal	270	198	241	232	238	132	222
Protein, g	7.5	8.1	7.6	7.1	13.90	13.51	12.50
Digestible carbohydrates, g	50	38.6	47.9	45.1	42.33	16.66	39.4
Fat, g	4.1	0.94	2.0	2.0	1.45	1.21	1.63
Total Dietary fiber, g	2.8	8.5	2.0	6.1	4.53	23.24	9.63
Soluble, g			0	4.3	1.28	2.79	2.65
Insoluble, g					2.84	19.37	6.79
Ash, g					1.69	2.08	1.57

(1) Includes wheat fiber VITACEL WF 101 from Rettenmaier & Söhne GMBH.
(2) Includes polydextrose Litesse from Danisco Sweeteners Ltd.
(3) Includes a mix of soluble and insoluble fibers. Patent Nr. 200601668. CSIC. 2006 (Santos 2010).
(4) Includes inulin and oat fiber (Santos 2010).

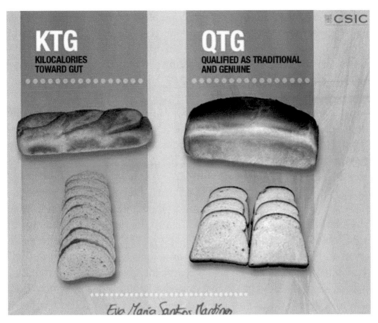

Figure 3. Designed experimental high-fiber (KTG, QTG) and light (KTG) breads (Santos 2010). Picture and photocomposition by Eva Santos Martínez, with permission.

(European Commission 2006). In addition to arabinoxylan, ß-glucan and cellulose, resistant starch, lignin and other phenolics associated with carbohydrate polymers are part of the cereal dietary fiber complex. Despite the known health effects, recommendations, labeling and communication campaigns, the majority of cereal foods consumed are made of refined flour, and contain less dietary fiber and other health-promoting compounds than are present in the whole grain raw material (Poutanen et al. 2014).

O'Connor (2012) considers in a recent review the health impact that the nutrients intake bread provides, reports evidences regarding the health benefits of specific macro and microcomponents of bread and describes the effect of bread consumption on satiety and appetite control. In this section, special emphasis is placed on the starch digestibility and starch nutritional fractions of breads. Glycaemic index (GI) is a characteristic of the rate at which sugar is absorbed from the bloodstream after eating a specific food. It is determined by comparing the blood glucose response to ingestion of 50 g of available carbohydrate from a test food with that of a reference food (typically either glucose or white bread that is made from wheat flour). A slow release and absorption of glucose may be generated in a food matrix according to the processing conditions and surrounding ingredients (Lehmann and Robin 2007), encompassing beneficial effects in the management of diabetes and hyperlipidemia (Jenkins 2007). Bread, like potatoes and white rice, is generally classified as a high GI food. However, the GI will vary, depending on a number of factors such as the type of grain (i.e., the use of barley and oats to make bread). Factors that influence gastric emptying and digestion rate include the physical structure of the bread, that is, the more compact the structure, the lower the glycaemic response (the particle size remains intact for longer, slowing down the digestive process); the fiber content; the type of starch in the bread (as RS slows gastric emptying); and the baking process (e.g., intensity of kneading) (Fardet et al. 2006). Adding fat to breadmixes reduces the GI but, of course, increases the fat and calorie content (Braaten et al. 1994). If bread is eaten with a meal, or in combination with other foods (such as a sandwich), the carbohydrate tends to be broken down more slowly and glucose enters the bloodstream at a slower rate (dependent on the macronutrient composition of the whole meal). The GI value given in the Foster–Powell et al. (2002) table for 95 types of bread varies widely from 27 (e.g., barley bread with 75% wholegrain-bread containing intact cereal grains is digested more slowly) to 95 (e.g., French baguette-starch is readily digested) (Foster–Powell et al. 2002). A low-to-moderate GI value would be < 70 and a high GI value would be in the range of 70–100. Increasing the content of fiber in bread has been shown to reduce the GI of bread in a recent dietary intervention trial (Broekaert et al. 2011), and by *in vitro* determinations (Angioloni and Collar 2011c). Given that white bread has a high GI value, recent advances in reformulating white bread by using composite flours (maize flour, barley flour or flours from cereal-free grains such as leguminous or pseudocereals) to produce novel bread products have improved glycaemic responses determined either *in vivo* or *in vitro* (Angioloni and Collar 2012; Burton et al. 2011; Collar et al. 2014a,b; Collar and Angioloni 2014a) (Table 3).

The *in vitro* determination of carbohydrate digestibility to predict the glycaemic response of complex foods is of great interest since *in vivo* evaluations are invasive, labor-intensive and costly (Lehmann and Robin 2007). In cereal products such as bread, the starch gelatinization extent, and the cooking time and temperature influence the formation of SDS (Englyst et al. 2003). In addition, amylose can complex with lipids hindering attack by hydrolytic enzymes more than its free carbohydrate. Characteristics such as solubility and the presence of fiber, fat and protein all contribute to the rate of digestion (Dona et al. 2010). Through the process of retrogradation, gelatinized or solubilized starch can be transformed from an unstructured into a more ordered or crystalline state. This large physical change causes heat processed starchy foods to harden or become stale as they spontaneously approach a metastable state of lower free energy. This has been reported to decrease the GI value, due to an increased resistance to amylase (Chung et al. 2006). Starch hydrolysis that follows first order kinetics (Frei et al. 2003), proceeded at different rate and extent for blended samples compared to the wheat flour counterparts (Table 3). The steadystate kinetic constant (k) of amylolysis that has been proposed as are liable index of the inherent susceptibility of flour starches to amylase hydrolysis (Frei et al. 2003) ranged from 0.042 for a mix of oat:rye:buckwheat:wheat to 0.1106 for teff:greenpea:buckwheat:wheat in blended samples *vs.* 0.0720 in control breads, evidencing from slower to faster hydrolysis kinetics, respectively, depending on bread formulation. C_∞ that corresponds to the equilibrium percentage of starch hydrolyzed after 16 h, varied from 60 to 91. Control breads underwent up to 81% of starch hydrolysis, so that major non-wheat replaced

Table 3. Starch hydrolysis kinetics, Expected glycaemic index and relevant Starch nutritional fractions of blended breads (Angioloni and Collar 2011b, 2012; Collar et al. 2014a,b; Collar and Angioloni 2014a).

Blended bread	Starch hydrolysis kinetics					Starch nutritional fractions (per 100 g bread, as is)				
	C_∞	k	H_{90}, %	HI, %	eGI	RDS g	SDS g	DS g	RS, g	TS, g
WT	81	0.072	81	100	94	68.5	7.5	76	1.8	78
T:GP:BK:WT, 7.5:7.5:7.5:77.5	74	0.0797	74	91	87	56.2	5.7	61.9	2.8	65
T:GP:BK:WT, 15:15:15:55	71	0.1106	71	88	84	60.0	2.3	62.3	2.5	65
T:GP:BK:WT, 15:7.5:15:62.5	76	0.0599	75	94	89	59.6	11.8	71.4	2.3	74
T:GP:BK:WT, 15:15:7.5:62.5	76	0.0821	76	93	89	54.3	4.5	58.8	2.2	61
YM-WT	71	0.074	71	89	85	52.3	8.1	60.5	4.7	65
WM-WT	67	0.055	67	86	82	45.9	12.5	58.4	5.5	64
YM-RS-WT	63	0.074	63	79	76	45.9	6.2	52.2	11.8	64
WM-RS-WT	60	0.046	59	74	72	37.1	16.3	53.4	11.6	65
O:R:BK:WT, 15:15:15:55	90	0.094	90	100	94	55	3.5	60	1.4	59
O:R:BK:WT, 20:20:20:40	91	0.042	89	97	92	42	16.0	61	3.2	61
O:R:BK:WT, 25:25:25:25	90	0.053	89	97	92	46	11.6	61	4.2	62
CP:GP:SB:WT:CMC:GL, 20:20:2:48:5:5	73	0.098	73	77	75	42.9	5.3	48	2.3	50
CP:GP:SB:WT:CMC:GL, 20:14:8:52:3:3	60	0.089	60	63	63	32.4	1.4	34	2.4	36
CP:GP:SB:WT:CMC:GL, 20:8:14:48:5:5	72	0.066	71	77	75	38	5.2	43	2.4	46
CP:GP:SB:WT:CMC:GL, 14:14:8:58:3:3	73	0.068	73	77	75	34.6	5.2	40	1.8	42
WT:CB, 60:40	79	0.094	79	96	91	53.1	3.4	57	4.4	61
WT:HBGB, 60:40	75	0.052	74	89	85	34.7	9.3	44	7	51

Flours and ingredients used in blends: WT, wheat; T, teff; GP, greenpea; BK, buckwheat; YM, yellow maize; WM, White maize; RS, resistant starch; O, oat; R, rye; CP, chickpea; SB, soybean; CMC, carboxymethylcellulose; GL, gluten; CB, comercial barley; HBGB, high ß-glucan barley; RDS: rapidly digestible starch, SDS: slowly digestible starch, eGI: expected glycaemic index, DS: digestible starch, TS: total starch. C_∞: equilibrium concentration, k: kinetic constant, H_{90}: total starch hydrolysis at 90 min, *HI*: hydrolysis index. A first order kinetic equation $[C = C_\infty(1-e^{-kt})]$ was applied to describe the kinetics of starch hydrolysis C concentration at t time; t time. TS = DS + RS; DS = RDS + SDS.

samples showed a lower extent of starch hydrolysis despite at 90 min of reaction time, the equilibrium is already reached in almost all blended samples with similar values for C_∞ and H_{90} (Table 3).

Calculation of the samples hydrolysis indices ($HI_\%$), the proportion of flourstarch that is theoretically digestible, by dividing the area under the hydrolysis curve of each blended sample by the corresponding area of the control sample

(Table 3) pointed out the lowest value in sample containing chickpea:greenpea:soybean in good accordance with the lowest equilibrium percentage of starch hydrolyzed C_∞, and hence leading to the lowest *eGI* (63). Categorized starch fractions based on the rate of glucose released and its absorption in the gastrointestinal tract include rapidly digestible starch (RDS), slowly digestible starch (SDS) and resistant starch (RS), defined here as the three consecutive nutritional fractions divided by reaction time when *in vitro* starch digestion takes place (Table 3). Simultaneous lower RDS and higher SDS and RS contents, are considered suitable nutritional trends for dietary starch fractions (Englyst et al. 2003). RDS is the fraction of starch granules that cause a rapid increase in blood glucose concentration after ingestion of carbohydrates. The fraction of starch that is said to be RDS *in vitro* is defined as the amount of starch digested in the first 20 min of a standard digestion reaction mixture. Although RDS is defined by experimental analysis of digestion *in vitro*, it has been reported that the rate of starch conversion to sugar follows similar kinetics in the human digestive system (Dona et al. 2010). Values for RDS (g/100 g bread, as is) were all lower in blended breads (from 32.4%–60.0%) than in control WT (68.5%) breads (Table 3). SDS is defined as the starch that is digested after the RDS but in no longer than 120 min under standard conditions of substrate and enzyme concentration. The ingestion of SDS has been proven to result in a smaller increase and longer sustained rise in plasma glucose (Sands et al. 2009). Blended breads explicited a wide range of SDS (g/100 g bread, as is) values ranging from 1.4% for complex leguminous flour formulations to 16.3% found in RS-enriched white maize flour blends, *vs.* control breads that contained intermediate amounts (7.5%) (Table 3). The fraction of starch that escapes digestion in the small intestine, and may be subject to bacterial fermentation in the large intestine, is termed RS. Blended breads with no added RS contained up to 7.0% of RS (g/100 g bread, as is) for matrices containing 40% of high ß-glucan barley flour (Collar and Angioloni 2014a); values are in general higher than the content found in control breads (1.8%) (Table 3). Simultaneous lower rapidly digestible starch (57.1%) and higher slowly digestible starch (12.9%) and resistant starch (2.8%) contents (g per 100 g fresh bread), considered suitable nutritional trends for dietary starch fractions (Englyst et al. 2003), were met by the blend formulated 7.5% teff, 15% greenpea, 15% buckwheat (Collar et al. 2014b). The associated mixture that replaced 37.5% of wheat flour (WF), showed a rather lower extent and slower rate of starch hydrolysis with medium-low values for C_∞, and *H90*, and lowest *k,* and intermediate eGI (86). Maize-based blended breads also showed most appealing nutritional quality than WF breads, in terms of lower digestible starch and RDS, higher SDS and RS contents of medium-high sensorially rated bread matrices (Collar et al. 2014a).

The incorporation of non-wheat flours into wheat bread formulation seems to reduce starch hydrolysis, probably because of their lower starch and higher fiber and protein contents (Tables 4 and 5). The reduced rate and overall reduced starch digestibility of barley mixed breads may be affected by high content of viscous soluble dietary fiber components like in legume matrices (Angioloni and Collar 2012; Collar and Angioloni 2014a) supported by the high amount of β-glucan determined in wheat–barley breads (Table 5). In addition, high protein content of barley flours (Table 5) can promote starch-protein interactions restricting enzyme attack.

Table 4. Chemical and nutritional information of single and blended cereal breads.

Nutrient	Oat (O)	Kamut®	Spelt	Rye (R)	Buck-wheat (BK)	Wheat (WT)	O:R:BK:WT, 20:20:20:40
	per 100 g bread, as is						
Moisture, g	33.6	31.6	29.7	30.2	29.6	28.1	38.9
Fat, g	3.26	0.33	0.47	0.34	0.80	0.33	1.01
Protein, g	13.57	11.26	10.36	6.99	12.59	9.60	9.43
Ash, g	1.73	1.40	1.79	1.26	1.78	1.10	1.40
Digestible carbohydrates, g	36	49	53	50	46	59	42
Total dietary fiber, g	11.91	6.23	5.02	11.30	9.65	1.88	7.29
Soluble dietary fiber, g	2.92	0.28	1.04	3.56	1.70	0.85	1.96
Insoluble dietary fiber, g	8.99	5.95	3.98	7.74	7.95	1.03	5.33
Resistant starch, g	4.28	1.11	1.08	4.31	4.77	0.94	3.15
β-glucans, g	2.30	0.17	0.42	0.92	0.62	0.10	0.81
Minerals, mg	444	377	542	388	438	336	396
Ca, mg	10.6	10.0	17.2	26.9	20.1	24.7	21,4
Cu, mg	0.2	0.2	0.2	0.1	0.2	0.1	0,2
Fe, mg	2.2	1.8	1.4	1.9	1.7	0.7	1,4
Mg, mg	78.3	52.4	61.2	30.5	20.9	24.9	35,9
Mn, mg	1.9	1.3	1.6	1.2	0.8	0.3	0,9
K, mg	199.9	147.4	201.2	155.4	197.4	62.8	136
Na, mg	149.2	162.6	258.2	170.8	195.6	241.9	200
Zn, mg	1.8	1.4	1.5	0.9	1.1	0.5	0.97
Total phenolics, mg	280	219	188	209	209	238	745
Phenolic bioavailability, %	9	16	17	16	17	17	74
Energy, kcal	225	242	267	228	237	278	292

Source: adapted from Angioloni and Collar (2011b), with permission.

6. Value-added breads

Although it would be expected this new decade to create some entirely new product templates, it should also be considered evolutions of existing product platforms. It raises a great deal of recent interest that minor cereals, ancient crops, pseudocereals and legumes, besides wheat, constitute highly nutritional and healthy grains with potential breadmaking applications. Indigenous foods from different cultures with ethnic eating habits are moving in a globalized world with strong immigration movements, encompassing the use of traditional local raw materials as novel ingredients in classic and highly consumed foods (fermented baked goods) somewhere else. In this dynamic and diverse context, the integration of non-breadmaking grains and seeds into viscoelastic breadmaking systems and fermented baked goods appear as a challenging

Table 5. Proximate chemical and nutritional composition of flours (per 100 g flour, d.b.) and blended breads (per 100 g fresh blended bread).

Sample code	Protein (g)	Total dietary fiber (g)	Insoluble dietary fiber (g)	Soluble dietary fiber (g)	Fat (g)	Ash (g)	Digestible Carbohydrates (g)	Energy kcal	Moisture (g)
Flours									
Wheat (WT)	14.13	2.19	1.20	0.99	1.56	0.63	82	-	14.32
Commercial barley (CB)	11.27	15.2	10.05	5.15	1.69	1.52	58		12.8
High ß-glucan barley (HBGB)	17.74	32.1	18.5	13.71	5.38	1.83	35		8.3
Yellow maize (YM)	5.68	3.55	0.99	2.55	2.16	0.66	88		12.99
White maize (WM)	5.25	4.31	0.77	3.54	1.56	0.56	88		13.54
Teff (T)	13.05	12.19	7.40	4.80	5.06	2.21	67	-	11.90
Chickpea (CP)	16.56	22.2			6.16	2.60	43		9.9
Soybean (SB)	49.68	13.6			3.24	5.81	17		10.5
Greenpea (GP)	25.12	14.56	8.50	6.05	1.27	2.58	57	-	8.17
Buckwheat (BW)	19.71	13.52	6.58	6.93	3.44	2.05	61	-	11.70
Breads									
T:GP:BK:WT, 7.5:7.5:7.5:77.5	11.6	2.9	1.63	1.24	3.6	-	50	283	32.3
T:GP:BK:WT, 15:15:15:55	12.2	4.3	2.42	1.88	3.8	-	48	283	31.9
T:GP:BK:WT, 15:7.5:15:62.5	11.7	3.8	2.13	1.67	3.8	-	51	295	29.3
T:GP:BK:WT, 15:15:7.5:62.5	12.2	3.8	2.21	1.63	3.7	-	48	282	32.2
CP:GP:SB:WT: CMC:GL, 20:20:2:48:5:5	11.58	8,18	3.46	4.72	1.28	0.80	31	201	46.5
CP:GP:SB:WT: CMC:GL, 20:14:8:52:3:3	12.33	7,52	3.78	3.74	1.46	0.99	34	217	42.9
CP:GP:SB:WT: CMC:GL, 20:8:14:48:5:5	14.42	8,79	3.84	4.95	1.52	1.12	30	216	42.3
CP:GP:SB:WT: CMC:GL, 14:14:8:58:3:3	12.93	7,24	3.43	3.81	1.36	0.98	42	249	34.8
WT:CB, 60:40	7,31	4.01	2,77	1,24	0,56	0,56	39	198	38,6
WT:HBGB, 60:40	8,1	11.91	8,22	3,69	1,11	0,96	25	166	40,5
WT, 100%	11.1	1.4	0.83	0.59	3.4	-	51	283	32.9

but promising strategy to create novel enhanced-value cereal-based goods (Collar 2014a,b). One of the current prioritized goals in cereal research is aimed at exploring and highlighting the competences and exploiting the suitability of non-breadmaking whole grains with unique nutritional components, to be included in mixed matrices with wheat to obtain novel and healthy fermented baked goods meeting the functional and sensory restrictions of viscoelastic breadmaking systems.

6.1 *Challenges and opportunities of grains and seeds with poor viscoelastic value in breadmaking*

The suitability of minor/ancient cereals (rye, oat, Kamut wheat, spelt wheat) and pseudocereals (buckwheat) was recently assessed in single (100% of wheat flour replacement) and multigrain (from 20 to 44% of wheat flour replacement) matrices (Angioloni and Collar 2011b). The research allowed the identification of the qualitative (oat, rye, buckwheat) and quantitative (up to 75% of wheat flour replacement) grains in the mixed matrices providing enhancement of nutritional quality (Table 4), and minimization of the techno-functional impairment and sensory depreciation of the resulting breads. Nutritional information on single grain breads showed in general superior nutritional quality for non-wheat breads (per 100 g bread) in terms of lower digestible starch (oat 36 g, buckwheat 46 g) and higher total dietary fiber (oat, rye, buckwheat), soluble (oat 3 g, rye 3.6 g) and insoluble (oat, rye, Kamut, buckwheat) subfractions, resistant starch (oat 4.28 g, rye 4.31 g, buckwheat 4.77 g) and minerals (oat 444 mg, buckwheat 438 mg). Higher amounts of bioactive components such as β-glucans (oat, rye) and phenolics (buckwheat) were also quantified. In addition, oat provided high-fat (3.3 g) and high-protein (13.6 g) bread with lower energy (225 kcal). Single cereals and pseudocereals (oat, rye, buckwheat) with enhanced nutritional features (high RS, minerals, bioactive components and dietary fiber contents, low *GI* and *HI*) gave tough and sensorially poorly acceptable breads. Quaternary blends based on oat, rye, buckwheat and common wheat flours with potentially improved nutritional profile were made. Wheat flour was replaced at (A) 15%, (B) 20% and (C) 25% by single oat, rye and buckwheat flours, giving a total wheat substitution level from 45 to 75% in quaternary mixtures.

The nutritional information of blended breads showed superior nutritional quality, as they contain from three to four times the dietary fiber (DF) of regular white wheat bread. Blended breads B and C can be labeled as high-fiber breads (> 6 g DF per 100 g food) according to Nutritional Claims for DF Foods (European Commission 2006). As the fiber content measured in breads derived only from the flours used (no fiber was added to the bread formulation), the total amount of dietary fiber in breads was principally determined by the insoluble dietary fiber fraction (Table 4). Better sensory-rated attributes in line with the higher performance for textural features during aging were observed for blend A and B breads. Blends A and B with low and intermediate wheat flour replacement respectively were slightly softer when freshly baked and followed a slower staling rate during storage when compared with blend C with the highest level of wheat substitution. The lowest RDS content, a high RS content and the highest SDS content, which are considered suitable nutritional trends for dietary starch fractions, were observed for blend B. Blends B and C showed a rather low extent of starch hydrolysis, with low values for k and H_{90}. Minor cereals and pseudocereals may reduce starch hydrolysis, probably because of their higher fiber content. In breadmaking, the interactions between fibers and endogenous biopolymers can lead to a very close and compact structure in restricted conditions of water availability, entrapping protein and starch granules. As a result, a delay in enzyme attack is observed. Food structure, degree of porosity and surface area accessibility to enzymes from the digestive tract seem to contribute to total degradability of food. The reduced HI measured for multigrain breads B and C provoked a slight but significant decrease in the *eGI* value. The quality profile of associated mixtures of oat, rye, buckwheat and common wheat flours (20:20:20:40 w/w/w/w) proved that blended flours are suitable to make highly nutritious, modern and innovative baked goods meeting functional and sensory standards in terms of nutritional added value, palatability, convenience and easy handling during processing (Angioloni and Collar 2011b).

In parallel, the suitability of oat, millet and sorghum in breadmaking was assessed in simple binary wheat flour matrices in which wheat flour was replaced from 0% to 60%. The research allowed the quantification of grains (up to 30% for millet and sorghum and up to 50% for oat of wheat flour replacement) to be incorporated into the binary blended matrices providing minimization of techno-functional impairment and sensory depreciation of breads (Angioloni and Collar 2013a). Combinations of gluten, vegetable fat and a commercial mix of surfactants, ascorbic acid and antistaling enzymes were used to make breads with 10% increased level of wheat flour replacement by single oat, millet and sorghum in binary mixed samples. The quality profile of binary mixtures of oat-wheat (60:40 w/w), millet-wheat (40:60 w/w) and sorghum-wheat (40:60 w/w) was significantly improved in terms of keepability during storage, mainly for oat-wheat blends which stale at a similar rate than 100% wheat breads. Overall acceptability of highly replaced wheat breads deserved higher scores for oat and sorghum composite breads (7/10) than control wheat breads (6/10). Oat, millet and sorghum represent a viable alternative to make aerated breads with mitigated technological and sensory constraints based on non-viscoelastic cereals.

The significance of grain (chickpea, pea) and oilseed (soybean) legumes on the nutritional and functional added value of wheat breads was investigated in composite matrices (from 18 to 54% of wheat flour replacement) (Angioloni and Collar 2012). Gluten (from 1 to 5% of wheat flour replacement) and carboxymethylcellulose (from 1 to 5% of wheat flour replacement) were used as structuring agents. The study allowed the identification of the qualitative (chickpea and pea) and quantitative legumes (up to 42% of wheat flour replacement), providing enhancement of nutritional value of sensorially accepted breads. Associated mixtures of legumes-wheat-structuring agents (42:52:6) have proven to make highly nutritious breads in terms of promoted dietary fiber fractions, lower and slower starch hydrolysis, decreased rapidly digestible starch and reduced expected glycaemic index. In addition, viscoelastic restrictions and sensory standards are met.

6.2 Breadmaking potential of high β-glucan barley flours and maize flours

The ability of high β-glucan barley (HBGB) flour *versus* regular commercial barley (CB) to make highly nutritious wheat (WT) blended breads meeting functional and sensory standards was investigated (Collar and Angioloni 2014a). Mixed breads obtained by 40% replacement of WT flour by HBGB flours are more nutritious than those replaced by CB flours and much more than regular WT flour breads in terms of elevated levels of dietary fiber fractions (soluble, insoluble, resistant starch and β-glucans), slowly digestible starch subfraction and bioaccessible polyphenols providing higher antiradical activity. WT/CB and WT/HBGB breads can be, respectively, labeled as source of fiber (3 g DF/100 g food) and high-fiber breads (6 g DF/100 g food), according to Nutritional Claims for dietary fiber foods. The consumption of 100 g of WT/HBGB can meet up to almost 50% the required dietary fiber, providing a β-glucan intake high enough to meet the requirements of the EFSA health claim (3 g/day), contributing a reduced blood cholesterol level. The techno-functional performance of fresh blended breads and the sensory appreciation were in general preserved or even improved.

The suitability of white (W) and yellow (Y) maize flours as basic ingredients to make nutritious and healthy breads were investigated (Collar et al. 2014a). Resistant starch (R) and common wheat flour (WF) were incorporated into formulations as single and associated extra ingredients, and dough machinability, bread nutritional and functional profiles, starch hydrolysis kinetics, and keeping behavior were assessed in blended maize matrices, and compared with the maize and wheat flour counterparts. Simultaneous replacement of maize flours by R and WF at 40% significantly modified textural profile, crumb grain features and firming kinetics, and free polyphenol pattern of breads thereof compared to the respective Y or W maize counterparts. Bigger specific volume (+28% Y-R-WF, +36% W-R-WF), softer crumb bread (–64% Y-R-WF, W-R-WF), more aerated structure and homogeneous crumb grain, and lower and slower staling kinetics are observed in composite Y and W maize-based breads, respectively. Nutritional information on maize-based blended breads showed most appealing nutritional quality than WF breads, in terms of lower digestible starch (up to –21% in Y-R-WF, W-R-WF, WR) and rapidly digestible starch (up to –37% in W-R-WF), higher slowly digestible starch (up to three times in WR), and resistant starch contents (from 5 to 6 times in Y-R-WF, W-R-WF, W-R, Y-R) of medium-high sensorially rated bread matrices. All single and blended maize-based breads can be labeled as high-fiber breads (6 g DF/100 g food). It has been substantiated that 6–12 g of resistant starch intake at a meal offers positive effects on postprandial glucose and insulin levels (Behall et al. 2006), whereas resistant starch intakes of approximately 20 g/day have been considered necessary to enhance health (e.g., increasing faecal bulk) (Murphy et al. 2008). Also, Commonwealth Scientific and Industrial Research Organization of Australia (CSIRO) has recommended that the total intake of RS should be 15–20 g/day to tackle bowel cancer in Australia (Baghurst et al. 1996). As a consequence, in terms of health-related benefits and prebiotic dosage of resistant starch (Homayouni et al. 2014), a daily intake of 100 g of single Y-R, W-R, W-R-WF and W-R-WF provides enough resistant starch to positively affect postprandial glucose and insulin levels, while 170 g covers the amount necessary to enhance health.

6.3 Composite bread matrices

The use of pseudocereals and ancient grains for breadmaking applications is receiving particular attention since they involve nutrient dense grains with proven health-promoting attributes. Dilution up to 20% of the basic rye/wheat flour blend by accumulative addition of amaranth, buckwheat, quinoa and teff flours (5% single flour) did positively impact either some dough visco-metric and visco-elastic features, or some techno-functional and nutritional characteristics of mixed bread matrices, and induced concomitant dynamics in lipid binding over mixing and baking steps (Collar and Angioloni 2014b). A preferential lipid binding to the gluten/non-gluten proteins and to the outside part of the starch granules takes place during mixing, in such a way that the higher the accumulation of bound lipids during mixing, the higher the bioaccessible polyphenol content in blended breads. During baking, lipids bind to the gluten/non-gluten proteins at the expenses of both a free lipid displacement and a lipid migration from the inside part of the starch granules to the protein active sites. It was observed that the higher the decrease of free lipid content during baking, the higher the pasting temperature and the lower the total setback on cooling and the dynamic moduli, but the higher the specific volume in blended breads. Wheat flour replacement from 22.5% up to 45% by incorporation of ternary blends of teff (T), green pea (GP) and buckwheat (BW) flours provided technologically viable and acceptable sensory rated multigrain breads with superior nutritional value compared to the 100% wheat flour (WT) counterparts (Collar et al. 2014b). Blended breads exhibited superior nutritional composition, larger amounts of bioaccessible polyphenols, higher anti-radical activity, and lower and slower starch digestibility. Simultaneous lower rapidly digestible starch (57.1%) and higher slowly digestible starch (12.9%) and resistant starch (2.8%) contents (g per 100 g fresh bread), considered suitable nutritional trends for dietary starch fractions, were met by the blend formulated 7.5% T, 15% GP and 15% BK. The associated mixture that replaced 37.5% WT, showed a rather lower extent and slower rate of starch hydrolysis with medium-low values for C_∞, and $H90$, and lowest k, and intermediate expected GI (86). All multigrain breads can be labeled as source of dietary fiber ($\geq$ 3 g dietary fiber/100 g bread).

7. Conclusions and future prospects

Although bread consumption has declined over the few past years, bread remains a staple food in many countries. Bread is an excellent carrier of macro, micronutrients and bioactive components, that fulfills an increasing number of nutritional and health claims. National and international health agencies worldwide encourage higher bread consumption, particularly whole grain versions, associated to a superior nutritional pattern, lower and slower glycaemic profile, and higher amount of phytochemicals with health promoting effects. Increasing the nutritional profile and promoting healthier attributes of bread encompass the inclusion into formulations of whole/ancient grains, minor cereals, pseudocereals, leguminous, oleaginous, all natural ingredients high in protein, dietary fiber, vitamins, minerals and antioxidants. The restoration of dough visco-elasticity in non-wheat matrices for breadmaking applications is still challenging. Cereal trends matching consumer's demands encompass (a) a move from traditional processing with a high value product and low value by-products towards a processing where almost every fraction of the raw material could be best exploited for optimal nutritional end use and (b) an increasing exploration and exploitation of the power of novel technologies, particularly those non-invasive and non-destructive, to create highly nutritious, sensorially accepted innovative cereal-based goods. The introduction of new processing techniques in breadmaking has not been largely achieved so far, although it will likely happen in a stepwise manner to maintain organoleptic properties of bread that will be acceptable to consumers.

Acknowledgements

Author gratefully acknowledges the financial support of the Spanish Institutions Ministerio de Economía y Competitividad (Project AGL2011-22669) and Consejo Superior de Investigaciones Científicas (CSIC).

Keywords: Bread, functionality, nutrition, health, chemical composition, amino acids, protein, lipids, vitamins, minerals, bioactives, antioxidants

References

Angioloni, A. and C. Collar. 2011a. Polyphenol composition and "*in vitro*" antiradical activity of single and multigrain breads. Journal of Cereal Science, 53: 90–96.

Angioloni, A. and C. Collar. 2011b. Nutritional and functional added value of oat, Kamut, spelt, rye, and buckwheat versus common wheat in breadmaking. Journal of the Science of Food and Agriculture, 91: 1283–1292.

Angioloni, A. and C. Collar. 2011c. Physicochemical and nutritional properties of reduced-caloric density high-fiber breads. LWT-Food Science and Technology, 44: 747–758.

Angioloni, A. and C. Collar. 2012. High legume-wheat matrices: an alternative to promote bread nutritional value meeting dough viscoelastic restrictions. European Food Research and Technology, 234/2: 273–284.

Angioloni, A. and C. Collar. 2013a. Suitability of oat, millet and sorghum in breadmaking. Food and Bioprocess Technology, 6: 1486–1493.

Baghurst, P.A., K.I. Baghurst and S.J. Record. 1996. Dietary fiber, non-starch polysaccharides and resistant starch—a review. Food, Australia, 48: S3–S35.

Behall, K.M., D.J. Scholfield, J.G. Hallfrisch and H.G.M. Liljebergelmståhl. 2006. Consumption of both resistant starch and ß-glucan improves postprandial plasma glucose and insulin in women. Diabetes Care, 29: 976–981.

Braaten, J.T., F.W. Scott, P.J. Wood et al. 1994. High beta-glucan oat bran and oat gum reduce postprandial blood glucose and insulin in subjects with and without type 2 diabetes. Diabetic Medicine, 11: 312–318.

Broekaert, W.F., C.M. Courtin, K. Verbeke, T. Van de Wiele, W. Verstraete and J.A. Delcour. 2011. Prebiotic and other health-related effects of cereal-derived arabinoxylans, arabinoxylan-oligosaccharides, and xylooligosaccharides. Journal of Agricultural and Food Chemistry, 51: 178–194.

Burton, P.M., J.A. Monro, L. Alvarez and E. Gallagher. 2011. Glycaemic impact and health: new horizons in white bread formulations. Critical Reviews in Food Science and Nutrition, 51: 965–982.

Chung, H.-J., H.S. Lim and S.-T. Lim. 2006. Effect of partial gelatinization and retro-gradation on the enzymatic digestion of waxy rice starch. Journal of Cereal Science, 43: 353–359.

Collar, C. 2008. Novel high fiber and whole grain breads. pp. 184–214. *In*: Bruce Hamaker (ed.). Technology of Functional Cereal Products. Woodhead Publishing Limited Abington Hall, Abington, Cambridge CB21 6AH, England.

Collar, C. 2009. The ICC Book of Ethnic Cereal-based Foods and Beverages Across the Continents. Quality Assurance and Safety of Crops & Foods, 1(4): 263–263.

Collar, C. 2014a. Barley, corn, sorghum and other cereal grains. pp. 107–126. *In*: Weibiao Zhou, Y.H. Hui, I. De Leyn, M.A. Pagani, C.M. Rosell, J.D. Selman and N. Therdthai (eds.). Bakery Products Science and Technology. 2nd ed. John Wiley and Sons, Ltd. Chichester, UK.

Collar, C. 2014b. New trends in cereal based products. pp. 293–310. *In*: Raquel De Pinho Ferreira Guine and Paula Maria Dos Correia (eds.). Engineering Aspects of Cereal and Cereal-based Products. CrcPr I Llc.

Collar, C. and A. Angioloni. 2014a. Nutritional and functional performance of barley flours in breadmaking: mixed breads vs wheat breads. European Food Research and Technology, 238: 459–469.

Collar, C. and A. Angioloni. 2014b. Pseudocereals and teff in complex breadmaking matrices: impact of lipid dynamics on the bread functional and nutritional profiles. Journal of Cereal Science, 59: 145–154.

Collar, C., F. Balestra and D. Ancarani. 2014a. Food and Bioprocess Technology. An International Journal, 7: 3579–3590.

Collar, C., T. Jiménez, P. Conte and C. Fadda. 2014b. Impact of ancient cereals, pseudocereals and legumes on starch hydrolysis and antiradical activity of technologically viable blended breads. Carbohydrate Polymers, 113: 149–158. DOI: 10.1016/j.carbpol.2014.07.020.

Collar, C. and C.M. Rosell. 2013. Bakery and confectioneries. pp. 554–582. *In*: M. Chandrasekaran (ed.). Valorization of Food Processing By-Products Series: Fermented Foods and Beverages Series. Valorization of By Products from Plant Based Food Processing Industries. CRC Press, Taylor & Francis Group.

Cracknell, R.L. and T. Watts. 2010. Western ethnic foods and their wheat requirements. *In*: J.R.N. Taylor and R.L. Cracknell (eds.). The ICC Book of Ethnic Cereal-Based Foods and Beverages across the Continents. The University of Pretoria, Lynnwood Road, Pretoria 0002, South Africa. Electronic version IBSN: 978-1-86854-739-5.

Cuniberti, M. and M.L. Seghezzo. 2009. Developments in wheat and other cereal-based local foods in the South America region. *In*: J.R.N. Taylor and R.L. Cracknell (eds.). The ICC Book of Ethnic Cereal-Based Foods and Beverages across the Continents. The University of Pretoria, Lynnwood Road, Pretoria 0002, South Africa. Electronic version IBSN: 978-1-86854-739-5.

Department of Health (DH). 1991. Nutrition and Bone Health with Particular Reference to Calcium and Vitamin D: Report of the Subgroup on Bone Health (Working Group on the Nutritional Status of the Population) of the Committee on Medical Aspects of Food and Nutrition Policy. The Stationary Office: London.

Dewettinck, K., F. Van Bockstaele, B. Kühne, D. Van de Walle, T.M. Courtens and X. Gellynck. 2008. Review. Nutritional value of bread: Influence of processing, food interaction and consumer perception. Journal of Cereal Science, 48: 243–257.

Dona, A.C., G. Pages, R.G. Gilbert and P.W. Kuchel. 2010. Digestion of starch: *In vivo* and *in vitro* kinetic models used to characterise oligosaccharide or glucose release. Carbohydrate Polymers, 80: 599–617.

Englyst, K.N., S. Vinory, H.N. Englyst and V. Lang. 2003. Glycaemic index of cereal products explained by their content of rapidly and slowly available glucose. British Journal of Nutrition, 89: 329–339.

Euromonitor. 2011. Euromonitor International. Passport, Bread in the U.S. (September, 2011).

European Commission. 2006. Regulation (EC) Nr. 1924/2006 of the European Parliament and of the Council on nutrition and health claims made on foods. Official Journal of the European Union 2006, L 404/9, 24. Online http://eur-lex.europa.eu/legal-content/EN/TXT/PDF/?uri=CELEX:32006R1924&from=EN.

Fardet, A., F. Leenhardt, D. Lioger, A. Scalbert and C. Rémésy. 2006. Parameters controlling the glycaemic response to breads. Nutrition Research Reviews, 19: 18–25.

Folloni, S. and R. Ranieri. 2013. Whole grain products in (Southern) Europe: consumer trends and technological implications. Proceedings Whole Grains Summit 2012. AACC Intl. CFW Plexus, 44–46.

Foster-Powell, K., S.H.A. Holt and J.C. Brand-Miller. 2002. International table of glycemic index and glycemic load values. American Journal of Clinical Nutrition, 76: 5–56.

Frei, M., P. Siddhuraju and K. Becker. 2003. Studies on the *in vitro* starch digestibility and the glycemic index of six different indigenous rice cultivars from the Philippines. Food Chemistry, 83: 395–402.

Henderson, L., K. Irving, J. Gregory, C.J. Bates, A. Prentice, J. Perks, G. Swan and M. Farron. 2003. National Diet and Nutrition Survey: Adults aged 19 to 64 years, Vol. 3: Vitamin and Mineral Intake and Urinary Analytes. The Stationary Office: London.

Homayouni, A., A. Amini, A.K. Keshtiban, A. Mohammad, A.M. Mortazavian, K. Karim Esazadeh and S. Pourmoradian. 2014. Resistant starch in food industry: a changing outlook for consumer and producer. Starch-Starke, 66: 102–114.

International Markets Bureau. 2012. American Eating Trends Report. Bread. Agriculture and Agri-Food Canada.

Jenkins A.L. 2007. The glycemic index: Looking back 25 years. Cereal Foods World, 52: 50–53.

Kyrø, C., G. Skeie, L.O. Dragsted, J. Chstensen, K. Overvad, G. Hallmans, I. Johansson, E. Lund, N. Slimani, N.F. Johnsen, J. Halkjær, A. Tjønneland and A. Olsen. 2011. Intake of whole grains in Scandinavia is associated with healthy lifestyle, socio-economic and dietary factors. Public Health Nutrition, 14/10: 1787–1795.

Koksel, H., D. Gocmen and S. Ozturk. 2009. Traditional turkish cereal-based foods and beverages. *In*: J.R.N. Taylor and R.L. Cracknell (eds.). The ICC Book of Ethnic Cereal-Based Foods and Beverages across the Continents. The University of Pretoria, Lynnwood Road, Pretoria 0002, South Africa. Electronic version IBSN: 978-1-86854-739-5.

Lehmann, U. and F. Robin. 2007. Slowly digestible starch–Its structure and health implications: A review. Trends in Food Science & Technology, 18: 346–355.

Martin, B.R., C.M. Weaver, R.P. Heaney, P.T. Packard and D.L. Smith. 2002. Calcium absorption from three salts and $CaSO_{(4)}$-fortified bread in premenopausal women. Journal of Agricultural and Food Chemistry, 50: 3874–3876.

Mattila, P., J.M. Pihlava and J. Hellstrom. 2005. Contents of phenolic acids, alkyl- and alkenyl-resorcinols, and avenanthramides in commercial grain products. Journal of Agricultural and Food Chemistry, 53: 8290–8295.

Murphy, M.M., J.S. Douglass and A. Birkett. 2008. Resistant starch intakes in the United States. Journal of American Dietetic Association, 108: 67–78.

National Diet and Nutrition Survey (NDNS): Adults Aged 19 to 64 Years, 2000–2001. Office for National Statistics. Social and Vital Statistics Division. Food Standards Agency. Department of Health. Persistent identifier: 10.5255/UKDA-SN-5140-1.

O'Connor, A. 2012. An overview of the role of bread in the UK diet. Review. Nutrition Bulletin, 37: 193–212.

Pellegrini, N., M. Serafini, S. Salvatore, D. Del Rio, M. Bianchi and F. Brighenti. 2006. Total antioxidant capacity of spices, dried fruits, nuts, pulses, cereals and sweets consumed in Italy assessed by three different *in vitro* assays. Molecular Nutrition and Food Research, 50: 1030–1038.

Poutanen, K. 2012. Past and future of cereal grains as food for health. Trends in Food Science and Technology, 25: 58–62.

Poutanen, K., N. Sozer and G. Della Valle. 2014. Review. How can technology help to deliver more of grain in cereal foods for a healthy diet? Journal of Cereal Science, 59: 327–336.

Rolls. 2005. The Volumetrics Eating Plan: Techniques and Recipes for Feeling Fuller on Fewer Calories. Harper Collins, New York.

Sands, A.L., H.J. Leidy, B.R. Hamaker, P. Maguire and W.W. Campbell. 2009. Consumption of the slow-digesting waxy maize starch leads to blunted plasma glucose and insulin response but does not influence energy expenditure or appetite in humans. Nutrition Research, 29: 383–390.

Santos, E. 2010. Incorporation of dietary fibers from different sources into improved cereal-based goods: design, development and viability. IATA-CSIC. PhD report. University of Valencia, Spain.

SENC. 2004. Sociedad Española de Nutrición Comunitaria. Guía de la alimentación saludable. http://www.nutricioncomunitaria.org/BDProtegidos/guia_alimentacion%20SENC_I_1155197988036.pdf.

Solah, V.A. 2009. Asian wheat-based foods: quality health foods for the future. *In*: J.R.N. Taylor and R.L. Cracknell (eds.). The ICC Book of Ethnic Cereal-Based Foods and Beverages across the Continents. The University of Pretoria, Lynnwood Road, Pretoria 0002, South Africa. Electronic version IBSN: 978-1-86854-739-5.

Taylor, J.R.N. and J. Taylor. 2009. Traditional and new east and southern African cereal-based foods and beverages. *In*: J.R.N. Taylor and R.L. Cracknell (eds.). The ICC Book of Ethnic Cereal-Based Foods and Beverages across the Continents. The University of Pretoria, Lynnwood Road, Pretoria 0002, South Africa. Electronic version IBSN: 978-1-86854-739-5.

Taylor, J.R.N. and R.L. Cracknell. (eds.). 2009. The ICC Book of Ethnic Cereal-Based Foods and Beverages across the Continents. The University of Pretoria, Lynnwood Road, Pretoria 0002, South Africa. Electronic version IBSN: 978-1-86854-739-5.

USDA. 2011, 2014. Economic Research Service, US Department of Agriculture. Loss adjusted food availability: grains per capita availability adjusted for loss. Available from: http://www.ers.usda.gov/ Data/FoodConsumption/ FoodGuideSpreadsheets.htm#grain (accessed November 12, 2011), http:// www.ers.usda.gov/data-products/food-availability-(per-capita)-data-system/ (accessed July 15, 2014) .

USDA. 2012. Department of Agriculture, Agricultural Research Service. 2012. USDA National Nutrient Database for Standard Reference, Release 25. Nutrient Data Laboratory Home Page, http://www.ars. usda.gov; Dietary Reference Intakes (DRIs): Recommended Dietary Allowances and Adequate Intakes. Elements. Food and Nutrition Board. Institute of Medicine. National Academies. http://www.nap.edu.

USDA Nutrient Database, 2004. Composition of Foods Raw, Processed, Prepared USDA National Nutrient Database for Standard Reference, Release 16-1.

WHO. 2003. World Health Organization. Diet, Nutrition and the Prevention of Chronic Disease. Report of a Joint WHO/FAO Expert Consultation. *In*: World Health Organization Technical Report Series, vol. 916. I-viii, 1–149.

Relevant websites (accessed August 2014)
wholegrainscouncil.org/
www.bakersfederation.org.uk/
www.dge.de/
www.eatforhealth.gov.au/
www.efsa. europa.ue
www.fuldkorn.dk/english/
www.hc-sc.gc.ca/fn-an/food-guide-aliment/index-eng.php
www.mypyramid.gov
www.norden.org/fi/julkaisut/julkaisut/nord-2013-009
www.nutritiondata.com

3

Sourdough Bread

Sudhanshu S. Behera[1,*] and *Ramesh C. Ray*[2,*]

1. Introduction

"Sourdough" is one of the oldest forms of cereal fermentation utilized primarily for baking purposes and it has been proven to be perfect for upgrading the shelf life, texture, palatability, and nutritional values of wheat and rye breads. Its main function is to leaven the dough to produce more aerated bread. In recent years, the traditional sourdough bread production has gained tremendous success with increasing demand by the consumers for more organic, tasty and healthy foods (Arendt et al. 2007; Mariotti et al. 2014; Torrieri et al. 2014).

Traditionally, sourdoughs are obtained by spontaneous fermentation of a mixture of flour (wheat or rye), water, and salt by the autochthonous culture of homo- and hetero-fermentative lactic acid bacteria (LAB), in association with yeasts; however, recent years have seen the use of defined allochthonous starters and control of the fermentation process. LAB produce a number of metabolites such as organic (lactic and acetic acid), exopolysaccharides (EPS), anti-microbial substances (i.e., bacteriocins) and a variety of species specific enzymes (i.e., α-amylase, pectinase, phytase, etc.) that have been shown to impart beneficial effects on the texture, nutritive values, and staling of bread. For example, EPS can stimulate the viscoelastic properties of dough, increase loaf volume, reduce crumb hardiness and enhance the shelf life (Torrieri et al. 2014). In this chapter, we discuss briefly the sourdough microflora, types of sourdough breads, nutritional implications of sourdough and gluten-free sourdough breads.

[1] Department of Biotechnology & Medical Engineering, National Institute of Technology, Rourkela-769008, India.
  Email: ssbehera.nitrkl2013@gmail.com
[2] ICAR- Central Tuber Crops Research Institute (Regional Centre), Bhubaneswar-751019, India.
  Email: rc_rayctcri@rediffmail.com
* Corresponding authors

2. History of sourdough

Sourdough was likely originated in ancient Egypt around 1500 BC and was the first form of leavening of dough available to the bakers (Wood 1996). It remained the usual form of leavening down into the European Middle ages until being replaced by barm (the foam, or scum, formed on the top of the liquor-fermented alcoholic beverages such as beer or wine from the brewing process), and then later by purpose-cultured yeast (Pollock and Cairns 1991).

Historically, the use of sourdough was necessary for rye bread production, because Baker's yeast is not suitable as a leavening agent for rye bread, as rye does not contain enough gluten. The rye bread is basically made from starch in the flour and a known carbohydrate (pentosans). However, rye amylase is active at significantly higher temperatures than wheat amylase, causing the structure of bread to deteriorate. The lower pH of the starter, therefore, inactivates the amylase and allows the carbohydrates in the bread to gel and set properly. In the 1920s, the first dough acidifier, a mixture of pre-gelatinized flour and lactic acid came to the market. Further, the development of dried sourdoughs as convenient bakery ingredients was also initiated in 1920s and 1930s and resulted finally in early 1970s in the development of naturally fermented organic dried sourdoughs (Brandt 2007).

The tradition of making sourdough wheat bread is widely used in the Mediterranean and the Middle East countries and also in the San Francisco bay in United States since 1849 (De Vuyst and Neysens 2005). In San Francisco sourdough bread, the predominant strain of *Lactobacillus* starter, is named as *Lactobacillus sanfranciscensis* (Jay et al. 2005).

3. Sourdough microflora

Sourdough is a combination of ground cereals (e.g., wheat or rye) and water that is spontaneously fermented with a stable culture of LAB and yeast. Broadly speaking, LAB and yeasts enact an important role in sourdough fermentation processes and the production of LAB:yeasts in sourdough are generally 100:1 (Ottogalli et al. 1996). In the process of bread making, yeast offers gas (CO_2) that leavens the dough and the LAB generate lactic acid that gives flavor and delay bread spoilage (De Vuyst et al. 2009). In general, homo-fermentative LAB play a significant role in most of the fermented foods, while hetero-fermentative LAB are prevalent in sourdough, exclusively when prepared conventionally (Corsetti et al. 2003). However, LAB, both homo- and hetero-fermentative species (Table 1) are mostly responsible for the process of dough acidification; but yeasts and hetero-fermentative species of LAB are responsible for the leavening (Gobbetti et al. 1995; Spicher and Brümmer 2001).

With recent improvements in the biodiversity study of sourdough LAB (Table 1), particularly sourdough ecosystems, several novel species have been isolated from traditional sourdough, such as *Lactobacillus mindensis, Lb. spicheri, Lb. rossiae, Lb. zymae, Lb. acidifarinae, Lb. hammesii,* and *Lb. nantensis* (De Vuyst et al. 2009; Rizzello et al. 2014). Isolation of novel taxa mainly depends on the cultivation in selective media and conditions while the distribution of the taxa of LAB is highly variable from one sourdough ecosystem to another (De Vuyst et al. 2009). So far,

Table 1. Fermenting sourdough species of bacteria (LAB).

Obligate homo-fermentative	Obligate hetero-fermentative	Facultative hetero-fermentative
Lactobacillus acidophilus *Lb. delbrueckii* *Lb. farciminis* *Lb. mindensis* *Lb. amylovorus* *Lb. johnsonii*	*Lb. sanfranciscensis Lb. brevis* *Lb. fermentum* *Lb. pontis* *Lb. reuteri* *Lb. fructivorans* *Lb. panis* *Lb. buchneri Lactobacillus* sp.	*Lb. plantarum* *Pediococcus pentosaceus*

Adopted from De Vuyst et al. 2009

a few less than 50 different species of LAB, including *Lactococcus, Leuconostoc, Enterococcus, Pediococcus, Streptococcus,* and *Weissella*, have been isolated from sourdough, *Lactobacillus* strains are the most frequently observed (Hammes et al. 2005), while *Leuconostoc* sp., and *Enterococcus* sp., are irregularly used or found in sourdough ecosystem. Among lactobacilli, *Lb. sanfranciscensis, Lb. planatarum* and *Lb. brevis* are most often isolated from sourdough ecosystem. In one report, Gänzle et al. (2007) communicated that two species of LAB species such as *Lactobacillus acidophilus* and *Lb. reuteri* may be of intestinal origin and, due to cross-contamination, are found in sourdough ecosystem.

More than 20 species of yeasts (Table 2) are found in sourdough (Gullo et al. 2003). *Saccharomyces cerevisiae* is the most commonly found yeast species (De Vuyst et al. 2014). But, the figure of *S. cerevisiae* may be overestimated due to the lack of reliable systems for identification and classification of yeasts from this habitat (Vogel 1997).

Table 2. Fermenting sourdough species of yeast.

Species	Synonyms
Candida glabrata	*Torulopsis glabrata*
Candida humilis	*Candida milleri*
Debaryomyce shansenii	*Torulopsis candida* *Candida famata*
Dekkera bruxellensis	*Brettanomyces custersii*
Issatchenkia orientalis	*Candida krusei*
Kluyveromyces marxianus	-
Saccharomyces bayanus	*Saccharomyces inusitatus*
Saccharomyces cerevisiae	*Saccharomyces fructuum*
Saccharomyces exiguous	*Torulopsis holmii* *Candida holmii* *Saccharomyces minor*
Saccharomyces kluyveri	-
Saccharomyces servazzi	-
Torulaspora delbrueckii	*Torulopsis colliculosa, Vandida colliculosa, Saccharomyces delbrueckii, Saccharomyces inconspicuous*

In particular, yeasts associated with LAB in sourdough are *Saccharomyces exiguus*, *Candida humilis* (formerly described as *Candida milleri*) and *Issatchenkia orientalis* (formerly described as *Candida krusei*) (Foschino et al. 1999). Moreover, other yeast species include *Pichia anomala* (also called *Hansenula anomala*), *Saturnispora saitoi* (also called *Pichiasaitoi*), *Torulaspora delbrueckii*, *Debaryomyce shansenii* and *Pichia membranifaciens* (Gobbetti et al. 1994; Succi et al. 2003; Hammes et al. 2005). The large instability in the number and type of yeast species found depends on several factors such as degree of dough hydration, type of cereal used, leavening temperature, and sourdough maintenance temperature (Gobbetti et al. 1994).

4. Classification of sourdough production processes

On the basis of the technology applied, three standard protocol of the sourdoughs fementation have been followed (Table 3):

- Type I (traditional sourdough),
- Type II (accelerated sourdough), and
- Type III (dried sourdough).

While artisanal and industrial technologies also largely use other conventional protocols (Gobbetti et al. 2005).

Table 3. Scheme of sourdough production process.

Type I (Traditional sourdough)	Type II (Accelerated sourdough)	Type III (Dried sourdough)
Flour, H_2O, starter (LAB & yeast), NaCl, sugar ↓ Mixing ↓← Fermentation at RT Bread dough ↓←(final pH at 3.8–4.5) Traditional sourdough **bread** (e.g., San Francisco sourdough)	Flour, H_2O, starter (LAB & yeast), NaCl, sugar ↓ Mixing ↓← Fermentation at >RT Bread dough ↓← Baking & final pH 3.5 Sourdough II ↓ **Bread**	Flour, H_2O, starter (LAB & yeast), NaCl, sugar ↓ Mixing ↓← Fermentation at >RT Bread dough ↓← Baking and drying Sourdough III ↓ **Bread**

Adopted from Corsetti and Settanni 2007

4.1 Type I sourdough or traditional sourdough

Type I sourdough is produced with traditional techniques and are characterized by continuous, daily refreshment to hold on the microorganisms in an active state and has very high metabolic activity. The fermentation is carried out in a temperature range of 20–30°C (68–86°F) and the matrix has a pH range of 3.8–4.5. Traditional San Francisco sourdough is an example of Type I sourdough and the LAB, *Lactobacillus sanfranciscensis* was named for its discovery in San Francisco sourdough starter, though it is not endemic to San Francisco (Jay et al. 2005; Komlenić et al. 2010).

The starter culture containing *Lb. sanfranciscensis* for production of San Francisco French bread is responsible for acid (acetic and lactic acid) production from maltose.

4.2 Type II sourdough or accelerated sourdough

The industrial action of the baking operation and the industrial appeal for faster, most competent and extensive sourdough fermentation processes resulted in the evolution of Type II sourdoughs. In the recent trend of industrial bakeries, several altered accelerated sourdough fermentation processes were present (Stolz and Bocker 1996). In the Type II sourdough, baker's yeast or *Saccharomyces cerevisiae* is incorporated to leaven the dough and obligate hetero-fermentative LAB such as *Lb. pontis*, *Lb. panis*, *Lb. sanfranciscensis*, *Lb. brevis*, *Lb. fermentum*, *Lb. reuteri*, *Weissela confuse* and *Lb. frumenti* as well as obligate homo-fermentative such as *Lb. acidophilus*, *Lb. delbrueckii*, *Lb. farciminis*, *Lb. amylovorus* (rye), *Lb. johnsonii* highlight the microflora (Table 4) (Jay et al. 2005; Arendt et al. 2007).

In the late stationary phase these microorganisms are commonly found and thus possess restricted metabolic activity. Moreover, the sourdoughs have a high acid content (pH less than 3.5) and are fermented within a temperature range of 30 to 50°C (86 to 122°F) for many days without feedings, which reduces the flora's metabolic activity (Sadeghi 2008). This process was adopted by some industry, in part, due to simplification of multiple-step build typical of Type I sourdoughs (Hui 2007).

Table 4. Classification of sourdough and their characteristics microflora.

Type I sourdough	Type II sourdough	Type III sourdough
Obligate hetero-fermentative *Lb. sanfranciscensis*, *Lactobacillus* sp. *Lb. brevis*, *Lb. buchneri*, *Lb. fermentum*, *Lb. fructivorans*, *Lb. pontis*, *Lb. reuteri*, *W. cibaria*.	**Obligate hetero-fermentative** *Lb. sanfranciscensis*, *Lb. brevis*, *Lb. fermentum*, *Lb. pontis*, *Lb. reuteri*, *W. confusa*, *Lb. panis*, *Lb. frumenti*.	**Obligate hetero-fermentative** *Lb. brevis*.
Obligate homo-fermentative *Lb. acidophils*, *Lb. delbrueckii*, *Lb. farciminis*, *Lb. mindensis*, *Lb. amylovorus*.	**Obligate homo-fermentative** *Lb. acidophilus*, *Lb. delbrueckii*, *Lb. farciminis*, *Lb. amylovorus*, *Lb. johnsonii*.	**Facultative hetero-fermentative** *Lb. plantarum*, *P. pentosaceus*.
Yeasts *Candida humilis* (*Candida milleri*), *Issatchenkia orientalis* (*Candida krusei*).	**Yeasts** No yeast, *S. cerevisiae* may be added.	-

Lb = Lactobacillus, P = Pediococcus, W = Weissela

4.3 Type III sourdoughs or dried sourdoughs

The type III sourdough is dried doughs in powder forms, which are initiated by defined starter cultures. They mostly contain LAB that are resistant to drying and are able to survive in that form. The LAB found in this conditions are either obligate hetero-fermentative such as *Lb. brevis* and/or facultative hetero-fermentative like *Pediococcus pentosaceus* and *Lb. plantarum* strains. The drying process such as spray-drying or drum-drying leads to an increased shelf life of the sourdough and turns it into a stock product until further use. The dried sourdoughs are easily distinguished in aroma, color and acid content and are convenient as well as simple in use, resulting in standardized end products (Stolz and Bocker 1996).

5. Biochemistry of sourdough fermentation

The utilization of carbohydrate source by the LAB, for the production of acetic and lactic acids are greatly influenced by the associated yeasts and availability of the types of sugars. Starting from glucose as carbohydrate sources, the homo-fermentative LAB specifically produce lactic acid through glycolysis/Embden-Meyerhof (EM) pathway (homo-lactic fermentation), whereas hetero-fermentative LAB produce, apart from lactic acids, CO_2, acetic acids and/or ethanol depending on the availability of substrates acting as electron acceptors (Ray and Joshi 2014). Gobbetti et al. (2005) reported that facultative (e.g., *Lb. plantarum* and *Lb. alimentarius*) and obligatory hetero-fermentative (e.g., *Lb. sanfranciscensis* and *Lb. pontis*) LAB follow the biochemical route of the EM pathway/glycolysis and through 6-phosphogluconate/phosphoketolase (6-PG/PK) pathway for hexose fermentation respectively, and are commonly found in the sourdoughs. The facultative hetero-fermentative LAB contains a constitutive, fructose-1, 6-diphosphate aldolase, the key enzyme of EM pathway/glycolysis that ferments hexose. The disaccharides cleaved by specific hydrolases (aldolases) and/ or phosphohydrolases to monosaccharides, which enter into EM/6-PG/PK pathways (Corsetti et al. 2003).

In general, the competitiveness of obligatory hetero-fermentative lactobacilli in sourdough is described by their integration of maltose and external electron acceptors (Vogel et al. 2002). At the same time, 6-phosphogluconate/phosphoketolase (6-PG/PK) pathway, additional energy yield may appear by the action of acetate kinase, which in the vicinity of electron acceptors, allows the recycling of NAD^+ without formation of ethanol as end product (Gobbetti et al. 2005).

Pentose such as xylulose and ribulose are phosphorylated and converted to xylulose-5-phosphate or ribulose-5-phosphate respectively, by the action of isomerases or epimerase and further metabolized through the lower half of the 6-PG/PK pathway (Ray and Joshi 2014). The pentoses are easily utilized by the obligatory hetero-fermentative LAB, since they possess a crucial enzyme of the 6-PG/PK pathway, the phosphoketolase. Further, fermentation of pentose results in the generation of equimolar quantities of acetic and lactic acids; after all no dehydrogenation steps are mandatory to reach the intermediate, xylulose-5-phosphate. There will be no evolution of CO_2, while acetyl phosphate undergoes substrate level phosphorylation with the help of acetate kinase, to produce acetate and ATP.

The LAB, *Lb. sanfranciscensis* mainly utilize fructose as an external electron acceptor and reduced to mannitol. The enzyme, mannitol dehydrogenase of *Lb. sanfranciscensis* catalyses for both the reduction of fructose to mannitol and the oxidation of mannitol to fructose in the presence of optimum temperature and pH of 35°C and 5.8–8.0, respectively (Korakli and Vogel 2003). The use of fructose as an extraneous electron acceptor was also shown in *Leuconostoc mesenteroides* (Erten 1998). In a nutshell, the practical importance of using extraneous acceptors of electrons is the change of fermentation quotient (i.e., lactate/acetate molar ratio), which enhance the baking, sensorial and shelf-life of sourdough breads (Gobbetti 1998; Spicher and Brümmer 2001).

6. Sourdough breads: traditional and novel types

6.1 Rye sourdough

Rye flours contain higher levels of pentosans than wheat flour; hence the baking properties differ significantly. The proteins in rye dough play a lesser role in the crumb forming process than in wheat dough, because the pentosans usually inhibit the gluten network. Further, the typical acidic characteristics of sourdough increase the solubility and swelling properties of pentosans as well as partially inactivate the α-amylase activity in rye flour. An excessive amount of α-amylase in rye flour produces not only a sticky crumb, but, at higher levels, it produces a very open grain and a reduction in loaf volume by making them more elastic and extensible and confers the acidic flavor characteristic of rye breads (Arendt et al. 2007).

6.2 Wheat sourdough

The use of sourdough in wheat breads has gained popularity in recent times as a means to improve the quality and flavor of wheat breads (Arendt et al. 2007). San Francisco sourdough French bread is an example of wheat products that rely on the process of souring. Several reports have also stated that the incorporation of LAB in the form of sourdough notably delays wheat bread staling.

6.3 Gluten-free sourdough

The majority of the gluten-free bakery products in the market are of poor quality as compared to their wheat counterparts (Arendt et al. 2007). This is mainly due to the unique properties of gluten, and the absence of a protein network in gluten-free products. Current research focuses to find out alternate substrates for rye and wheat such as barley flour and jackfruit seed flour for making bread that celiac patients can tolerate. The other approach involves the use of such flour with the sourdough starter to improve the quality of gluten-free matrix. The effects of addition of sourdough produced using a mixture of brown rice flours, corn starch, buckwheat and soya flour to a gluten-free bread recipe were investigated (Moore et al. 2007).

6.4 Novel sourdough

There are large number of studies to find alternate substrates, apart from rye and wheat, to make functional bread using sourdough. Few recent works have been cited in the following paragraph.

Consumption of whole grain barley foods reduces blood cholesterol and glycemic index, and promotes weight loss by increasing satiety. However, barley has only been marginally exploited by the baking industry, due to its deteriorating effect on bread quality. The use of sourdough can be a strategy to improve the quality of barley bread. In a recent study, two sourdoughs, made with sole hull-less barley flour or with a mixture of 50 g/100 g barley and 50 g/100 g wheat flours, were characterized from a microbiological and technological point of view, in comparison with a sole wheat flour sourdough. Overall, the results showed that the barley sourdoughs investigated could be used to obtain barley bread with enhanced nutritional value (Mariotti et al. 2014). Likewise, the use of sourdough fermentation and mixture of wheat, chickpea, lentil and bean flours was found to enhance the nutritional, texture and sensory characteristics of white bread (Rizzello et al. 2012).

Lactobacillus plantarum C48 and *Lactococcus lactis* subsp. *lactis* PU1, were reported to synthesize γ-aminobutyric acid (GABA) (Coda et al. 2010). These *Lactobacillus* strains were used as starter for sourdough fermentation of chickpea, amaranth, quinoa and buckwheat flours (ratio 5:1:3:1) to enrich the bread with GABA. The results were compared with wheat flour bread fermented with conventional baker's yeast. The non-conventional sourdough bread had the highest concentration of free amino acids and GABA (ca. 4467 and 504 mg/kg, respectively) concomitant with high concentration of phenolics and antioxidant activity, and the glycemic index was lower than the wheat bread (Coda et al. 2010).

7. Nutritional implications

Sourdough fermentation has proved useful in improving the texture and palatability of whole grain and fiber-rich or gluten-free products and it may stabilize or increase the levels of bioactive compounds (Katina et al. 2005). The effects of sourdough on the nutritional quality of bread are shown in Fig. 1.

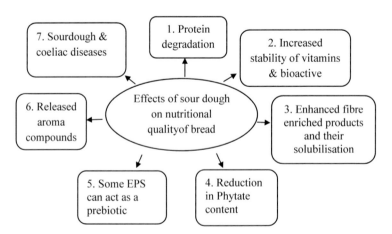

Figure 1. Effect of sourdough on the nutritional quality of bread (Arendt et al. 2007; updated).

7.1 Proteolysis

The degradation of protein during sourdough fermentation is one of the key features that influence the overall quality of sourdough bread (Gänzle et al. 2008). LAB or yeast proteinases (either intracellular or extracellular) do not play a major role in protein hydrolysis in sourdough (Wieser et al. 2008). Instead, proteolysis (breakdown of proteins into peptides) during sourdough bread fermentation is initiated by wheat or rye endogenous proteinases that are activated by the low pH. Further hydrolysis of peptides into amino acids is carried out by intracellular/extracellular peptidases of LAB (Di Cagno et al. 2004). In addition, most sourdough LAB, and in particular *Lb. sanfranciscensis,* prefer peptides uptake rather than amino acids transport (Thiele et al. 2004).

7.2 Sourdough on the stability of vitamins and bioactive compounds

Intake of whole grain food products is believed to have many health benefits, such as low starch digestibility, improved blood sugar regulation and lessened risk of diabetes, cancer, and cardiovascular diseases (Jacobs et al. 1998; Liu et al. 2000; Pereira et al. 2002).

There are mixed reports on either enhancing or decreasing effects of sourdough fermentation on the bio-availability of minerals and vitamins in the final products depending on the types of the sourdough process (Liukkonen et al. 2003). For example, sourdough fermentation has been reported to increase the folate content of both wheat and rye breads (Liukkonen et al. 2003; Kariluoto et al. 2004), and in rye fermentation the levels of folate is found more than double (Kariluoto et al. 2004). Similarly, a decrease in tocopherol and tocotrienol (Wennemark and Jägerstad 1992) and decrease/increase in thiamine content were reported depending on the fermentation process (Ternes and Freund 1988). The presence of yeast assume to support for the formation of thiamine and folates, especially after long fermentation time (Batifoulier et al. 2005), but the content of thiamine has also been reported to decrease in the baking process, more in wheat than in rye baking (Martinez-Villaluenga et al. 2009). Overall, the fermentation step can affect the retention of vitamins in the baking process. For example, in whole-wheat baking, a short baking process was shown to decrease the vitamin B1 content, while a prolonged yeast or sourdough fermentation maintained the content of above vitamins. In the long fermentation process, whole-wheat bread making with yeast resulted in a 30 percent enrichment in riboflavin (vitamin B2), but the use of mixed fermentations (yeast with sourdough) did not have a synergistic effect on B vitamin levels (Batifoulier et al. 2005). It has been observed that during sourdough preparation vitamin E content had declined.

Sourdough fermentation has been also shown to increase the anti-oxidativity (DPPH radical scavenging) in the methanol extracted fraction of rye sourdough, contemporaneously increased the levels of easily extractable phenolic compounds (Liukkonen et al. 2003). Katina et al. (2005) reported that fermentation of rye bran with yeast was also shown to increase the level of free ferulic acid. Anson et al. (2012) reported that wheat bran bio-processed with yeast fermentation in combination with cell wall hydrolytic enzymes increased the *in vitro* bio-accessibility of phenolic compounds as well as the colonic end metabolites 3-phenylpropionic in breads.

7.3 Sourdough in fiber enriched products and solubilisation

Recently, the health benefits of dietary fibers (DF) in food matrices have generated huge interest because of the several either proven or hypothetical health benefits. As a consequence, the markets are nowadays flooded with many new high-fiber food products. In the process of rye sourdough fermentation, endogenous rye proteases, especially aspartic proteases, hydrolyze rye proteins, mainly secalins. This generates amino acids and small peptides, which act as flavor precursor (Tuukkanen et al. 2005).

Salmenkallio-Marttila et al. (2001) proposed that pre-fermentation of the wheat barn with yeast alone or in symbiotic association with LAB improves the loaf volume and crumb softness of bread during storage. Moreover, the potential activity of endogenous enzymes of flour especially, the amylases and proteases, assumed efficient in sourdough fermentation (Hansen et al. 2002).

7.4 Reduction in phytate (anti-nutritional factors) content

The cereal grains, legumes and oilseeds generally constitute 1–4 percent by weight of phytic acid [myo-inositol hexakis (dihydrogen-phosphate) or myo-inositol hexakiphosphate (IP6)], being a source of myo-inositol (Pandey et al. 2001). It acts as the major storage form of phosphorous and it strongly chelates metallic cations such as Ca, Fe, K, Mg, Mn and Zn making them insoluble and thus unavailable for nutrition (Moroni et al. 2009). Therefore, phytic acid is considered to be an anti-nutritional factor in humans and animals. Its anti-nutritional properties are due to the presence of the central hexaphosphate ring, and being the highly charged (contains six anionic groups) it acts as a chelator of dietary minerals. Moreover, phytic acid complexes basic amino groups of proteins, subsequently reduced bioavailability of basic amino acids (Wodzinski and Ullah 1996).

Any type of fermentation process including sourdough promotes degradation of phytic acid by creating optimal pH for activation of phytases. For example, sourdough fermentation has been shown to enhance phytate hydrolysis that favors mineral solubility in case of whole wheat bread as compared to traditional yeast fermentation (Lopez et al. 2000). Another study has revealed that *Lb. sanfranciscensis* has phytase activity and when used as starter for sourdough fermentation in wheat flour, a major reduction of over 50 percent of the phytate level was found in comparison to un-started dough (De Angelis et al. 2003).

7.5 Some EPS can act as prebiotic

Lactobacilli produce EPS that have many beneficial effects on technological properties of bread, including water absorption of the dough, dough machinability, increased loaf volume and retarded bread staling (Tieking et al. 2005). LAB during sourdough fermentation also produces other metabolites such as mannitol, glucose and acetate that can improve bread quality (Korakli et al. 2003). Further, some of the EPS produced by LAB have prebiotic properties (Roberfroid et al. 1998). In particular, the levan produced by *Lb. sanfranciscensis* LTH2590 is metabolized by bifidobacteria (Korakli et al. 2003). In a recent study, Torrieri et al. (2014) showed that the addition of 30 g/100 g of sourdough, obtained using selected EPS producing-LAB, had a positive effect on bread volume and crumb texture. Shelf life was improved substantially. Further, the EPS producing LAB sourdough showed higher moisture content, better mechanical properties during storage and had a protective effect on bread staling.

There are two classes of EPS extra-cellularly produced by LAB: homo-polysaccharides and hetero-polysaccharides. Homo-polysaccharides are composed of only one type of monosaccharide and are synthesized by glucan and fructo-syltransferases using sucrose as the glycosyl donor (Brandt 2007). The lactobacilli such as *Lb. sanfranciscensis* (producing fructan)*, Weissellacibaria* MG1 (producing dextran) and *Lactobacillus reuteri* VIP (producing reuteran) have positive effect on dough rheology and bread texture (Korakli et al. 2003; Brandt 2007; Sandra et al. 2012).

7.6 Aroma compounds

The flavor of leavened baked goods is influenced by several factors such as raw materials, sourdough process, type of starters, and proofing and baking conditions. Microbial and enzymatic conversions of carbohydrates, proteins, peptides, and lipids in the dough result in the formation of alcohols, esters and carbonyls creating flavor compounds relevant for the crumb odor. The crust odor is influenced by the thermal reactions during the process of baking (Hansen and Schieberle 2005).

The ratio between lactic acid and acetic acid is an important factor affecting the aroma of the final bread (Corsetti and Settanni 2007). It is influenced by the fermenting microorganism, the fermentation temperature and the type of flour (Hansen and Schieberle 2005). LAB can catalyze reactions such as deamidation, transamination and decarboxylation, and their amino acid metabolism also contribute to the flavor. For example, glutamine is converted to glutamate during sourdough fermentation that imparts taste to the bread (Gänzle et al. 2007). The expression of the arginine deaminase pathway in *Lactobacillus* sp. promotes higher production of ornithine, and thus enhances the formation of 2-acetyl pyrroline that is responsible for the roasty note of wheat bread crumb (Gänzle et al. 2007).

Similarly proteins as well as lipids also affect the bread quality. Lipids oxidation, which occurs during flour storage and mixing of the dough, induces the formation of (E)-2-nonenal and other aldehydes which are key aroma compounds in wheat and rye breads (Hansen and Schieberle 2005; Vermeulen et al. 2007; Moroni et al. 2009).

7.7 Sourdough and Coeliac disease

Coeliac or celiac disease (CD) is a condition, where the victim's body reacts to the gliadin fraction of wheat and the prolamins of rye (secalins), barley (hordeins) and oats (avidins) (Murray 1999). The inflammation of small intestine due to ingestion of gluten, leads to the mal-absorption of several important nutrients such as iron, folic acid, calcium and fat-soluble vitamins.

The Codex Alimentarius Commission (1994, 2000) of the World Health Organization (WHO) and the Food and Agricultural Organization (FAO) communicate in a draft revised standard for 'gluten-free foods' as:

- Consisting of, or made only from, ingredients which do not contain any prolamins from wheat or all *Triticum* species such as spelt (*Triticum speltra* L.), kamut (*Triticum polonicum* L.) or durum wheat, rye, barley, oats or their crossbreed varieties with a gluten level not exceeding 20 ppm, or
- Consisting of ingredients from wheat, rye, barley, oats, spelt or their crossbreed varieties which are branded as 'gluten free', with a gluten level not exceeding 200 ppm, or
- Any mixture of two ingredients as mentioned above with a level not exceeding 200 ppm (Katina et al. 2005; Arendt et al. 2007).

8. Future perspectives

Sourdough is established technology in improving and diversifying the sensory quality of bread, and especially in whole grain type baking it is finding good use. The concept of bran fermentation has also been introduced to assist in bringing more bran in palatable form for high-fiber baked goods. Fermentation and acid production have been consistently shown to bring about improved mineral bioavailability. Sourdough baking is also consistently shown to deliver breads with slow starch digestibility and hence low glycemic responses, and has shown promise in improving texture of gluten-free bread for celiac patients. In the future, it can be anticipated that sourdough processing could be used to design foods with specific gut-mediated health effects, such as demonstrated changes in composition or activity of intestinal microbiota. The extracellular polysaccharides produced by lactic acid bacteria could act as selective or functional substrates for gut microbiota. Production of bioactive peptides remains a yet quite unexplored potential, which could be accomplished by utilizing the proteolytic activity of the acidified cereal system. As with other food processing, the challenge in fermenting cereal raw materials lies in the ability to combine good sensory quality with demonstrated nutritional and health benefits.

Acknowledgements

The authors thank Dr. Cristina M. Rosell, Food Science Department, Institute of Agrochemistry and Food Technology, Valencia, Spain and Prof. A.F. El Sheikha, Department of Biology, Al-Baha University, Al-Baha, Saudi Arabia, for their suggestions and critically going through the manuscript.

Keywords: Sourdough, spontaneous fermentation, lactic acid bacteria, exopolysaccharides, bacteriocins, lactic acid, yeasts, Rye sourdough, Wheat sourdough, Gluten-free sourdough, γ-aminobutyric acid (GABA), DPPH radical scavenging, Coeliac disease

References

Anson, N.M., Y.M. Hemery, A. Bast and G.R. Haenen. 2012. Optimizing the bioactive potential of wheat bran by processing. Food & function, 3: 362–375.

Arendt, E.K., L.A. Ryan and F. Dal Bello. 2007. Impact of sourdough on the texture of bread. Food Microbiology, 24: 165–174.

Batifoulier, F., M.A. Verny, E. Chanliaud, C. Remesy and C. Demigne. 2005. Effect of different breadmaking methods on thiamine, riboflavin and pyridoxine contents of wheat bread. Journal of Cereal Science, 42: 101–108.

Brandt, M.J. 2007. Sourdough products for convenient use in baking. Food Microbiology, 24: 161–164.

Coda, R., C.G. Rizzello and M. Gobbetti. 2010. Use of sourdough fermentation and pseudo-cereals and leguminous flours for the making of a functional bread enriched of γ-aminobutyric acid (GABA). International Journal of Food Microbiology, 137: 236–245.

Corsetti, A. and L. Settanni. 2007. Lactobacilli in sourdough fermentation. Food Research International, 40: 539–558.

Corsetti, A., M. De Angelis, F. Dellaglio, A. Paparella, P.F. Fox, L. Settanni and M. Gobbetti. 2003. Characterization of sourdough lactic acid bacteria based on genotypic and cell-wall protein analyses. Journal of Applied Microbiology, 94: 641–654.

De Angelis, M., G. Gallo, M.R. Corbo, P.L. McSweeney, M. Faccia, M. Giovine and M. Gobbetti. 2003. Phytase activity in sourdough lactic acid bacteria: Purification and characterization of a phytase from *Lactobacillus sanfranciscensis* CB1. International Journal of Food Microbiology, 87: 259–270.

De Vuyst, L. and P. Neysens. 2005. The sourdough microflora: Biodiversity and metabolic interactions. Trends in Food Science & Technology, 16: 43–56.

De Vuyst, L., G. Vrancken, F. Ravyts, T. Rimaux and S. Weckx. 2009. Biodiversity, ecological determinants, and metabolic exploitation of sourdough microbiota. Food Microbiology, 26: 666–675.

De Vuyst, L., S. Van Kerrebroeck, H. Harth, G. Huys, H.M. Daniel and S. Weckx. 2014. Microbial ecology of sourdough fermentations: Diverse or uniform? Food microbiology, 37: 11–29.

Di Cagno, R., M. De Angelis, S. Auricchio, L. Greco, C. Clarke, M. De Vincenzi, C. Giovannini, M. D'Archivio, F. Landolfo, G. Parrilli, F. Minervini, E. Arendt and M. Gobbetti. 2004. Sourdough bread made from wheat and nontoxic flours and started with selected Lactobacilli is tolerated in celiac sprue patients. Applied and Environmental Microbiology, 70: 1088–1096.

Erten, H. 1998. Metabolism of fructose as an electron acceptor by *Leuconostoc mesenteroides*. Process Biochemistry, 33: 735–739.

Foschino, R., R. Terraneo, D. Mora and A. Galli. 1999. Microbial characterization of sourdoughs for sweet baked products. Italian Journal of Food Science, 11: 19–28.

Gänzle, M.G., J. Loponen and M. Gobbetti. 2008. Proteolysis in sourdough fermentations: mechanisms and potential for improved bread quality. Trends in Food Science & Technology, 19: 513–521.

Gänzle, M.G., N. Vermeulen and R.F. Vogel. 2007. Carbohydrate, peptide and lipid metabolism of lactic acid bacteria in sourdough. Food Microbiology, 24: 128–138.

Gobbetti, M. 1998. The sourdough microflora: Interactions of lactic acid bacteria and yeasts. Trends in Food Science & Technology, 9: 267–274.

Gobbetti, M., A. Corsetti, J. Rossi, F. La Rosa and S. De Vincenzi. 1994. Identification and clustering of lactic acid bacteria and yeasts from wheat sourdoughs of central Italy. Italian Journal of Food Science, 6: 85–94.

Gobbetti, M., M. De Angelis, A. Corsetti and R. Di Cagno. 2005. Biochemistry and physiology of sourdough lactic acid bacteria. Trends in Food Science & Technology, 16: 57–69.

Gobbetti, M., M.S. Simonetti, A. Corsetti, F. Santinelli, J. Rossi and P. Damiani. 1995. Volatile compound and organic acid production by mixed wheat sourdough starters: influence of fermentation parameters and dynamics during baking. Food Microbiology, 12: 497–507.

Gullo, M., A.D. Romano, A. Pulvirenti and P. Giudici. 2003. *Candida humilis* dominant species in sourdoughs for the production of durum wheat bran flour bread. International Journal of Food Microbiology, 80: 55–59.

Hammes, W.P., M.J. Brandt, K.L. Francis, J. Rosenheim, M.F. Seitter and S.A. Vogelmann. 2005. Microbial ecology of cereal fermentations. Trends in Food Science & Technology, 16: 4–11.

Hansen, A. and P. Schieberle. 2005. Generation of aroma compounds during sourdough fermentation: applied and fundamental aspects. Trends in Food Science & Technology, 16: 85–94.

Hansen, H.B., M. Andreasen, M. Nielsen, L. Larsen, B.K. Knudsen, A. Meyer, L. Meyer and Á. Hansen. 2002. Changes in dietary fibre, phenolic acids and activity of endogenous enzymes during rye bread-making. European Food Research and Technology, 214: 33–42.

Hui, Y.H. (ed.). 2007. Handbook of Food Products Manufacturing: Health, Meat, Milk, Poultry, Seafood, and Vegetables (Vol. 1). John Wiley & Sons, Inc., Hoboken, New Jersey.

Jacobs, D., K. Meyer, L. Kushi and A. Folsom. 1998. Whole-grain intake may reduce the risk of ischemic heart disease death in post-menopausal women: The Iowa women's health study. American Journal of Clinical Nutrition, 68: 248–257.

Jay, J.M., M.J. Loessner and D.A. Golden. 2005. Modern Food Microbiology, 7th Ed. Springer, New York.

Kariluoto, S., L. Vahteristo, H. Salovaara, K. Katina, K.H. Liukkonen and V. Piironen. 2004. Effect of baking method and fermentation on folate content of rye and wheat breads. Cereal Chemistry, 81: 134–139.

Katina, K., E. Arendt, K.H. Liukkonen, K. Autio, L. Flander and K. Poutanen. 2005. Potential of sourdough for healthier cereal products. Trends in Food Science & Technology, 16: 104–112.

Komlenić, D.K., Ž. Ugarčić-Hardi, M. Jukić, M. Planinić, A. Bucić-Kojić and I. Strelec. 2010. Wheat dough rheology and bread quality affected by *Lactobacillus brevis* preferment, dry sourdough and lactic acid addition. International Journal of Food Science & Technology, 45: 1417–1425.

Korakli, M. and R.F. Vogel. 2003. Purification and characterisation of mannitol dehydrogenase from *Lactobacillus sanfranciscensis*. FEMS Microbiology Letters, 220: 281–286.

Korakli, M., M. Pavlovic, M.G. Gänzle and R.F. Vogel. 2003. Exopolysaccharide and kestose production by *Lactobacillus sanfranciscensis* LTH2590. Applied and Environmental Microbiology, 69: 2073–2079.

Liu, S., J. Manson, M. Stampfer, F. Hu, E. Giovannucci, G. Colditz, C. Hennekens and W. Willett. 2000. A prospective study of whole-grain intake and risk of type 2 diabetes mellitus in US women. American Journal of Public Health, 90: 1409–1415.

Liukkonen, K.H., K. Katina, A. Wilhelmsson, O. Myllymaki, A.M. Lampi, S. Kariluoto, P. Vieno and K. Poutanen. 2003. Process-induced changes on bioactive compounds in whole grain rye. Proceedings of the Nutrition Society, 62: 117–122.

Lopez, H.W., A. Ouvry, E. Bervas, C. Guy, A. Messager, C. Demigne and C. Remesy. 2000. Strains of lactic acid bacteria isolated from sourdoughs degrade phytic acid and improve calcium and magnesium solubility from whole wheat flour. Journal of Agricultural and Food Chemistry, 48: 2281–2285.

Mariotti, M., C. Garofalo, L. Aquilanti, A. Osimani, L. Fongaro, S. Tavoletti, A. Hager and F. Clementi. 2014. Barley flour exploitation in sourdough bread-making: a technological, nutritional and sensory evaluation. LWT-Food Science and Technology, 59: 973–980.

Martinez-Villaluenga, C., A. Horszwald, J. Frias, M. Piskula, C. Vidal-Valverde and H. Zieliński. 2009. Effect of flour extraction rate and baking process on vitamin B1 and B2 contents and antioxidant activity of ginger-based products. European Food Research and Technology, 230: 119–124.

Moore, M.M., B. Juga, T.J. Schober and E.K. Arendt. 2007. Effect of lactic acid bacteria on properties of gluten-free sourdoughs, batters, and quality and ultrastructure of gluten-free bread. Cereal Chemistry, 84: 357–364.

Moroni, A.V., F. Dal Bello and E.K. Arendt. 2009. Sourdough in gluten-free bread-making: An ancient technology to solve a novel issue? Food Microbiology, 26: 676–684.

Murray, J.A. 1999. The widening spectrum of celiac disease. The American Journal of Clinical Nutrition, 69: 354–365.

Ottogalli, G., A. Galli and R. Foschino. 1996. Italian bakery products obtained with sourdough: Characterization of the typical microflora. Advances in Food Science, 18: 131–144.

Pandey, A., G. Szakacs, C.R. Soccol, J.A. Rodriguez-Leon and V.T. Soccol. 2001. Production, purification and properties of microbial phytases. Bioresearch and Technology, 77: 203–214.

Pereira, M., D. Jacobs, J. Pins, S. Raatz, M. Gross, J. Slavin and E. Seaquist. 2002. Effect of whole grains on insulin sensitivity in overweight hyperinsulinemic adults. American Journal of Clinical Nutrition, 75: 848–855.

Pollock, C.J. and A.J. Cairns. 1991. Fructan metabolism in grasses and cereals. Annual Review of Plant Biology, 42: 77–101.

Ray, R.C. and V.K. Joshi. 2014. Fermented foods: Past, present and future. pp. 1–36. *In*: R.C. Ray and D. Montet (eds.). Food Biology Series: 1. Microorganisms and Fermentation of Traditional Foods. CRC Press, Taylor & Francis Group, LLC, Florida.

Rizzello, C.G., M. Calasso, D. Campanella, M. De Angelis and M. Gobbetti. 2014. Use of sourdough fermentation and mixture of wheat, chickpea, lentil and bean flours for enhancing the nutritional, texture and sensory characteristics of white bread. International Journal of Food Microbiology, 180: 78–87.

Rizzello, C.G., R. Coda, F. Mazzacane, D. Minervini and M. Gobbetti. 2012. Micronized by-products from debranned durum wheat and sourdough fermentation enhanced the nutritional, textural and sensory features of bread. Food Research International, 46: 304–313.

Roberfroid, M.B., J.A. Van Loo and G.R. Gibson. 1998. The bifidogenic nature of chicory inulin and its hydrolysis products. The Journal of Nutrition, 128: 11–19.

Sadeghi, A. 2008. The secrets of sourdough: A review of miraculous potentials of sourdough in bread shelf life. Biotechnology (Faisalabad), 7: 413–417.

Salmenkallio-Marttila, M., K. Katina and K. Autio. 2001. Effect of bran fermentation on quality and microstructure of high-fibre wheat bread. Cereal Chemistry, 78: 429–435.

Sandra, G., C. Schwab, F.D. Bello, A. Coffey, M. Gänzle and E. Arendt. 2012. Comparison of the impact of dextran and reuteran on the quality of wheat sourdough bread. Journal of Cereal Science, 56: 531–537.

Spicher, G. and J.M. Brümmer. 2001. Baked goods. pp. 239–319. In: H.J. Rehm and G. Reed (eds.). Biotechnology Set, 2nd Ed. Wiley-VCH Verlag GmbH, Weinheim.

Stolz, P. and G. Bocker. 1996. Technology, properties and applications of sourdough products. Advances in Food Science, 18: 234–236.

Succi, M., A. Reale, C. Andrighetto, A. Lombardi, E. Sorrentino and R. Coppola. 2003. Presence of yeasts in Southern Italian sourdoughs from *Triticumaestivum* flour. FEMS Microbiology Letters, 225: 143–148.

Ternes, W. and W. Freund. 1988. Effects of different doughmaking techniques on thiamin content of bread. Getreide Mehl und Brot, 42: 293–297.

Thiele, C., S. Grassl and M. Gänzle. 2004. Gluten hydrolysis and depolymerization during sourdough fermentation. Journal of Agricultural and Food Chemistry, 52: 1307–1314.

Tieking, M., M.A. Ehrmann, R.F. Vogel and M.G. Gänzle. 2005. Molecular and functional characterization of a levansucrase from the sourdough isolate *Lactobacillus sanfranciscensis* TMW 1.392. Applied Microbiology and Biotechnology, 66: 655–663.

Torrieri, E., O. Pepe, V. Ventorino, P. Masi and S. Cavella. 2014. Effect of sourdough at different concentrations on quality and shelf life of bread. LWT-Food Science and Technology, 56: 508–516.

Tuukkanen, K., J. Loponen, M. Mikola, T. Sontag-Strohm and H. Salovaara. 2005. Degradation of secalins during rye sourdough fermentation. Cereal Chemistry, 82: 677–682.

Vermeulen, N., M.G. Gaenzle and R.F. Vogel. 2007. Glutamine deamidation by cereal-associated lactic acid bacteria. Journal of Applied Microbiology, 103: 1197–1205.

Vogel, R.F. 1997. Microbial ecology of cereal fermentations. Food Technology and Biotechnology, 35: 51–54.

Vogel, R.F., M.A. Ehrmann and M.G. Gaenzle. 2002. Development and potential of starter lactobacilli resulting from exploration of the sourdough ecosystem. Antonie van Leeuwenhoek International Journal of General and Molecular Microbiology, 81: 631–638.

Wennemark, B. and M. Jägerstad. 1992. Bread making and storage of various wheat fractions affect vitamin E. Journal of Food Science, 57: 1205–1209.

Wieser, H., N. Vermeulen, F. Gaertner and R.F. Vogel. 2008. Effects of different Lactobacillus and Enterococcus strains and chemical acidification regarding degradation of gluten proteins during sourdough fermentation. European Food Research and Technology, 226: 1495–1502.

Wodzinski, R.J. and A.H.J. Ullah. 1996. Phytase. Advances in Applied Microbiology, 42: 263–302.

Wood, E.D. 1996. Back to the first sourdough. pp. 7–17. In: E.D. Wood (ed.). World Sourdough from Antiquity. Ten Speed Press, California, Berkeley.

4

Fermentation Process and Bioavailability of Phytochemicals from Sourdough Bread

Maciej Kuligowski,[1,*] *Jacek Nowak*[1] and
Iwona Jasińska-Kuligowska[2]

1. Introduction

The fermentation process during sourdough production depends on several factors—the type of milled product (most popular are wheat and rye) and technology. The term sourdough bread refers to various products: from crispy bread from Scandinavia (Menzel et al. 2012), typical (soft) bread (Andersson et al. 2010) to steamed sourdough from China (Kim et al. 2009). Technology affects the time of microbial activity. For example, some authors described a three-stage procedure as a traditional wheat sourdough bread production process (Paramithiotis et al. 2005). One-stage and two-stage methods of wheat sourdough bread production are also used (Gąsiorowski 2004). Four- or five-stage fermentation procedures are used for rye sourdough bread production (Gąsiorowski 1994). The fermentation time of sourdough varies from 2 hr when using a commercial starter (Ostasiewicz et al. 2009) to 144 hr in case of panettone (Brandt 2007; Gänzle 2014) if this product is to be treated as bread. The

---

[1] Poznań University of Life Sciences, Faculty of Food Science and Nutrition, Institute of Food Technology of Plant Origin, Department of Fermentation and Biosynthesis, ul. Wojska Polskiego 31, 60-637 Poznań.
  Emails: maciek@up.poznan.pl; jacnow@up.poznan.pl
[2] Poznań University of Economics, Faculty of Commodity Sciences, Department of Food Commodity Science.
  Email: iwona.jasinska-kuligowska@ue.poznan.pl
* Corresponding author

time of microbial activity influences changes of chemical compounds. Breads popular in central Europe are made from a blend of wheat and rye flour. Their fermentation depends on the proportion of rye to wheat flour (Röcken 1996). Some regions have traditional breads produced from different flours. For example broa from Northern Portugal is produced by mixing maize and rye flours (Rocha and Malcata 2012). The type of medium, i.e., flour, is the next factor, which can determine changes of chemical compounds in fermented material. In many countries and regions different types and strains of microorganisms (lactic acid bacteria and yeasts) are used to produce sourdough (Hansen 2006; Nionelli et al. 2014; De Vuyst et al. 2014). Different microbial populations are connected with different fermentation temperatures and therefore some changes in phytochemicals may not be the same in sourdough from different countries.

2. Phytic acid and phytates

The term phytochemicals is not precisely defined. It is used for compounds originating from plants, which often have some more or less important effect on the human organism. Examples of such compounds are phytic acid. This acid strongly binds metallic cations of Ca, Fe, K, Mg, Mn and Zn, making them insoluble and thus unavailable for nutrition, called phytates (Bohn et al. 2008; Hansen 2006). Phytic acid is recognized as an antinutritional factor (Poutanen et al. 2009), which can be significant breakdown during sourdough fermentation. Some researchers found that during growth of lactic acid bacteria and decrease of environmental pH, endogenous phytase from grain was activated. Acidification of the dough with sourdough addition provides a significant phytates breakdown (70 percent of the initial flour content compared to 40 percent without any leavening agent or acidification) (Leenhardt et al. 2005; Gänzle 2014). Different authors found that sourdough fermentation was more efficient than yeast fermentation in reducing the phytate content in whole wheat bread (62 and –38 percent, respectively) (Lopez et al. 2001). Other important research proved that phytate contents in yeast and sourdough bread were lower than in whole wheat flour (–52 and –71 percent, respectively). As a result sourdough bread was a better source of available minerals, especially magnesium, iron and zinc in experiments on rats. Copper absorption increased significantly when rats were fed sourdough bread, whereas unprocessed whole flour depressed copper absorption (Lopez et al. 2003). Levels of blood hemoglobin, hematocrit, serum ferritin and serum iron as well as excreted iron significantly decreased in mice when they were fed sourdough bread as compared to yeast bread and non-fermented bread (Chaoui et al. 2006). Yeasts seem to have no important effect on phytic acid, although some authors described that high phytase-active yeasts were isolated from Danish and Lithuanian sourdoughs (Nuobariene et al. 2012).

Phytic acid is concentrated in the aleurone layers of grains (Poutanen et al. 2009) and the type of flour used in dough production determines the amount of this compound in bread. Fermentation time is also important. Prolonged fermentation of whole wheat sourdough reduces phytate content by almost 90 percent, whereas 40 percent of phytate remains in traditional French bread (Lopez et al. 2001). Prolonged fermentation with sourdough still leads to improved Mg and P solubility due to the decreased phytate content and acidification.

However, phytic acid and its salts may also have a positive influence on the human body. Several studies in the medical literature have reported phytate as a broad-spectrum anti-neoplastic agent. Colon cancer cells, human leukaemic hematopoietic cells and erythroleukemia cells were inhibited by the administration of phytate. Phytate could also limit the proliferation of breast cancer cells, cervical cancer, prostate cancer and hepatoma cell in humans (Shamsuddin et al. 1992; Kumar et al. 2010).

3. Alkylresorcinols

Cereal alkylresorcinols, phenolic lipids are 1,3-dihydroxybenzene compounds with an alkyl chain substituted at position 5 of the phenolic ring. Alkyl chains possess from 15 to 27 carbons. Alkylresorcinols represent a significant proportion of the phytochemicals present in wheat and rye and they are concentrated in the bran fraction of these cereals. These compounds are therefore significant components of food products rich in whole grain wheat and rye, but not in products containing only refined cereal flour (Ross et al. 2004). Alkylresorcinols are attributed a role in the modification of the structure and function of phospholipid membranes (Kozubek and Tyman 1999) and enzyme inhibition, suppression of adipocyte lipolysis and inhibition of colon cancer tumor growth (Landberg et al. 2014). Spontaneous fermentation and fermentation only with yeasts *Saccharomyces cerevisiae* has no effect on changes in these compounds. Although the use of a fermentation starter composed of *S. cerevisiae*, *Lactobacillus plantarum* and *Lactobacillus brevis* decreases the level of alkylresorcinols on about 14 percent (Katina et al. 2007b). However, with the use of the same microorganisms under different fermentation conditions the reducing effect was not observed (Liukkonen et al. 2003). Alkylresorcinols are heat stable during baking (Gunenc et al. 2013). Approximately 40 percent of alkylresorcinols were recovered in effluent from the human small intestine, indicating that 60 percent of alkylresorcinols are taken up from or converted in the small intestine (Ross et al. 2003). Alkylresorcinols possess antioxidant properties and exhibit an ability to protect cellular lipid components from oxidative processes (Dziki et al. 2014). However, no correlation was found between total amounts of alkylresorcinols in bread and *in vitro* antioxidant properties (Korycińska et al. 2009). In turn, alkylresorcinols content showed a small positive correlation with total phenolic content. Additionally, some authors concluded that other phenolics, such as ferulic acid, have more pronounced effect on antioxidant activity of wheat bran in comparison with alkylresorcinols (Gunenc et al. 2013).

4. Polyphenols

Polyphenols, defined as plant secondary metabolites, contain one or more aromatic rings with more than one hydroxyl group (Martínez et al. 2014). The major phenolic acid in rye is ferulic acid, which accounts for about 50 percent of total phenolic acids. Caffeic, dihydrobenzoic and sinapic acids are also present (Shewry et al. 2010). Phenolic acids in wheat and rye occur predominantly in the bound form and as dimers. The concentration of free phenolic acids is low (Boskov Hansen et al. 2002; Shewry et al. 2010). Some studies showed that yeast fermentation of wheat bran significantly increases the total free phenolic content and *in vitro* antioxidant activity, mainly resulting from the increase in soluble free syringic, p-coumaric, and ferulic acids (Moore et al. 2007). Nevertheless the amount of free vanillic acid was decreased (Moore et al. 2007), because yeasts *Saccharomyces cerevisiae* are able to biotransform a variety of phenolic acids, such as vanillic acid derivatives, into other compounds (Priefert et al. 2001). Lactic acid bacteria during cereal grain fermentation possess an ability to liberate phenolic acids (Hole et al. 2012). Sourdough fermented bread contains the higher content of free ferulic acid in comparison to yeast bread. Crumb of sourdough bread from whole meal rye contained 33.2 μg/g free ferulic acid, whereas prepared with the same method whole wheat bread contained only 5.9 μg/g. Free ferulic acid contents were 5.7 and 13.8 μg/g in whole meal rye and bread from this flour, respectively, when the breads were fermented only by yeast (Konopka et al. 2014). Rye bran bread intake elevates urinary excretion of ferulic acid in humans and it was shown that this compound from such kind of bread is bioavailable. In a study on humans, within the period of intervention (2 × 6 weeks with 4 weeks washout), the elevated ferulic acid did not produce a measurable antioxidative effect on the subjects' LDL (Harder et al. 2004).

Cereal products are important sources of antioxidants in the human diet. The antioxidants of cereal grains are a large group of compounds with various chemical structures (Konopka et al. 2014). Sourdough fermented samples contain more soluble proteins, phenolic acids, lipid degradation products (diene and triene compounds), and tocochromanols than flour and yeast fermented products (Konopka et al. 2014). Although, some studies present that level of phenolic compounds was higher in dough fermented by *S. cerevisiae* in comparison with sourdough obtained by starter (*S. cerevisiae*, *L. plantarum* and *L. brevis*) and spontaneous fermentation (Katina et al. 2007b). However, total antioxidant properties of sourdough bread, defined as the sum of lipophilic and hydrophilic compound activities, were significantly higher than for yeast bread (Konopka et al. 2014). Different authors obtained similar effects, total phenolics and antioxidant activities were higher in dough fermented by *L. rhamnosus* when compared to yeast fermented dough (Đorđević et al. 2010). Furthermore, some authors observed that, in comparison to baker's yeast wheat bread, sourdough wheat bread offers more antioxidant protection for rats during 7-week experimental diets (Gianotti et al. 2011).

Phenolic acids in cereals are mostly present in the bound form through ester bonds to arabinoxylan chains or through ether bonds to lignin (Hole et al. 2012). The antioxidant activities of phenolic acids are well documented; however, phenolic acid bioaccessibility in high-fiber cereal products is low and does not exceed 5 percent (Jenner et al. 2005; Anson et al. 2009; Konopka et al. 2014). Hydrophilic monomeric forms are more accessible and are probably partially absorbed in the upper alimentary tract, particularly in the stomach. The bound forms of phenolic acids, which are prevalent in bread, become bioaccessible only after enzymatic hydrolysis (Andreasen et al. 2001; Anson et al. 2009; Konopka et al. 2014). Esterases produced by microflora in the large intestine (Jenner et al. 2005) and naturally occurring esterases in the mucous membrane of the small intestine (Andreasen et al. 2001) show the ability to release the bound forms of phenolic acids.

Cereal fermentation with sourdough microflora can lead to a significant increase in the content of free phenolic acids, thereby improving their bioavailability (Hole et al. 2012). It was found that bioavailability of free phenolic compounds from bran was higher in both *in vitro* (Anson et al. 2009) and human studies (Anson et al. 2011). A presumable mechanism for fermentation-induced increase in bioaccessibility and bioavailability of phenolic compounds in cereal grains is that degrading enzymes present in both grains and microbes result in the structural breakdown of the cell wall matrix, which increases accessibility of bound and conjugated phenolic compounds to enzymatic activity (Wang et al. 2014).

5. Polysaccharides and oligosaccharides

Arabinoxylan, lignin and other compounds classified as fiber can improve the function of the intestinal tract and stimulate the growth of probiotics. The physiological effect of dietary fiber depends on its chemical and physical characteristics such as the degree of polymerization of polysaccharides, the presence of side chains and the degree of cross-linking, particle size and cell wall integrity (Raninen et al. 2011). Dietary fiber mainly consists of plant polysaccharides and lignin (Gobbetti et al. 2014). Some of them are intensively changed during fermentation, that is the case of fructans, which have prebiotic properties. Fructans found in cereals contain up to approx. 20 molecules of hexose; they are highly soluble non-reducing oligosaccharides. Fructans have been detected in grain of many cereal species. The richest source of fructans is rye grain, in which the content of these compounds is from 1.7 to 6.6 g/100 g d.m. Wheat grain contains much lower amounts of fructans, ranging from 0.9 to 2.3 g/100 g d.m. (Glitsø and Bach Knudsen 1999; Fretzdorff and Welge 2003; Karppinen et al. 2003; Haskå et al. 2008; Andersson et al. 2009). The content of fructans in cereal grain depends on such factors as genotype, climatic conditions of culture, physiological condition of grain, etc. (Boskov Hansen et al. 2003). Fermentation using starters and yeasts contributes to degradation of these compounds (Boskov Hansen et al. 2003; Jasińska-Kuligowska et al. 2013).

Fructans are hydrolyzed to fructose by yeast invertase, as such they may partly replace sucrose in bread production; thus their content in the final product is reduced (Escrivá and Martínez-Anaya 2000). Changes in the levels of fructans were described in the production of rye bread using different methods. The highest decrease of fructans content from 5 to 1.9 percent were observed during fermentation with a simultaneous use of bacteria and yeasts, while at the application of yeasts alone these changes were much smaller, from 5 to 3.4 percent (Andersson et al. 2009). Reduction in fructan contents was also reported by other authors, from 6.2 g/100 g d.m. in wholegrain rye flour to 4.1 g/100 g d.m. in dough and 3.4 g/100 g d.m. in bread crumb (Boskov Hansen et al. 2002). Differences in the contents of fructans were described in commercially available rye breads, depending on the production method and the type of used flour. In bread the content of fructans (g/100 g product) was 1.05 in light bread, 1.42 in dark bread, while in bread produced with sourdough it was 1.07 (Biesiekierski et al.

2011). Other authors did not detect fructooligosaccharides in rye and wheat breads produced using sourdough with an addition of baker's yeast, purchased at traditional, local Polish bakeries (Król and Grzelak 2006).

Another group of physiologically important compounds included in the dietary fiber consists of pentosans. In the studies it was found that pentosans contained in bread may improve physiological intestinal function (Gråsten et al. 2003). In the course of rye bread production using sourdough the total pentosan content was found to decrease, while the content of soluble pentosans increased and baking caused no further degradation of these compounds (Boskov Hansen et al. 2002). Other reports described a two-fold increase in the amounts of soluble pentosans in fermented rye bran in relation to non-fermented raw material (Katina et al. 2007a).

Beta-glucans have shown positive health benefit in several clinical trials, mainly reduction of LDL cholesterol level and glycemic response. These physiological effects have been highly correlated with β-glucan viscosity and molecular weight. Some authors described that sourdough bread showed better potential over yeast-fermented breads in terms of preserving β-glucan molecular weight and viscosity during the baking process when a blend of whole wheat flour and oat bran was used (Gamel et al. 2014).

6. Folate

Folate compounds belong to the vitamin B group, and folate is a generic term referring to derivatives of folic acid. Folate in food exists as various vitamers differing in oxidation status and single carbon substituents, and with a variable number of glutamyl residues (Kariluoto et al. 2006; Kariluoto 2008). The essential B-vitamin folate is required for DNA synthesis and a good folate status prevents against neural tube defects. Folate nutritive is also associated with cardiovascular diseases, colon cancer and certain anemia. Since humans cannot synthesize folates, they must obtain them from foods. Cereals—especially whole grain products—are major contributors to folate in the diet. Bread is an important folate source in several countries (Kariluoto et al. 2006; Kariluoto 2008; Öhrvik et al. 2010).

The quantity of certain compounds found in cereal grains can be significantly increased by the use of the fermentation process. This effect is not only associated with the breaking of a bond and the release of bioactive compounds from complex matrices, but also related to the biosynthesis by the microorganisms. The released compounds are more easily absorbable by the human digestive system.

Such biosynthesis for folate during bread making was also observed. Although some *Lactobacillus* spp. consumed folates, their effect on folate contents in sourdough was minimal (Kariluoto et al. 2006). Sourdough fermentation of whole rye grains more than doubles the increase in folate levels. Losses of folates during the baking stage at 220–240°C were very low (Liukkonen et al. 2003). It was concluded that the increase of folate content during fermentation is mainly due to folate synthesis by yeasts. Some authors reported that the total native folate content in rye flour expressed as folic acid was 29 µg/100 g dry basis and during fermentation with baker's yeast raised to 46 µg/100 g (proofed dough) and then decreased to 34 µg/100 g as a result of baking treat (Gujska and Majewska 2005). Moreover, spontaneous fermentation seems to possess more potential to increase folate amount. Spontaneous fermentation resulted in a three-fold increase in the folate contents. Two folate producing bacteria *Enterobacter cowanii* and *Pantoea agglomer* were isolated from flour (Kariluoto et al. 2006). The presence of these bacteria in commercial sourdough starters was not described. During baking some forms of folates change, the level of 10-HCO-folic acid increased, but contents of other forms of this compound decreased. The duration of the baking process had an effect on the amounts of [6S]-5-CH$_3$-H$_4$-folate. Folate bioaccessibility, as estimated by the gastrointestinal model, in different wholemeal breads was above 75 percent (Öhrvik et al. 2010).

7. Summary

Fermentation using lactic acid bacteria and/or yeast substantially affect the nutritional and health-promoting value of bread. Not all bioactive phytochemicals during sourdough fermentation and their bioavailability have been fully described. For example plant sterols was described as quantitatively stable (Liukkonen et al. 2003), but in different studies a slight increase was observed (Katina et al. 2007b). In available literature during sourdough fermentation, lignans did not show any significant change (Katina et al. 2007b; Jasińska 2011), while the level of tocopherols and tocotrienols decreased (Liukkonen et al. 2003). Information about the bioavailability of some compounds from sourdough bread are still insufficient and incomplete.

Sourdough application has been extensively increased in the recent years due to the consumers' demand for food without the addition of chemical preservatives (Plessas et al. 2011). New fermentation methods, fermentation parameters (Katina et al. 2006) and new microbial strains (Settanni et al. 2013) are being tested to yield certain properties. In the future, specific and strictly defined changes in sourdough bread will be provided by those factors. Management changes and food production dedicated to people with a certain demand for health-promoting ingredients will become possible. With the use of new raw materials, e.g., tempeh, teff, leguminous seeds (Kuligowski et al. 2008; Alaunyte et al. 2012; Rizzello et al. 2014) for the production of sourdough, or modified composition of traditional products (Kawka et al. 2005), it may be an effective way to prevent certain diseases.

Keywords: Sourdough, bread, phytochemicals, bioavailability, fermentation process

References

Alaunyte, I., V. Stojceska, A. Plunkett, P. Ainsworth and E. Derbyshire. 2012. Improving the quality of nutrient-rich Teff (Eragrostis tef) breads by combination of enzymes in straight dough and sourdough breadmaking. Journal of Cereal Science, 55: 22–30.

Andersson, A.A.M., P. Åman, M. Wandel and W. Frølich. 2010. Alkylresorcinols in wheat and rye flour and bread. Journal of Food Composition and Analysis, 23: 794–801.

Andersson, R., G. Fransson, M. Tietjen and P. Åman. 2009. Content and molecular-weight distribution of dietary fiber components in whole-grain rye flour and bread. Journal of Agricultural and Food Chemistry, 57: 2004–2008.

Andreasen, M.F., P.A. Kroon, G. Williamson and M.T. Garcia-Conesa. 2001. Intestinal release and uptake of phenolic antioxidant diferulic acids. Free Radical Biology & Medicine, 31: 304–314.

Anson, N.M., A.-M. Aura, E. Selinheimo, I. Mattila, K. Poutanen, R. Van den Berg, R. Havenaar, A. Bast and G.R.M.M. Haenen. 2011. Bioprocessing of wheat bran in whole wheat bread increases the bioavailability of phenolic acids in men and exerts antiinflammatory effects *ex vivo*. Journal of Nutrition, 141: 137–143.

Anson, N.M., E. Selinheimo, R. Havenaar, A.-M. Aura, I. Mattila, P. Lehtinen, A. Bast, K. Poutanen and G.R.M.M. Haenen. 2009. Bioprocessing of wheat bran improves *in vitro* bioaccessibility and colonic metabolism of phenolic compounds. Journal of Agricultural and Food Chemistry, 57: 6148–6155.

Biesiekierski, J.R., O. Rosella, R. Rose, K. Liels, J.S. Barrett, S. Shepherd, P.R. Gibson and J.G. Muir. 2011. Quantification of fructans, galacto-oligosaccharides and other short-chain carbohydrates in processed grains and cereals. Journal of Human Nutrition and Dietetics, 24: 154–176.

Bohn, L., A. Meyer and S. Rasmussen. 2008. Phytate: impact on environment and human nutrition. A challenge for molecular breeding. Journal of Zhejiang University—Science, B 9, 165–191.

Boskov Hansen, H., M.G. Andreasen, M.M. Nielsen, L.M. Larsen, K.E. Bach Knudsen, A.S. Meyer, L.P. Christensen and Å. Hansen. 2002. Changes in dietary fibre, phenolic acids and activity of endogenous enzymes during rye bread-making. European Food Research and Technology, 214: 33–42.

Boskov Hansen, H., C.V. Rasmussen, K.E. Bach Knudsen and Å. Hansen. 2003. Effects of genotype and harvest year on contents and composition of dietary fibre in rye (*Secale cereale* L.) grain. Journal of the Science of Food and Agriculture, 83: 76–85.

Brandt, M.J. 2007. Sourdough products for convenient use in baking. Food Microbiology, 4: 161–164.

Chaoui, A., M. Faid and R. Belahsen. 2006. Making bread with sourdough improves iron bioavailability from reconstituted fortified wheat flour in mice. Journal of Trace Elements in Medicine and Biology, 20: 217–220.

De Vuyst, L., S. Van Kerrebroeck, H. Harth, G. Huys, H.M. Daniel and S. Weckx. 2014. Microbial ecology of sourdough fermentations: Diverse or uniform? Food Microbiology, 37: 11–29.

Đordević, T.M., S.S. Šiler-Marinković and S.I. Dimitrijević-Branković. 2010. Effect of fermentation on antioxidant properties of some cereals and pseudo cereals. Food Chemistry, 119: 957–963.

Dziki, D., R. Różyło, U. Gawlik-Dziki and M. Świeca. 2014. Current trends in the enhancement of antioxidant activity of wheat bread by the addition of plant materials rich in phenolic compounds. Trends in Food Science & Technology (in press).

Escrivá, C. and M.A. Martínez-Anaya. 2000. Influence of enzymes on the evolution of fructosans in sourdough wheat processes. European Food Research and Technology, 210: 286–292.

Fretzdorff, B. and N. Welge. 2003. Fructan and raffinose contents in cereals and pseudo-cereal grains. Getreide, Mehl und Brot, 57: 3–8.

Gamel, T.H., E.-S.M. Abdel-Aal and S.M. Tosh. 2014. Effect of yeast-fermented and sour-dough making processes on physicochemical characteristics of β-glucan in whole wheat/oat bread. LWT—Food Science and Technology (in press).

Gänzle, M.G. 2014. Enzymatic and bacterial conversions during sourdough fermentation. Food Microbiology, 37: 2–10.

Gąsiorowski, H. 1994. Technologia produkcji chleba żytniego. pp. 223–245. *In*: H. Gąsiorowski (ed.). Żyto chemia i technologia. Państwowe Wydawnictwo Rolnicze i Leśnie, Poznań.

Gąsiorowski, H. 2004. Produkcja pieczywa pszennego. pp. 395–458. *In*: H. Gąsiorowski (ed.). Pszenica chemia i technologia. Państwowe Wydawnictwo Rolnicze i Leśnie, Poznań.

Gianotti, A., F. Danesi, V. Verardo, D.I. Serrazanetti, V. Valli, A. Russo, Y. Riciputi, N. Tossani, M.F. Caboni, M.E. Guerzoni and A. Bordoni. 2011. Role of cereal type and processing in whole grain *in vivo* protection from oxidative stress. Frontiers in Bioscience, 16: 1609–1618.

Glitsø, L.V. and K.E. Bach Knudsen. 1999. Milling of whole grain rye to obtain fractions with different dietary fibre characteristics. Journal of Cereal Science, 29: 89–97.

Gobbetti, M., C.G. Rizzello, R. Di Cagno and M. De Angelis. 2014. How the sourdough may affect the functional features of leavened baked goods. Food Microbiology, 37: 30–40.

Gråsten, S., K.-H. Liukkonen, A. Chrevatidis, H. El-Nezami, K. Poutanen and H. Mykkänen. 2003. Effects of wheat pentosan and inulin on the metabolic activity of fecal microbiota and on bowel function in healthy humans. Nutrition Research, 23: 1503–1514.

Gujska, E. and K. Majewska. 2005. Effect of Baking Process on Added Folic Acid and Endogenous Folates Stability in Wheat and Rye Breads. Plant Foods for Human Nutrition, 60: 37–42.

Gunenc, A., H. Tavakoli, K. Seetharaman, P.M. Mayer, D. Fairbanks and F. Hosseinian. 2013. Stability and antioxidant activity of alkylresorcinols in breads enriched with hard and soft wheat brans. Food Research International, 51: 571–578.

Hansen, A. 2006. Sourdough bread. pp. 1–21. *In*: Y.H. Hui (ed.). Handbook of food science, technology and engineering, CRC Press, Boca Raton.

Harder, H., I. Tetens, M.B. Let and A.S. Meyer. 2004. Rye bran bread intake elevates urinary excretion of ferulic acid in humans, but does not affect the susceptibility of LDL to oxidation *ex vivo*. European Journal of Nutrition, 43: 230–236.

Haskå, L., M. Nyman and R. Andersson. 2008. Distribution and characterisation of fructan in wheat milling fractions. Journal of Cereal Science, 48: 768–774.

Hole, A.S., I. Rud, S. Grimmer, S. Sigl, J. Narvhus and S. Sahlstrom. 2012. Improved bioavailability of dietary phenolic acids in whole grain barley and oat groat following fermentation with probiotic *Lactobacillus acidophilus, Lactobacillus johnsonii*, and *Lactobacillus reuteri*. Journal of Agricultural and Food Chemistry, 60: 6369–6375.

Jasińska, I. 2011. The study on possibility of use milling rye fraction to obtain products with higher content of bioactive compounds. PhD Thesis, Poznań University of Life Sciences, Poznań, Poland.

Jasińska-Kuligowska, I., M. Kuligowski, P. Kołodziejczyk and J. Michniewicz. 2013. Wpływ procesów fermentacji, ekstruzji i wypieku na zawartość fruktanów w produktach żytnich (Effect of fermentation, extrusion and baking processes on content of fructans in rye products). Żywność. Nauka. Technologia. Jakość, 90: 129–141.

Jenner, A.M., J. Rafter and B. Halliwell. 2005. Human fecal water content of phenolics: the extent of colonic exposure to aromatic compounds. Free Radical Biology & Medicine, 38: 763–772.

Kariluoto, S. 2008. Folates in rye: Determination and enhancement by food processing. PhD Thesis, University of Helsinki, Finland.

Kariluoto, S., M. Aittamaa, M. Korhola, H. Salovaara, L. Vahteristo and V. Piironen. 2006. Effects of yeasts and bacteria on the levels of folates in rye sourdoughs. International Journal of Food Microbiology, 106: 137–143.

Karppinen, S., O. Myllymäki, P. Forssell and K. Poutanen. 2003. Fructan content of rye and rye products. Cereal Chemistry, 80: 168–171.

Katina, K., R.L. Heiniö, K. Autio and K. Poutanen. 2006. Optimization of sourdough process for improved sensory profile and texture of wheat bread, LWT—Food Science and Technology, 39: 1189–1202.

Katina, K., A. Laitila, R. Juvonen, K.-H. Liukkonen, S. Kariluoto, V. Piironen, R. Landberg, P. Aman and K. Poutanen. 2007a. Bran fermentation as a means to enhance technological properties and bioactivity of rye. Food Microbiology, 24: 175–186.

Katina, K., K.H. Liukkonen, N.A. Kaukovirta, H. Adlercreutz, S.M. Heinonen, A.M. Lampi, J.M. Pihlava and K. Poutanen. 2007b. Fermentation-induced changes in the nutritional value of native or germinated rye. Journal of Cereal Science, 46: 348–355.

Kawka, A., A. Liczbańska and J. Łapa. 2005. Wpływ całoziarnowej mąki jęczmiennej i wybranych dodatków technologicznych na jakość pieczywa pszenno-jęczmiennego (The effects of wholegrain barley flour and selected technological additives on the quality of wheat-barley bread). Żywność. Nauka. Technologia. Jakość, 43: 33–46.

Kim, Y., W. Huang, H. Zhu and P. Rayas-Duarte. 2009. Spontaneous sourdough processing of Chinese Northern-style steamed breads and their volatile compounds. Food Chemistry 114: 685–692.

Konopka, I., M. Tańska, A. Faron and S. Czaplicki. 2014. Release of free ferulic acid and changes in antioxidant properties during the wheat and rye bread making process. Food Science and Biotechnology, 23: 831–840.

Korycińska, M., K. Czelna, A. Jaromin and A. Kozubek. 2009. Antioxidant activity of rye bran alkylresorcinols and extracts from whole-grain cereal products. Food Chemistry, 116: 1013–1018.

Kozubek, A. and J.H.P. Tyman. 1999. Resorcinolic lipids, the natural non-isoprenoid phenolic amphiphiles and their biological activity. Chemical Reviews, 99: 1–25.

Król, B. and K. Grzelak. 2006. Qualitative and quantitative composition of fructooligosaccharides in bread. European Food Research and Technology, 223: 755–758.

Kuligowski, M., Ł. Nowak and J. Nowak. 2008. Enrichment of cereal products with tempeh-fermented legume seeds. 7th European Young Cereal Scientists and Technologists Workshop, Lithuania, 7: 28.

Kumar, V., A.K. Sinha, H.P.S. Makkar and K. Becker. 2010. Dietary roles of phytate and phytase in human nutrition: A review. Food Chemistry, 120: 945–959.

Landberg, R., M. Marklundc, A. Kamal-Eldind and P. Åman. 2014. An update on alkylresorcinols— Occurrence, bioavailability, bioactivity and utility as biomarkers. Journal of Functional Foods, 7: 77–89.

Leenhardt, F., M.A. Levrat-Verny, E. Chanliaud and C. Rémésy. 2005. Moderate decrease of pH by sourdough fermentation is sufficient to reduce phytate content of whole wheat flour through endogenous phytase activity. Journal of Agricultural and Food Chemistry, 53: 98–102.

Liukkonen, K.H., K. Katina, A. Wilhelmsson, O. Myllymäki, A.M. Lampi, S. Kariluoto, V. Piironen, S.M. Heinonen, T. Nurmi, H. Adlercreutz, A. Peltoketo, J.M. Pihlava, V. Hietaniemi and K. Poutanen. 2003. Process-induced changes on bioactive compounds in whole grain rye. Proceedings of the Nutrition Society, 62: 117–122.

Lopez, H., V. Krspine, C. Guy, A. Messager, C. Demigne and C. Remesy. 2001. Prolonged fermentation of whole wheat sourdough reduces phytate level and increases soluble magnesium. Journal of Agricultural and Food Chemistry, 49: 2657–2662.

Lopez, H.W., V. Duclos, C. Coudray, V. Krespine, C. Feillet-Coudray, A. Messager, C. Demigné and C. Rémésy. 2003. Making bread with sourdough improves mineral bioavailability from reconstituted whole wheat flour in rats. Nutrition, 19: 524–530.

Martínez, V., M. Mitjans and M.P. Vinardell. 2014. Cytoprotective effects of polyphenols against oxidative damage. pp. 275–288. *In*: R.R. Watson, V.R. Preedy and S. Zibadi (eds.). Polyphenols in Human Health and Disease. Academic Press.

Menzel, C., A. Kamal-Eldin, M. Marklund, A. Andersson, P. Åman and R. Landberg. 2012. Alkylresorcinols in Swedish cereal food products. Journal of Food Composition and Analysis, 28: 119–125.

Moore, J., Z. Cheng, J. Hao, G. Guo, J.G. Liu, C. Lin and L. Yu. 2007. Effects of solid-state yeast treatment on the antioxidant properties and protein and fiber compositions of common hard wheat bran. Journal of Agricultural and Food Chemistry, 55: 10173–10182.

Nionelli, L., N. Curri, J.A. Curiel, R. Di Cagno, E. Pontonio, I. Cavoski, M. Gobbetti and C.G. Rizzello. 2014. Exploitation of Albanian wheat cultivars: Characterization of the flours and lactic acid bacteria microbiota, and selection of starters for sourdough fermentation. Food Microbiology, 44: 96–107.

Nuobariene, L., Å.S. Hansen and N. Arneborg. 2012. Isolation and identification of hytase-active yeasts from sourdoughs. LWT—Food Science and Technology, 48: 190–196.

Öhrvik, V., H. Öhrvik, J. Tallkvist and C. Witthöft. 2010. Folates in bread: retention during bread-making and *in vitro* bioaccessibility. European Journal of Nutrition, 49: 365–372.

Ostasiewicz, A., A. Ceglińska and S. Skowronek. 2009. Jakość pieczywa żytniego z dodatkiem zakwasów (Quality of rye bread with leavens addend). Żywność. Nauka. Technologia. Jakość, 63: 67–74.

Paramithiotis, S., Y. Chouliaras, E. Tsakalidou and G. Kalantzopoulos. 2005. Application of selected starter cultures for the production of wheat sourdough bread using a traditional three-stage procedure. Process Biochemistry, 40: 2813–2819.

Plessas, S., A. Alexopoulos, I. Mantzourani, A. Koutinas, C. Voidarou, E. Stavropoulou and E. Bezirtzoglou. 2011. Application of novel starter cultures for sourdough bread production. Anaerobe, 17: 486–489.

Poutanen, K., L. Flander and K. Katina. 2009. Sourdough and cereal fermentation in a nutritional perspective. Food Microbiology, 26: 693–699.

Priefert, H., J. Rabenhorst and A. Steinbuchel. 2001. Biotechnological production of vanillin. Applied Microbiology and Biotechnology, 56: 296–314.

Raninen, K., J. Lappi, H. Mykkänen and K. Poutanen. 2011. Dietary fiber type reflects physiological functionality: comparison of grain fiber, inulin, and polydextrose. Nutrition Reviews, 69: 9–21.

Rizzello, C.G., M. Calasso, D. Campanella, M. De Angelis and M. Gobbetti. 2014. Use of sourdough fermentation and mixture of wheat, chickpea, lentil and bean flours for enhancing the nutritional, texture and sensory characteristics of white bread. International Journal of Food Microbiology, 180: 78–87.

Rocha, J.M. and F.X. Malcata. 2012. Microbiological profile of maize and rye flours, and sourdough used for the manufacture of traditional Portuguese bread. Food Microbiology, 31: 72–88.

Röcken, W. 1996. Applied aspects of sourdough fermentation. Advances in Food Science, 18: 212–218.

Ross, A.B., A. Kamal-Eldin and P. Åman. 2004. Dietary alkylresorcinols: absorption, bioactivities, and possible use as biomarkers of whole-grain wheat- and rye-rich foods. Nutrition Reviews, 62: 81–95.

Ross, A.B., A. Kamal-Eldin, E.A. Lundin, J.X. Zhang, G. Hallmans and P. Åman. 2003. Cereal alkylresorcinols are absorbed by humans. Journal of Nutrition, 133: 2222–2224.

Settanni, L., G. Ventimiglia, A. Alfonzo, O. Corona, A. Miceli and G. Moschetti. 2013. An integrated technological approach to the selection of lactic acid bacteria of flour origin for sourdough production. Food Research International, 54: 1569–1578.

Shamsuddin, A.M., A. Baten and N.D. Lalwani. 1992. Effects of inositol hexaphosphate on growth and differentiation in K-562 erythroleukemia cell line. Cancer Letters, 64: 195–202.

Shewry, P.R., V. Piironen, A.M. Lampi, M. Edelmann, S. Kariluoto, T. Nurmi, R. Fernandez-Orozco, A.A. Andersson, P. Aman, A. Fraś, D. Boros, K. Gebruers, E. Dornez, C.M. Courtin, J.A. Delcour, C. Ravel, G. Charmet, M. Rakszegi, Z. Bedo and J.L. Ward. 2010. Effects of genotype and environment on the content and composition of phytochemicals and dietary fiber components in rye in the Healthgrain diversity screen. Journal of Agricultural and Food Chemistry, 58: 9372–9383.

Wang, T., F. He and G. Chen. 2014. Improving bioaccessibility and bioavailability of phenolic compounds in cereal grains through processing technologies: A concise review. Journal of Functional Foods, 7: 101–111.

5

Phytochemicals as Functional Bread Compounds: Physiological Effects

Sylwia Mildner-Szkudlarz[1],* and *Joanna Bajerska*[2]

1. Introduction

As the role of diet in the prevention of human diseases such as cancer, atherosclerosis, heart disease, osteoporosis, and obesity has become more evident, many consumers increasingly seek functional food to improve their diets. Recent studies have suggested that plant food phytochemicals, including phenolic compounds (PCs), might have potential beneficial health effects, mainly related to their antioxidant capacity (Llobera and Cañellas 2008). A large number of epidemiological investigations have established an association between diets rich in PC and a decrease in the risk of suffering from many of the diseases of civilization (Rice-Evans et al. 1996). Moreover, several investigators have reviewed the importance of dietary fiber (DF) in recent years. It is well known that DF promotes beneficial physiological effects, including improvement in gastrointestinal function, the moderation of postprandial insulin response, and reductions in total and low-density lipoprotein (LDL) cholesterol (Davidson and McDonald 1998). Consequently, there is a trend towards searching for natural raw materials rich in DF and high in antioxidant capacity as functional ingredients for the food industry.

[1] Department of Food Science and Nutrition, Poznań University of Life Sciences, Wojska Polskiego 28, PL-60-637, Poznań, Poland.
Email: mildners@up.poznan.pl
[2] Department of Human Nutrition and Hygiene, Poznań University of Life Sciences, Wojska Polskiego 28, PL-60-637, Poznań, Poland.
Email: joanna.bajerska@up.poznan.pl
* Corresponding author

Bread is a staple processed food that dates back over 12,000 years, and is arguably one of the oldest functional foods developed by humans. Because of recommendations that bread—and especially whole-grain rye bread—should be an integral part of the diet, it may serve as a convenient food for delivering DF and phenolic antioxidants in high concentrations. Moreover, cereals are the best vehicle for fortification in most developing countries, because 95% of the population consumes cereals as a dietary staple. These are also relatively inexpensive to grow and are consumed worldwide at all economic levels. There have been many investigations into enhancing the nutritive value of cereal-based products, which have involved the supplementation of bread with DF or PC (Table 1). However, bioactive ingredients added to bread to enhance their nutritive value may adversely affect the viscoelastic properties of dough and the quality of bread, giving smaller bread volume, sensory panel scores, and a harder crumb. Thus, it is necessary to consider the chemical composition of the bioactive ingredients used in breadmaking, with a specific focus on the impact of added DF and PC on dough rheology and bread quality.

2. The effect of added phytochemicals

Gluten properties are largely responsible for the end-use quality of wheat in many food products. Understanding the factors affecting gluten properties is therefore of great importance. The addition of materials rich in DF may modify (improve or worsen) wheat dough properties. Dough development time (DDT) and dough stability (DS) are indicators of flour strength, with higher values indicating stronger dough (Wang et al. 2002). Decreased DS and prolonged DDT (from 4.2 to 5.8 min) were possible after the use of mango peel powder to replace flour at 10% (w/w) (Ajila et al. 2008). However, Mildner-Szkudlarz et al. (2013a) and Wang et al. (2002) found that the addition of grape by-products (GPs) from 4 to 10%, and of carob and pea (at 3% w/w) did not alter the DDT. Recently, Sudha et al. (2007) have reported an increase in DDT and a decrease in DS in wheat flour upon the addition of apple pomace. Such increases in DDT and decreases in DS indicate that the decrease in dough strength may be due to the dilution of gluten proteins in wheat flour upon the addition of fibrous materials. It is also known that not only the structure of gluten protein, but also the bonding within the protein plays important roles in the dough formation. The covalent and noncovalent bonds in the protein play important roles in the development and functionality of the dough (Bushuk 1998). Although hydrogen bonds are individually weak, they create stability in the dough when large numbers of them are established during dough development. Thus, the chemical structure of fiber determines its impact on DS and DDT, probably due to the number of hydroxyl groups of the fiber that interact with water through hydrogen bonding (Wang et al. 2002).

Ingredients rich in DF can lead to strict dough, which requires long mixing times. This was observed upon addition of GP (Mildner-Szkudlarz et al. 2013a), apple pomace (Sudha et al. 2007), and mango peel powder (Ajila et al. 2008). However, addition of hazelnut testa (Anil 2007), inulin, pea fiber, and carob fiber (Wang et al. 2002) decreased the mixing tolerance index (MTI). Changes in MTI are due to the dilution of gluten protein with fibrous materials. This could also be explained by the interaction

Table 1. Effects of different sources of bioactive ingredients on physical, sensory, and nutritional properties of bread.

Phytochemical source	Addition levels (% flour)	Physical and sensory properties	Nutritional properties			Acceptable level (%)	References
			TPC[a]	AA[b]	Other		
			Pseudocereals				
Buckwheat	15–30	Improves color, taste and odor, decreases the gummy taste	1.2–1.6	1.7–2.4[g]	—	30	Chlopicka et al. (2012)
	15 (common buckwheat, husked and unhusked)	Does not change the volume or sensory scores; slightly decreases lightness and increases redness and yellowness; however, these color differences are not recognized in sensory evaluation	0.9–1.8[c] 0.03–004[d]	1.8–3.8[h]	—	15	Lin et al. (2009)
Amaranth	15–30	Impairs color and taste, increases the gummy taste; has a bad, strange, difficult-to-taste taste	1.0–1.5	1.2–1.8[g]	—	Does not seem to be a favorable modification	Chlopicka et al. (2012)
	10–20	Decreases loaf volume and crumb elasticity; increases water absorption and crumb hardness; contributes to denser crumb structure and more uniform porosity; improves crust color and flavor	—	—	Increases: 43%–75% in zinc, 52%–91% in manganese, 76%–88% in magnesium, 57%–171% in calcium; 700%–1129% in squalene	15	Bodroža-Solarov et al. (2008)
	0–50	Increases water absorption and moisture content; decreases loaf volume and sensory scores for odor, taste, color, and texture	—	—	—	15	Ayo (2001)

Table 1. contd....

Table 1. contd.

Phytochemical source	Addition levels (% flour)	Physical and sensory properties	Nutritional properties			Acceptable level (%)	References
			TPC[a]	AA[b]	Other		
Quinoa	15–30	Impairs color; has an interesting, delicate, crusty taste	1.1–1.5	1.1–1.2[g]	—	30	Chlopicka et al. (2012)
	6	Very acceptable, with an overall linking score of 5.8 (in a scale of 7)	—	—	To achieve 100% of the daily allowance of omega-6 and omega-3 fatty acids, 23 and 55 slices, respectively, of quinoa bread would need to be consumed	6	Calderelli et al. (2010)
Barley flours	5–20	Improves the flavor only up the 10% level; thereafter, decreases the taste score and overall acceptability, changing the crust color from creamy white to dull brown	1.04–1.1	—	Increases: 2%–19% in phytic acid, 5%–7% in amylase inhibitor activity, 276%–437% in total β-glucan decreases: 2%–6% in *in vitro* starch digestibility	15	Dhingra and Jood (2001)
	40 (three different hulled varieties)	Significantly differs in sensory scores from the control bread; sensory attributes, such as bitterness, off-odor, and off-flavor, correspond well with the phenolic content	Significant increases, though this depends on the barley variety	Significant increases, though this depends on the barley variety	—	—	Holtekjølen et al. (2008)
Plant by-products							
Grape pomace	4–10 (without seeds)	Decreases overall acceptability; increases alcohol and sharp odor; increases crumb hardness	2.2–4.0	2.0–2.7[i] 5.2–10.8[g]	10%–39% increase in TDF	6	Mildner-Szkudlarz et al. (2011)
Grape pomace	2.5–10 (grape seed flour)	Decreases brightness, volume, acceptance of astringency and sweetness taste, as well as overall acceptability; increases hardness and porosity	18.3–70.8	—	—	5	Hoye and Ross (2011)

Coconut flour	10–30	Increase parameters (dough development time farinographic, arrival time, and stability), decrease water absorption, appearance, texture, and overall acceptability	—	—	20	Gunathilake et al. (2009)
	10	—	1.1	Increases (times): 3.1–3.5 × TDF, 1.9–2.8 × iron, 1.1–1.2 × zinc, 2.1–12.4 × calcium	—	Trinidad et al. (2006)
Hazelnut testa	5–10	Increases farinographic (water absorption, development time, stability, time to breakdown) and extensographic parameters (energy, resistance to extension, maximum resistance); decreases mixing tolerance index and extensibility; slightly reduces volumes, total sensory scores, and degree of softening	—	—	10	Anil (2007)
Plant extracts						
Green tea extract (GTE)	0.15–0.5	Decrease the brightness, sweetness and volume, increase the hardness, stickiness and astringency	—	—	0.5% is the threshold level of GTE for astringency, sweetness, porosity and hardness; 0.15% is the threshold level of GTE for brightness and stickiness	Wang et al. (2007)

Table 1. contd....

Table 1. contd.

Phytochemical source	Addition levels (% flour)	Physical and sensory properties	Nutritional properties			Acceptable level (%)	References
			TPC[a]	AA[b]	Other		
Plant extracts							
	0.5–1.1	Impair flavor and general acceptability, do not change the texture	282.7–663.3[e]	6.8–13.1[i]		0.8	Bajerska et al. (2010)
Saffron extract	0.08–0.16	Decrease overall acceptability, rise phenolic and sharp taste and flavor, impair the color	1.4–1.6	1.4–1.7[g]	—	0.12	Bajerska et al. (2013)
Grape seed extract	0.09–0.29	Favorable change the color without causing significant changes in other sensory properties, do not change the texture	—	~ 2.8–5.8[j]	Reduces CML content (30%–50%)	0.29	Peng et al. (2010)
Buckwheat extract	2.5–5 (green part of Tartary buckwheat)	Affect the quality of the bread in a negative way, decrease the volume, and impair sensory acceptance, give slightly less aromatic bread	1.2–2.1[f]	~ 1.8–4[fi]	—	2.5	Gawlik-Dziki et al. (2010)

[a] Times increase in total phenolic compounds (TPC) between control samples and samples with the smallest and greatest enhancements
[b] Times increase in antioxidant activity (AA) between control samples and samples with the smallest and greatest enhancements
[c] Content of rutin, expressed as mg rutin/100 g DM
[d] Content of quercetin, expressed as mg quercetin/100 g DM
[e] Total phenol content, expressed as mg catechin/100 g DM
[f] Bread after the action of simulated saliva (stage I) and simulated intestinal juice (stage III)
[g] Antioxidant activity determined by FRAP assay
[h] Antioxidant activity determined by the conjugated diene method
[i] Antioxidant activity determined by DPPH˙ assay
[j] Antioxidant activity determined by ABTS method

between DF and gluten, influencing the dough mixing properties as suggested by Chen et al. (1988). The disruption of bread crumb structure is due to the impairment of gas retention. The addition of fiber lowers resistance to dough extension, and increased concentrations of insoluble and soluble cell wall materials have been shown to partially disrupt the gluten network (Collar et al. 2007).

Phytochemicals (PCs) affect bread quality by interfering with dough formation (Wang et al. 2004). It has been reported that ferulic acid affects overmixing in a way similar to that of thiol-blocking reagents, increasing the rate of dough breakdown and making the dough sticky. Furthermore, in the presence of ferulic acid, the dough does not recover, even after a resting period (Okada et al. 1987). Moreover, Labat et al. (2000) declared that the addition of ferulic acid to wheat flour can shorten the DDT, increase the rate of dough breakdown, and make the dough sticky. The study of Wang and Zhou (2004) showed that the resistance-to-extension ratio of the dough was greatly decreased by the addition of green tea extract. The authors suggested that tea catechins react with wheat protein by scavenging free radicals (GS$^{\cdot}$), resulting in changes in dough rheology. PCs added to food formulations containing proteins have been also shown to bind protein molecule residues, resulting in lower food quality and lower bioavailability of the affected proteins, although data here are limited. The main mechanism of polyphenol–protein binding is considered to be the noncovalent interaction of the amino, hydroxyl, and carboxyl groups of the protein with gallate and hydroxylate benzol groups of polyphenols (Huang et al. 2004). The complexation of polyphenols, as well as their enzymatic and nonenzymatic oxidation products, with protein in seed, meals, or flours has been reputed to reduce the nutritional value of proteins from these sources (Haslam 1989). Moreover, oxidized phenols reacting with amino acids and proteins might inhibit the activity of proteolytic enzymes and lipases (Milic et al. 1968). This proteolytic splitting is influenced by the amino acid composition, the native structure of the proteins, structural changes following upon derivatization with PCs, molecular size, conformational flexibility of phenolic antioxidants, and water solubility of the phenols (Kroll and Rawel 2001).

As the bread matrix is a complex system, the mechanism responsible for the increase in bread hardness on the addition of ingredients rich in PCs and DF still remains unknown. The decrease in loaf volume and the increase in hardness might be attributable to the higher water absorption (WA) of fiber-rich incorporated doughs. This observation is explained by an interaction between the water and hydroxyl groups of polysaccharides through hydrogen bonding. Thus, less water is available for the development of the starch-gluten network, causing an underdeveloped gluten network and reduced loaf volume (Brennan and Cleary 2007). Although Sudha et al. (2007), Ajila et al. (2008) and Anil (2007) all reported an increase, Artz et al. (1990) and Mildner-Szkudlarz et al. (2013a) reported a decrease in WA, with increasing phytochemical contents. Furthermore, Vernaza et al. (2011) and Sobczyk et al. (2010) did not observe any variation in WA with the incorporation of different bioactive ingredients. Clearly, differences in WA depend on the chemical structure of the fibers added, the association between molecules, the size of the particles and the porosity of the fibers (Thebaudin et al. 1997). For example, grape by-products consist mainly of cellulose, hemicelluloses, and lignin. The lignin fraction in grape by-products is the most abundant fraction, contributing nearly 46% of the total DF. Lignin is insoluble in water and has hydrophobic binding capacity, so, if this fraction predominates, WA might decrease (Eastwoood 1973). Furthermore, Camire and Flint (1991) found no correlation between nonstarch polysaccharides and hydration capacity, suggesting that other components, such as starches, may be responsible for changes in hydration capacity. Thus, the varied hardness and volume in breads supplemented with phytochemicals might be also explained by the affected enzyme activity and yeast activity (Wang et al. 2007). Zhang and Kashket (1998) suggest that the activities of amylases in dough might be restricted by the PCs, leading to inadequate maltose for yeast activity during proofing. Moreover, Turchetti et al. (2005) reported that catechins were capable of inhibiting the activity of yeast, causing poorer gassing power. Subsequently, a smaller volume of bread with a relatively harder, denser texture is obtained.

An attractive aroma, which includes both taste and flavor, and overall consumer acceptance, are also very important, as this ensures the marketing success of any novel food. It is known that high levels of added PCs in a food product might be significantly involved in the taste sensation of bread and include astringency, bitterness, and sweetness (Wang et al. 2007; Bajerska et al. 2010; Mildner-Szkudlarz et al. 2011). Astringency is a chemically induced complex of tactile sensations, and occurs when praline-rich proteins, such as salivary proteins, are precipitated in the mouth, causing the loss of their lubricating effect (Kallithraka et al. 2001). Scharbert and Hofmann (2005) reported that catechins are responsible for the astringent sensation. The lowest threshold concentration for the astringency in liquids is exhibited by epigallocatechin gallate; the other catechins are also responsible for astringency, but at relatively higher threshold concentrations. On the other hand, Robichaud and Noble (1990) found that catechin and gallic acid were more bitter than astringent. The extent to which phenolic antioxidants are responsible for the sensory characteristics associated with bread quality, as well as with consumers' perceptions, is unknown at the present time. Hence, there is a need to carry out a sensory study on the quality of bread with the addition of bioactive ingredients.

3. Impact of baking on the level and stability of bioactive compounds

The stability of bioactive components during the baking process should be taken into consideration to ensure optimum retention in new products, as well as in the commercialization of functional ingredients. The stability of PCs is affected by pH, water activity, exposure to light, oxygen, temperature, and enzymatic activities; moreover, temperature is the most decisive factor in their decomposition. However, heating may alter the phenolic antioxidants in bread to different extents and in different ways. Moreover, regardless of the amount of PCs added, the percentage loss might also depend on structural factors, as well as on processing conditions.

The results obtained by Bajerska et al. (2010) and by Wang and Zhou (2004) show that green tea catechins are relatively stable during baking. According to Bajerska et al. (2010), the most stable catechin during the breadmaking process is (–)-EGC, which shows average losses of 6–7%. For the other major catechins, EGCG and ECG, losses of about 18% and 35%, respectively, were observed during baking. Wang and

Zhou (2004), when adding 0.05%, 0.1%, and 0.15% GTE to bread dough, indicated that 17% of the (−)-EGCG and 34% of the (−)-EGC was lost in bread, while only 9% of the (−)-ECG was lost. According to Mildner-Szkudlarz et al. (2013a), the most stable PC during the baking of biscuits with the addition of 10%, 20%, and 30% white grape pomace were γ-resorcylic acid and gallic acid, with average losses of 11% and 18%, respectively. The percentage loss of catechin was about 31%, while procyanidins B1 and B2, which were identified in white grape pomace at 6.74 and 5.48 mg/100 g DM respectively, were not retained after the baking process. Sharma and Zhou (2011) also found considerable loss of catechins during biscuit baking. The amount of ECG and EGCG at the end of the baking process for 0.3% green tea extract was about 30% and 21%, respectively. Rupasinghe et al. (2008), when adding 4%, 8%, 16%, 24%, and 32% apple skin powder to muffins, reported that flavonols and favan-3-ol are relatively more resistant to thermal degradation during baking than anthocyanins and phenolic acids. Furthermore, these authors found about a 39% loss of quercetin glycosides, and significant increased free quercetin and phloretin levels. They suggested that quercetin and phloretin aglycones were produced during the baking process through the thermohydrolysis or deglycosylation of the glycosides of quercetin and phloretin. This observation was supported by Rohn et al. (2007), who reported that the main product of thermal degradation of onion quercetin glucosides is their aglycone quercetin, which remained stable during roasting at 180°C. On the other hand, it is known that glycosylated structures of betacyanins are more stable than aglycons, probably because of the higher oxidation–reduction potentials of the former (von Elbe and Attoe 1985). At high temperatures, cyanidin glycosides are hydrolyzed to cyanidin aglycone, which undergoes spontaneous degradation to various products (Seeram et al. 2001). Concerning the structural aspects, according to Hrazdina and Franzese (1974), in acidic solution, malvidin 3,5-diglucoside was oxidized more rapidly than acylated malvidin analogue—an effect ascribed to the decreased activity of the C2 position or to steric hindrance.

The thermal process may also result in the synthesis of Maillard reaction products (MRPs), mainly melanoidins, which possess some antioxidant activity. For example, Michalska et al. (2008) found a good correlation between advanced MRPs and Trolox Equivalent Antioxidant Capacity (TEAC) and Oxygen Radical Antioxidant Capacity ($ORAC_{FL}$) assays during the process of baking rye bread. Gawlik-Dziki et al. (2009) suggested that the antioxidant activity of bread enriched with 2.5% and 5% extract from the green parts of Tartary buckwheat was mainly due to synergistic effects between MRPs and buckwheat extract compounds.

Despite the structural aspect and temperature of the process, the loss of PCs could be also due to the combined effect of the pH of the system, the interactions of the phenols with certain components in the dough during preparation (especially wheat proteins via hydrogen bonding), and the degradation of PCs during the various stages of breadmaking (including mixing). It seems that the oxidation of phenols induced by active oxygen must play a very minor role, due to addition of yeast which assimilate oxygen during the mixing process (Wang and Zhou 2004). It is well known that degradations of phenols in aqueous systems also depend strongly on pH values. In the case of wheat bread dough, the pH is in the range of 5–6. Friedman and Jürgens (2000) have studied the stability of the natural polyphenols in pH values between 3 and 11, demonstrating that caffeic, chlorogenic, and gallic acids are not stable to high pH, while (–)-catechin, (–)-epigallocatechin, ferulic acid, rutin, and *trans*-cinnamic acid resisted major pH-induced degradation. The stability of anthocyanins and their colors is also highly dependent on pH, due to changes in the concentration of four species: flavylium cation, quinonoidal base, pseudobase, and carbinol and chalcone. Conversion of one species to another is typically accompanied by dramatic changes in color and stability. Among the four species, the red flavylium cation present at pH 1.0–2.4 is the most stable (Cabrita et al. 2000). According to Sharma and Zhou (2011), tea catechins are less stable in alkaline pH and more stable in acidic pH.

4. Addition of plant by-products to bread

The food industry generates many millions of tons per year of plant processed by-products, particularly in the fruit and cereal processing sectors. Fruit and cereal processing by-products are currently only partially valorized at different value-added levels and are extensively managed as a waste of environmental concern with the relevant negative effects on the overall sustainability of the food processing industry. Such wastes are quite unstable, due to their propensity to microbiological spoilage and oxidation, which limits their potential for use. The treatment and disposal of waste is thus a serious environmental problem, and new technologically and economically viable strategies for converting by-products to high-value food would prevent their disposal as waste and would increase remarkably both the sustainability and competitiveness of the worldwide food industry. Many authors' results indicate that food industry waste exhibits considerable antioxidant properties. Thus, it is advisable to search for other potential uses of by-product—not only those that might be economically sensible, but also for those that might improve the wholesomeness and range of food products. Calculations for agrifood chains show that the exploitation of the by-products of food processing represents one of the most effective means of reducing their carbon footprints.

Grapes are one of the world's largest fruit crops, and approximately 80% of their yield is utilized for winemaking. The winemaking industry thus generates large quantities of waste which, because of their high pollution load, considerably increase the chemical and biochemical oxygen demand (Lafka et al. 2007). For that reason, treatment of winemaking wastes is a serious environmental problem, and uses (other than as fertilizers) need to be found for these by-products (Lafka et al. 2007). Grape by-products (GP) have drawn increased attention in recent years because of their potential health benefits, not only as an antioxidant agents, but also as antibacterial, antiobesity, antithrombotic, and anticarcinogenic agent; they also display inhibitory effects against atherosclerosis and hypercholesterolemia (Jayaprakasha et al. 2003; Park et al. 2008; Mildner-Szkudlarz and Bajerska 2013). These various biological properties are believed to be due to the functions of GP polyphenols and DF, because, even after contact with the fermenting wine, they still contain a large amount of such phytochemicals. According to Llobera and Cañellas (2007), grape pomace and steam are valuable sources of SDF and Klason lignin. Generally, fruit DF has greater nutritive value than DF derived from cereals, because they contain significant amounts of bioactive compounds, such as PCs and carotenoids. Moreover, GP are a good source of many health-enhancing phytonutrients, including flavanols, phenolic acids, and anthocyanins (Lafka et al. 2007; Mildner-Szkudlarz et al. 2010). PCs from GP have been shown to be potent scavengers of free radicals and to inhibit cancer cell proliferation through (at least) the induction of apoptosis (Parry et al. 2011). Additionally, DF from grape pomace protects healthy colon tissue against tumor development and reduces the risk of cancer (Lizarraga et al. 2011); it has also been shown to be effective in protecting against oxidative damage due to lipid peroxidation by improving the antioxidant defense system in rats fed a high-fat diet, as well as in those fed a low-fat diet (Lee et al. 2009).

Mildner-Szkudlarz et al. (2011) have examined the soluble (SDF) and insoluble (IDF) DF, PCs, antioxidant activity, and organoleptic characteristics of sourdough mixed rye bread with GP at four different levels: 4%, 6%, 8%, and 10%. The addition of GP significantly improves dietary fraction contents, as bread with a 10% addition of GP contains 39% and 37% higher contents of IDF and SDF than does control bread. The assay of radical-scavenging activity (DPPH˙) and reducing ability (FRAP) showed that the addition of GP greatly enhances the antioxidant properties of mixed rye breads. DPPH˙ levels in five types of mixed rye breads ranged from 5.55 to 15.02 mM TRE/g DM, while the FRAP value ranged from 4.44 to 48.14 mM Fe^{II}/g DM. The PC profiles of supplemented breads were dominated by procyanidin B1 and B2, catechin, epicatechin, caffeic acid, and myricetin. However, with an increase in the level of GP, the hardness and gumminess of the bread significantly increased. The authors also observed slight differences in the concentrations of volatile compounds. Sensory evaluation of bread samples showed that, as the level of GP increased, bread volume, porosity, and overall acceptance decreased. Moreover, breads with greater levels of GP were described as having stronger alcoholic and sharp (astringent) notes. Sensory evaluation of GP-enhanced breads demonstrated that a maximum of 6% GP could be incorporated in preparing acceptable products. Hoye and Ross (2011) examined the consumer acceptance and physical properties, including total phenolic content (TPC), of bread made with varying levels of grape seed flour (2.5–10%), as well as the impact of frozen storage on the consumer acceptance and TPC of these breads. The replacement of 10% of the wheat flour by grape seed flour increased the bread TPC from 0.064 mg tannic acid/g DM to 4.25 mg tannic acid/g DM. However, replacement of 5% decreased the loaf's brightness and volume, with an increase in hardness and porosity. The authors observed an increase in the astringent note and a reduction in the overall acceptance of bread containing $\geq 7.5\%$ grape seed flour. Therefore, the replacement of 5% with grape seed flour was recommended for the production of fortified breads with acceptable physical and sensory properties and high TPC activity, compared to the control bread.

Coconut flour is the residue remaining after the extraction of coconut milk or of virgin coconut oil. Trinidad et al. (2006) reported that coconut flour can provide not only added value in the industry, but also a nutritious and healthy source of dietary fiber. Coconut flour contains 60.9% TDF, with IDF being the major fraction at 56.8%. Coconut flour may play a role in controlling cholesterol and sugar levels in blood and in preventing colon cancer. Moreover, studies show that consumption of high-fiber coconut flour increases fecal bulk (Gunathilake et al. 2009). Trinidad et al. (2006)

have determined the effectiveness of the dietary fiber component of coconut flour as a functional food; they supplemented cereal-based products, including cinnamon bread and multigrain loaves, with 10% coconut flour, and determined the dietary fiber composition and fermentability characteristics of the coconut flour, as well as the effect of coconut flour on mineral availability, and the contents of phytic and tannic acid. Compared with white bread, the addition of 10% coconut flour to cinnamon bread and multigrain loaves increased the phytic acid content from 2.05 mg/g to 2.27 and 2.23 mg/g, respectively, while tannic acid content was raised from 1.14 mg/g to 2.66 and 1.85 mg/g, respectively. The control white bread contained 3.1% TDF, while the cinnamon bread and multigrain bread had 9.5 and 10.8% TDF—an approximately threefold increase. Increasing the amount of coconut flour DF in the test foods did not affect mineral availability. The multigrain loaves were the best source of calcium, containing nearly 12.4 times as much as white bread. Gunathilake et al. (2009) have found that blending wheat flour with coconut flour at different levels alters the organoleptic and rheological properties of different blends, even though the addition of as much as 20% coconut flour to white bread is possible for producing products with acceptable qualities.

Hazelnut testa is obtained by brushing hazelnuts following a roasting process. Hazelnut testa includes some phenolic substances, such as gallic, *p*-hydroxyl benzoic, sinapic, and caffeic acids, as well as epicatechin and quercetin, which have antioxidant properties, and dietary fiber (Yurttas et al. 2000). In the study of Anil (2007), hazelnut testa was added to wheat flour bread in fine and coarse forms, at 5% and 10% levels, as dry (not hydrated) and hydrated to increase the dietary fiber content. Percentage added, particle size, and hydration process were found to affect certain quality parameters of doughs and breads significantly. Farinograph and extensograph results show that the addition of hazelnut testa has significant effect on dough's rheological properties. Breads enriched with hazelnut testa had similar, or slightly smaller, loaf volumes than the control. Hydration of hazelnut testa prior to its addition to wheat flour increased the detrimental effects on bread loaf volume. The use of hazelnut testa caused the crumb to darken. Increasing levels of hazelnut testa and hydration caused slight decreases in total sensory scores. Results showed that 5–10% additions of fine or coarse hazelnut testa received the best scores in sensory evaluation, and can be recommended in breadmaking as a source of dietary fiber.

5. Addition of pseudocereals to bread

Pseudocereals are defined as starchy food grains other than those classified as cereals (barley, corn, maize, millet, oat, rice, rye, sorghum), legumes (fenugreek, amaranth, quinoa, lupin), oilseeds (soybean, flaxseed, safflower seed, sesame seed), and nuts (Fletcher 2004). Pseudocereals are being used extensively in the development of functional foods. Whole pseudocereal grains are rich in a wide range of compounds— such as flavonoids, phenolic acids, trace elements, fatty acids, vitamins, saponins, phytosterols, squalene, and fagopyritols—that have known effects on human health (Kalinova and Dadakova 2009). Pseudocereals can provide beneficial health effects, so bread supplemented with them, if used as a staple food, could diversify the daily model of nutrition (Martirosyan et al. 2007).

Buckwheat is an important functional food in some countries including, China, Japan and Taiwan, where it is used to prepare noodles (Lin et al. 2009). Common buckwheat seeds contain rutin and isovitexin, while the hulls contain rutin, orientin, vitexin, quercetin, isovitexin, and isoorientin (Tian et al. 2002). Compared with most grain crops, as well as with fruits and vegetables, buckwheat contains more rutin, which possess antioxidant, anti-inflammatory, and anticarcinogenic effects, and can also thicken the walls of blood vessels, reducing their permeability and preventing arteriosclerosis (Sun and Ho 2005). It is also important that buckwheat seeds are a rich source of six fagopyritols (B1, B2, B3, A1, A2, A3), which are the galactosyl derivatives of D-*chiro*-inositol. Fagopyritols are structurally similar to galactosamine D-*chiro*-inositol, which is related to a pH 2.0 (type P) putative insulin mediator (Larner et al. 1988). The consumption of Tartary buckwheat as flour or in biscuits has been demonstrated to have hypoglycemic effects in diabetic patients (Lu et al. 1992). Thus, the potential of the consumption of buckwheat, and particularly the consumption of fagopyritols, in reducing symptoms of NIDDM is of considerable interest. Chlopicka et al. (2012) have determined the effect on the antioxidant properties and sensory value of breads of adding buckwheat flour at two different levels (15 and 30%). Their results show that the addition of buckwheat flour at levels of up to 15% or 30% to wheat flour improved satisfactory bread properties and attributes, such as color, odor, and taste. Bread with the addition of 30% buckwheat flour had an interesting, natural taste and was crustier than both the control bread and bread with 15% buckwheat flour. Moreover, buckwheat flour at 30% reduced the gummy attribute, which could otherwise decrease value of bread. The control white bread had 1.7 mg GAE/g DM, while bread with 15% and 30% of buckwheat had 2.1 and 2.65 mg GAE/g DM—approximately 1.2 and 1.6 as much. FRAP assay of the breads ranged from 0.64 (control bread) to 1.51 (30% addition of buckwheat flour) mg TRE/g DM. Lin et al. (2009) produced buckwheat-enhanced wheat breads by substituting 15% of the wheat flour with common buckwheat (*Fagopyrum esculentum* Moench), with or without the husk. Enhancing of wheat flour in the formula with buckwheat would not interfere with bread specific volume and overall acceptance. The supplemented breads characterized better flavor and mouth feel sensory attributes. Buckwheat-enhanced wheat bread contained more functional components rutin and quercetin as expected and was good in antioxidant activity, reducing power and scavenging ability on DPPH radicals with unhusked buckwheat-enhanced wheat bread being the most effective. Moreover, husky buckwheat has a higher content of insoluble β-glucans, which stimulate immune system polysaccharides (Hozová et al. 2007). Therefore, buckwheat breads have extra functionality and health effects for consumers.

Amaranth is an excellent source of high-quality balanced protein, composed mainly of globulins and albumins, which have high bioavailability (Escudero et al. 2004). Moreover, amaranth is a good source of vitamins and minerals especially, riboflavin, vitamin E, calcium, magnesium, zinc, and iron. According to Klimczak et al. (2002), the main PC found in amaranth seeds are caffeic, *p*-hydroxybenzoic, and ferulic acids. The lipids in amaranth are rich in squalene, tocotrienols, and phytosterols. Amaranth seed oil contains approximately 6% squalene (Escudero et al. 2004), which is a strong antioxidant and anticancerogen that reduces cholesterol levels (Martinez-Correa et al. 2010). Several studies have shown that the nutritional quality of bakery products is improved when wheat flour is supplemented with amaranth. In the study of Chlopicka et al. (2012), amaranth flour added at 30% increases the TPC and FRAP activity from 1.7 mg GAE/g DM and 63.8 mg TRE/100 g DM, respectively, in the control bread to 2.65 mg GAE/g DM and 150.8 mg TRE/100 g DM, respectively, in the enhanced bread. However, significant negative observations of changes in sensory attributes associated with the quantity of amaranth were found. Thus, the authors indicated that the addition of amaranth flour to wheat bread does not seem to be a favorable modification. Moreover, Bodroža-Solarov et al. (2008) produced amaranth-enhanced wheat bread by substituting 10%–20% wheat flour with expanded amaranth grain. The addition of the expanded grain significantly increased ash, protein, and crude fiber. They found about 43%–75%, 52%–91%, 76–88% and 57–171% increases in zinc, manganese, magnesium, and calcium contents, respectively. Compared to white bread, the addition of 20% amaranth grain increased the squalene content from 3.5 mg/100 g to 43 mg/100 g. However, the higher doses of supplementation affects the physical and sensory characteristics of bread, decreasing loaf volume and crumb elasticity, while increasing WA and crumb hardness. Although the addition of amaranth contributes to a denser crumb structure with more uniform porosity, it improved crust color and flavor. The authors reported that supplementation levels up to 15% were sensorially acceptable. Ayo (2001) has also reported that amaranth flour could be used up to 15% in production of wheat–amaranth grain composite bread without significant effects on the physical or sensory qualities, or on consumer acceptance of the product. Higher levels of amaranth flour (25–30%) are possible only in the production of wheat–amaranth cookies (Sindhuja et al. 2005).

Quinoa is a good source of high-quality protein, vitamins (riboflavin, thiamine, and folic acid), and minerals (magnesium, zinc, and iron). Moreover, quinoa seeds are an abundant source of flavonoids, which consist mainly of glycosides of the flavonols kaempferol and quercetin (Dini et al. 2004). Quinoa lipids are characterized by a high degree of unsaturation, with linoleic acid being predominant (at 50% of total fatty acids) (Alvarez-Jubete et al. 2009). Furthermore, high α-linolenic acid content (3.8–8.3%) is also found in quinoa seeds (Alvarez-Jubete et al. 2009), which have an important role in the prevention and regulation of cardiovascular diseases, cancer, osteoporosis, and inflammatory and autoimmune diseases (Simopoulos 2001). Other interesting components in quinoa include saponins and glycosides with one or more sugar chains on a triterpene or steroid aglycone backbone, which might possess anticarcinogenic and cholesterol lowering properties (Guclu-Ustundag and Mazza 2007). Chlopicka et al. (2012) studied the characteristics of breads with the addition of 15% and 30% quinoa flour. In that study, the TPC increased from 1.7 mg GAE/g DM (in the control white bread) to 2.54 mg GAE/g DM in the bread enhanced with 30% quinoa flour. There was thus an almost one-and-a-half-fold increase in bioactive compounds in the 30% quinoa flour-enriched breads. Sensory analysis of the breads showed that the addition of quinoa flour to the dough produced bread very much appreciated by the testers, with an interesting, delicate, crusty taste. In another study, Calderelli et al. (2010) produced a functional bread by mixing wheat flour, sugar, salt, bread improver, soya oil, yeast, water, and 6% powdered quinoa grains. The quinoa bread was characterized by low levels of saturated fatty acids and a ratio between the sum of the polyunsaturated and saturated fatty acids of over 0.45—which is recommended for bread to be considered healthy in terms of cardiac diseases. The authors showed that quinoa breads could be regarded as standard breads, as they enjoyed high acceptance among customers.

Barley grains have also been investigated for several potential new applications as a whole grain and for its value-added products. The cell walls in the barley kernel, as well as in the endosperm, contain large amounts of β-glucans (Newman and McGuire 1985). In human diets, β-glucans function as food fiber, and are known to have beneficial effects, such as decreasing serum cholesterol (Kalra and Jood 2000). Barley is mostly known for its high levels of dietary fiber, but it also contains measurable amounts of catechins and some dimer and trimer procyanidins (McMurrough and Baert 1994). *In vitro* studies have indicated that TPC of an 80% methanolic extract from whole barley grains ranged from 24.34 to 26.90 μg/mg of lyophilizate, while the antioxidant activity, based on the relative abilities of the extracts to scavenge ABTS$^{·+}$, range from 0.054 to 0.150 μM TRE/mg of lyophilizate (Zdunczyk et al. 2006). These values are approximately 2.7 and 2.3 times greater than for wheat grains. According to Dhingra and Jood (2001), additions of 15% barley flour to wheat flour produces acceptable breads. However, the substitution of barley flours to wheat at 20% levels produced organoleptically unacceptable bread, with dull brown crust color and lower scores for texture, flavor, and taste. Increasing the barley flour in the blends to acceptable levels (15%) significantly increases levels of phytic acid (225.6–268 mg/100 g), polyphenols (315–346 mg/100 g), total β-glucans (0.41–2.20 g/100 g DM), and amylase inhibitor activity (68.3–73.2 AIU/g), while decreasing the *in vitro* starch digestibility (42.8–40.38 mg maltose released/g meal), as compared with the control. The antioxidant properties and sensory profile of bread enhanced with 40% barley flour from three different hulled varieties have been studied by Holtekjølen et al. (2008). The sensory evaluation showed clear differences between the breads baked with the different barley varieties and the control. Moreover, sensory scores for bitterness, off-odor, and off-flavor correlated well with TPC, in accordance with the study of Wang et al. (2007) and Scharbert and Hofmann (2005). On the other hand, according to Wang et al. (1998), β-glucan-rich fractions may play a role in the improvement of crumb grain by stabilizing air cells in the dough and preventing their coalescence.

6. Addition of plant extracts to bread

Antioxidants are mainly used as food additives, with the aim of prevention oxidative deterioration of fats and oils in processed foods. Synthetic antioxidants, such as 3-tertbutyl-4-methoxyphenol (that is, butylated hydroxyanisole, BHA), 2,6-di-tert-butyl-4-methylphenol (that is, butylated hydroxytoluene, BHT), and tert-butylhydroquinone (TBHQ), have been typically used as antioxidants for foods since the beginning of the twentieth century (Pokorný 1991; Byrd 2001). Although these synthetic antioxidants are efficient and relatively cheap, their use is questionable, due to their health risks and toxicity (Pokorný 1991; Byrd 2001). Recently, special attention has been paid to the isolation of antioxidant compounds from natural sources, and particularly from plant source, such as rosemary, oregano, green pepper, tea, mango, grape skin and seeds, blackcurrant seeds, tomato seeds, and amaranth peel (Pizzale et al. 2002; Samotyja and Malecka 2007; Mildner-Szkudlarz et al. 2009). The antioxidant properties of these plant extracts have been chiefly attributed to their polyphenol contents. PCs, which are plant secondary metabolites, have many positive effects on human health, including antiallergenic, antiviral, antioxidant, anti-inflammatory, anticarcinogenic properties, and their ability to prevent cardiovascular diseases. They are found frequently in food products, such as fruits, vegetables and grains. Thus, these natural antioxidants play a major role in enhancing shelf life, as well as preserving the nutritional and organoleptic qualities, of bakery products.

Tea leaves (*Camellia sinensis* L.) are a good source of polyphenols (mainly flavonoids) that possesses various pharmacological effects, such as antihypertensive, antiarteriosclerotic, hypoglycemic, and hypocholesterolemic properties (Karori et al. 2007). There are six main catechins in tea leaves: (+)-catechin, (−)-epicatechin, (−)-epicatechin gallate, (−)-epigallocatechin, (−)-epigallocatechin gallate, and (−)-gallocatechin (Peterson et al. 2005). Among these, EGCG is primarily responsible for the beneficial effects of green tea (Siró et al. 2008). There is some evidence for the possible preventive role of green tea and its active components in CVD and other diet-dependent diseases (Siró et al. 2008). The levels of the different tea catechins, and their ratios, are mainly linked with the degree of fermentation of the leaf. During black tea fermentation, the oxidation of catechins causes the formation of catechin quinones, which subsequently react with the two main pigments, the theaflavins and thearubigens (Leung et al. 2001). In the preparation of green tea, the leaves are first steamed and then dried relatively rapidly. This stops the enzyme-catalyzed oxidation of tea-leaf catechins. Therefore, the main differences between black and green tea are associated with the levels of catechins and the oxidized condensation products. Sensory analysis and instrumental analyses were used to investigate the effect produced on crumb appearance, texture properties, and taste profile of new functional breads by green tea extracts (GTE) at 0.15 and 0.5% (Wang et al. 2007).

The concentration levels of total tea catechins were approximately 0.53 and 1.78 mg/g (wet basis) in the dough, for GTE at 1.5 and 5.0 g/kg flour, respectively. These results indicate that GTE is significantly involved in the taste sensation of bread, as well as its hardness, stickiness, astringency, and sweetness. It was found that GTE decreases the brightness, sweetness, and volume, while increasing the hardness, stickiness, and astringency of the enhanced breads. According to the authors, the threshold level of GTE for the astringent and sweet notes was 0.5%, while for brightness, hardness, and stickiness, the threshold was 0.15%. The effects of GTE at 0.5%–1.1% on catechin stability, antioxidant properties, and the sensory profiles of sourdough rye breads were also analyzed by Bajerska et al. (2010), who showed that the breadmaking process was optimal for the stability of tea catechins and caffeine. According to these authors, one slice of rye bread (40 g) with GTE at 0.5% and 1.1% provides 18.7 mg and 47.6 mg total tea catechins, respectively. The amount of EGCG and caffeine ranged from 11.0 mg to 26.9 mg, and from 7.2 mg to 17.6 mg, per slice of fresh rye bread, with 0.5% and 1.1% GTE, respectively. However, sensory scores for taste, flavor, and overall acceptability were significantly lower when bread was prepared with 1.1% GTE than in the case of the control bread. The level of GTE should thus be limited to 0.8%. The significantly higher enhancement found here, as compared with study of Wang et al. (2007), is probably related to the masking effect of the flavor bouquet produced during the sourdough fermentation process.

Since ancient times, saffron has been used as a medicinal plant and a culinary spice. Saffron contains carbohydrates, minerals, vitamins, carotenes, and flavonoids (Winterhalter and Straubinger 2000). According to Caballero-Ortega et al. (2007), *trans*-crocin 4 is the most abundant ingredient in commercial saffron, followed by *trans*-crocin 3 and *cis*-crocin 4. There is evidence that the bioactive ingredients of saffron, such as crocetin, safranal, picrocrocin, and crocins, may possess antihyperglycemic effects (Bathaie and Mousavi 2010). For example, investigations have shown that crocins inhibit different types of tumor cell growth (Abdullaev 1993, 2002), which could suggest that saffron with a high concentration of carotenoid may be a source for antitumor agents. Bajerska et al. (2013) studied the characteristics of sourdough rye breads with addition of saffron extract (containing 2% safranal) 0.08–0.16%. Both the TPC and antioxidant activity measured by FRAP assay of the experimental breads increased gradually and significantly with increasing saffron extract level: TPC rose from 2.2 to 2.6 mg CE/g DM, and FRAP assay from 5.5–0.12 to 9.3–0.31 mg of Fe^{II}/g DM for the control and the enriched bread with 0.16% saffron extract breads, respectively. The addition of saffron extract worsened the color of all the breads, and in sourdough rye bread led to a significant darkness in the bread crumb. Moreover, the results indicate that the yellowness varied significantly and proportionally to the amount of saffron extract added. The decreases in bread volumes were observed only for the samples with the highest enhancement. The control bread had the best odor in terms of the typical aroma of freshly baked breads, and the addition of 0.16% saffron extract to the bread formula significantly decreased this aroma. That bread was characterized by unpleasant astringent and phenolic tastes and flavors. The authors thus concluded that a dose of 0.12% could be maximally included in the bread formula in order to avoid altering consumer acceptability.

Grape seeds are a rich source of PCs. Tannins in grape seeds tend to be in monomeric form, rather than polymerized. The seed tannins mainly consist of epicatechin units, along with smaller amounts of catechin, epicatechin gallate, and epigallocatechin. According to Souquet et al. (2000), the levels of gallates in the seeds are about 30% higher than those in the skin and stems. Moreover, procyanidin B1, B2, quercetin 3-glucuronide, astilbin, gallic and caftaric acids have been also detected (Guendez et al. 2005). Peng et al. (2010) have used commercial grape seed extract containing 95% proanthocyanidins at 0.09%, 0.17%, and 0.29% as functional ingredients. They also evaluated the antioxidant activity, antiglycation, and physical properties of new breads. Their results show that the antioxidant activity of bread increases proportionally with the amount of extract added. However, the breadmaking process reduced the extract's antioxidant capacity by about 30–40%. Heat treatment of foods is a key operation in the industry, resulting in the development of a large range of flavors and tastes through Maillard reactions. Nevertheless, through the Schiff base and Amadori product, advanced MRPs called AGEs are also formed (Maillard 1912). Among the better known AGEs is N^ε-(carboxymethyl) lysine (CML), a biomarker associated with oxidative stress, atherosclerosis, and diabetes in humans (Nerlich and Schleicher 1999). Although the breadmaking process shows significant thermal degradation of extract, there is excellent inhibition of CML. Adding 0.17%

and 0.29% grape seed extract to bread leads to over 30% and 50% reduction in crust CML content, respectively. Despite the changes in color, which were accepted by about 70% of the panelists, the sensory properties did not show differences with the control bread. Moreover, the authors did not find differences in the hardness of bread samples with and without the addition of extract.

Two types of buckwheat are used around the world: common buckwheat (*Fagopyrum esculentum*) and Tartary buckwheat (*Fagopyrum tataricum*). Tartary buckwheat has the disadvantages of bitter taste, small seed size, and tight seed coat that make dehulling difficult. Although common buckwheat has a sweeter taste, larger seed size, and easier dehulling, it contains less rutin in the seed than does Tartary buckwheat (Jiang et al. 2007). The green parts of buckwheat, used as a vegetable, are abundant in rutin, 3-flavonols, phenolic acids, and their derivatives. Gawlik-Dziki et al. (2009) examined the antioxidant activity and physical properties of functional bread enriched with 2.5% and 5% extract from the green parts of Tartary buckwheat. The prepared bread samples were also subjected to *in vitro* digestion with simulated saliva, gastric, and intestinal fluids. Increasing the buckwheat extract in the blends to 5% significantly increased the TPC (0.62–0.90 mg GAE/mL), total flavonoids (0.21–0.46 mg QE/mL), and total phenolic acids (0.31–1.51 µg CAE/mL), compared to the control (for the samples after digestion with the simulated intestinal juice). The free radical scavenging activity, measured by DPPH˙ assay, increased with the increasing level of buckwheat extract and in the progress of the *in vitro* digestion. The reducing and chelating power also increased with increasing level of extract, and the highest values were observed after simulated gastric digestion (reducing power) and after simulated intestinal digestion (chelating power). Additionally, the results showed that the higher the buckwheat extract, the lower the volume of the bread. Crust and crumb color of the enriched bread was darker, while its taste and smell had less aromatic compounds. Therefore, the 2.5% extract was the best level for achieving optimum taste, smell, elasticity, and the appropriate volume of bread.

7. Conclusions

There is no doubt that cereal-based functional products constitute some of the most promising and dynamically developing segments of the food industry. In today's world, the development and utilization of new functional breads is a challenging task. The results here have shown that the addition of functional ingredients, including DF and PC rich ingredients, to breads not only enhances their nutritional value and antioxidant status, but also affects the rheological, physical, and sensory properties of baked products. Thus, for successful product development, attention should be paid both to consumer demands and technological process conditions. The invention of newer breadmaking technologies aimed at improving nutritional value vis-à-vis the acceptability of the new functional breads will be the focal area in the near future. The stability of bioactive components during the baking process should also be taken into consideration to ensure their optimum retention in new products. Commercialization of functional ingredients should also be pursued. Further studies are needed to determine the optimal method (for example, encapsulation) of improving the stability and bioavailability of active components in the food matrices. Moreover, there are the challenges of more deeply investigating the interaction mechanisms of functional ingredients within breads constituents, and thus of improving their nutritional values and safety in potential industrial applications.

Keywords: Acceptability, by-products, functional foods, phytochemicals, plant extracts, pseudocereals, stability

References

Abdullaev, F.I. 1993. Biological effects of saffron. BioFactors, 4: 83–86.

Abdullaev, F.I. 2002. Cancer chemopreventive and tumoricidal properties of saffron (*Crocus sativus* L.). Exp. Biol. Med., 227: 20–25.

Ajila, C.M., K. Leelavathi and U.J.S. Prasada Rao. 2008. Improvement of dietary fiber content and antioxidant properties in soft dough biscuits with the incorporation of mango peel powder. J. Cereal Sci., 48: 319–326.

Alvarez-Jubete, L., E.K. Arendt and E. Gallagher. 2009. Nutritive value and chemical composition of pseudocereals as gluten-free ingredients. Int. J. Food Sci. Nutr., 60 (Suppl. 4): 240–257.

Anil, M. 2007. Using of hazelnut testa as a source of dietary fiber in breadmaking. J. Food Eng., 80: 61–67.

Artz, W.E., C.C. Warren and R. Villota. 1990. Twin screw extrusion modification of corn fiber. J. Food Sci., 55: 746–754.

Ayo, J.A. 2001. The effect of amaranth grain flour on the quality of bread. Int. J. Food Properties, 4: 341–351.

Bajerska, J., S. Mildner-Szkudlarz, J. Jeszka and A. Szwengiel. 2010. Catechin stability, antioxidant properties and sensory profiles of rye breads fortified with green tea extracts. J. Food Nutr. Res., 49: 104–111.

Bajerska, J., S. Mildner-Szkudlarz, T. Podgórski and E. Oszmatek-Pruszyńska. 2013. Saffron (*Crocus sativus* L.) powder as an ingredient of rye bread: an anti-diabetic evaluation. J. Med. Food, 16: 847–856.

Bathaie, S.Z. and S.Z. Mousavi. 2010. New applications and mechanisms of action of saffron and its important ingredients. Critical Rev. Food Sci. Nutr., 50: 761–786.

Bodroža-Solarov, M., B.E.V. Filipč, Z. Kevrešan, A. Mandić and O. Šimurina. 2008. Quality of bread supplemented with popped Amaranthus cruentus grain. J. Food Process Eng., 31: 602–618.

Brennan, C.S. and L.J. Cleary. 2007. Utilisation Glucagel_R in the [beta]-glucan enrichment of breads: a physicochemical and nutritional evaluation. Food Res. Int., 40: 291–296.

Bushuk, W. 1998. Interactions: the keys to cereal quality. Minnesota, U.S.A. American Association of Cereal Chemists, Inc.

Byrd, S.J. 2001. Using antioxidants to increase shelf life of food products. Cereal Foods World, 46: 48–53.

Caballero-Ortega, H., R. Pereda-Miranda and F.I. Abdullaev. 2007. HPLC quantification of major active components from 11 different saffron (*Crocus sativus* L.) sources. Food Chem., 100: 1126–1131.

Cabrita, L., T. Fossen and Ø.M. Andersen. 2000. Colour and stability of the six common anthocyanins 3-glucosides in aqueous solutions. Food Chem., 68: 101–107.

Calderelli, V.A.S., D.T. Benassi, J.V. Visentainer and G. Matioli. 2010. Quinoa and flaxseed: potential ingredients in the production of bread with functional quality. Braz Archives Biol. Technol., 53: 981–986.

Camire, M.E. and S.I. Flint. 1991. Thermal processing effects on dietary fiber composition and hydration capacity in corn meal, oat meal, and potato peels. Cereal Chem., 68: 645–647.

Chen, H., G.L. Rubenthaler and E.G. Schanus. 1988. Effect of apple fiber and cellulose on the physical properties of wheat flour. J. Food Sci., 53: 304–305.

Chlopicka, J., P. Pasko, S. Gorinstein, A. Jedryas and P. Zagrodzki. 2012. Total phenolic and total flavonoid content, antioxidant activity and sensory evaluation of pseudocereal breads. LWT—Food Sci. Technol., 46: 548–555.

Collar, C., E. Santos and C.M. Rosell. 2007. Assessment of the rheological profile of fibre enriched bread doughs by response surface methodology. J. Food Eng., 78: 820–826.

Davidson, M.H. and A. McDdonald. 1998. Fibre: forms and functions. Nutr. Res., 18: 617–624.

Dhingra, S. and S. Jood. 2001. Organoleptic and nutritional evaluation of wheat breads supplemented with soybean and barley flour. Food Chem., 77: 479–488.

Dini, I., G.C. Tenore and A. Dini. 2004. Phenolic constituents of Kancolla seeds. Food Chem., 84: 163–168.

Eastwoood, M.A. 1973. Vegetable fibre: its physical properties. Proc. Nutr. Soc., 32: 137–143.

Escudero, N.L., M.L. de Arellano, J.M. Luco, M.S. Giménez and S.I. Mucciarelli. 2004. Comparison of the chemical composition and nutritional value of Amaranthus cruentus flour and its protein concentrate. Plant Foods Human Nutr., 59: 15–21.

Fletcher, R.J. 2004. Pseudocereals, overview. pp. 488–493. *In*: G. Wrigley, H. Corke and C.E. Walker (eds.). Encyclopedia of Grain Science Elsevier, Oxford.

Friedman, M. and H.S. Jürgens. 2000. Effect of pH on the stability of plant phenolic compounds. J. Agric. Food Chem., 48: 2101–2110.

Gawlik-Dziki, U., D. Dziki and B. Baraniak. 2009. The effect of simulated digestion *in vitro* on bioactivity of wheat bread with Tartary buckwheat flavones addition. LWT—Food Sci. Technol., 42: 137–143.

Guclu-Ustundag, O. and G. Mazza. 2007. Saponins: properties, applications and processing. Critical Rev. Food Sci. Nutr., 47: 231–258.

Guendez, R., S. Kallithraka, D.P. Makris and P. Kefalas. 2005. Determination of low molecular weight polyphenolic constituents in grape (*Vitis vinifera* sp.) seed extracts: Correlation with antiradical activity. Food Chem., 89: 1–9.

Gunathilake, K.D.P.P., C. Yalegama and A.A.N. Kumara. 2009. Use of coconut flour as a source of protein and dietary fibre in wheat bread. Asian J. Food Agro-Industry, 2: 382–391.

Haslam, E. 1989. Plant polyphenols. Practical polyphenolic. From structure to molecular recognition and physiological action. Cambridge University Press.

Holtekjølen, A.K., A.B. Bævre, M. Rødbotten, H. Berg and S.H. Knutsen. 2008. Antioxidant properties and sensory profiles of breads containing barley flour. Food Chem., 110: 414–421.

Hoye, C.J. and C.F. Ross. 2011. Total phenolic content, consumer acceptance, and instrumental analysis of bread made with grape seed flour. J. Food Sci., 76: 428–436.

Hozová, B., L. Kuniak, P. Moravčíková and A. Gajdošová. 2007. Determination of water-insoluble β-D-glucan in the whole-grain cereals and pseudocereals. Czech J. Food Sci., 25: 316–324.

Hrazdina, G. and A.J. Franzese. 1974. Oxidation products of acylated anthocyanins under acidic and neutral conditions. Phytochem., 13: 231–234.

Huang, H.H., K.C. Kwok and H.H. Liang. 2004. Effects of tea polyphenols on the activities of soybean trypsin inhibitors and trypsin. J. Agric. Food Chem., 84: 121–126.

Jayaprakasha, G.K., T. Selvi and K.K. Sakariah. 2003. Antibacterial and antioxidant activities of grape (*Vitis vinifera*) seed extracts. Food Res. Int., 36: 117–122.

Jiang, P., F. Burczynski, C. Campbell, G. Pierce, J.A. Austria and C.J. Briggs. 2007. Rutin and flavonoid contents in three buckwheat species *Fagopyrum esculentum, F. tataricum,* and *F. homotropicum* and their protective effects against lipid peroxidation. Food Res. Int., 40: 356–364.

Kalinova, J. and E. Dadakova. 2009. Rutin and total quercetin content in amaranth (*Amaranthus* spp.). Plant Foods Human Nutr., 64: 68–74.

Kallithraka, S., J. Bakker, M.N. Clifford and L. Vallis. 2001. Correlations between saliva protein composition and some T–I parameters of astringency. Food quality Pref., 12: 145–152.

Kalra, S. and S. Jood. 2000. Effect of dietary barley β-glucan on cholesterol and lipoprotein fractions in rats. J. Cereal Sci., 31: 141–145.

Karori, S.M., F.N. Wachira, J.K. Wanyoko and R.M. Ngure. 2007. Antioxidant capacity of different types of tea products. African J. Biotechnol., 6: 2287–2296.

Klimczak, I., M. Malecka and B. Pacholek. 2002. Antioxidant activity of ethanolic extracts of amaranth seeds. Nahrung/Food, 46: 184–186.

Kroll, J. and H.M. Rawel. 2001. Reactions of plant phenols with myoglobin: Influence of chemical structure of the phenolic compounds. J. Food Sci., 66: 48–58.

Labat, E., M.H. Morel and X. Rouau. 2000. Effect of lactase and ferulic acid on wheat flour dough. Cereal Chem., 77: 823–828.

Lafka, T.I., V. Sinanoglou and E.S. Lazos. 2007. On the extraction and antioxidant activity of phenolic compounds from winery waste. Food Chem., 104: 1206–1214.

Larner, J., L.C. Huang, C.F.W. Schwartz, A.S. Oswald, T.Y. Shen, M. Kinter, G. Tang and K. Zeller. 1988. Rat liver insulin mediator which simulates pyruvate dehydrogenase phosphatase contains galactosamine and D-chiro-ilnositol. Biochem. Biophys. Res. Com., 151: 1416–1426.

Lee, S.J., S.K. Choi and J.S. Seo. 2009. Grape skin improves antioxidant capacity in rats fed a high fat diet. Nutr. Res. Practice, 3: 279–285.

Leung, L.K., Y. Su, R. Chen, Z. Zhang, Y. Huang and Z.Y. Chen. 2001. Theaflavins in black tea and catechins in green tea are equally effective antioxidants. J. Nutr., 131: 2248–2251.

Lin, L., H. Liu, Y. Yu, S. Lin and J. Mau. 2009. Quality and antioxidant property of buckwheat enhanced wheat bread. Food Chem., 112: 987–991.

Lizarraga, D., M.P. Vinardell, V. Noé, J.H. van Delft, G. Alcarraz-Vizán, S.G. van Breda, Y. Staal, U.L. Günther, M.A. Reed, C.J. Ciudad, J.L. Torres and M. Cascante. 2011. A lyophilized red grape pomace containing proanthocyanidin-rich dietary fiber induces genetic and metabolic alterations in colon mucosa of female C57BL/6J mice1–3. J. Nutr., 141: 1597–1604.

Llobera, A. and J. Cañellas. 2008. Antioxidant activity and dietary fibre of Prensal Blanc white grape (*Vitis vinifera*) by-products. Int. J. Food Sci. Technol., 43: 1953–1959.

Llobera, A. and J. Cañellas. 2007. Dietary fibre content and antioxidant activity of Manto Negro red grape (*Vitis vinifera*): pomace and stem. Food Chem., 101: 659–666.

Lu, C., J. Xu, P. Zho, H. Ma, H. Tong, Y. Jin and S. Li. 1992. Clinical application and therapeutic effect of composite Tartary buckwheat flour on hyperglycemia and hyperlipidemia. pp. 20–26. *In*: R. Lin, M. Zhou, Y. Tao, J. Li and Z. Zhang (eds.). Proceedings of the 5th International Symposium on Buckwheat, Aug, 1992, Taiyuan, China. Agriculture Publishing House, Beijing, China, 458–464

Maillard, L.-C. 1912. Action des acides aminés sur les sucres. Formation des Mélanoidins par voieméthodique. Compt. Rend., 154: 66–68.

Martinez-Correa, H.A., D.C.A. Gomes, S.L. Kanehisa and F.A. Cabral. 2010. Measurements and thermodynamic modeling of the solubility of squalene in supercritical carbon dioxide. J. Food Eng., 96: 43–50.

Martirosyan, D.M., L.A. Miroshnichenko, S.N. Kulakova, A.V. Pogojeva and V.I. Zoloedov. 2007. Amaranth oil application for coronary heart disease and hypertension. Lipids Health Dis., 6: 1–12.

McMurrough, I. and T. Baert. 1994. Identification of proanthocyanidins in beer and their direct measurement with a dual electrode electrochemical detector. J. Inst. Brew., 100: 409–416.

Michalska, A., M. Amigo-Benavent, H. Zielinski and M.D. del Castillo. 2008. Effect of bread making on formation of Maillard reaction products contributing to the overall antioxidant activity of rye bread. J. Cereal Sci., 48: 123–132.

Mildner-Szkudlarz, S. and J. Bajerska. 2013. Protective effect of grape by-product-fortified breads against cholesterol/cholic acid diet-induced hypercholesterolaemia in rats. J. Sci. Food Agric., 93: 3271–3278.

Mildner-Szkudlarz, S., J. Bajerska, R. Zawirska-Wojtasiak and D. Górecka. 2013a. White grape pomace as a source of dietary fibre and polyphenols and its effect on physical and nutraceutical characteristics of wheat biscuits. J. Sci. Food Agric., 93: 389–395.

Mildner-Szkudlarz, S., R. Zawirska-Wojtasiak and M. Gośliński. 2010. Phenolic compounds from winemaking waste and its antioxidant activity towards oxidation of rapeseed oil. Int. J. Food Sci. Technol., 45: 2272–2280.

Mildner-Szkudlarz, S., R. Zawirska-Wojtasiak, W. Obuchowski and M. Gośliński. 2009. Evaluation of antioxidant activity of green tea extract and its effect on the biscuits lipid fraction oxidative stability. J. Food Sci., 74: S362–S370.

Mildner-Szkudlarz, S., R. Zawirska-Wojtasiak, A. Szwengiel and M. Pacyński. 2011. Use of grape by-product as a source of dietary fibre and phenolic compounds in sourdough mixed rye bread. Int. J. Food Sci. Technol., 46: 1485–1493.

Milic, B., S. Stojanovic, N. Vucureuic and M. Turcic. 1968. Chlorogenic and quinic acids in sunflower meal. J. Sci. Food Agric., 19: 108.

Nerlich, A.G. and E.D. Schleicher. 1999. Nℇ-(Carboxymethyl)lysine in atherosclerotic vascular lesions as a marker for local oxidative stress. Atherosclerosis (Shannon, Ireland), 144: 41–47.

Newman, C.W. and C.F. McGuire. 1985. Nutritional quality of barley. pp. 403–456. *In*: C.W. Newman and C.F. McGuire (eds.). Barley. American Society of Agronomy, Madison, WI.

Okada, K., Y. Negishi and S. Nagao. 1987. Factors affecting dough breakdown during overmixing. Cereal Chem., 64: 428–434.

Park, S.-H., T.-S. Park and Y.-S. Cha. 2008. Grape seed extract (*Vitis vinifera*) partially reverses high fat diet-induced obesity in C57BL/6J mice. Nutr. Res. Practice, 2: 227–233.

Parry, J.W., H. Li, J.-R. Liu, K. Zhou, L. Zhang and S. Ren. 2011. Antioxidant activity, antiproliferation of colon cancer cells, and chemical composition of grape pomace. Food Nutr. Sci., 2: 530–540.

Peng, X., J. Ma and K. Cheng. 2010. The effect of grape seed extract fortification on the antioxidant activity and quality attributes of bread. Food Chem., 119: 49–53.

Peterson, J., J. Druyer, S. Bhagwat, D. Haytowitz, J. Holden, A.L. Eldridge, G. Beecher and J. Ala-Desamni. 2005. Major flavonoids in dry tea. J. Food Comp. Anal., 18: 487–501.

Pizzale, L., R. Bortolomeazzi, S.U. Vichi, E. Uberegger and L.S. Conte. 2002. Antioxidant activity of sage (*Salvia offcinalis* and *S. fructicosa*) and oregano (*Origanum onites* and *O. indercedens*) extracts related to their phenolic compound content. J. Sci. Food Agric., 82: 1645–1651.

Pokorńy, J. 1991. Natural antioxidants for food use. Trends Food Sci. Technol., 9: 223–226.

Rice-Evans, C.A., N.J. Miller and G. Paganga. 1996. Structure antioxidant activity relationships of flavonoids and phenolic acids. Free Rad. Biol. Med., 20: 933–956.

Robichaud, J.L. and A.C. Noble. 1990. Astringency and bitterness of selected phenolics in wine. J. Sci. Food Agric., 53: 343–353.

Rohn, S., N. Buchner, G. Driemel, M. Rauser and L.W. Kroh. 2007. Thermal degradation of onion quercetin glucosides under roasting conditions. J. Agric. Food Chem., 55: 1568–1573.

Rupasinghe, H.P.V., L. Wang, G.M. Huber and N.L. Pitts. 2008. Effect of baking on dietary fibre and phenolics of muffins incorporated with apple skin powder. Food Chem., 107: 1217–1224.

Samotyja, U. and M. Małecka. 2007. Effects of blackcurrant seeds and rosemary extracts on oxidative stability of bulk and emulsified lipid substrates. Food Chem., 104: 317–323.

Scharbert, S. and T. Hofmann. 2005. Molecular definition of black tea taste by means of quantitative studies, taste reconstitution, and omission experiments. J. Agric. Food Chem., 53: 5337–5384.

Seeram, N.P., L.D. Bourquin and M.G. Nair. 2001. Degradation products of cyaniding glycosides from tart cherries and their bioactivities. J. Agric. Food Chem., 49: 4924–4929.

Sharma, A. and W. Zhou. 2011. A stability study of green tea catechins during the biscuit making process. Food Chem., 126: 568–573.

Simopoulos, A.P. 2001. Evolutionary aspects of diet, the omega-6/omega-3 ratio and genetic variation: nutritional implications for chronic diseases. Biomed. Pharmacotherapy, 60: 502–507.

Sindhuja, A., M.L. Sudha and A. Rahim. 2005. Effect of incorporation of amaranth flour on the quality of cookies. Eur. Food Res. Technol., 221: 597–601.

Siró, I., E. Kápolna, B. Kápolna and A. Lugasi. 2008. Functional food. Product development, marketing and consumer acceptance—a review. Appetite, 51: 456–467.

Sobczyk, M., T. Haber and K. Witkowska. 2010. The influence of an addition of oat flakes on the quality of dough and wheat bread. Acta. Agrophysica., 16: 423–433.

Souquet, J.-M., B. Labarbe, C. Le Guernevé, V. Cheynier and M. Moutounet. 2000. Phenolic composition of grape stems. J. Agric. Food Chem., 48: 1076–1080.

Sudha, M.L., R. Vetrimani and K. Leelavathi. 2007. Influence of fibre from different cereals on the rheological characteristics of wheat flour dough and on biscuit quality. Food Chem., 100: 1365–1370.

Sun, T. and C.-T. Ho. 2005. Antioxidant activity of buckwheat extracts. Food Chem., 90: 743–749.

Thebaudin, J.Y., A.C. Lefebvre, M. Harrington and C.M. Bourgeois. 1997. Dietary fibres: nutritional and technological interest. Trends Food Sci. Technol., 8: 41–48.

Tian, Q., D. Li and B.S. Patil. 2002. Identification and determination of flavonoids in buckwheat (*Fagopyrum esculentum* Moench, Polygonaceae) by high performance liquid chromatography with electrospray ionization mass spectrometry and photodiode array ultraviolet detection. Phytochem. Anal., 13: 251–256.

Trinidad, T.P., A.C. Mallillin, D.H. Valdez, A.S. Loyola, F.C. Askali-Mercado, J.C. Castillo, R.R. Encabo, D.B. Masa, A.S. Maglaya and M.T. Chua. 2006. Dietary fiber from coconut flour: A functional food. Innovative Food Sci. Emerg. Technol., 7: 309–317.

Turchetti, P., P. Pinelli, P. Buzzinin, A. Romani, D. Heimler, F. Franconi and A. Martini. 2005. *In vitro* antimycotic activity of some plant extracts towards yeast and yeast-like strains. Phytotherapy Res., 19: 44–49.

Vernaza, M.G., M.A. Gularte and Y.K. Chang. 2011. Addition of green banana flour to instant noodles: rheological and technological properties. Ciênc Agrotecnol Lavras, 35: 1157–1165.

von Elbe, J.H. and E.L. Attoe. 1985. Oxygen involvement in betanine degradation—Measurement of active oxygen species and oxidation reduction potentials. Food Chem., 16: 49–67.

Wang, J., C.M. Rosell and C. Benedito de Barber. 2002. Effect of the addition of different fibres on wheat dough performance and bread quality. Food Chem., 79: 221–226.

Wang, L., R.A. Miller and R.C. Hoseney. 1998. Effects of (1-3) (1-4)-β-D-glucans of wheat flour on breadmaking. Cereal Chem., 75: 629–633.

Wang, M.W., T. van Vliet and R.J. Hamer. 2004. How gluten properties are affected by pentosans. J. Cereal Sci., 39: 395–402.

Wang, R. and W. Zhou. 2004. Stability of tea catechins in the breadmaking process. J. Agric. Food Chem., 52: 8224–8229.

Wang, R., W. Zhou and M. Isabelle. 2007. Comparison study of the effect of green tea extract (GTE) on the quality of bread by instrumental analysis and sensory evaluation. Food Res. Int., 40: 470–479.

Winterhalter, P. and M. Straubinger. 2000. Saffron-renewed interest in an ancient spice. Food Rev. Int., 16: 39–59.

Yurttas, H.C., H.W. Schafer and J.J. Warthesen. 2000. Antioxidant activity of nontocopherol hazelnut (*Corylus* spp.) phenolics. J. Food Sci., 65: 276–280.

Zdunczyk, Z., M. Flis, H. Zielinski, M. Wroblewska, Z. Antoszkiewicz and J. Juskiewicz. 2006. *In vitro* antioxidant activities of barley, husked oat, naked oat, triticale, and buckwheat wastes and their influence on the growth and biomarkers of antioxidant status in rats. J. Agric. Food Chem., 54: 4168–4175.

Zhang, J. and S. Kashket. 1998. Inhibition of salivary amylase by black and green teas and their effects on the intraoral hydrolysis of starch. Caries Res., 32: 233–238.

6

Production of Selenium-enriched Breads and Their Nutritional and Nutraceutical Properties

Sergio O. Serna-Saldivar[1,a,*] and *Marco A. Lazo-Vélez*[1,b]

1. Introduction

Cereals, fish/shellfish, meat and dairy products are the main foods that provide dietary Se for the world population. These food items vary in their relevance as major contributors of total Se intake in different countries around the planet due to differences in consumer behavior and food convenience. For inhabitants of developing countries around the globe, cereals are undoubtedly the major source of Se because they provide most of the calories provided in the diet. The daily dietary consumption of Se depends mainly on its concentration in food and the amount of food consumed (Şlencu et al. 2012).

Cereal plants can effectively store Se in their caryopses, mainly in the form of SeM. However, the ambient especially in terms of soil fertility greatly affects concentration. According to Mehdi et al. (2013) Se concentration in wheat kernels greatly varies depending on the growing area. In deficient Se soils of Sweden and New Zealand kernels contain only 0.006 ppm whereas in some parts of Canada more than 3 ppm. The 500 times difference is mainly attributed to the amount and bioavailability of Se in the soil.

---

[1] CIDPRO. Centro de Biotecnología-FEMSA. Escuela de Ingeniería y Ciencias. Tecnológico de Monterrey. Av. Eugenio Garza Sada 2501 Sur, C.P. 64849, Monterrey, N.L. México.
[a] Head and Professor, CIDPRO.
[b] PhD Student
* Corresponding author: sserna@itesm.mx

Several investigations dealing with the contribution of food sources to the dietary daily Se intake in different countries around the world clearly demonstrate that cereals and their products, mainly bread and breakfast items, provide up to 50% of the daily consumption although these grains have relatively low Se concentrations (between 10 and 550 µg Se/kg) (Aras et al. 2001; Combs et al. 2011; Galinha et al. 2012; Javier et al. 2013). Among the extensive array of cereal-based foods, bread is still considered the main staple for most cultures around the globe. Lazo-Vélez et al. (2014) summarized the contribution of bread to the dietary intake of Se for people of selected countries around the world. For instance, bread is among the three top food groups that provide most of the dietary Se for the Australians, Spaniards, Turkish, Danish, Irish, New Zealanders, Egyptians, North Americans and Englishmen.

The production of Se-enriched breads can represent a new niche within the bakery market aimed towards health consensus people. The potential is good because health and wellness bakeries in North America and Western Europe experienced sales that surpassed US$74 billion in 2011 with an estimated yearly growth rate of approximately 3% from 2010. The Asian and Latin American markets have also experienced an important growth in sales of fortified/functional and high-fiber bakery items that grew between 11 and 15%. These bakeries are forecasted to grow at 3% of Compound Annual Growth Rate and should account for around 17% of the predicted total bakery sales in year 2015 whereas the future global bakery market is estimated in US$492 billion by 2016 (Euromonitor International 2012).

Selenium is obtained through the diet in both inorganic and organic forms, the organic moieties being the most bioactive. The main organic sources are SeM and SeC (Combs et al. 2011) which are homologous of methionine and cysteine correspondingly. By a large amount, SeM is considered the chief organic form in wheat flour and yeast-leavened bread (Hart et al. 2011).

Se is considered an essential mineral because it is required for the synthesis of glutathione peroxidase (GPx) and other related selenoproteins (Rayman 2012). The different sorts of GPx protects mammalian systems from oxidative stress, cancer and CVD (Beckett and Arthur 2005; Combs et al. 2011; Park et al. 2011; Rayman 2012; Şlencu et al. 2012).

The aim of this chapter is to review factors involved in the presence of Se species in bakery products as affected by agronomic practices, wheat dry-milling, sprouting, fermentation and other baking operation units. Emphasis is made to the production of breads enriched with inorganic and organic Se and their nutritional and health benefits and implications.

2. Human selenium consumption around the globe

According to Lazo-Vélez et al. (2014) yeast-leavened breads are the best sources of dietary Se for most of the world population. Bakery products are the most relevant for Europeans, Americans, Asians and North Africans (Choi et al. 2009; De M. Souza et al. 2013; Durán et al. 2013; Fairweather-Tait et al. 2011; Ferreira et al. 2002; Hussein and Bruggeman 1999; Lazo-Vélez et al. 2014; Navia et al. 2014; Pappa et al. 2006;

Waegeneers et al. 2013). Figure 1 depicts per capita bread selenium consumption for people living in different continents around the globe and the average Se content of bread produced in selected countries. Approximately 50 kg/yr of baked goods are still consumed for each individual in the planet. The breads clearly differ in Se content in different countries around the world. The USA bread contains about 230 µg/kg whereas breads produced in European countries with poor Se in the soil only 20 µg/kg.

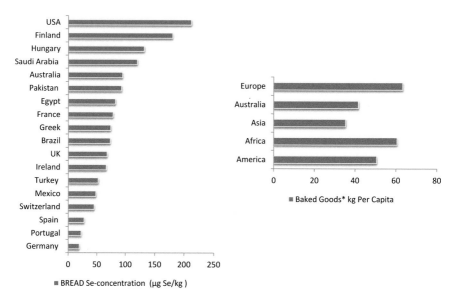

Figure 1. Per capita wheat and bread selenium consumption in selected countries around the globe. *The baked goods category includes bread, pastries and cakes. Wheat production in year 2012 according to the FAOSAT (FAO 2014); Baked goods consumed in 2013 by Euromonitor (2014); and Se concentration by several authors cited by Lazo-Vélez et al. (2014).

3. Selenium in foods with special emphasis in breads

Table 1 summarizes the average Se contents plus the standard deviations commonly assayed in the most popular animal and vegetable foods consumed by an average human being. The animal products like meats, shrimp, tuna fish and eggs are good sources of Se; however, their intake is inadequate in groups of people with limited purchasing power. On the other hand, the vegetable derived products usually contain lesser amounts of this trace mineral. Fruits and vegetables are practically devoid of Se whereas cereal and legume grains contain adequate amounts. However, yeast-leavened breads contain higher amounts due to the effectiveness of the fermenting media in transforming inorganic selenium into bioavailable organic forms. The different sorts of breads commonly contain from 0.2 to 0.4 mg Se/kg. Generally speaking, whole grain and fermented bakery products contain more Se compared to refined flour and

Table 1. Comparison of selenium concentration of breads with other animal and vegetable selected foods.

Animal food item	Se concentration (mg/kg)	Vegetable food item	Se concentration (mg/kg)
Whole milk, fluid	0.032 ± 0.006	Beans, refried	0.063 ± 0.017
Cheese, american	0.194 ± 0.052	Corn flakes	0.054 ± 0.023
Beef, ground pan cooked	0.228 ± 0.058	Corn, cooked hominy grits	0.018 ± 0.006
Ham, cured	0.336 ± 0.084	Bread, white enriched	0.212 ± 0.086
Pork sausage	0.268 ± 0.056	Bread, whole wheat	0.312 ± 0.081
Turkey breast, oven roasted	0.355 ± 0.103	Bread, rye	0.242 ± 0.044
Eggs boiled	0.333 ± 0.077	Bread, cracked wheat	0.300 ± 0.067
Beef steak, broiled	0.328 ± 0.087	Bagel	0.306 ± 0.079
Shrimp	0.026 ± 0.064	Muffin, plain	0.091 ± 0.023
Yogurt, plain	0.036 ± 0.008	Noodles, boiled	0.293 ± 0.102
Salmon fillet, baked	0.332 ± 0.056	Rice, white, cooked	0.064 ± 0.019
Tuna, canned in water	0.604 ± 0.081	Banana, raw	0.006 ± 0.014
Ice cream, regular, vanilla	0.033 ± 0.013	Tortilla, flour	0.249 ± 0.075

chemically-leavened counterparts. Food products derived from cereal grains still provide about 60% and 50% of the total caloric and protein consumption for an average world inhabitant (FAO 2014). The Se supply by cereal-based products in developing countries is more relevant. For instance for Eritreans and Burkina Faso people cereals provide more than 80% of the Se intake (Joy et al. 2013).

Most of the Se assayed in bakery products is contributed by the amount originally associated to the flour (Hart et al. 2011). Nevertheless, other sources of Se are generally incorporated during the bread making procedure such as the fermenting media (yeast or bacteria), and minerals associated to yeast food, salts and other ingredients such as eggs and milk products.

Production of high Se breads can be efficiently achieved using one or more strategies. The Se content can be controlled in the wheat kernel maturing in the field through the use of fertilizers containing Se or purposely adding inorganic selenium salts to the wheat flour at the conclusion of the milling process. The most effective way to achieve high levels of Se is through the use of sprouted wheat which was germinated with the presence of selenium salts or the direct use of selenized yeast or LAB or supplementing inorganic Se as part of the yeast food. Table 2 depicts different alternatives or strategies to produce breads with high levels of Se. The combination of two or more strategies can result in breads containing supranutritional levels of organic Se that is less toxic compared to the inorganic counterparts.

Table 2. Strategies to enhance selenium in wheat kernels, flours and yeast-leavened and sour breads.

Source	Dose tested	Grain (mg Se/kg)	Flour (mg Se/kg)	Suppl. (%)	Bread (dw) (mg Se/kg)	Reference
Plant growth in selenium-rich soils						
Wheat	Se-high soil	0.53	0.36–1.40	100	0.36–1.40	Garvin et al. (2011)
Wheat	Se-low soil	7.56	5.86–10.29	100	0.47–1.03	Garvin et al. (2011)
Wheat	High-Se/low-Se blended flour	–	–	–	1.2–3	Haug et al. (2007)
Selenium fertilization						
Wheat	10 g Se/ha (SeO$_4^{2-}$)		0.22–0.25 *	100	0.22 0.26 *	Hart et al. (2011)
Spring wheat	8 g Se/ha (SeO$_3^{2-}$)	0.25	0.17	100	0.18	Eurola et al. (1990)
Wheat	4, 20, 100 g Se/ha	0.4, 0.6, 1.2				Lyons et al. (2005)
Wheat	4, 20, 100 g Se/ha	0.15, 0.6, 2.1				Galinha et al. (2011)
Sprouting in presence of selenium						
Rye seedlings	10 mg Se/L (SeO$_3^{2-}$)		55.27	4	3.56	Bryszewska et al. (2005)
Yeast/Lactic acid bacteria fermentation						
Sponge dough	4.33 mg Se/kg flour (SeO$_3^{2-}$)				2.0	Lazo-Vélez et al. (2013)
Se-enriched yeast	5 mg Se/L (NaHSeO$_3$)			1.5	0.5 (as SeM)	Stabnikova et al. (2008)
Sourdough fermentation	Rye, Se-sprouts		485	2.5	0.3	Diowizka et al. (2014)

* Wholemeal bread

4. Selenium in wheat

The main factor affecting the amount of Se present in flours is the one present originally in wheat kernels followed by genotype. The Se assayed in wheat kernels varies according to the level of this mineral in the soil and the application of Se-containing fertilizers. According to Aro et al. (1998), the environmental conditions and the low pH and high iron content of the soil favor the deposition of reduced insoluble Se compounds (i.e., selenites and selenides) that are poorly available to plants. The Se form is important for bioavailability: selenate is less strongly adsorbed to minerals in the soil and more readily taken up by plants compared to selenite. Many factors such as dry climate, low organic matter concentration in the soil, high temperature, high pH and no water-logging may give a high ratio between selenate and selenite in the soil. Selenite, however, is the dominant form of inorganic Se in soils with high concentrations of organic matter, as in the Nordic European countries (because of low soil temperatures causing much slower degradation of soil organic matter than in tropical countries), and most likely also in waterlogged soils (Haug et al. 2007). Se is acquired by plants mainly in the form of selenate and selenite, and selenate is less toxic to plants than selenite (Lyons et al. 2005). The wheat plant absorbs Se from the soil and incorporates this mineral into proteins mainly in the form of SeM followed by SeC (Fig. 2). The pathway for the synthesis of SeM in plants and a large number of bacteria and yeast is greatly enhanced when methionine is deficient. In this case, SeM can replace methionine from 50 to 99% (Ouerdane and Mester 2008).

Barclay and MacPherson (1992) assayed Se of the 1989 harvest of bread wheats in Scotland and amounts ranged from 0.028 μg/g dry weight for home-grown wheat to 0.518 μg/g for Canadian import wheat, which constituted about 13.8% of the wheat used in bread.

According to Alfthan et al. (1991) and Eurola et al. (1990), the enrichment of fertilizers with Se has been effective to increase levels in wheat, rye and oat kernels and the amounts present in meat and milk of domestic animals fed forages grown in Se-fertilized soils. As a result of the proposed Se enriched fertilization program, the Finnish increased its mean dietary intake from 40 to 100 μg/d in 1987 with the improvement of Se plasma levels. Eurola et al. (1990) explain that in order to raise Se content of agricultural products in Finland, Se-enriched fertilizers have been applied since 1984. The intervention has been successful because Se contents of spring and winter wheats, rye and oats greatly improved. These investigators documented that spring wheats contained 20 to 30 fold increase in Se. Aro et al. (1998) documented that the Finland Se fertilization program initially included the addition of 16 mg/kg of sodium selenate to the fertilizers destined for grain production with the goal of increasing Se in grains by tenfold. Later on the level was reduced and adjusted to 6 to 8 mg/kg fertilizer.

5. Selenium in wheat flour

It is well known that the physical removal of the wheat anatomical parts for production of refined flours greatly affect chemical composition and functionality. Refined flours

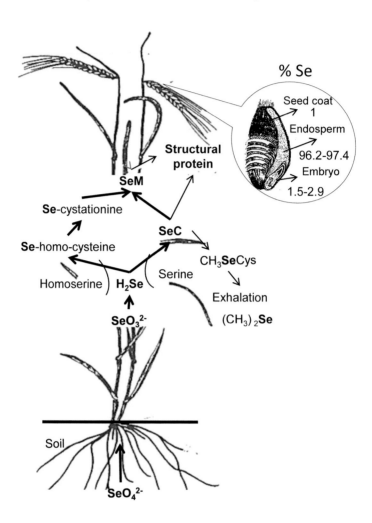

Figure 2. Transformation of selenium in the wheat plant and distribution of selenium in the wheat kernel. Adapted from Lyons et al. (2005), Rayman (2008) and Terry et al. (2000).

usually contain less protein, minerals, lipids and vitamins compared to the kernel. An excellent indicator of the flour extraction rate is the ash content because kernels with approximately 1.7% ash loose most minerals when milled into white flour that usually contains from 0.3 to 0.4% ash (Serna-Saldivar 2010). As a result, commercial refined wheat flours contain lower amounts of Se compared to the whole kernel. According to Moore et al. (2010) in wheat kernels, Se concentrates in the protein surrounding the starch granules in the starchy endosperm cells and more homogeneously in the aleurone cells. In an early research, Lorenz (1978) studied commercial flours milled from hard and soft wheats harvested from different states and provinces of the USA and Canada and concluded that the Se content ranged from 5 to 109 µg/100 g and from

2 to 13 µg/100 g, respectively. The refined flour contained about 50% Se compared to its respective wheat sample indicating that the bran and shorts rich in aleurone and germ tissues contained higher amounts compared to the starchy endosperm. Se content in hard wheat flour ranged from 3 to 78 µg/100 g and in soft wheat flours from 1 to 2 µg/100 g.

Likewise, Barclay and MacPherson (1986) determined that Se contents of various wheat flours used chiefly for bread production in the UK were significantly correlated with the flour protein content. More recently, Garvin et al. (2011) researched the fate of Se after dry milling of low and high-Se wheats and concluded that the amount of Se present in the original kernels and retained in refined flours was 71.2 and 66.4% for the low and high-Se wheats, respectively.

Hart et al. (2011) researched the retention and speciation of Se in flour after the experimental application of Se fertilizer to a wheat crop. The Se concentration of flour ranged from 30 ng/g in white flour and 35 ng/g in whole meal flour from untreated plots up to > 1800 ng/g in white and > 2200 ng/g in whole meal flour processed from grain treated with selenium fertilizer (as selenate) applied at the highest rate of 100 g/ Ha. Interestingly, the relationship between the quantity of Se applied to the crop and the amount of this mineral assayed in flour was approximately linear. SeM accounted for most of the total extractable Se species in enriched flours.

Se grain fortification, depending on wheat genotype, affected the pasting viscosity properties of wheat flour and the end-use quality of wheat (Gong et al. 2014). Studies of Garvin et al. (2011) with high-Se flours (> 5.8 µg Se/g) obtained through agronomic fortification schemes negatively affected farinograph dough stability and bread volume. The volume of the high-Se loaves was about 10% less compared to counterparts baked with patent-flours. However, the high-Se blended with low-Se wheat (0.36–1.40 µg Se/g) to a desired concentration yielded good quality breads. The same authors suggest that replacement of methionine residues with SeM in wheat proteins alter gluten and functional properties necessary for proper dough development and gas retention during fermentation.

Another strategy to increase Se in refined wheat flours is by the direct addition of sodium selenite along with the vitamin and mineral premix usually dosed during the last stage of the milling process. The strategy could be effective but processors need to carefully monitor the amounts of Se in the finished flour because inorganic Se can be toxic when overdosed and consumed at high levels.

6. Effect of sprouting on selenium concentration

There have been several research studies of the use of sprouted or germinated grains to produce Se-enriched flours and breads. Cereal grains such as wheat, rye and oats and legumes such as soybeans and common beans have the ability to assimilate and accumulate significant amounts of supplemented Se during the physiological event of germination (Bryszewska et al. 2005; Diowksz et al. 2000; Lintschinger et al. 2000; Liu and Gu 2009). Sugihara et al. (2004) germinated for 5 to 8 days in a Se rich media 28 plant species including *Triticum aestivum* and concluded that the wheat kernel assimilated between 68 and 98% of the originally supplemented Se. Chemical analysis of selenium showed that the main species in all the sprouts was *Se*-methylselenocysteine followed by SeM, non-metabolized selenite and γ-glutamyl-*Se*-methylselenocysteine. Lintschinger et al. (2000) confirmed that the biotransformation rate of Se in wheat sprouts germinated for 5 and 7 days in solutions containing selenate. Metabolism of the absorbed Se was analyzed by determination of Se species in extracts of the sprouts using anion exchange HPLC coupled to ICP-MS. Wheat assimilated and converted efficiently Se since the inorganic Se was less than 20% of the 1.2 mg Se/kg originally supplemented during germination. Wheat contained 100 mg of Se/kg of dry mass. The metabolism of the selenate was inversely related to the total uptake rates. At low and high Se enrichment less than 20% and 40 to 50% of the total Se content within the sprouts remained as inorganic. Diowksz et al. (2014) composited Se-enriched flour from sprouted wheat kernels with regular wheat flour for production of sourdough breads. The proposed enrichment increased the rate of fermentation and allowed the reduction of the fermentation time by 8 to 16 h. Sourdough breads elaborated with Se-fortified sprouted rye flour composited with wheat flour at a ratio of 1:25 increased concentration to 3.5 mg/kg bread. As expected, the major Se organic source was SeM (Bryszewska et al. 2005). Interestingly, the dosage of 2.5% did not deteriorate the sensory attributes of the enriched bread (Diowksz et al. 2014).

A problem related to the use of flour milled from sprouted kernels is its high enzymatic activity especially in terms of α- and β-amylases and proteases. In most bread formulations, the wheat flour is usually supplemented with diastatic malt (0.5 to 1.25%) in order to adjust the total diastatic power so to provide substrate for yeast and achieve better bread volume and crumb characteristics. However, for proper dough development, the level of α-amylase is critical. An excess enzyme activity fosters a sticky dough and low extensibility resulting in a sticky bread crumb containing undesirable large loci.

7. Selenium in breads

7.1 Effect of Se-enriched yeast and/or lactic acid bacteria

The most popular and easy way to produce Se-enriched leavened breads is by the use of yeast (*Saccharomyces cerevisiae*). The generation of high levels of SeM with yeast is often more used than other biological sources such as the utilization of high Se grains or LAB (Ponce de León et al. 2002). Yeast allows the efficient incorporation of inorganic Se and massive biosynthesis of related organic compounds (Nagodawithana and Gutmanis 1985; Ouerdane and Mester 2008). Miroshnychenko and Miroshychenko (2008) patented a process for preparing Se-enriched yeast containing high amounts of organically bound selenium (content between approximately 3,000 and 5,000 ppm). It was achieved by adding Se to the nutrient medium wherein formation of multiple enzyme-metal complexes was optimized. This media increased the maximum rate of the fermentation and boosted the concentration of organic selenium moieties. The invention also provided a means for the production of practically non-toxic selenium-enriched yeast products for use in foods, dietary supplements, or drugs. Esmaeili et al. (2012) also produced Se-enriched yeast by growing it in Se-rich media. The aim of their study was to determine the optimum conditions to maximize yeast Se levels. Fermentation was carried out at different temperatures (28–30°C), initial pH values (4.5–5.8), shaking speed (130–160 rpm), fermentation times (24–48 h), size of inoculums (30–60 g/L), Se concentration (15–25 µg/mL) and time of Se addition (0–9 h). Results showed total Se accumulation and organic Se formation which ranged from 107.9 to 287.6 mg/kg and 93.27 to 269.05 mg/kg, respectively. The most suitable conditions for total and organic Se incorporation in yeast were: addition of sodium selenite 25 µg/mL, at 9 h after inoculation, inoculums size of 30 g/L, temperature of 28°C, initial pH value of 5.8, shaking speed of 130 rpm and incubation time of 48 h.

Both yeast and LAB have biochemical pathways that promote organic selenium formation. Bakery yeast is capable of metabolizing up to 3000 µg Se/g converting approximately 90% of the Se into SeM; thus leaving only traces of the inorganic form (Schrauzer 2000). According to the biosynthetic pathways of sulfur amino acids in *Saccharomyces cerevisiae* Se is metabolized by first reducing $SeO_4^{2-} \rightarrow SeO_3^{2-}$ to adenosine-50-phosphoselenate (APSe) and then the SeO_3^{2-} to selenide (H_2Se) by a non-enzymatically process. This non-enzymatic reduction generates intermediate metabolites commonly known as glutathione-S-selenite ($GSSeO_2^{3-}$) and glutathione-conjugated selenide ($GSSe^-$) (Mehdi et al. 2013). The resulting H_2Se is subsequently converted to SeC from serine and this amino acid effectively incorporated to selenoproteins or further converted to the most popular and abundant form of SeM. Alternatively, homoserine can also be transformed into SeM (Schrauzer 2000). Interestingly, mammalian systems lack the ability to biosynthesize the essential amino acid methionine and SeM and therefore these amino acids should be acquired from the diet.

Similarly, it has been reported that various species of LAB used for production of sour breads convert efficiently inorganic Se into organic forms (Pophaly et al. 2014). Selenium accumulation in LAB was first reported by Calomme et al. (1995) and since then this property has been reported in strains of *Lactobacillus plantarum, Lactobacillus delbrueckii* subsp. *bulgaricus, Lactobacillus casei, Lactobacillus rhamnosus LB3, Lactobacillus fermentum LB7, Lactobacillus reuteri, Lactobacillus brevis, Lactobacillus sanfranciscensis* and *Lactobacillus buchneri*. Calomme et al. (2008) found a high correlation between the bacterial Se concentration and the levels of Se in the medium. The Se concentration in biomass was respectively 253 ± 50, 375 ± 33 and 407 ± 108 µg/g dry weight for *Lactobacillus delbrueckii* subsp. *bulgaricus, L. plantarum* and *L. casei* subsp. *casei* when 1 mg/L of Se was present in the medium. The characterization of the bacterial seleno compounds revealed that ^{75}Se was generally incorporated, as selenocysteine, into protein of *Lactobacillus delbrueckii* subsp. *bulgaricus.* Addition of L-cysteine to the medium decreased the bacterial Se content. It was concluded that *L. delbrueckii* subsp. *Bulgaricus* incorporated Se non-specifically into bacterial protein. The application of Se-enriched *lactobacillus* in Se supplementation would be an interesting approach since SeM is the major seleno compound in commercialized Se-yeast. Interestingly SeM was not detected in lactobacilli. The conversion rate is related to the type of fermenting microorganism and the length of fermentation. Bacteria such as *L. plantarum, L. sanfrancisco,* and *Lb. brevis* cultured with regular yeast stimulated growth and the accumulation of Se. Also, both kinds of microorganisms fermenting sprouted flours had been successfully used to produce high Se breads containing from 28 to 32 µg Se/100 g (Diowksz et al. 2000).

Pophaly et al. (2014) indicate that LAB are capable of delivering a number of nutritive, safe and more bioavailable Se compounds like SeC, SeM and methylated selenium species for mammalians. Selenium-enriched probiotics have been shown to confer several health benefits on the host for their antioxidative, antipathogenic, antimutagenic, anticarcinogenic and anti-inflammatory activities. The LAB, besides transforming inorganic Se to organic forms, concentrate this essential mineral in their biomass, which represents a detoxification mechanism against its toxic effects. Selenocysteine, one of the major products of transformation may further be incorporated into selenoproteins, although neither SeC insertion assembly nor any of the several known selenoproteins have yet been reported in LAB.

The retention and speciation of Se in bread was determined following experimental applications of Se fertilizers to a high-yielding wheat crop grown in the United Kingdom (Hart et al. 2011). Total Se was measured using ICP-MS and the profile of Se species in bread was determined using HPLC-ICP-MS. The relationship between the amount of Se applied to the crop and the amount present in bread was approximately linear, indicating minimal loss of Se during bread production. On average, application of Se at 10 g/ha increased total Se in white and wholemeal bread by 155 and 185 ng/g, respectively, equivalent to 6.4 and 7.1 µg Se per average slice of white and wholemeal bread, respectively. SeM accounted for 65–87% of total extractable Se species in bread. The rest of the Se moieties were SeC, Se-methylselenocysteine, selenite and selenate. This study clearly indicated that Se present in bread is highly related to the amount present in wheat kernels.

Selenized yeast cultures, which were grown in media cultures containing from 2 to 5 µg Se/mL, did not have any adverse effects in terms of fermentation quantified by the rate of CO_2 generation. Se-enriched breads produced from Se-enriched yeast had similar quality properties compared to the control. The only adjustment needed in order to produce equally quality breads was in the optimum dough proofing time which increased from 8 to 17% when using selenized yeast (Stabnikova et al. 2008).

7.2 Effect of dough fermentation

The supplementation of Se to yeast food increases the levels of organic Se assayed in the bread. Se-enriched yeast-leavened breads produced with sodium selenite (< 5 µg/g flour) added directly to sponge doughs fermented for 24 h contained higher levels of SeM compared to counterparts produced by the straight dough procedure (Lazo-Vélez et al. 2013). Baking tests demonstrated that Se supplementation did not affect rate of fermentation, the organoleptic properties of breads and the general baking production scheme. Two slices of Se-enriched bread can supply 200 µg SeM, the dose recommended to prevent cancer and oxidative stress. The physical features (water absorption, bread weight, bread volume, color, density, oven spring, etc.) and organoleptic evaluations for the enriched loaves were evaluated. In all these parameters, the experimental breads had practically identical attributes compared to the control. Thus, breads rich in SeM can be used as functional foods because this amino acid is effectively used to metabolize GPx, which protects mammalian systems against oxidative stress, most sorts of cancers and chronic diseases (Lazo-Vélez et al. 2013).

The addition of 0.5% more regular instant dry yeast (Lazo-Vélez et al. 2013) or 2% more sugar (Stabnikova et al. 2008) helped to counteract low bread volumes when using flours that contained less than 5 µg Se/g. In addition, it helped to offset the negative yeast activity effects due to the addition of the inorganic Se salts.

7.3 Effect of oxidation of selenium-species in bread making

Reduction to elemental Se associated to Na_2SeO_3 has been observed due to the acidity generated during dough fermentation and the presence of other reducing agents such as ascorbic acid. The reduced Se causes pink or red color formation. Colored dots are observed in microorganism culture, dough and bread crumb after baking (Diowksz et al. 2000; Lazo-Vélez et al. 2013; Stabnikova et al. 2008). This phenomenon has been observed in concentrations over 10 mg Se/L microorganism culture or 7 mg Se/kg flour used for baking purposes. SeM added directly to flour might be oxidized to methionine selenoxide and this reaction generally occurs during baking. Additionally, it has been shown that methionine selenoxide may be easily reduced back to SeM by glutathione (GSH). On the other hand, SeM found in biofortified or sprouted wheat may not be oxidized by the heat treatment because the SeM is forming part of the polypeptides of wheat proteins (Haug et al. 2007).

7.4 Utilization of selenium rich ingredients for production of specialty breads

An array of food ingredients rich in Se have been used for the production of specialty breads. There are different strategies to increase Se in breads through the addition of non-flour ingredients. For instance, the utilization of Se-enriched eggs or milk is feasible through the supplementation of this essential mineral to lying hens and dairy cows, respectively (Bennett and Cheng 2010; Cobo-Angel et al. 2014). Other possible approach is through the use of Se-enriched salt especially in areas where this mineral is deficient (Haug et al. 2007).

On the other hand, non-traditional ingredients with high Se contents have been proposed for the production of breads. Within this group is broccoli seed sprouts and powdered onion which contain high amounts of Se especially if the plants grew in soils fertilized with this trace mineral. These two sources have been proposed to produce nutraceutical breads with antioxidant and anticarcinogenic properties. Gawlik-Dziki et al. (2013, 2014) indicated that 2% substitution with broccoli seed or 3% with powdered onion skin significantly improved the nutritional and nutraceutical properties without affecting the sensory attributes of the breads. Zeng et al. (2006) concluded that the low molecular weight methylselenol is one of the most effective anticarcinogenic compounds and this metabolite is mainly found in broccoli. Therefore, broccoli-enriched breads can contain both SeM and methylselenol as protective agents.

Several species of fungi such as mushrooms have been also proposed as ingredients for bread making (Corey et al. 2009; Ulziijargal et al. 2013). These fungi have the capacity to accumulate Se when cultured along with a media high in this trace mineral (Milovanović et al. 2014). Corey et al. (2009) used Portobello (*Agaricus bisporus*) mushrooms that substituted 5, 10 or 20% of wheat flour with dehydrated mushroom flour. Results indicated that with higher replacement levels decreased bread volume and increased bread firmness. Interestingly, these fungi contain high protein and lysine contents so they are ideally suited to improve protein quality (Corey et al. 2009). Thus, *de novo* research is needed in order to determine these deleterious effects. These investigations open the opportunity to produce Se-enriched mushrooms and then use them as partial substitution of wheat flour for bread making. The high Se-mushrooms will additionally provide good quality protein rich in lysine, chromium and other essential trace minerals.

8. Nutritional and human health implications of selenium

8.1 Absorption, metabolism and bioavailability of selenium

Human dietary Se is acquired through the food chain by eating plants or processed foods such as breads (Fig. 3) (Haug et al. 2007; Rayman 2008). Table 1 depicts Se concentrations in common animal and plant foods. The post-absorptive metabolism of Se depends on whether it is consumed in organic or inorganic forms (Finley 2006). The inorganic selenite uptake is by simple diffusion whereas the organic SeM absorption occurs through the amino acid active transport system (Mehdi et al. 2013). Most investigators agree that SeM is more bioavailable than selenite although both forms are well absorbed in both the duodenum and caecum of the gastrointestinal tract (Mehdi et al. 2013). Furthermore, these two Se sources appear to provide different reserves in the organism. There are two main reserves of Se in the body. The first is known as exchangeable metabolic reserve, in this via Se is incorporated by reducing $SeO_4^{2-} \rightarrow SeO_3^{2-}$ and may be accessed by Se-amino acids (Fig. 3). The second major reserve consists of SeM (Daniels 1996) that is metabolized in similar manner than Met and it is also stored in body tissues. Se can be subsequently released by catabolism to maintain adequate levels (Fig. 3, EFSA 2009; Swanson et al. 1991).

Bread SeM is easily incorporated into body tissues (structural selenoproteins) or metabolized to other forms such as selenium hydride (H_2Se) by two key mechanisms: a trans-selenization of SeC followed by a reaction of β-lyase, or directly by a reaction of γ-lyase forming methylselenol (CH_3SeH) and a subsequent demethylation (Fig. 3) (Brozmanová et al. 2010; Ganther 1999; Rayman 2005).

In contrast, inorganic selenium can be excreted in the urine, and only small amounts incorporated into functional Se-proteins (selenoproteins) (Finley 2006). This is because selenoprotein expression is tightly regulated (Finley 2006) and animals, unlike plants, do not possess the ability to biosynthesize SeM (Schrauzer 2000). H_2Se is formed from Na_2SeO_3 by Se-digluthation pathway (GSSeSG) through thiol

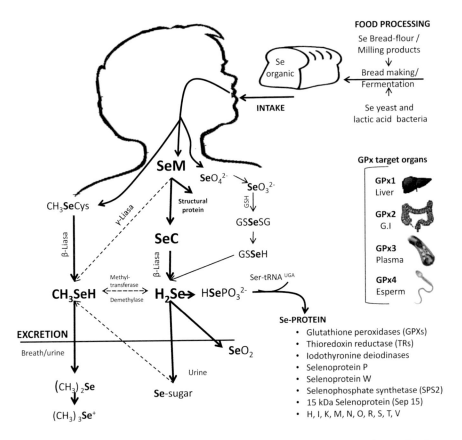

Figure 3. Human metabolic pathways of biologically important Se compounds yeast-leavened and sour breads. Adapted from Beckett and Arthur (2005), Brozmanová et al. (2010) and Rayman (2008).

reduction and NADPH dependent reductases. On the other hand, CH$_3$SeCys, which can be also supplied by bread (Cubadda et al. 2010; Hart et al. 2011; Şlencu et al. 2012), is converted via the action of β-lyase to CH$_3$SeH (Fig. 3) (Brozmanová et al. 2010; Ganther 1999; Rayman 2005).

The CH$_3$SeH is the key intermediate for the production of H$_2$Se, in selenized methylated compounds, the balance between H$_2$Se and CH$_3$SeH depends on methylation/demethylation activities. Methylation is a major route for the Se metabolism in microorganisms, plants and animals but the demethylation to inorganic Se can only occur in animals. H$_2$Se generated during metabolism of either organic or inorganic compounds is necessary to provide the source for biosynthesis of selenoproteins after the activation of Se-phosphate (HSeP$_3$O^{2-}) (Brozmanová et al. 2010; Ganther 1999; Rayman 2005). Also, CH$_3$SeH is an intermediate for methylated metabolites such as di-methyl-selenide [(CH$_3$)$_2$Se] and tri-methyl-selenide [(CH$_3$)$_3$Se$^+$], which are excreted by different ways. Likewise, compounds derived from H$_2$Se in the form of selenized proteins and Se-glycosides are excreted in the urine (Brozmanová et al. 2010) (Fig. 3).

8.2 Implications in nutrition

The deficiency of Se affects approximately 15% of the world population, which is attributed to the consumption of food crops with inherently low Se concentration (White and Broadley 2009). The lower limit of the safe range of dietary Se daily intake estimated by the WHO is 40 and 30 µg for men and women, respectively (Rayman 2004). These requirements were calculated from the dietary amounts needed to achieve two-thirds of the maximal GPx3 activity, assuming an interindividual variability of normal dietary Se intake of 16% (Allen et al. 2006; Levander 1997). The WHO (Allen et al. 2006) established RDA's of 10, 15 and 25 µg for children aged 1 to 3 years, 4 to 6 years or 7 to 10 years, respectively and 35 to 45 µg for adolescents aged 11 to 14 years or 15 to 17 years, respectively. The same organization established Se daily intakes of 55 µg for adults and geriatrics and 55 and 70 µg for pregnant and lactating women, respectively (EFSA 2009).

The Se levels and the GPx activity of whole blood and of erythrocytes, respectively, were determined in 139 normal Danes and related to sex and smoking habits (Clausen and Nielsen 1988). No differences were found in relation to sex apart from a higher GPx activity of females. Smokers showed significantly lower Se values compared to non-smokers counterparts, but the two groups had identical GPx activities. Individuals were divided into four experimental groups, receiving daily oral doses of 200 µg of Se for three months in the form of selenite, selenate, L-SeM or selenium contained in yeast. Both the inorganic Se compounds and the organic derivatives gave rise to steady state levels of GPx after one month of supplementation. However, the Se levels in the groups receiving organic Se showed a steady rise during the whole period, whereas those supplemented with inorganic Se leveled off after a period of one to three months. However, selenite gave rise to significantly higher Se levels and GPx activities in smokers than in non-smokers. By taking both the Se level and the GPx activity into consideration, organic Se (i.e., L-SeM) was concluded to be more bioavailable than the inorganic forms.

The basal requirement or Se needed to prevent signs of nutrient deficiency for adult males and females are 21 and 16 µg, respectively. These requirements were derived from the amount needed to protect against Keshan disease plus the body weight correction factor. On the other hand, daily doses lower than 11 µg lead to deficiency and health problems such as cardiomyopathies, Keshan disease and an increased vulnerability to free radicals or oxidative stress, associated to cancer initiation (Letavayová et al. 2006).

The Europeans are considered to have deficient Se intake although varies from country to country (Lener et al. 2013). A previous European nutritional and health report by Elmadfa et al. (2009) observed that the Se intake in children and teenagers was not within the recommendation in all participating countries except for Finnish females in whom the intake was slightly above the recommended daily intake range of 30 to 70 µg. This condition is due among other things to physicochemical factors associated to soils such as redox status, pH and soil microbiological activity that affect Se assimilation and concentration in plants/foods (Mehdi et al. 2013) which consequently lowers Se-serum levels in humans (Bryszewska et al. 2005; Haug et al. 2007).

According to Alfthan et al. (1991) and Aro et al. (1998) the average dietary Se intake in Finland increased from 40 to 100 µg/d in 1987 because of the addition in 1985 of Se to fertilizers. A Se-supplementation study was performed in 1987 on the same men as were followed in a 1981 study that had a similar design (200 µg Se/d) (Eurola et al. 1990). Selenite and selenate, but not selenium yeast increased platelet GPx activity by 30% compared with placebo. Selenium yeast and selenite increased plasma Se after 11 wk from 1.39 µmol/L to peak values of 2.15 and 1.58 µmol/L, respectively. Only yeast selenium was incorporated into red cells. From a regression plot based on present and literature data, it was estimated that the plasma Se concentration needed to achieve maximal platelet GPx activity was 1.25–1.45 µmol/L. At the present Se intake of 100 µg/d in Finland, GPx activity is saturated in plasma and erythrocytes and almost saturated in platelets (Alfthan et al. 1991).

The Se daily intake from bread in France, UK and other countries is narrow due to the poor quantities associated to this staple (Arnaud et al. 2007). Se intakes declined in several European countries during the past 30 years mainly because these countries are no longer importing high-Se wheat from North America (Adams et al. 2002; Allen et al. 2006; Hart et al. 2011; Támas et al. 2010). For example, a relationship between body Se status and Se levels in bread is considerable in the UK (Johnson et al. 2010). The daily amount of Se declined from > 60 µg in 1974 to 29 to 39 µg in 1997 and is currently estimated to be between 48 and 58 µg (Hart et al. 2011). Currently, the UK population obtains only 6 µg a day from bread (Broadley et al. 2009). In UK, bread and cereals were claimed to be the major source (43%) of dietary Se back in 1985 (Barclay and MacPherson 1992) and these staple only provided 13% of the dietary Se 17 years later (Adams et al. 2002). Likewise, Barclay and MacPherson (1992) concluded that the Scottish ingested 31 µg Se/d which is well below the recommended levels of 70 and 55 µg for adult males and females, respectively. The average GPx level in 478 samples of human wholeblood was 6.08 units/mL and this increased to 6.65 in 62 subjects consuming wholemeal bread.

Dietary Se deficiencies can be addressed through dietary diversification, food fortification, supplementation and/or by crop biofortification (White and Broadley 2009). Strategies for biofortification of wheat plants to produce Se-enriched flour have been the most researched. Among wheat products, bread making is the process that yields higher amounts of bioavailable Se. Breads and other bakery products have been proposed as the ideal vehicle for Se-supplementation programs (Stabnikova et al. 2008). Se-biofortification programs have been executed especially in countries containing Se-deficient soils like New Zealand, Finland and UK. Interestingly, the population of these countries has shown a significant positive effect in terms of improving Se status due to the consumption of products manufactured from Se-enriched wheat flour (Djujić et al. 2000; Lyons 2010; Poblaciones et al. 2014).

Notwithstanding, the response of the supplementation program is quite different in countries with low endogenous levels of Se in comparison to counterparts containing higher levels (Lener et al. 2013). It is necessary to carefully assess the risk of Se-supplementation although no toxic effects were observed when daily Se doses of 20–388 µg associated to wheat bread were provided to healthy males for six weeks (California Environmental Protection Agency 2010).

Se toxicosis, named Selenosis, induces DNA damage that occurs with daily doses between 3,200 and 5,000 µg (Brozmanová et al. 2010). Several recent studies have evidenced the potential adverse effects of Se supplementation with increased risk of developing type-2 diabetes mellitus and cardio-metabolic effects (Al-Othman et al. 2012; Rayman 2012). The daily intakes of up to 3.4 µg Se per $kg^{0.75}$ (plasma total Se level of 147 ng/mL) was associated with the risk of these chronic diseases (Combs et al. 2011). The effects may depend on genotype variations due to common polymorphisms in key genes controlling the synthesis of GPx, selenoprotein-P and thioredoxin reductase-1 (Wu et al. 2009). These adverse effects are observed mainly in individuals with adequate-to-high Se status and therefore the administration of Se supplements is contraindicated (Rayman 2012).

The Se levels in human subjects can be assessed by determining concentrations in whole blood or serum, hair, nails and urine. The Se status can be also determined by the selenoprotein-P and GPx activity in plasma and other blood compartments (Ashton et al. 2009; Djujić et al. 2000; Johnson et al. 2010; Fairweather-Tait et al. 2011). Al-Othman et al. (2012) reported an important collection of data comparing the mean Se concentration of blood serum in patients of several countries.

Human dietary intervention studies have demonstrated the potential of Se-enriched wheat and bread products to increase its biomarkers (Hart et al. 2011). Se intake (0.04 to 200 µg/g) in wheat/bread administered for several weeks (1 to 9 weeks) was highly bioavailable because it increased both blood Se and GPx levels (Belobrajdic and Bird 2013; Bryszewska et al. 2007; Gudmundsdottir et al. 2012; Hurst et al. 2013). The Se associated to bread has been particularly well retained by various body tissues (Hart et al. 2011; Thiry et al. 2012). Subjects consuming whole wheat bread containing high levels of Se increased blood GPx levels by 10% (Belobrajdic and Bird 2013; Thomson et al. 1985).

Bryszewska et al. (2007) investigated the potential of Se-enriched rye/wheat sourdough bread as a route for supplementing dietary selenium intakes. In addition to their regular diets, 24 female volunteers were fed daily for four weeks either Se-enriched bread or non-enriched bread (68.02 and 0.84 µg Se/d respectively). 42% of the Se was present as SeM. Plasma Se levels and platelet GPx activity were measured in the volunteers during six weeks. A highly significant difference was observed in the average plasma Se whereas platelet GPx activity was not significant. Two weeks after cessation of the intervention, the average Se plasma levels in the enriched group was still significantly elevated, suggesting that the absorbed Se had been incorporated into the body's reserves and was then being slowly released back into the blood.

Meltzer et al. (1992) investigated in 18 healthy Norwegians how the consumption of different doses of wheat Se affected serum levels. The experimental subjects were given Se-rich bread providing daily 100, 200 or 300 µg Se for six weeks. Serum Se increased significantly by 20, 37 and 53 µg/L in the three groups, respectively. The blood response and renal clearance results compared well with data obtained from less Se-replete populations, and support the hypothesis that dietary SeM was incorporated into a non-specific amino acid pool. This clinical study concluded that the intake of wheat Se was the main determinant of blood Se levels in Norwegians.

8.3 Role of selenium in human health

Low Se status has been associated with increased risk of mortality, poor immune function, and cognitive decline. On the other hand, higher Se status has proven antiviral effects, it is essential for successful male and female reproduction, and reduces the risk of autoimmune thyroid disease. Furthermore, prospective investigations have shown some benefits of higher Se status on the risk of prostate, lung, colorectal, and bladder cancers, but findings from other trials have been contradictory (Rayman 2012).

Se-deficiency (< 30 µg/d) is associated with various pathological conditions including increased oxidative stress, infertility, immune dysfunction, cognitive impairment, and increased risk for specific cancers such as prostate, colon, lung and others (Adams et al. 2002; Wu et al. 2009; Chen et al. 2013) as Keshan and Kashin-Beck diseases which are endemic to some regions of Asia (Şlencu et al. 2012). Worldwide, between 0.5 and 1 billion people have Se deficiency (Haug et al. 2007; Hu et al. 2014). Se-intake in the majority of countries is relatively low in comparison with the recommendation of the WHO of 50–70 µg/d (Allen et al. 2006). Worldwide, Se values ranges from 17 to 224 µg/d excluding the values corresponding to selenosis in Keshan areas (Şlencu et al. 2012).

Despite the many potential health benefits of Se, the mechanisms of action by which this mineral promotes better health are beginning to be elucidated. Se-supplementation can modify the genome stability by nutrient-nutrient and nutrient-gene interaction protecting against DNA damage events such as increase in DNA strand oxidation and telomere shortening (Fenech 2010). Another proposed mechanism is that the 20 known selenoproteins in mammals (Gladyshev and Kryukov 2001) exert health benefits. These proteins are divided into three groups: proteins into which Se is incorporated nonspecifically, specific Se-binding proteins, and proteins that contain this metal in the form of selenocysteine (Hatfield and Gladyshey 2002). In the last group, the relevant enzymes GPx and superoxide dismutase are included. These are considered the most relevant enzymes of the cell antioxidant defense system. Se incorporated as methylselenic acid might participate in cell cycle arrest, caspases/apoptosis, antiangiogenesis and other mechanisms for cancer prevention (Kong 2013). Additional information suggested that Se may have an important role in immune function, mammalian development and male reproduction, and in slowing the aging process (Hatfield and Gladyshev 2002; Rayman 2012). According to Pophaly et al. (2014) Se associated to LAB rich in SeC confers several health benefits on the host due to its antioxidative, antipathogenic, antimutagenic, anticarcinogenic and anti-inflammatory activities.

8.3.1 Prevention of aging and mortality

In at least three prospective studies, high Se status has been associated with low overall mortality (Rayman 2012). A non-linear association was noted between Se status and all-cause and cancer mortality in 13,887 adult participants followed up for up to 12 years in the US Third National Health and Nutrition Examination Survey

(Bleys et al. 2008). In the 9-year longitudinal Epidemiology of Vascular Aging study of 1389 elderly French individuals, low plasma Se at baselin, that averaged 87 µg/L, was associated with increased overall and cancer mortality (Akbaraly et al. 2005). Moreover, in the Baltimore Women's Health and Aging Study low serum Se was a significant independent predictor of all-cause five-year mortality in older women (Ray et al. 2006).

8.3.2 Role of selenium in the immune response and viral diseases

Selenium is known as an immune stimulant because it increases the proliferation of T cells, the cytotoxic lymphocyte and natural killer cell activity usually compromised in geriatric people and cancer patients (Rayman 2012). Selenoproteins are essential for activating T cell function, which are especially sensitive to oxidative stress. Broome et al. (2004) researched how Se supplementation (50 and 100 µg/d as sodium selenite) of UK patients challenged with an oral attenuated poliovirus affected Se plasma concentration and lymphocyte phospholipid and cytosolic GPx activities. Selenium supplements augmented the cellular immune response through an increased production of interferon gamma and other cytokines, an earlier peak T cell proliferation, and an increase in T helper cells. Selenium-supplemented subjects also showed more rapid clearance of the poliovirus recovered from feces. Wood et al. (2000) investigated selenium yeast supplementation (400 µg/d) of geriatric volunteers and found that the intervention increased total cell count by 27% mainly due to an increase of CD4[+] T cells and cytotoxicity of natural killer cells. Kiremidjian-Schumacker et al. (2000) conducted a clinical study of sodium selenite supplementation (200 µg/d) for eight weeks of patients with squamous head and neck carcinoma and concluded that supplementation significantly enhanced cell mediated immune response both during and after therapy. Se supplementation resulted in the ability of the patient's lymphocytes to respond to stimulation with mitogen to generate cytotoxic lymphocytes and to destroy tumor cells. The enhanced responsiveness was evident during therapy and following conclusion of therapy.

Selenium has great implications in functioning of the thyroid gland which possesses the highest Se concentration of all tissues (Rayman 2012). The main role of selenium in this gland is the synthesis of iodothyronine deiodinases which produce the active thyroid hormone triiodothyronine or T3. Selenium in the form of GPx3 protects thyroid cells from hydrogen peroxide and is related to prevention of thyroid tissue damage, cancer and goiter (Derumeaux et al. 2003; Glattre et al. 1989; Rayman 2012). Furthermore, several clinical studies have shown that supplementation of 80 to 200 µg/d as sodium selenite or SeM was effective against autoimmune thyroid disease (Nacamulli et al. 2010; Rayman 2012).

Low serum Se levels have been associated with decreased survival of HIV-infected patients (Rayman 2000, 2012). Two randomized clinical trials have shown that supplementation of 200 µg/d of Se benefits HIV-positive patients. Burbano et al. (2002) evaluated the impact of Se chemoprevention on hospitalizations in 186 HIV-infected individuals participating in a randomized, double-blind, placebo-controlled clinical trial during 1998–2000. Clinical evaluations were conducted every six months. Inpatient hospitalizations, hospitalization costs, and rates of hospitalization were determined two years before and during the trial. At enrollment, no significant differences in CD4 cell counts or viral burden were observed between the two study arms. Interestingly, the total number of hospitalizations declined from 157 before the trial to 103 during the two year study. A marked decrease in total admission rates (RR = 0.38; p = 0.002) and percent of hospitalizations due to infection for those receiving Se was observed. As a result, the cost for hospitalization decreased 58% in the Se supplemented group, compared to a 30% decrease in the placebo group. Authors concluded that Se supplementation appears to be a beneficial adjuvant treatment to decrease hospitalizations as well as the cost of caring for HIV-1-infected patients. In another trial with HIV-positive patients a higher plasma Se concentration decreased viral load even after adjustment of the antiretroviral therapy HIV disease stage and duration and hepatitis C co-infection.

8.3.3 Role of selenium on brain functioning

Selenium has been recognized as one of the most relevant nutraceuticals for brain functioning. Its deficiency causes irreversible brain damage. Selenoprotein-P has a special role in delivering Se to the brain by binding to a receptor. When this selenoprotein is not synthesized, mammalians including humans develop spontaneous seizures, lack of coordination, Parkinson's disease and cognitive decline. Thus, this selenoprotein has a relevant neuroprotective role enhancing neuronal survival (Rayman 2012). Human studies link the risk of Alzheimer disease and dementia to bodily Se levels (Rayman 2012).

Shahar et al. (2010) investigated the association between plasma Se concentrations and the presence of weak neurological signs related the *striato nigral* system. Plasma Se concentration was assessed in 1012 geriatric participants in the InCHIANTI study, a population-based cohort study in Tuscany, Italy. Investigators noted a significant trend towards increased prevalence of Parkinson's disease in the lower Se quartiles. Furthermore, there were a strong association between plasma Se and timed performance-based assessments. Lower levels of Se were significantly associated with decreased performance in neurological tests of coordination.

8.3.4 Role of selenium in fertility and reproduction

Se deficiency impairs fertility and reproduction. Deficiency of this mineral and its selenoproteins such as GPx4 negatively affects spermatogenesis and fertility. Women who had first trimester or recurrent miscarriages or higher incidence of preterm babies contain significantly lower levels of Se. A low Se status, characterized by low plasma and toenail Se levels and placental GPx, is also linked to preeclampsia. Selenoproteins could counteract preeclampsia symptoms by reducing oxidative stress and inflammation and regulating the vascular tone (Rayman et al. 2011, 2012; Urisini et al. 1999).

8.3.5 Role of selenium in cardiovascular disease and cholesterolemia

Selenium has positive effects against CVD because of its antioxidant properties, inhibition of platelet aggregation and inflammation and lowering serum cholesterol levels (Rayman 2012). Meta-analysis human studies have shown a significant inverse association between Se status and risk of CVD particularly in individuals with low Se intake or status (Rayman 2012). Yeast selenium supplementation (100, 200 or 300 µg/d) of approximately 500 geriatric people with low Se status increased plasma Se levels and lowered both total and non-HDL cholesterol suggesting a potentially beneficial effect on CVD risk. According to Rayman (2012), the effectiveness of Se supplementation is related to Se status and erythrocyte GPx activity is an effective predictor of the risk of CVD.

8.3.6 Role of selenium in cancer prevention

The role of Se in cancer prevention has been demonstrated in numerous *in vitro* cellular models, a diversity of animal studies and in several clinical trials (Chen et al. 2013; Combs et al. 2011; Etminan et al. 2005; Lener et al. 2013; Peters and Takata 2008; Rayman 2009, 2012). However, controversy remains on the possible advantages and risks of selenium in cancer prevention. According to Lippman et al. (2009) the renowned SELECT human trial concluded that Se supplementation did not provide an eminent benefit. On the other hand, the daily intake of supranutritional levels of Se (200–300 µg/d) stimulated antioxidant protection mechanisms principally associated to GPx activity. These levels can reduce risk of colorectal, lung, bladder, liver, esophageal, gastric thyroid and prostate cancers. Combs et al. (2011) showed that the daily consumption of 1.2 µg Se per $kg^{0.75}$ (plasma total Se level of 106 ng/mL) safely reduced the risk of cancer.

Peters and Takata (2008) concluded after intervention and observational studies that Se possesses chemopreventive effects against prostate and colorectal cancers. Several cancer preventive mechanisms have been described and it is likely that Se acts through multiple pathways. In particular, the antioxidative and antiinflammatory effects mediated through activity of selenoenzymes. Wei et al. (2004) examined the relationship between baseline serum Se levels and the subsequent risk of death from esophageal and gastric cancers, heart disease and total death over 15 years in China. These authors found significant inverse associations between serum Se and death from esophageal and gastric cancers and trends toward inverse associations due to heart disease.

A study investigated the protective effects of yeast-leavened breads with supra-nutritional levels of dietary SeM using immune-suppressed mice (SCID CB.17) bearing human colorectal adenocarcinoma HT-29. The supra-nutritional levels of SeM synthesized by yeast during dough fermentation provided necessary amounts to assure a proper GPx activity and the protective effects against colon cancer comparable to the one provided by the SeM pure standard (Gutierrez 2011). However, other studies of Se-fortified wheat products are not so encouraging. Wu et al. (2009) observed that Se-biofortified wheat used for the elaboration of puffed wheat biscuits did not substantially modify the selected biomarkers of degenerative diseases and health status in healthy

South Australian males. Thus, in future studies it will be necessary to observe whether any specific genotypes react differently to Se biofortification.

The molecular mechanisms by which Se is considered as chemopreventive are not fully elucidated. However, it is known that the form and dosage of organic and inorganic Se forms are determinants of the biological and cancer preventive activities. The antioxidant protection of selenoproteins, the specific inhibition of tumor cell growth by Se metabolites, the modulation of cell cycle and apoptosis, and the effect on DNA repair have been proposed as the main mechanism of action by which Se is chemoprotective against various forms of cancer (Brozmanová 2010).

8.3.7 Se-enriched breads in human health prospects

There is an overwhelming evidence of the positive and health promoting effects of Se supplementation especially when serum levels are low. Therefore, the production and consumption of Se-enriched breads could be used as a vehicle to increase serum values that in turn will improve the general health of the average population. For example, the potential supplementation of Se in breads and other foods in Estonia and Poland, where epidemiological studies recommend raising blood Se levels (Lener et al. 2013), could be a strategy to reduce the risk of colorectal cancer. Moreover, Wada (2011) suggests that Se supplementation through regular foods has a great advantage over the oral administration especially in terms of safety. Se-supranutritional programs might help to combat diseases that have become endemic in many countries. These programs could be emulated in South African countries where HIV is endemic and particularly virulent in populations with low Se intakes (Otieno et al. 2014).

Vegetarian and lactovegetarian diets are based in foods low in Se and therefore people following these dietary regimes are more prone to develop deficiency (Adams et al. 2002; MacGrath et al. 2014; Navarro-Alarcon and Cabrera-Vique 2008; Şlencu et al. 2012). A UK dietary study, conducted in 2000, found that Se intakes of vegetarians were indeed lower than those of the general population (MAFF 2000). Thus, Se-enriched breads have a special significance in the diet of a predominantly vegetarian population. Likewise, Millan et al. (2012) found a positive correlation between plasma Se concentration and the level of physical activity. Therefore, people or athletes that practice intense physical activity will be benefited by the consumption of Se-enriched breads.

Public programs aimed to increase Se levels in regular and sourdough breads could be implemented in developing countries such as Brazil, Ecuador and Bolivia where cereals are the main energy source and the general population has low purchasing power and therefore low consumption of animal foods (Ferreira et al. 2002; Sempértegui et al. 2003). In these areas, Se deficiency is especially prevalent among children with protein and caloric deficiencies (Sempértegui et al. 2003). Therefore, Se-enrichment programs associated to traditional and popular cereal foods is a potentially powerful tool for the prevention of Se-deficiency and combating common diseases especially in countries where regular or sourdough breads are considered as the most affordable foods, such as Latin America, Europe and Arab countries.

Conclusions

Breads can serve as vehicles for Se supplementation. Se-enriched breads can be elaborated by several and easy strategies. The consumption of these bakery products may counterbalance deficiencies in blood Se levels especially in countries with poor Se content in soil or in those that have deficient consumption of animal products. Public programs may be carried out in countries with high risk of Se-deficiency, cancer, other oxidative stress diseases and VIH. On the other hand, Se-enriched baked goods can increase further their nutraceutical value adding high quality proteins, dietary fibers, vitamins and minerals (Ca, Fe, Zn), β-glucans and DHA/EPA. Finally, more research is needed to determine the effects of selenized flours in terms of baking properties and product characteristics especially in terms of organoleptic properties.

Acknowledgements

Authors would like to express their sincere gratitude to the Nutrigenomic Research Chair of Tecnologico de Monterrey for funding research activities throughout the years.

Keywords: Bread, bread making, cancer, cardiovascular disease, flour, HIV, immune response, inflammation, lactic acid bacteria, oxidative stress, selenium, selenoproteins, sourdough, wheat, yeast

Abbreviations

APSe	:	adenosine 50-phosphoselenate
CVD	:	cardiovascular diseases
FDA	:	U.S. Food and Drug Administration
GPx	:	glutathione peroxidase
HIV	:	human immunodeficiency virus
HPLC	:	high performance liquid chromatography
ICP-MS	:	inductively coupled plasma mass spectrometry
LAB	:	*lactic acid bacteria*
RDA	:	recommended daily allowance
Se	:	selenium
SeC	:	selenocysteine
SeM	:	selenomethionine
WHO	:	World Health Organization of the United Nations

References

Adams, M.L., E. Lombi, F.-J. Zhao and S.P. McGrath. 2002. Evidence of low selenium concentrations in UK bread-making wheat grain. Journal of the Science of Food and Agriculture, 82: 1160–1165.

Akbaraly, N.T., J. Arnaud, I. Hininger-Favier, V. Gourlet, A.M. Roussel and C. Berr. 2005. Selenium and mortality in the elderly: results from the EVA study. Clinical Chemistry, 51: 2117–2123.

Alfthan, G., A. Aro, H. Arvilommi and J.K. Huttunen. 1991. Selenium metabolism and platelet glutathione peroxidase activity in healthy Finnish men: effects of selenium yeast, selenite and selenate. American Journal of Clinical Nutrition, 53: 120–125.

Allen, L., B. Benoist, O. De Dary and R. Hurrell. 2006. WHO/FAO guidelines on food fortification with micronutrients. WHO Press, Geneva, Switzerland.

Al-Othman, A.M., Z.A. Al-Othman, G.E. El-Desoky, M. Aboul-Soud, M.A. Habila and J.P. Giesy. 2012. Daily intake of selenium and concentrations in blood of residents of Riyadh City, Saudi Arabia. Environmental Geochemistry and Health, 34: 417–431.

Aras, N.K., A. Nazli, W. Zhang and A. Chatt. 2001. Dietary intake of zinc and selenium in Turkey. Journal of Radioanalytical Nuclear Chemistry, 249: 33–37.

Arnaud, J., S. Bertrais, A.M. Roussel, N. Arnault, D. Ruffieux, A. Favier, S. Berthelin, C. Estaquio, P. Galan, S. Czernichow and S. Hercberg. 2007. Serum selenium determinants in French adults: the SU.VI.M.AX study. British Journal of Nutrition, 95: 313–320.

Aro, A., P. Ekholm, G. Alfthan and P. Varo. 1998. Effects of selenium supplementation of fertilizers on human nutrition and selenium status. pp. 81–97. *In*: W.T. Frankenberger and R.A. Engbert (eds.). Environmental Chemistry of Selenium. Marcel Dekker, New York.

Ashton, K., L. Hooper, L.J. Harvey, R. Hurst, A. Casgrain and S.J. Fariweather-Tait. 2009. Methods of assessment of selenium status in humans: a systematic review. American Journal of Clinical Nutrition, 89: 2025–2039.

Barclay, M.N.I. and A. Macpherson. 1986. Selenium content of wheat flour used in the UK. Journal of the Science of Food and Agriculture, 37(11): 1133–1138.

Barclay, M.N.I. and A. MacPherson. 1992. Selenium content of wheat for bread making in Scotland and the relationship between glutathione peroxidase (E.C. 1.11.1.9) levels in whole blood and bread consumption. British Journal of Nutrition, 68: 261–270.

Beckett, G.J. and J.R. Arthur. 2005. Selenium and endocrine systems. Journal of Endocrinology, 184: 455–465.

Belobrajdic, D.P. and A.R. Bird. 2013. The potential role of phytochemicals in wholegrain cereals for the prevention of type-2 diabetes. Nutrition Journal, 12: 62.

Bennett, D.C. and K.M. Cheng. 2010. Selenium enrichment of table eggs. Poultry Science, 89(10): 2166–2172.

Bleys, J., A. Navas-Acien and E. Guallar. 2008. Serum selenium levels and all-cause, cancer, and cardiovascular mortality among US adults. Archives Internal Medicine, 168: 404–410.

Brozmanová, J., D. Mániková, V. Vlcková and M. Chovanec. 2010. Selenium: a double edged sword for defense and offence in cancer. Archives of Toxicology, 84: 919–938.

Broadley, M., J. Alcock, J. Alford, P. Cartwright, I. Foot, S.J. Fairweather-Tait, D.J. Hart, R. Hurst, P. Knott, S.P. McGrath, M.C. Meacham, K. Norman, H. Mowat, P. Scott, J.L. Stroud, M. Tovey, M. Tucker, P.J. White, S.D. Young and F-J. Zhao. 2009. Selenium biofortification of high-yielding winter wheat (*Triticum aestivum* L.) by liquid or granular Se fertilisation. Plant Soil, 332: 5–18.

Broome, C.S., F. McArdle, J.A. Kyle, F. Andrews, N.M. Lowe, C.A. Hart, J.R. Arthur and M.J. Jackson. 2004. An increase in selenium intake improves immune function and poliovirus handling in adults with marginal selenium status. American Journal of Clinical Nutrition, 80: 154–162.

Bryszewska, M.A., W. Ambroziak, A. Diowksz, M.J. Baxter, N.J. Langford and D.J. Lewis. 2005. Changes in the chemical form of selenium observed during the manufacture of a selenium-enriched sourdough bread for use in a human nutrition study. Food Additives and Contaminants, 22: 135–140.

Bryszewska, M.A., W. Ambroziak, N.J. Langford, M.J. Baxter, A. Colyer and D.J. Lewis. 2007. The effect of consumption of selenium enriched rye/wheat sourdough bread on the body's selenium status. Plant Foods for Human Nutrition, 62: 121–126.

Burbano, X., M.J. Miguez-Burbano, K. McCollister, G. Zhang, A. Rodriguez, P. Ruiz, R. Lecusay and G. Shor-Posner. 2002. Impact of a selenium chemoprevention clinical trial on hospital admissions of HIV-infected participants. HIV Clinical Trials, 3: 483–491.

California Environmental Protection Agency. 2010. Pesticide and environmental toxicology branch. Office of Environmental Health Hazard Assessment, pp. 76–100.

Calomme, M.R., J. Hu, K. Van den Branden and D.A.Vanden Berghe. 1995. Seleno-lactobacillus. An organic selenium source. Biology Trace Element Research, 47: 379–383.

Calomme, M.R., K. Van den Branden and D.A. Vanden Berghe. 2008. Selenium and *Lactobacillus* species. Journal of Applied Bacteriology, 79(3): 331–340.

Chen, Y.-C., K. Prabhu and A. Mastro. 2013. Is selenium a potential treatment for cancer metastasis? Nutrients, 5(4): 1149–1168.

Choi, Y., J. Kim, H.-S. Lee, C. Kim, I.K. Hwang, H.K. Parka and C.H. Oh. 2009. Selenium content in representative Korean foods. Journal of Food Composition and Analysis, 22: 117–122.

Clausen, J. and S.A. Nielsen. 1988. Comparison of whole blood selenium values and erythrocyte glutathione peroxidase activities of normal individuals on supplementation with selenate, selenite, L-selenomethionine and high selenium yeast. Biology of Trace Elements Research, 15: 125–138.

Cobo-Angel, C., J. Wichtel and A. Ceballos-Marquez. 2014. Selenium in milk and human health. Animal Frontiers, 4(2): 38–43.

Combs, G., J. Watts, M. Jackson, L. Johnson, H. Zeng, A. Scheett, E. Uthus, L. Schomburg, A. Hoeg, C. Hoefig, C. Davis and J. Milner. 2011. Determinants of selenium status in healthy adults. Nutrition Journal, 10: 75.

Corey, M., R. Beelman and K. Seetharman. 2009. Potential for nutritional enrichment of whole-wheat bread with Portabella mushroom powder (*Agaricus bisporus* (J. Lge) Imbach, Agaricomycetideae). International Journal of Medicinal Mushrooms, 11(2): 157–166.

Cubadda, F., F. Aureli, S. Ciardullo, M. D'Amato, A. Raggi, R. Acharya, R.A.V. Reddy, and N.T. Prakash. 2010. Changes in selenium speciation associated with increasing tissue concentrations of selenium in wheat grain. Journal of Agriculture and Food Chemistry, 58: 2295–2301.

Daniels, L.A. 1996. Selenium metabolism and bioavailability. Biological Trace Element Research, 54: 185–189.

De M. Souza, A., R.A. Pereira, E.M. Yokoo, R.B. Levy and R. Sichieri. 2013. Alimentos mais consumidos no Brasil : inquérito nacional de alimentação 2008–2009 [Most consumed foods in Brazil : national dietary survey 2008–2009]. Revista de Saúde Pública, 47: 190–199.

Derumeaux, H., P. Valeix, K. Castetbon, M. Bensimon, M.C. Boutron-Ruault, J. Arnaud and S. Hercberg. 2003. Association of selenium with thyroid volume and echostructure in 35 to 60 year old French adults. European Journal of Endocrinology, 148: 309–315.

Diowksz, A., E. Kordialik-Bogacka and W. Ambroziak. 2014. Se-enriched sprouted seeds as functional additives in sourdough fermentation. LWT-Food Science and Technology, 56(2): 524–552.

Diowksz, A., B. Pęczkowska, M. Włodarczyk and W. Ambroziak. 2000. Bacteria/yeast and plant biomass enriched in Se via bioconversion process as a source of Se supplementation in food. Progress in Biotechnology, 17: 295–300.

Djujić, I.S., O.N. Jozanov-Stankov, M. Milovac, V. Janković and V. Djermanović. 2000. Bioavailability and possible benefits of wheat intake naturally enriched with selenium and its products. Biology Trace Element Research, 77: 273–285.

Durán, P., J.J. Acuña, M.A. Jorquera, R. Azcón, F. Borie, P. Cornejo and M.L. Mora. 2013. Enhanced selenium content in wheat grain by co-inoculation of selenobacteria and arbuscular mycorrhizal fungi: A preliminary study as a potential Se biofortification strategy. Journal of Cereal Science, 57: 275–280.

EFSA. 2009. Scientific opinion of the panel on food additives and nutrient sources added to food on L-selenomethionine as a source of selenium added for nutritional purposes to food supplements, following a request from the European Commission. The EFSA Journal, 1082: 1–38.

Elmadfa, I., A. Meyer, V. Nowak, V. Hasenegger, P. Putz, R. Verstraeten, A.M. Remaut-DeWinter, P. Kolsteren, J. Dostálová, P. Dlouhý, E. Trolle, S. Fagt, A. Biltoft-Jensen, J. Mathiessen, M. Velsing Groth, L. Kambek, N. Gluskova, S. Voutilainen, A. Erkkilä, M. Vernay, C. Krems, A. Strassburg, A.L. Vasquez-Caicedo, C. Urban, A. Naska, E. Efstathopoulou, E. Oikonomou, K. Tsiotas, V. Bountziouka, V., Benetou, A. Trichopoulou, G. Zajkás, V. Kovács, E. Martos, P. Heavey, C. Kelleher, J. Kennedy, A. Turrini, G. Selga, M. Sauka, J. Petkeviciene, J. Klumbiene, T. Holm Totland, L.F. Andersen, E. Halicka, K. Rejman, B. Kowrygo, S. Rodrigues, S. Pinhão, L.S. Ferreira, C. Lopes, E. Ramos, M.D. Vaz Almeida, M. Vlad, M. Simcic, K. Podgrajsek, L. Serra Majem, B. Román Viñas, J. Ngo, L. Ribas Barba, W. Becker, H. Fransen, B. Van Rossum, M. Ocké, B. Margetts, A. Rütten, K. Abu-Omar, P. Gelius and A. Cattaneo. 2009. European nutrition and health report 2009. Annals of Nutrition and Metabolism, 55(2): 1–40.

Esmaeili, S., K. Khosravi-Darani, R. Pourahmad and R. Komeili. 2012. An experimental design for production of selenium-enriched yeast. World Applied Sciences Journal, 19 (1): 31–37.

Etminan, M., J.M. FitzGerald, M. Gleave and K. Chambers. 2005. Intake of selenium in the prevention of prostate cancer: a systematic review and meta-analysis. Cancer Causes Control, 16: 1125–1131.

Eurola, M., P. Ekholm, M. Ylien, P. Koivistoinen and P. Varo. 1990. Effects of selenium fertilization on the selenium content of cereal grains, flour, and bread produced in Finland. Cereal Chemistry, 67: 334–337.

Euromonitor International. 2012. Conundrums in global bakery: a simultaneous quest for health and indulgence. Available in http://blog.euromonitor.com/2012/08/conun drums-in-global-bakery-a-simultaneous-quest-for-health-and-indulgence.html.

Euromonitor International. 2014. Related analysis of baked goods per capita, 2013. Passport GMID. Database.

Fairweather-Tait, S., Y. Bao, M.R. Broadley, R. Collings, D. Ford, J.E. Hesketh and R. Hurst. 2011. Selenium in human health and disease. Antioxidant Redox Signal, 14: 1337–1383.

FAO (Food and Agriculture Organization). 2014. Corporate Statistical Database. Rome, Italy. Electronic page: faostat.fao.org.

Fenech, M.F. 2010. Dietary reference values of individual micronutrients and nutriomes for genome damage prevention: current status and a road map to the future. American Journal of Clinical Nutrition, 91: 1438–1454.

Finley, J.W. 2006. Bioavailability of selenium from foods. Nutrition, 62(3): 146–151.

Ganther, H. 1999. Selenium metabolism, selenoproteins and mechanisms of cancer prevention: complexities with thioredoxin reductase. Carcinogenesis, 20(9): 1657–1666.

Galinha, C., M.C. Freitas, A. Pacheco, J. Coutinho, B. Maçãs and A.S. Almeida. 2012. Selenium supplementation of Portuguese wheat cultivars through foliar treatment in actual field conditions. Journal of Radioanalytical and Nuclear Chemistry, 297(2): 227–231.

Galinha, C., M.C. Freitas, M.G. Pacheco, J. Coutinho, B. Maçãs and A.S. Almeida. 2011. Determination of selenium in bread-wheat samples grown under a Se-supplementation regime in actual field conditions. Journal of Radioanalytical and Nuclear Chemistry, 291: 231–235.

Garvin, D.F., G. Hareland, B.R. Gregoire and J.W. Finley. 2011. Impact of wheat grain selenium content variation on milling and bread baking. Cereal Chemistry, 88: 195–200.

Gawlik-Dziki, U., M. Swieca, D. Dariusz, L. Swczyk, Z. Urszula, R. Rózylo, K. Kaszuba, D. Ryszawy and J. Czyz. 2014. Anticancer and Antioxidant Activity of Bread Enriched with Broccoli Sprouts. BioMed Research International, In Press.

Gawlik-Dziki, U., M. Świeca, D. Dziki, B. Baraniak, J. Tomiło and J. Czyz. 2013. Quality and antioxidant properties of breads enriched with dry onion (*Allium cepa* L.) skin. Food Chemistry, 138: 1621–1628.

Gladyshev, V.N. and G.V. Kryukov. 2001. Evolution of selenocysteine-containing proteins: significance of identification and functional characterization of selenoproteins. Biofactors, 14: 87–92.

Glattre, E., Y. Thomassen, S.O. Thoresen, T. Haldorsen, P.G. Lund-Larsen, L. Theodorsen and J. Aaseth. 1989. Prediagnostic serum selenium in a case-control study of thyroid cancer. International Journal of Epidemiology, 18: 45–49.

Gong, P., T. Li, A. Wang, F. Sun, S. Gu, X. Yin and W. Guan. 2014. Selenium biofortification and its effects on flour paste viscosity properties in wheat. pp. 55–61. *In*: G.S. Bañuelos, Z-Q. Lin and X. Yin (eds.). Selenium in the environment and human health. Taylor and Francis Group, London.

Gudmundsdottir, E., I. Gunnarsdottir, A. Thorlacius, O. Reykdal, H. Gunnlaugsdottir, I. Thorsdottir and L. Steingrimsdottir. 2012. Blood selenium levels and contribution of food groups to selenium intake in adolescent girls in Iceland. Food Nutrition Research, 56: 176–184.

Gutierrez, V.A. 2011. Evaluación *in vivo* del efecto quimiopreventivo en cancer de colon de SeMet biosintetizada por *S. cerevisiae* en pan. M., Tecnologico de Monterrey, Campus Monterrey, Monterrey, N.L., Mexico.

Hart, D.J., S.J. Fairweather-Tait, M.R. Broadley, S.J. Dickinson, I. Foot, P. Knott, S.P. McGrath, H. Mowat, K. Norman, P.R. Scott, J.L. Stroud, M. Tucker, P.J. White, F.J. Zhao and R. Hurst. 2011. Selenium concentration and speciation in biofortified flour and bread: Retention of selenium during grain biofortification, processing and production of Se-enriched food. Food Chemistry, 126: 1771–1778.

Hatfield, D.L. and V.N. Gladyshev. 2002. How selenium has altered our understanding of the genetic code. Molecular Cell Biology, 22(11): 3565–3576.

Haug, A., R.D. Graham, O.A. Christophersen and G.H. Lyons. 2007. How to use the world's scarce selenium resources efficiently to increase the selenium concentration in food. Microbial Ecology in Health and Disease, 19: 209–228.

Hu, J., Q. Zhao, X. Cheng, C. Selomulya, C. Bai, X. Zhu, X. Li and H. Xiong. 2014. Antioxidant activities of Se-SPI produced from soybean as accumulation and biotransformation reactor of natural selenium. Food Chemistry, 146: 531–537.

Hurst, R., E. Siyame, S. Young, A. Chilimba, E. Joy, C. Black, E.L. Ander, M.J. Watts, B. Chilima, J. Gondwe, D. Kang'ombe, A. Stein, S. Fairweather-Tait, R. Gibson, A. Kalimbira and M.R. Broadley.

2013. Soil-type influences human selenium status and underlies widespread selenium deficiency risks in Malawi. Scientific Reports, 3: 1425.

Hussein, L. and J. Bruggeman. 1999. Selenium analysis of selected Egyptian foods and estimated daily intakes among a population group. Food Chemistry, 65: 527–532.

Javier, F., L. Garrido and L. López. 2013. Selenio y salud; valores de referencia y situación actual de la población española. Nutrición Hospitalaria, 28: 1396–1406.

Johnson, C.C., F.M. Fordyce and M.P. Rayman. 2010. Symposium on "Geographical and geological influences on nutrition": Factors controlling the distribution of selenium in the environment and their impact on health and nutrition. Proceedings Nutrition Society Journal, 69: 119–132.

Joy, E., E.L. Ander, S.D. Young, C.R. Black, M.J. Watts, A.D.C. Chilimba, B. Chilima, E.W. Siyame, A.A. Kalimbira, R. Hurst, S.J. Fairweather-Tait, A.J. Stein, R.S. Gibson, P.J. White and M.R. Broadley. 2013. Dietary mineral supplies in Africa. Physiologia Plantarum, 151(3): 208–229.

Kiremidjian-Schumacker, L., M. Roy, R. Glickman, K. Schneider, S. Rothstein, J. Cooper, H. Hochster, M. Kim and R. Newman. 2000. Selenium and immunocompetence in patients with head and neck cancer. Biology Trace Element Research, 73: 97–111.

Kong, A.T. 2013. Inflammation, oxidative stress, and cancer: dietary approaches for cancer prevention. CRC Press, Taylor & Francis Group, Boca Raton, FL, pp. 477–479.

Lazo-Vélez, M., V. Gutiérrez-Díaz, A. Ramírez-Medrano and S.O. Serna-Saldívar. 2013. Effect of sodium selenite addition and sponge dough fermentation on selenomethionine generation during production of yeast-leavened breads. Journal of Cereal Science, 58: 164–169.

Lazo-Vélez, M., A. Chavez-Santoscoy and S.O. Serna-Saldívar. 2014. Selenium-enriched breads and their benefits in human nutrition and health as affected by agronomic, milling and baking factors. Cereal Chemistry, http://dx.doi.org/10.1094/CCHEM-05-14-0110-RW.

Lener, M.R., S. Gupta, R.J. Scott, M. Tootsi, M. Kulp, M-L. Tammesoo, A. Viitak, A. Metspalu, P. Serrano-Fernández, J. Kładny, K. Jaworska-Bieniek, K. Durda, M. Muszyńska, G. Sukiennicki, A. Jakubowska and J. Lubiński. 2013. Can selenium levels act as a marker of colorectal cancer risk? BMC Cancer, 13: 214.

Letavayová, L., V. Vlcková and J. Brozmanová. 2006. Selenium: from cancer prevention to DNA damage. Toxicology, 227: 1–14.

Levander, O.A. 1997. Nutrition and newly emerging viral diseases: an overview. Journal of Nutrition, 127(suppl.): 948S–950S.

Lintschinger, J., N. Fuchs, J. Moser, D. Kuehnelt and W. Goessler. 2000. Selenium-enriched sprouts. A raw material for fortified cereal-based diets. Journal of Agriculture and Food Chemistry, 48: 5362–5368.

Lippman, S.M., E.A. Klein, P.J. Goodman, M.S. Lucia, I.M. Thompson, L. Ford, G. Parnes, H.L. Minasian, L.M. Gaziano, J.M. Hartline, J.A. Parsons, J.K. Bearden, J.D. Crawford 3rd, E.D. Goodman, G.E. Claudio, J. Winquist, E. Cook, E.D. Karp, D.D. Walther, P. Lieber, M.M. Kristal, A.R. Darke, A.K. Arnold, K.B. Ganz, P.A. Santella, R.M. Albanes, D. Taylor, P.R. Probstfield, J.L. Jagpal, T.J. Crowley, Jr., J.J. Meyskens F.L. Baker and L.H.C.A. Coltman Jr. 2009. Effect of selenium and vitamin E on risk of prostate cancer and other cancers: the Selenium and Vitamin E Cancer Prevention Trial (SELECT). The Journal of the American Medical Association, 301: 39–51.

Liu, K. and Z. Gu. 2009. Selenium accumulation in different brown rice cultivars and its distribution in fractions. Journal of Agriculture and Food Chemistry, 57: 695–700.

Lorenz, K. 1978. Selenium in wheats and commercial wheat flours. Cereal Chemistry, 55: 287–294.

Lyons, G.H., Y. Genc, J.C.R. Stangoulis, L.T. Palmer and R.D. Graham. 2005. Selenium distribution in wheat grain, and the effect of post-harvest processing on wheat selenium content. Biological Trace Element Research, 103: 155–168.

Lyons, G. 2010. Selenium in cereals: improving the efficiency of agronomic biofortification in the UK. Plant Soil, 332: 1–4.

MacGrath, S.P., M.J. Poblaciones and S.M. Rodrigo. 2014. Biofortification of field crops with selenium in Mediterranean conditions. pp. 55–61. *In*: G.S. Bañuelos, Z.-Q. Lin and X. Yin (eds.). Selenium in the environment and human health. Taylor and Francis Group, London.

Mehdi, Y., J.-L. Hornick, L. Istasse and I. Dufrasne. 2013. Selenium in the environment, metabolism and involvement in body functions. Molecules, 18: 3292–3311.

Meltzer, H.M., G. Noerheim, E. Bjorgeloken and H. Holm. 1992. Supplementation with wheat selenium induces a dose-dependent response in serum and urine of a Se-replete population. British Journal of Nutrition, 67: 287–294.

Millan, A., D. Florea, L. Sáenz, J. Molina, B. López-González, A. Pérez de la Cruz and E. Planells. 2012. Deficient selenium status of a healthy adult Spanish population. Nutrision Hospitalaria, 27(2): 524–528.

Milovanović, I., I. Brčeski, M. Stajić, A. Korać, J. Vukojević and A. KneDević. 2014. Potential of Pleurotus ostreatus mycelium for selenium absorption. TSWJ, http://dx.doi.org/10.1155/2014/681834.

Miroshnychenko, O. and Z. Miroshychenko. 2008. A method of producing selenium-enriched yeast products, and uses thereof. CA 2649145 C.

MAFF (Ministry of Agriculture, Fisheries and Food, UK) 2000. Duplicate diet study of vegetarians-dietary exposures to 12 metals and other elements. Food Surveillance Info Sheet No. 193.

Moore, K.L., M. Schroder, E. Lombi, F.J. Zhao, S.P. McGrath, M.J. Hawkesford, P.R. Shewry and C.R.M. Grovenor. 2010. NanoSIMS analysis of arsenic and selenium in cereal grain. New Phytologist, 185: 434–445.

Nacamulli, D., C. Mian, D. Petricca, F. Lazzarotto, S. Barollo, D. Pozza, S. Masiero, D. Faggian, M. Plebani, M.E. Girelli, F. Mantero and C. Betterle. 2010. Influence of physiological dietary selenium supplementation on the natural course of autoimmune thyroiditis. Clinical Endocrinology, 73: 535–539.

Nagodawithana, T. and F. Gutmanis. 1985. Method for the production of selenium yeast. U.S. patent 4530846.

Navarro-Alarcon, M. and C. Cabrera-Vique. 2008. Selenium in food and the human body: a review. Science of the Total Environment, 400: 115–141.

Navia, B., R.M. Ortega, J.M. Perea, A. Aparicio, A.M. López-Sobaler and E. Rodríguez-Rodríguez. 2014. Selenium status in a group of schoolchildren from the region of Madrid, Spain. Journal of Human Nutrition and Dietetics, 27: 239–246.

Ouerdane, L. and Z. Mester. 2008. Production and characterization of fully selenomethionine-labeled *Saccharomyces cerevisae*. Journal of Agricultural and Food Chemistry, 56: 11792–11799.

Otieno, S.B., F. Were, E. Kabiru and K. Waza. 2014. Study of selenium content in foods in high HIV prevalence community: A case study in Pala-Bondo district, Kenya. pp. 55–61. *In*: G.S. Bañuelos, Z-Q. Lin and X. Yin (eds.). Selenium in the environment and human health, Taylor and Francis Group, London.

Pappa, E.C., A.C. Pappas and P.F. Surai. 2006. Selenium content in selected foods from the Greek market and estimation of the daily intake. Science of the Total Environment, 372: 100–108.

Park, K., E. Rimm, D. Siscovick, D. Spiegelman, J.S. Morrisc and D. Mozaffarian. 2011. Demographic and lifestyle factors and selenium levels in men and women in the U.S. Nutrition Research and Practice, 5: 357–364.

Peters, U. and Y. Takata. 2008. Selenium and the prevention of prostate and colorectal cancer. Molecular Nutrition Food Research, 52: 1261–1272.

Poblaciones, M.J., S. Rodrigo, O. Santamaría, Y. Chen and S.P. Mcgrath. 2014. Agronomic selenium biofortification in *Triticum durum* under Mediterranean conditions: From grain to cooked pasta. Food Chemistry, 146: 378–384.

Ponce de León, C.A., M.M. Bayoán and J.A. Caruso. 2002. Selenium incorporation into *Saccharomyces cerevisiae* cells: a study of different incorporation methods. Journal of Applied Microbiology, 92: 602–610.

Pophaly, S.D., P.S. Poonam, H. Kumar, S. Kumar Tomar and R. Singh. 2014. Selenium enrichment of lactic acid bacteria and bifidobacteria: A functional food perspective. Trends in Food Science and Technology, 39: 135–145.

Ray, A.L., R.D. Semba, J. Walston L. Ferrucci, A.L., Cappola, M.O. Ricks, X.L. Xue and L.P. Fried. 2006. Low serum selenium and total carotenoids predict mortality among older women living in the community: the women's health and aging studies. Journal of Nutrition, 136: 172–176.

Rayman, M.P. 2000. The importance of selenium to human health. Lancet, 356: 233–241.

Rayman, M.P. 2004. The use of high-selenium yeast to raise selenium status: how does it measure up? British Journal of Nutrition, 92: 557–573.

Rayman, M. 2005. Selenium in cancer prevention: a review of the evidence and mechanism of action. Proceedings of the Nutrition Society, 64: 527–542.

Rayman, M.P. 2008. Food-chain selenium and human health: emphasis on intake. British Journal of Nutrition, 100: 254–268.

Rayman, M.P. 2009. Selenoproteins and human health: insights from epidemiological data. Biochimica et Biohysica Acta, 1790: 1533–1540.

Rayman, M.P., S. Stranges, B.A. Griffin, R. Pastor-Barriuso and E. Guallar. 2011. Effect of supplementation with high selenium yeast on plasma lipids: a randomized, controlled trial. Annals Internal Medicine, 154: 656–665.

Rayman, M.P. 2012. Selenium and human health. Lancet, 379: 1256–1268.

Schrauzer, G.N. 2000. Selenomethionine: a review of its nutritional significance, metabolism and toxicity. Journal of Nutrition, 130(7): 1653–1656.

Sempértegui, F., B. Estrella, W. Vallejo, L. Tapia, D. Herrera, F. Moscoso, G. Cerón, J. Griffiths and D. Hamer. 2003. Selenium serum concentrations in malnourished Ecuadorian children: a case-control study. Int. J. Vitam. Nutr. Res., 73: 181–186.

Serna-Saldivar, S.O. 2010. Cereal grains: properties, processing and nutritional attributes. CRC Press/ Taylor & Francis, Boca Raton, FL.

Serna-Saldivar, S.O. and R. Abril-Dominguez. 2011. Production and nutraceutical properties of breads fortified with DHA- and omega-3-containing oils. pp. 313–323. In: V.R. Preedy, R. Ross Watson and V.B. Patel (eds.). Flour and breads, and their fortification in health and disease prevention. Academic Press, London.

Shahar, A., K.V. Patel, R.D. Semba, S. Bandinelli, D.R. Shahar, L. Ferrucci and J.M. Guralnik. 2010. Plasma selenium is positively related to performance in neurological tasks assessing coordination and motor speed. Movement Disorders, 25: 1909–1915.

Şlencu, B.G., C. Ciobanu and R. Cuciureanu. 2012. Selenium content in foodstuffs and its nutritional requirement for humans. Clujul Medical, 85: 139–145.

Stabnikova, O., V. Ivanov, I. Larionova, V. Stabnikov, M. Bryszewska and J. Lewis. 2008. Ukrainian dietary bakery product with selenium-enriched yeast. LWT-Food Science and Technology, 41: 890–895.

Sugihara, S., M. Kondo, Y. Chihara, M. Yuji, H. Hattori and M. Yoshida. 2004. Preparation of selenium-enriched sprouts and identification of their selenium species by high-performance liquid chromatography-inductively coupled plasma mass spectrometry. Bioscience Biotechnology Biochemistry, 68(1): 193–199.

Swanson, C., B. Patterson, O. Levander, C. Veillon, P. Taylor, K. Helzlsouer, P. Adam and L. Zech. 1991. Human [74Se] selenomethionine metabolism: a kinetic model. The American Journal of Clinical Nutrition, 54: 917–926.

Támas, M., Z. Mándoky and J. Csapó. 2010. The role of selenium content of wheat in the human nutrition. A literature review. Acta Univ. Sarpientiae Alimentaria, 3: 5–34.

Terry, N., A. Zayed and M. De Souza. 2000. Selenium in higher plants. Annual Review of Plant Physiology and Plant Molecular Biology 51: 401–432.

Thiry, C., A. Ruttens, L. De Temmerman, Y-J. Schneider and L. Pussemier. 2012. Current knowledge in species-related bioavailability of selenium in food. Food Chemistry, 130(4): 767–784.

Thomson, C.D., L.K. Ong and M.F. Robinson. 1985. Effects of supplementation with high-selenium wheat bread on selenium, glutathione peroxidase and related enzymes in blood components of New Zealand residents. American Journal of Clinical Nutrition, 41: 1015–1022.

Ulziijargal, E., J.-H. Yang, L.-Y. Lin, C.-P. Chen and J.-L. Mau. 2013. Quality of bread supplemented with mushroom mycelia. Food Chemistry, 138(1): 70–76.

Urisini, F., S. Heim, M. Kiess, M. Maiorino, A. Roveri, J. Wissing and L. Flohe. 1999. Dual function of the selenoprotein PHGPx during sperm maturation. Science, 285: 1393–1396.

Ventura, M.G., M.-C. Freitas, A. Pacheco, T. Meerten and H.T. Wolterbeek. 2006. Selenium content in selected Portuguese foodstuffs. European Food Research and Technology 224: 395–401.

Wada, S. 2011. Colorectal cancer and the preventive effects of food components. pp. 207–222. In: A.G. Georgakilas (ed.). Cancer Prevention—From Mechanisms to Translational Benefits. InTech.

Waegeneers, N., C. Thiry, L. De Temmerman and A. Ruttens. 2013. Predicted dietary intake of selenium by the general adult population in Belgium. Food Additives & Contaminants Part A, 30(2): 278–285.

Wei, W.Q., C.C. Abnet, Y.L. Qiao, S.M. Dawsey, Z.W. Dong, X.D. Sun, J.H. Fan, E.W. Gunter, P.R. Taylor and S.D. Mark. 2004. Prospective study of serum selenium concentrations and esophageal and gastric cardia cancer, heart disease, stroke and total death. American Journal of Clinical Nutrition, 79: 80–85.

White, P.J. and M.R. Broadley. 2009. Biofortification of crops with seven mineral elements often lacking in human diets–iron, zinc, copper, calcium, magnesium, selenium and iodine. New Phytologist., 182: 49–84.

Wood, S.M., C. Beckham, A. Yosioka, H. Darban and R.R. Watson. 2000. β-carotene and selenium supplementation enhances immune response in aged humans. Integrative Medicine, 2: 85–92.

Wu, J., C. Salisbury, R. Graham, G. Lyons and M. Fenech. 2009. Increased consumption of wheat biofortified with selenium does not modify biomarkers of cancer risk, oxidative stress, or immune function in healthy Australian males. Environmental Molecular Mutagenesis, 50(6): 489–501.

Zeng, H., M. Briske-Anderson, J.P. Idso and C.D. Hunt. 2006. Nutrition and disease. the selenium metabolite methylselenol inhibits the migration and invasion potential of HT1080 tumor cells. Journal of Nutrition, 136(6): 1528–1532.

7

Microorganisms Involved in Spoilage of Bread and Its Control Measures

P. Saranraj[1,*] and *P. Sivasakthivelan*[2]

1. Introduction

Bread is a food product that is universally accepted as a very convenient form of food that has desirability to all population rich—and poor, rural and urban. Its origin dates back to the Neolithic era and is still one of the most consumed and acceptable staple in all parts of the world. It is a good source of nutrients, such as macronutrients and micronutrients that are all essential for human health (Potter and Hotchkiss 2006).

Bread and other bakery products are subjected to various spoilage problems, viz., physical, chemical and microbial; the latter is the most serious one particularly bacterial (*Bacillus* sp.) and mold growth. Various molds involved in spoilage of bread include *Rhizopus, Mucor, Penicillium, Eurotium, Aspergillus* and *Monilia* (Saranraj and Geetha 2012). Likewise, yeast spoilage known as "Chalk mold" is caused by *Pichia butonii*. In this chapter, the types of microbial spoilage, various methods for detection of these spoilage and appropriate control measures are described.

[1] Asstt. Professor, Sacred Heart College, Tirupattur, India.
  Email: microsaranraj@gmail.com
[2] Department of Microbiology, Annamalai University, Chidambaram – 608 002, Tamil Nadu, India.
  Email: plantdoctorsiva@yahoo.co.in
* Corresponding author

2. Bacterial rope spoilage

Rope spoilage is a bread disease consisting in bacterial decomposition of the bread crumb. Spoilage organisms are heat-resistant spores of bacteria belonging to *Bacillus* genera, which survive the baking process. Members of the *Bacillus* genus that bring about bacterial spoilage of bread are known as rope. This is of major economic concern to the baking industry. Ropiness, which is the most important spoilage of bread after moldiness, occurs particularly in summer when the climatic conditions favor the growth of bacteria. It is mainly caused by *Bacillus subtilis* but *Bacillus licheniformis*, *Bacillus megaterium* and *Bacillus cereus* have also been associated with ropy bread. Most important rope formers are *B. subtilis*, *B. licheniformis* and *B. mesentericus*, also known as *B. pumilus*. The incidence of wheat bread spoilage caused by *Bacillus* has increased during the last few years presumably because more bread is produced without preservatives and often raw materials such as bran and seeds are added. Spoilage of bread by rope formation may constitute a health risk, high numbers of *B. subtilis* and *B. licheniformis* in foods may cause a mild form of food illness. Consumption of ropy bread has been associated with food-borne illness in reports from Canada and the United Kingdom (Ybar et al. 2012; Rumeus and Turtoi 2013).

Sources of rope spores microorganisms in bread products are mostly present in the ingredients, especially flour and yeasts. Unlike molds that are destroyed when exposed to baking temperatures, rope spores microorganisms are able to form spores and survive the baking process, germinate, and continue to grow. Optimum growth conditions for rope formers are 35°C to 45°C, humid environment (e.g., packed bread) and pH values higher than 5.3 (Rumeus and Turtoi 2013).

The origins of the *Bacillus* species are reported to be raw materials, particularly flour, and from the bakery atmosphere, equipment surfaces and other raw materials. Spores found in flour and other raw materials are resistant to heat and some of them can survive the baking process where temperatures in the center of the crumb remains at a maximum of 97–101°C for only a few minutes. Failure to reach this temperature in all parts of the bread greatly increases the proportion of surviving spores. It has been found that all baking flours are contaminated with *Bacillus* spores as a result of cultivation and processing methods. As this type of spoilage only affects the central portions of the loaf in its initial stages it is seldom evident to consumers at the time of purchase (Certel et al. 2009).

Rope spoilage can first become noticeable 12–24 hr after the loaf has been removed from the oven and is characterized by a distinctive sweet, fruit odor which has been likened to that of rotting pineapple or rotting melons. A discolored, sticky and soft breadcrumb subsequently follows this. Degradation of the breadcrumb is caused by the combined effects of microbial proteolytic and amylolytic enzymes breaking down the starch. Its sticky nature is due to the slime, extracellular polysaccharides, formed by certain rope-inducing strains. At this stage web-like strands are visible when the crumb is broken. The problem of rope spoilage of bread has been minimized in the Western countries through the application of good manufacturing practices, advanced process control, high hygiene standards and the use of chemical preservatives according to specified legal limits. However, the international trends towards the elimination of chemical preservatives, for example calcium propionate, from bread and other foodstuffs are expected to increase the risk of bread spoilage by rope-inducing *Bacillus* strains.

Ropiness occurs in non-acidified breads and consists in breaking down bread components and leaving behind a sticky, pasty, stringy mass which has a fruity, melon-type odor. Ropiness is referred to when the bread is pressed together and then pulled apart. If it is ropey then it will stretch into long, sticky, web-like strands. It is only visible for a short period of time; some strains do not even form ropes at all. The main characterization is therefore a fruity, melon-type odor. Discoloration of the crumb and a bitter taste may also be other symptoms. Packed wheat bread with a long shelf-life such as toast bread is highly susceptible (Rumeus and Turtoi 2013).

Ropiness prevention can be done through chemical or biological methods. Rope forming bacteria are very sensitive to low pH values, therefore their growth is inhibited when chemicals are added to dough. The most efficient chemicals used in bread making are propionic acid, calcium propionate, acetic acid, and calcium hydrogen phosphate. A dose of 1–5 g/kg of flour leads to a delay of ropiness of 3 to 21 d. Biological methods consist in the use of starter cultures of propionic bacteria (e.g., *Propionibacterium shemanii*), which have antagonistic behavior towards rope forming bacteria of *Bacillus* genera due to the synthesis of propionic acid and some substances with antibiotic effect. Other biological methods are the use of sourdough, liquid yeast, lactic-acid culture containing *Lactobacillus plantarum*, *Lactobacillus brevis*, *Lactobacillus fermenti*, etc. (Saranraj and Geetha 2012).

Valerio et al. (2008) worked with four fermentation products of the lactic acid bacterium *Lb. plantarum* ITM21B and obtained baked products with no ropy symptoms after three days and an enhancement of the *Bacillus*-free shelf-life of yeast leavened bread for seven days.

Valerio et al. (2012) examined the diversity of spore-forming bacteria isolated from raw materials and bread using molecular methods along with a rapid and innovative technology, the FT-NIR (Fourier transform near-infrared) spectroscopy. They found 13 bacterial species belonging to *Bacillus* (ten) and *Paenibacillus* (three) genera. The most frequent species was *Bacillus amyloliquefaciens*, found also in ropy bread. The screening test performed for rope production indicated that mainly *Bacillus amyloliquefaciens*, together with *B. subtilis* and *B. pumilus*, could cause spoilage in bread, even if the last two species were represented by a low number of isolates. The *Bacillus cereus* group and *B. megaterium* showed a lower percentage of isolates potentially able to cause the rope. However, considering the high number of *B. cereus* group isolates detected in the study of Valerio et al. (2012), this bacterial group should also be considered important in rope spoilage.

3. Fungal spoilage

Bakery products, especially bread, are intermediate moisture content products which are highly perishable. The most common forms of bread deterioration are moisture loss and microbiological spoilage. Spoilage of wheat bread and other bakery products by colonization and growth of fungi represents more than 90 percent of the total microbial contamination. Currently, such food matrices are preserved by the addition of weak organic acids such as calcium propionate. In recent years, there has been pressure from both legislation and consumers to reduce the amounts of preservatives added to food products. However, a reduction in the dose of preservatives used to control mold spoilage in bakery products may lead, under certain conditions, to a reduction in the shelf-life of the product (Magan and Aldred 2006).

Mold spoilage in bread is a serious economic concern. Losses due to mold spoilage vary between 1 and 5 percent of products depending on season, type of product and method of processing. Mold spoilage of bakery products has been the subject of many studies, and a number of species have been implicated. The most widespread and most important in bakery products are species of *Eurotium*, *Aspergillus* and *Penicillium*. Other genera isolated from bakery products have included *Cladosporium*, *Mucor* and *Rhizopus*, but due to their high a_w requirement for germination and growth, it is unlikely that bakery products will be spoiled by these fungi.

In addition to the economic losses associated with bakery products, another concern is the possibility of mycotoxin production. *Eurotium* species are usually the first fungi to colonize improperly dried, stored commodities, and when they grow, they increase the level of available water allowing other species (e.g., *Aspergillus* sp. and *Penicillium* sp.) to thrive. *Eurotium* sp. does not produce any significant mycotoxins, but it is important to know the conditions under which species of *Aspergillus* and *Penicillium* can grow and spoil the bakery products, because several species produce mycotoxins. For example, toxigenic *Aspergillus flavus* has been isolated from 3 of 15 home-stored bakery products and toxigenic *Penicillium* sp. have been isolated from wheat flour and bread in the USA. Several species of *Penicillium* produce mycotoxins, including *Penicillium chrysogenum* (Girardin 1997).

Problems due to spoilage yeasts in bread usually result from post-baking contamination. Slicing machines, bread coolers, conveyor belts and racks have been identified as sources. Yeast spoilage is characterized by visible growth on the surface of products (white or cream patches). The most frequent and troublesome yeast is *Pichia butonii*, which is known as "chalk mold". This yeast can multiply rapidly on bread, with visible growth often apparent some time before mold occurs. Filamentous fungi are more common than yeasts on British breads. However, since filamentous fungi are more easily recognized than yeasts they generate the majority of complaints.

4. Early detection and differentiation of bread spoilage

Early detection of food spoilage is important because of the legislative and consumer pressure to reduce the use of preservatives, particularly those based on organic acids, in intermediate moisture bakery products. Food spoilage causes large economic losses due to waste of raw materials or product. Microbial spoilage is the major problem causing deterioration of bread products but there is also a problem with physiological spoilage such as enzymatic spoilage. Mold spoilage accounts for between 1 and 5 percent of product losses depending on the season, type of product being produced and the method of processing. In the past, control of the safety of foods has mainly been performed by product testing of both raw materials and end products. The main problem with performing end product testing is the high number of samples to be examined before one can decide on the safety of a product batch, especially when the microorganisms are assumed to be heterogeneously distributed within the batch. In the last decade the rapid advances made in the development of electronic nose technology has attracted much interest in applications for the detection of spoilage microorganisms (Needham et al. 2005).

There is potential to differentiate between different types of bread spoilage using a Bloodhound BH-114 electronic nose. Microbial spoilage caused by bacteria, yeast and fungi, and enzymatic spoilage caused by lipoxygenase can be differentiated from one another and from unspoiled bread analogues after 48 hr using cluster analysis, prior to signs of visible spoilage. Analysis of the bread analogues with gas chromatography-mass spectrometry identified volatiles produced by the different spoilage types and unspoiled bread analogues. Microbial analysis showed that the levels of each microorganism used increased with time (Needham et al. 2005).

Traditional cultural detection of most microorganisms requires growth of the organism on selective media, which can take a number of days from isolation to identification. These methods are sensitive, inexpensive and give qualitative information on the number and the nature of the microorganisms present in a food sample. However, conventional methods require several days to produce results because they rely on the ability of microorganisms to multiply to visible colonies. Moreover, culture medium preparation, inoculation of plates, colony counting and biochemical characterization make these methods labor intensive. Traditional methods are of limited value especially for the analysis of perishable foods since the foods are sold and eaten before the results of the tests are known. Rapid methods can reduce the time taken to achieve results from days to a few hours or even minutes.

Rapid methods commercially available include DNA probes, the Polymerase Chain Reaction (PCR), latex agglutination tests, direct epifluorescent filter techniques, Enzyme Linked Immunosorbant Assay (ELISA), conductance, impedance, bioluminescence, immunomagnetic beads and biochemical assays such as API 20E and Micro ID. Methods currently available for measuring mold contamination in food include: microscopic examination, culture on agar, electrical measurements of conductance and other changes in the electrical properties of the contaminated food substratum and detection of fungal metabolites such as chitin, ergosterol or ATP. The applications of these methods are described below.

4.1 Colony forming units

Counting of Colony Forming Units (CFU) has been the traditional method used to quantify fungal and bacterial populations. The simplicity of this method is however outweighed by its drawbacks. The method requires long incubation times on selective media, is labor intensive and measures only culturable organisms. Counting of CFU is also not related to actual activity. Despite these drawbacks, CFU are used as the standard method in the food industry.

4.2 Conductance and impedance methods

Conductance is the ability of a system to conduct an electrical charge. Microbial growth and metabolism produce a change in conductivity by metabolizing substrates of low conductivity into smaller, mobile products of higher conductivity. An example of this, described by Silley and Forsythe (1996), is the conversion of glucose to two molecules of lactic acid with an increase in conductivity. Further metabolism converts the lactic acid and three oxygen molecules to carbonic acid, which is an even more effective electrical conductor. The smaller ions decrease the impedance, resistance to flow and therefore the conductance increases. Problems are encountered with some selective media, e.g., those with a high salt concentration. This can be overcome by using the indirect method, which is used for yeasts, which produces a negative change in conductance. The indirect method detects production of carbon dioxide by detecting changes in a potassium hydroxide solution, as carbon dioxide dissolves in it. Deak and Beuchat (1993) examined fruit juice concentrates containing an average microbial population of 35 CFU/ml by traditional plating techniques and direct and indirect impedance. The indirect method produced results 10–20 hr before the direct method with detection after approximately 50 hr. The detection time was shortened to an average of 14 hr if the samples were incubated for 24 hr at 25°C (Girardin 1997; Needham et al. 2005).

4.3 DNA probes

DNA probes were the first nucleic acid based assays for the detection of food-borne pathogens and were introduced for food analysis in the early 1980s. Commercially available kits target ribosomal RNA (rRNA). The technique exploits the species specific signatures encoded by nucleic acid sequences using nucleic acid segments called probes. The method can be as quick as 45 min but requires overnight cultures, which can present some problems with the use of selective broths. DNA probes have been found to be highly specific (Samadpour et al. 1990; Ingianni et al. 2001). Samadpour et al. (1990) used DNA probes to detect *shiga* toxin producing *Escherichia coli* in a range of food samples. They were able to detect 1.3 CFU/g of sample with results obtained within 48 hr even with an enrichment step incorporated into the method. DNA probes can be combined with other detection methods, which are described in the following sections.

4.4 Polymerase chain reaction

The Polymerase Chain Reaction (PCR) is used more for identification of organisms than enumeration. Short segments of DNA, or primers, are used in a thermocycler to amplify enzymatically a specific segment of the bacterial genome. The usefulness applied directly to foods is limited by the complex composition of food components, which inhibit PCR amplification. Only a few PCR assays have been developed into commercial kits. Ingianni et al. (2001) combined DNA probes with PCR for the detection of *Listeria monocytogenes* in a range of foods including bread. PCR combined with DNA probes produced more positive results and was more sensitive than PCR alone or traditional cultural methods. Results were also obtainable within a working day after an enrichment step of 68 hr, which improved results (Girardin 1997; Needham et al. 2005).

4.5 Direct epifluorescent filter technique

The direct epifluorescent filter technique (DEFT) is an extremely rapid microbiological analytical method, which has been used for many years for the direct quantification of microbial load in a variety of applications including predicting the shelf-life of foods. The method has gained acceptance for use with milk and milk-based products. The basic principles are that microorganisms are trapped on a membrane filter, which is stained with a fluorescent dye, e.g., acridine orange, and then examined using epifluorescent microscopy. The total microbial population can then be rapidly enumerated using image analysis. DEFT only takes between 2–30 min to perform and provides the ability to distinguish between viable and non-viable bacteria. This is due to the use of acridine orange, which fluoresces different colors in cells during different phases of growth. A disadvantage of DEFT is that it only allows presumptive identification on morphology. A completely automated DEFT system has been developed. The method incorporates the use of three computers to attend to the sample preparation, staining, filtration, drying and image analysis stages (Giardin 1997; Ingianni et al. 2001).

4.6 Latex agglutination tests

Latex agglutination tests (LAT) incorporate the use of antibody coated colored beads to agglutinate specific antigens, the bacterial cells. LAT are also available for analysis of bacterial toxins, which are sometimes known as reverse passive latex agglutination (RPLA) because the antibodies are attached (reverse) to latex beads (passive matrix) and used to detect soluble antigens (toxins). LAT are simple to perform, very specific and yield results quickly. LATs are available for a range of bacteria. Mold latex agglutination tests (MLA) depend on recognition of mold antigens. Two MLA tests specific for *Aspergillus* and *Penicillium* exopolysaccharide antigens have been developed (Girardin 1997). These have however been removed from the market due to poor sales (Giardin 1997).

4.7 Adenosine Triphosphate (ATP) bioluminescence

ATP bioluminescence is based on the reaction that naturally occurs in the North American firefly, *Photinus pyralis*. The reaction, catalyzed by the enzyme luciferase, uses the chemical energy contained within ATP molecules to drive the oxidative decarboxylation of the co-factor luciferin. The resultant production of yellow-green light is detected using a luminometer. A linear relationship exists between the concentration of ATP and light output, because one photon of light is emitted for every ATP molecule consumed. ATP is however the source of energy for all living organisms and therefore separation of bacterial or fungal ATP is the main problem encountered.

ATP is predominately used for hygiene testing in the food industry. Samkutty et al. (2001) used ATP bioluminescence for the rapid assessment of bacteriological quality of bread. They found that ATP could be useful in predicting standard plate counts in bread.

4.8 Enzyme Linked Immunosorbent Assay (ELISA)

Enzyme Linked Immunosorbent Assays (ELISA) involves absorbing specific antibodies onto wells of microtitre plates and the addition of complementary antigens. The enzyme-linked antibody specific for a test antigen then binds to the antigen forming a double antibody sandwich. A visible color change is produced by the addition of the substrate, which is measured spectrophotometrically. Several sandwich ELISAs have been developed for detecting the most frequently isolated fungal food contaminants: *Aspergillus, Penicillium*, *Fusarium*, *Mucor* and *Rhizopus, Cladosporium, Geotrichium* and *Botrytis*. Using the ELISA protocol, a number of food samples can be tested simultaneously and automatically (Giardin 1997; Needham et al. 2005).

4.9 Chitin assay

Chitin, a polymer of *N*-acetyl-D-glucosamine, is a major constituent of the walls of fungal spores and mycelium. It is not present in bacteria or foods. The assay as described by Pitt and Hocking (1994) involves alkaline hydrolysis of the sample causing partial depolymerization of chitin to produce chitosan. Subsequent treatment with nitrous acid then causes partial solubilization and deamination of glucosamine residues to produce 2,5-anhydromannose, which is estimated colorimetrically using 3-methyl-2-benzothiazolone hydrazone hydrochloride as the principle reagent. Improved assay sensitivity has been achieved by derivisation of glucosamine and other products with *o*-phtalaldehyde, separated by high performance liquid chromatography (HPLC) and detection of fluorescent compounds. The disadvantages of the assay are that it is rather complex requiring sophisticated and expensive equipment, the process is slow taking about 5 hr, and it lacks sensitivity. Also chitin does not increase proportionally with fungal growth and the assay lacks sensitivity so the results can be misleading. Discrimination between viable and non-viable cells is also not possible (Magan 1993; Eikenes et al. 2005).

4.10 Ergosterol assay

Ergosterol is the major steroid produced by fungi. It occurs as a lipid of fungal cell membranes, so is inherently likely to be correlated with hyphal growth and biomass. For estimation, samples are blended with methanol, saponified with strong alkali, extracted with petroleum ether, and fractionated by HPLC. Ergosterol is detected by ultraviolet absorption, optimally at 282 nm, a wavelength at which other sterols exhibit little or no absorbance. Determination of the ergosterol content is a reliable measure of fungal growth and is a more sensitive measure of biomass than chitin content. A new method, as described by Eikenes et al. (2005) called μSERS is a new biochip technology being developed for label-free detection of pathogens and their toxins. Another area being studied is the use of various biosensors (Pitt and Hocking 1994; Eikenes et al. 2005).

5. Sodium chloride and magnesium chloride in bread preservation

Sodium chloride (NaCl) has long been used for the preservation of food products and as a condiment. NaCl is a versatile compound that also contributes to the functional properties of several food products and is the primary dietary source of the essential mineral Na^+. In many populations, the dietary NaCl intakes well exceed the recommended maximum daily intakes of 5–6 g NaCl (= 2000–2400 mg Na^+) (FSA 2009). These include mean intakes as high as 9 g (3540 mg Na^+) in France and 11.7 g NaCl (4600 mg of Na^+) per day for men in Canada, Colombia, Hungary, Ladakh (India), Bassiano (Italy), Poland, Portugal and the Republic of Korea. The well-established association of high dietary sodium (Na^+) intake with the development of hypertension has prompted public health and regulatory authorities to recommend reduction of the dietary intake of NaCl. In addition to causing illness cardiovascular diseases (CVD) are of significant economic consequences worldwide, costing the EU approximately V169 billion per year. The combined estimated direct and indirect costs of CVD for the US in 2006 were $403.1 billion. Bibbins-Domingo et al. (2010) determined that it is more cost-effective to reduce NaCl intake compared to treatment of hypertension with medications. These reasons combined form an important part of the rationale for reducing salt levels in food products.

Due to the diverse and important roles of NaCl in food products, the reduction of NaCl levels combined with full or partial replacement may have an impact on the shelf stability (Bidlas and Lambert 2008) and functional properties of a food product. Growth related parameters such as the minimum a_w for growth have also been found to be influenced by the nature of the solute indicating that different solutes may have additional antimicrobial or even growth stimulating effects on both bacteria and fungi which are not accounted for by their a_w lowering effects. A_w depressing capacities of salts also differ (Samapundo et al. 2010), implying that the application of NaCl replacers may also influence the microbial stability and safety of food products as a_w of the altered products could be different to those with NaCl alone.

To date most of the studies found in literature on NaCl reduction and replacement have explored the functional and sensorial consequences in food products with very few considering the impact on the microbiological stability and safety. Mold spoilage is a serious and costly problem for the bakery industry. Although, studies have been done regarding salt reduction and replacement in bread and bakery products, none of these specifically mention the impact of salt reduction and/or replacement on the microbial stability or safety of these products. The influence of the solute responsible for a_w depression on the growth of bacteria has been observed for fungi by Suleman et al. (2001) who determined that at equivalent solute potentials within the range of 1.15 to 4.25 MPa, NaCl had the greater effects than either KCl or glycerol on the radial growth of *Chalara radicicola* and *Chalara paradoxa*, fungi associated with disease in date palms.

The influence of the compound responsible for a_w depression on the growth parameters of *Aspergillus niger* has also been reported by Parra et al. (2004). They reported that *Aspergillus niger* had an optimum water activity (a_w) for growth of 0.965 at 35°C on malt extract agar when glycerol was used to adjust the a_w and 0.990 when NaCl was used (Parra et al. 2004). Parra and Megan (2004) also reported a_w of 0.97 for two *Aspergillums niger* strains on malt extract agar whose a_w had been adjusted by glycerol. A_w reported by Parra et al. (2004) for growth on media with NaCl.

Samapundo et al. (2010) evaluated the effect of NaCl and various NaCl replacers ($CaCl_2$, $MgCl_2$, KCl and $MgSO_4$) on the growth of *Penicillium roqueforti* and *Aspergillus niger* at 22°C. In addition, challenge tests were performed on white bread to determine the consequences of NaCl reduction with or without partial replacement on the growth of *Penicillium roqueforti*. It can be concluded that at equivalent water phase concentrations the isolates exhibited differing sensitivities to the salts evaluated with NaCl and $MgCl_2$ having the greatest inhibitory action on the growth of *Aspergillus niger* and *Penicillium roqueforti*, respectively. The $MgSO_4$ had the least antifungal activity. At equivalent molalities, $CaCl_2$ had in general the largest antifungal activity. Although, the water activity (a_w) lowering effects of the compounds studied play a large role in explaining the trends observed, at equivalent water phase concentrations $MgCl_2$ was found to have a smaller inhibitory effect on *Aspergillus niger* than that expected from its a_w depressing effect. The challenge tests revealed that no difference occurred in the growth of *Penicillium roqueforti* on standard white bread, bread with 30 percent less NaCl and bread in which 30 percent of the NaCl has been partially replaced by a mixture of KCl. Their results are of importance in assessing the possible microbiological consequences of NaCl reduction or replacement in bread and similar bakery products.

The NaCl and $MgCl_2$ have in general the largest antimicrobial activities on *Aspergillus niger* and *Penicillium roqueforti*, respectively, at equivalent water phase concentrations as they gave rise to the slowest colony growth rates and the longest lag phase durations. This would imply that the replacement of NaCl with the salt replacers studied would probably give rise to products of reduced microbial stability with regards to *Aspergillus niger*. Whilst this is also true for *Penicillium roqueforti* for the majority of the salt replacers studied, replacement of NaCl by $MgCl_2$ would imply a product even more stable to *Penicillium roqueforti*. When comparisons were made on an equivalent molality basis $CaCl_2$ was found to generally have a consistently large antimicrobial activity on the growth of both fungi, whereas $MgCl_2$ had the largest effects on the growth of *Penicillium roqueforti*. $MgSO_4$ was determined to have the least antifungal activity from both an equivalent water phase concentration and molality point of view. Therefore its use as a NaCl replacer will also most likely result in products of reduced stability (Samapundo et al. 2010).

Although, a_w plays a very large role in the trends observed the differing sensitivities of the fungal isolates to $MgCl_2$ partially highlights the occurrence of species specific additional effects of the molecule itself other than its a_w lowering effects. The results obtained in this study imply that the microbial consequences of reduction will also largely depend on the initial NaCl level, the nature of the replacer and the fungal species encountered. At low initial NaCl levels (< 2 percent) such as those encountered in the challenge tests performed in this study, NaCl reduction with or without partial replacement did not affect the stability of white bread to *Penicillium roqueforti*. Future experiments should preferentially be in the form of challenge tests which help to provide important data on the real life consequences of NaCl reduction and partial replacement on the microbiological stability and safety of food products (Samapundo et al. 2010).

6. Weak preservatives in control of bread spoilage

Mold spoilage is a serious and costly problem for bakeries and use of preservatives is therefore an attractive means to diminish spoilage and insure food safety. However, consumers today are not in favor of additives as preservatives and an urge to reduce the quantities used exists within the bakery industry. Reduction of preservatives to sub-inhibitory levels has nevertheless been shown to stimulate growth of spoilage fungi in some cases and stimulate mycotoxin production (Membre et al. 2001).

Spoilage of bakery products is caused mainly by molds and yeasts and occasionally by bacteria such as the rope-causing heat-resistant endospore forming *Bacillus subtilis*. Mold spores are killed in the baking process, leaving after contamination to be the source of spoilage problems. Contaminants of wheat bread are mainly *Penicillium* sp. (90–100 percent), but *Clodosporium* and *Aspergillus* sp. also occur, the latter especially in warmer climates. Under favorable conditions molds can grow on a large variety of substrates. In bakery processing, the most common type of microbial spoilage is mold growth and in many cases it is the major factor governing shelf-life. The most widespread and probably most important molds, in terms of biodeterioration of bakery products, are species of *Eurotium*, *Aspergillus* and *Penicillium*. An aid in preventing fungal spoilage of foodstuffs would be the application of the combined preservation factors method.

The most important mold species on bread are *Penicillium commune*, *Penicillium crustosum*, *Penicillium brevicompactum*, *Penicillium chrysogenum*, *Penicillium roqueforti*, *Aspergillus versicolor* and *Aspergillus sydowii*. On rye bread *Penicillium roqueforti* is the major contaminant. In a four-year investigation of rye bread in Denmark *Penicillium roqueforti* (27%), *Penicillium corylophilum* (20%) and *Eurotium* sp. (15%) (*Eurotium repens* and *Eurotium rubrum*) were identified as the most important species. Varieties of *Penicillium roqueforti* have later been elevated to species; *Penicillium paneum* and *Penicillium carneum*. On cakes with low water activity *Eurotium* sp., *Aspergillus* sp. and *Wallemia sebi* are expected spoilage organisms. Yeast contaminants—also known as 'chalk molds'—are most common on sliced bread, and on rye bread *Endomyces fibuliger* and *Hyphopichia burtonii* have been reported as dominant species (Saranraj and Geetha 2012).

Consumers require high quality, preservative-free, safe foods with an extended shelf-life. A reason why consumers are especially concerned about additives and contaminants is that these are not seen to be intrinsic to the food but are considered as added extras. Ever since, the massive Anti-E Number lobby of the mid 1980's, the bread industry has been working to reduce the number of additives and so called synthetic preservatives in a genuine effort to make bread as natural and as fresh as possible. Alternatives to preservatives have been sought, that allow products to be presented in essentially the same form, but with modifications that make the product acceptable to a larger proportion of consumers. An example of this is the use of acetic acid as a preservative in place of propionic acid, vinegar being almost as effective as propionic acid as an antimycotic and more acceptable on the ingredient list. In the UK, when acetic acid is used as the bread preservative, it is added as vinegar. Both vinegar and calcium propionate are used as preservatives in British bread. Preservation of bakery products commonly involves the use of propionates and sorbates, and sometimes benzoates and is added in concentrations that do not exceed 0.3 percent (Marin et al. 2003).

Propionic, sorbic and benzoic acids are among the most commonly used food preservatives. Propionic acid inhibits molds and *Bacillus* spores, but not yeasts to the same extent, and has therefore been the traditional choice for bread preservation. Sorbic acid is considered to be more effective than propionic acid. It inhibits both molds and yeasts, and is used in a broad variety of food products, including fine bakery products, confectionary and bread. According to the European Parliament and Council Directive No. 95/2/EC, propionic and sorbic acid may be added to bakery wares in concentrations up to 3000 and 2000 ppm, respectively. Benzoic acid is used in many types of acidic food products, although it is mainly associated with fruit preservation. It is also used in combination with sorbic acid for confectionary and other types of products. Benzoic acid is allowed in concentrations of up to 1500 ppm (Saranraj and Geetha 2012).

Common methods of preservation of bakery products include weak-acid preservatives, such as benzoates, propionates and sorbates. These preservatives have, however, come under criticism because of their known toxicity when administered to test animals at high doses. As a response to increasing consumer pressure an effort is being made by producers to reduce the amounts of preservatives added to their products. The preservatives are often added as a salt of the acid because salts are more soluble in aqueous solution. The effectiveness of the preservatives is dependent on the pH of the product, as the antimicrobial effect of the undissociated acid is much stronger than the dissociated acid. The pKa values of propionic acid, sorbic acid and benzoic acid are 4.88, 4.76 and 4.18, respectively. Maximum pH for activity is around 6.0–6.5 for sorbate, 5.0–5.5 for propionate and 4.0–4.5 for benzoate (Saranraj and Geetha 2012).

Preliminary work on the effect of low doses of weak-acid preservatives on these and some other fungal isolates (*Eurotium* sp.) had been carried out on a wheat-flour agar. In that study, the same preservatives were assayed but in doses ranging from 0.003 to 0.3 percent. Results obtained showed that a 0.003 percent dose was completely useless under any pH level, while a 0.03 percent concentration would only be useful at a pH of 4.5. In the work of Marin et al. (2003), an analog of Madeira cake was used. Its usual pH is slightly basic (7.0 to 8.0). That's the reason why pH levels used in the experiment were 6.0 and 7.5 in order to keep the cake near to its common organoleptic features. Referring to water activity (a_w) in the initial experiment 0.80, 0.85, 0.90 and 0.95 were tested. In this case however, and as the common a_w of these products is 0.75 to 0.85 under normal conditions, the levels chosen for the assay were 0.80, 0.85 and 0.90, as it was known that none of the isolates tested was able to grow at 0.75 a_w.

Antimicrobials of the type of weak acids such as propionic, benzoic and sorbic acids are used as one of the numerous hurdles employed in food preservation. In recent years, this approach has, however, come under increased criticism as customers demand "more natural" and "fresh foods". Previous studies dealing with the prevention of growth of common molds spoiling bakery products have emphasized the interaction among factors such as a_w, temperature, pH and preservatives addition. Guynot et al. (2002) stated that by choosing the appropriate pH and equilibrium relative humidity (ERH) to maximize the effect of sorbic acid, the amount of acid needed to produce a specific increase in shelf-life could be minimized.

It is well established that low pH favor the activity of weak-acid preservatives. Organic acids, such as sorbic, are more effective in inhibiting microorganisms in their undissociated forms, which increase in concentration as the pH decreases. At low pH values, undissociated sorbic acid is thought to permeate the cell membrane altering the internal pH of the microorganisms, causing denaturation and inactivation of enzymes. In this study of Guynot et al. (2002), the dependence of potassium sorbate activity with the pH of the medium was confirmed, as fungal growth inhibition was much higher at pH 4.5 than at 5.5. At pH 4.5, depending on the isolate, concentrations in the range of 0.15–0.30 percent were effective in preventing fungal growth regardless of water activity. However, at pH 5.5, only *Aspergillus* sp. and *Penicillium corylophilum* were inhibited for up to four weeks, and higher concentrations were required. On the other hand, *Eurotium* sp. was totally inhibited only for one incubation week, after that time a considerable increase in analogues spoilage was observed.

Torres et al. (2003) studied the efficacy of single and mixtures of butylated hydroxy anisole (BHA) and propyl paraben (PP) on growth and production of the mycotoxin fumonisin and hydrolytic enzyme production by *Fusarium verticilliodes* and *Fusarium proliferatum in vitro* on maize-based media. They found that a mixture of BHA and PP showed potential for control of growth and fumonisin production over a range of a_w levels. Other natural solutions for use as preservatives have been researched including bateriocins, particularly from lactic acid bacteria and various essential oils.

7. Lactic acid bacteria as biopreservative in bread

Lactic acid bacteria (LAB) have been used in food fermentations for more than 4000 years. It is important to acknowledge that the widespread term "Lactic acid bacteria" have no official status in taxonomy and is only a general term of convenience used to describe the group of functionally and genetically related bacteria. Lactic acid bacteria consist of bacterial genera within the *Firmicutes* comprised of about 20 genera. The main members of the lactic acid bacteria are genera *Lactococcus*, *Lactobacillus*, *Streptococcus*, *Leuconostoc*, *Pediococcus*, *Carnobacterium*, *Aerococcus*, *Enterococcus*, *Oenococcus*, *Tetragenococcus*, *Vagococcus* and *Weissella*. *Lactobacillus* is the largest genus of this group, comprising around 80 recognized species. Lactic acid bacteria have a long history of use in a variety of cereal fermentations, especially in the manufacture of baked goods. It has been reported that around 50 different species of lactic acid bacteria have been isolated from sourdough. *Lactobacillus* strains are the most frequently observed bacteria in this matrix, but the species belonging to the genera *Leuconostoc*, *Weissella*, *Pediococcus*, *Lactococcus* or *Enterococcus* have been isolated as well (Petrulakova et al. 2010).

In recent years, biopreservation has gained increasing interest due to consumers' demands. Lactic acid bacteria as bio-preservation organisms are of particular interest: they have been used for centuries as starter cultures in the food industry and are able to produce different kind of bioactive molecules, such as organic acids, fatty acids, hydrogen peroxide and bacteriocins. The antifungal activity of LAB was documented. Authors also reported that lactic acid bacterial strains are able to inhibit mold growth in bread and bakery products. Numerous studies have described the isolation and characterization of antifungal components from LAB cultures but limited applications of the antifungal strains in baking have been reported. In the work of Dal Bello et al. (2007), *Lactobacillus reuteri*, *Lb. plantarum* and *Lb. brevis* (regarded as antifungal positive strains) were used in the formulation of a mixed starter culture and used together with *Saccharomyces cerevisiae* (commercial yeast) in bread elaboration.

Lactic acid bacteria used in sourdough fermentation lower the pH of bread dough, inhibit *Bacillus* spore germination and improve the flavor of the baked product. The desirable effects of LAB can also be exploited in bread-making processes that use *S. cerevisiae* as the leavening agent. Lactic acid bacteria are known to produce various antimicrobial compounds, including organic acids, hydrogen peroxide and bacteriocins. Lactic acid produced by LAB play a key role in inhibiting bacterial growth, but phenyllactic acid (PLA) and p-OH-phenyllactic acid (OH-PLA) which are produced by some strains of LAB also have antimicrobial activity. Some strains of *Lb. plantarum* produce both metabolites (Makras et al. 2006).

Phenyllactic acid (PLA) production by *Lb. plantarum* strain can be improved by increasing the concentration of its precursor, phenylalanine, in the culture medium, and simultaneously reducing the tyrosine concentration. Other workers have found that α-ketoglutaric acid influences PLA and OH-PLA production by LAB. This compound is the main α-keto acid acceptor for aminotransferase reactions, and it enhances the degradation of amino acids to metabolites such as aldehydes, alcohols, carboxylic acids, or hydroxy acids. The addition of α-ketoglutaric acid to the culture medium of LAB has been investigated mainly in cheese manufacturing, in which it enhances flavor by stimulation of amino acid catabolism (Vermeulen et al. 2006).

In general, LAB play a crucial role in the preservation and microbial safety of fermented foods, thus promoting the microbial stability of the final products of fermentation. Since, LAB naturally occur in various food products, they have traditionally been used as natural food biopreservatives. Protection of foods is due to the production of organic acids, carbon dioxide, ethanol, hydrogen peroxide and diacetyl, antifungal compounds such as fatty acids or phenyllactic acid, bacteriocins and antibiotics such as reutericyclin. Messens and De Vuyst (2002) have extensively reviewed the inhibitory substances produced by *Lactobacillus*. A fundamental feature of an antimicrobial substance to be active under food conditions is that it is produced at active concentrations and that the effect is not masked by food component.

8. Lactic acid bacteria and shelf-life of bread

Bread is a perishable commodity, whose shelf-life is normally limited by physiochemical deterioration called staling, leading to a hard and crumbly texture and a loss of fresh-bake flavor. The staling phenomenon has been intensively studied for decades, but a scientific and technological understanding of the mechanism of staling, however, is far from clear. Contamination of bread occurs after baking and airborne distribution of dust and mold spores is the main cause for bread spoilage. In addition to economical losses, bread spoilage also represents a health hazard for the consumers, especially when bread is contaminated with mycotoxigen molds. Modified atmosphere packaging, irradiation and addition of preservatives are among the most commonly used tools for prevention of bread spoilage. However, there is a definite need for other safe and efficient ways for preventing bread spoilage in order to respond to the increasing demand for natural, high quality products. Over the last decade, several studies have described the antifungal compounds produced by LAB and their activities against common bread spoilage organisms.

Lactic acid bacteria produce many antimicrobial substances, such as organic acids, CO_2, ethanol, hydrogen peroxide, diacetyl, fatty acids, phenyllactic acid, reuterin and fungicins. Among the organic acids, acetic and propionic acids produced by heterofermentative LAB are more effective than lactic acid. Caproic acid produced by *Lactobacillus sanfranciscensis*, together with a mixture of acetic, formic, propionic, butyric and N-valeric acids, play a key role in inhibiting *Fusarium*, *Penicillium*, *Aspergillus* and *Monilia* growth on bread. Also, *Lb. plantarum* shows a very broad antimicrobial activity, and the antifungal compounds 4-hydroxyphenyllactic and especially phenyllactic acids were identified as responsible for fungal inhibition (Ryan et al. 2009).

A synergistic effect was found when sourdough fermented with antifungal *Lb. plantarum* strains was used in combination with calcium propionate for production of wheat bread (Ryan et al. 2009). In particular, the presence of sourdough allowed reducing calcium propionate levels by around 30 percent, without affecting the shelf-life of bread. *Lactobacillus reuteri* was shown to produce in active concentrations reutericyclin, a low molecular weight antibiotic acting against Gram positive LAB and yeasts. *Lb. reuteri* strains have also been shown to produce reuterin, an antimicrobial substance active against bacteria, yeasts and fungi. Lactic acid bacteria are also effective against rope spoilage of bread induced by *Bacillus* sp., probably due to production of organic acids and other still unknown antibacterial substances.

Moore et al. (2008) used the antifungal strain *Lb. plantarum* to produce gluten-free sourdough from a mixture of brown rice, corn starch, buckwheat and soya flours. Fermenting 20 percent of the gluten-free flours with *Lb. plantarum* resulted in delaying the onset of staling in respect to chemically acidified gluten-free control breads. Furthermore, the antifungal activity of *Lb. plantarum* was retained during fermentation of gluten-free flours, and when 20 percent sourdough was added in the bread formulation, the growth of *Fusarium culmorum* was retarded up to 3 d in comparison to the control breads. The production of antifungal gluten-free sourdough can be regarded as a promising and valuable alternative to the use of additives for prolonging shelf-life and retarding staling of gluten-free breads. However, further research is needed to identify the optimal starters and fermentation conditions for achieving gluten-free bread of extended shelf-life and high quality.

9. Conclusions and perspectives

The present chapter concludes the predominant efficacy of sodium chloride, magnesium chloride, weak-acid preservatives and biopreservatives in bread. Mold spoilage and rope spoilage is still a major problem limiting the shelf-life of many high and intermediate moisture bread and bakery products. Losses due to mold spoilage have been resulting in lost revenue to the baking industries. Therefore, methods to control mold growth and to extend the shelf-life of bread is of great economic importance to the baking industry where an increased demand in global consumption exists. Other measures as good hygiene in the bakeries and if necessary complementary post packaging heat treatments or modified atmosphere packaging is the best alternatives. Effective alternatives would need to be sort before this can be effectively achieved. The future perspectives includes:

- Cleaning plans should be made which include all rooms, machines and appliances.
- Rules should be made to guarantee that the risk of foreign bodies in the bakery is drastically reduced (no glass in production rooms, no other small items that could fall in the dough).
- Hygiene training must be conducted regularly to show employees the possible consequences of acting unhygienically.
- All appliances which come into contact with non-baked fillings (cream mixers, Savoy bags, pots, etc.) must be washed hot or disinfected.

Keywords: Bakery products, bio-preservatives, bread, lactic acid bacteria, magnesium chloride, mold spoilage, rope spoilage, sodium chloride, weak preservatives

References

Bibbins Domingo, K., G.M. Chertow, P.G. Coxson, A. Moran, J.M. Lightwood, M.J. Pletcher and L. Goldman. 2010. Projected effect of dietary salt reductions on future cardiovascular disease. English Journal of Medicine, 362: 590–599.

Bidlas, E. and R.J.W. Lambert. 2008. Comparing the antimicrobial effectiveness of NaCl and KCl with a view to salt/sodium replacement. International Journal of Food Microbiology, 124: 98–102.

Certel, M., F. Erem and B. Karakas. 2009. Variation of microbiological properties, water activity and ropiness of white and whole meal bread under different storage conditions. GIDA—Journal of Food, 34: 351–358.

Dal Bello, F., C.I. Clarke, L.A. Ryan, H. Ulmer, T.J. Schober and K. Strom. 2007. Improvement of the quality and shelf-life of wheat bread by fermentation with the antifungal strain *Lactobacillus plantarum*. Journal of Cereal Science, 45: 309–318.

Deak, T. and L.R. Beuchat. 1993. Comparison of conductimetric and traditional plating techniques for detecting yeasts in fruit juices. Journal of Applied Bacteriology, 75: 546–550.

Eikenes, M., A.M. Hietala, G. Alfredsen, C.G. Fossdal and H. Solheim. 2005. Comparison of quantitative real-time PCR, chitin and ergosterol assays for monitoring colonization of *Trametes versicolor* in birch wood. Holzforschung, 59: 568–573.

FSA. 2009. Health effect of NaCl. pp. 115–120. Lyons & Burford, New York.

Girardin, H. 1997. Detection of filamentous fungi in foods. Science Des Aliments, 17: 3–19.

Guynot, M.E., A.J. Ramos, D. Sala, V. Sanchis and S. Marin. 2002. Combined effects of weak acid preservatives, pH and water activity on growth of *Eurotium* species on a sponge cake. International Journal of Food Microbiology, 76: 39–46.

Ingianni, A., M. Floris, P. Palomba, M.A. Madeddu, M. Quartuccio and R. Pompei. 2001. Rapid detection of *Listeria monocytogenes* in foods by a combination of PCR and DNA probe. Molecular and Cellular Probes, 15: 275–280.

Magan, N. 1993. Early detection of fungi in stored grain. International Biodeterioration and Biodegradation, 32: 145–160.

Magan, N. and D. Aldred. 2006. Managing microbial spoilage in cereal and bakery products. pp. 194–212. *In*: C.W. Blackburn (ed.). Food Spoilage Microorganisms. Woodhead Publications, Cambridge.

Makras, L., V. Triantafyllou, D. Fayol-Messaoudi, T. Adriany, G. Zoumpopoulou, E. Tsakalidou, A. Servin and L. De Vuyst. 2006. Kinetic analysis of the antibacterial activity of probiotic *Lactobacillus* sp. towards *Salmonella enterica* serovar *typhimurium* reveals a role for lactic acid and other inhibitory compounds. Research in Microbiology, 157: 241–247.

Marin, S., M. Abellana, M. Rubinat, V. Sanchis and A.J. Ramos. 2003. Efficacy of sorbates on the control of the growth of *Eurotium* species in bakery products with near neutral pH. International Journal of Food Microbiology, 87: 251–258.

Membre, J.M., M. Kubaczka and C. Chene. 2001. Growth rate and growth-no-growth interface of *Penicillium brevicompactum* as functions of pH and preservative acids. Food Microbiology, 18: 531–538.

Messens, W. and L.De Vuyst. 2002. Inhibitory substances produced by *Lactobacillus* isolated from sourdoughs–a review. International Journal of Food Microbiology, 72: 31–43.

Moore, M., F. Dal Bello and E. Arendt. 2008. Sourdough fermented by *Lactobacillus plantarum* improves the quality and shelf-life of gluten-free bread. European Food Research and Technology, 226: 1309–1316.

Needham, R., J. Williams, N. Beales, P. Voysey and N. Magan. 2005. Early detection and differentiation of spoilage of bakery products. Sensors and Actuators, B 106: 20–23.

Parra, R., D. Aldred, D.B. Archer and N. Magan. 2004. Water activity, solute and temperature modify growth and spore production of wild type and genetically engineered *Aspergillus niger* strains. Enzyme Microbial Technology, 35: 232–237.

Parra, R. and N. Megan. 2004. Modeling of the effect of temperature and water activity on growth of *Aspergillus niger* strains and applications for food spoilage molds. Journal of Applied Microbiology, 97: 429–438.

Petrulakova, Z., E. Hybenova, P. Gerekova, M. Kockov and E. Sturdik. 2010. Opatija—Proceedings of the 5th International Congress Flour-Bread `09: 409–415.

Pitt, J.I. and A.D. Hocking. 1994. Modern methods for detecting and enumerating food borne fungi. pp. 232–254. *In*: P.D. Patel (ed.). Rapid Analysis Techniques in Food Microbiology. Blackie Academic and Professional, London.

Potter, H. and I. Hotchkiss. 2006. Food Science (5th Edition). CBS Publishers and Distributors, New Delhi.

Rumeus, I. and M. Turtoi. 2013. Influence of sourdough use on rope spoilage of wheat bread. Journal of Agroalimentary Processes and Technologies, 19: 94–98.

Ryan, L.A.M., F.D. Bello, M. Czerny, P. Koehler and E.K. Arendt. 2009. Quantification of phenyllactic acid in wheat sourdough using high resolution Gas Chromatography-Mass Spectrometry. Journal of Agricultural and Food Chemistry, 57: 1060–1064.

Samadpour, M., J. Liston, J.E. Ongerth and P.I. Tarr. 1990. Evaluation of DNA probes for detection of shiga-like-toxin-producing *Escherichia coli* in food and calf fecal samples. Applied and Environmental Microbiology, 56: 1212–1215.

Samapundo, S., N. Deschuyffeleer, D. Van Laere, I. De Leync and F. Devlieghere. 2010. Effect of NaCl reduction and replacement on the growth of fungi important to the spoilage of bread. Food Microbiology, 20: 1–8.

Samkutty, P.J., R.H. Gough, R.W. Adkinson and P. McGrew. 2001. Rapid assessment of the bacteriological quality of bread using ATP bioluminescence. Journal of Food Protection, 64: 208–212.

Saranraj, P. and M. Geetha. 2012. Microbial spoilage of bakery products and its control by preservatives. International Journal of Pharmaceutical and Biological Archives, 3: 38–48.

Silley, P. and S. Forsythe. 1996. Impedance microbiology: a rapid change for microbiologists. Journal of Applied Bacteriology, 80: 233–243.

Suleman, P., A. Al-Musallam and C.A. Menezes. 2001. The effect of solute potential and water stress on Black scorch caused by *Chalara paradoxa* and *Chalara radicicola* on date palms. Plant Disease, 85: 80–83.

Torres, A.M., M.L. Ramirez, M.L. Arroyo, S.N. Chulze and N. Magan. 2003. Potential use of antioxidants for control of growth and fumonisin production by *Fusarium verticilliodes* and *Fusarium proliferatum* on wheat maize grain. International Journal of Food Microbiology, 83: 319–324.

Valerio, F., P. De Bellis, S.L. Lonigro, A. Visconti and P. Lavermicocca. 2008. Use of *Lactobacillus plantarum* fermentation products in bread-making to prevent *Bacillus subtilis* ropy spoilage. International Journal of Food Microbiology, 122: 328–332.

Valerio, F., P. De Bellis, M. Di Biase, S.L. Lonigro, B. Giussani, A. Visconti, P. Lavermicocca and A. Sisto. 2012. Diversity of spore-forming bacteria and identification of *Bacillus amyloliquefaciens* as a species frequently associated with the ropy spoilage of bread. International Journal of Food Microbiology, 156: 278–285.

Vermeulen, N., M.G. Ganzle and R.F. Vogel. 2006. Influence of peptide supply and co-substrates on phenylalanine metabolism of *Lactobacillus sanfranciscensis* and *Lactobacillus plantarum*. Journal of Agricultural Food Chemistry, 54: 3832–3839.

Ybar, A., F. Cetinkaya and G.E. Soyutemiz. 2012. Detection of rope-producing *Bacillus* in bread and identification of isolates to species level by Vitek 2 System. Journal of Biological and Environmental Sciences, 6: 243–248.

8

Bread Fungal Contamination: Risk of Mycotoxins, Protection of Anti-fungal and Need to Fungal Identification

Yehia A.-G. Mahmoud[1,2,*] and *Aly F. El Sheikha*[3,4]

1. Introduction

Mold is a term used to commonly describe the wooly growth that occurs on damp or decaying organic matter caused from the growth of fungi. There are more than a million species of fungi. Fungi are plant-like organisms that lack chlorophyll. Since fungi do not produce chlorophyll for food, fungi must absorb food from other sources. Fungi are able to grow in damp and dark places. Fungi generally consume dead matter such as paper, leaves, cardboard and wood (Moore et al. 2011).

Molds are able to grow on all kinds of food: cereals, meat, milk, fruit, vegetables, nuts, fats and products of these. The mold growth may result in several kinds of food-spoilage: off-flavors, toxins, discoloration, rotting and formation of pathogenic or allergenic propagules (Wareing 2012).

[1] Tanta University, Faculty of Science, Botany and Microbiology Department, Mycology Research, Laboratory, 31527 Tanta, Egypt.
[2] Al-Baha University, Faculty of Science, Department of Biology, P.O. Box 1988, Al-Baha, Saudi Arabia. Email: yehiamah@gmail.com
[3] Minufiya University, Faculty of Agriculture, Department of Food Science and Technology, 32511 Shibin El Kom, Minufiya Government, Egypt.
[4] Al-Baha University, Faculty of Science, Department of Biology, P.O. Box 1988, Al-Baha, Saudi Arabia. Email: elsheikha_aly@yahoo.com
* Corresponding author

Several mycotoxins have very significant antibiotic activity as well, which in time may give rise to bacteria with a cross-resistance to the most important antibiotic used today, like penicillin. The mycotoxins are formed during growth of molds on foods. Some of mycotoxins are only present in the mold, while most of them are excreted in the foods. In liquid foods and in fruits like peaches, pears and tomatoes the diffusion of mycotoxins can be very fast, leaving no part of the product uncontaminated (Scott 1991).

Organisms that cause food spoilage—molds, yeasts and bacteria—are always present in the air, water and soil. Enzymes that may cause undesirable changes in flavor, color and texture are present in raw fruits, bakery products, like many processed foods, and are subject to physical, chemical and microbiological spoilage (Smith et al. 2004). The major problem for long-term shelf life of baked goods is contamination with fungi (Coda et al. 2011). Molds attack many foods and produce potent toxic substances known as mycotoxins that are very dangerous to human health and life.

This chapter will highlight through its parts the risk posed by fungi that contaminate the bread on the health and will try to answer for the following questions: How you can identify those fungal species? What are the latest and the fastest and most efficient methods used in this purpose? and how the determination of fungus-contaminated species will reflect on the dangers that would result? What are the methods used to prevent or avoid fungal contamination of bread?

2. The fungal contamination in bread

Bread is the major component in the overall consumption of grains, particularly whole grains. There is an increasing variety of organic, "natural," and conventional bread—white, wheat, whole wheat, sprouted wheat, and gluten-free. Bakery products and cereals are a valuable source of nutrients in our diet providing us with most of our food calories and approximately half of our protein requirements. Cereals have been a basic food of man since prehistoric times and were consumed long before bread making was developed. Variety breads and other bakery products have increased in sales volume within the past decades. The nutrients in bakery products are carbohydrates, proteins, lipids, vitamins and minerals (Chavan and Kadam 1993).

Storage of bread under conditions of low humidity retards mold growth. In addition to the economic losses associated with bakery products, another concern is the possibility of mycotoxins production. *Eurotium* species are usually the first fungi to colonize improperly water allowing other species, *Aspergillus* and *Penicillium,* which can produce toxins to thrive. Losses of bakery products due to mold spoilage vary between 1–5 percent depending on seasons, type of products and methods of processing (Abellana et al. 1997). Since, filamentous fungi are more easily recognized than yeast, they generate the majority of complaints. Longer shelf life enables a greater variety of products to be kept in store and in the home (Abellana et al. 2000). Spoilage from microbial growth causes economic loss for both manufacturers and consumers. These losses could be due to many individual cases such as packaging, sanitary practice in manufacturing, storage conditions and product turnover. Needham et al. (2005) tested the microbial spoilage caused by bacteria, yeast and fungi and enzymic spoilage caused by lipoxygenase can be differentiated from one another and from unspoiled bread analogues after 48 hr using cluster analysis, prior to signs of visible spoilage.

Figure 1 illustrates that the several species of fungi can grow on different types of bread.

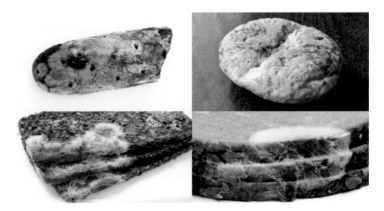

Figure 1. Diversity of fungi that grow on the different types of bread.

All details concerning the fungal spoilage in bread have been discussed before in Chapter 7 of this book (Microorganisms Involved in Spoilage of Bread and Its Control Measures).

Consumers today are not in favor of additives as preservatives and an urge to reduce the quantities used exists within the bakery industry (Membre et al. 2001). In general, most molds prefer high water potential (a_w values > 0.8) while a few xerophilic molds prefer to grow at a_w values as low as 0.65. Mold growth on bakery products is a serious problem that results in economic losses. Furthermore, losses of products due to mold spoilage are between 1 and 5 percent depending on the type of product, season, and the method of processing (Malkki and Rauha 2000). According to Hickey (1998), losses due to mold spoilage in the bakery industry average about 200 million pounds of product each year. Mold spores are generally killed by the baking process in fresh bread and other baked products. Therefore, for bread to become moldy, it must be contaminated either from the air, bakery surfaces, equipment, food handlers or raw ingredients after baking during the cooling, slicing or wrapping operations. This means that all spoilage problems caused by molds must occur after baking. Furthermore, moisture condensation on a product's surface, due to packaging prior to being completely cooled, may be conductive to mold growth. Jarvis (2001) found that mold spoilage caused undesirable odors and is often found on the surface of the product. Bakery products once considered as sick man's diet have now become essential food items of the vast majority of population (Saranraj and Geetha 2012).

3. Physical factors influence the fungal growth

Physical factors are the important factors governing mold-free shelf life of bakery products. It plays a decisive role when molds compete with bacteria to spoil high moisture foods (Ponte et al. 1993). Molds tend to be less fastidious in their relationships to pH than bacteria. Generally, molds are tolerant of acid conditions and favor an acidic pH (3.5–5.5). Therefore, foods with pH value < 4.5 are not usually spoiled by bacteria but are more susceptible to mold spoilage.

3.1 Water activity (a_w)

Abellana et al. (1999) obtained a method for studying the growth of xerophilic fungi on bakery products, and to determine the effect of water activity (a_w), temperature, isolates and their interaction on mycelial growth of *Eurotium* sp. The results showed that there were intra-isolate differences (P, 0.001) due to water activity (a_w), temperature, isolate, and two- and three-way interaction. Optimum growth of all isolates over water activity (a_w) temperature range tested showed optimum at 0.90 a_w and 30°C, with an interval of growth rate of 3.8–5.1 mm.d^{-1} at 0.75 a_w, growth was less than 0.15 mm.d^{-1}. *Aspergillus flavus* was able to grow at 0.90 a_w when the temperature was above 15.8°C. They showed that fungal growth by these species on a sponge cake analogue, with a composition similar to usual bakery products, was prevented if the a_w is kept at 0.85. Vytřasová et al. (2002) detected, isolated and identified xerophilic fungi *Eurotium amstelodami*, *Eurotium chevalieri*, *Eurotium herbariorum*, *Eurotium rubrum* and *Wallemia sebi*. Water activity at levels of 0.80 to 0.90 had a significant influence on fungal growth and determined the concentration of CO_2 needed to prevent cake analogue spoilage. At a_w level of 0.85, lag phases increased two-fold when the level of CO_2 in the headspace increased from 0 to 70 percent. In general, no fungal growth was observed for up to 28 d of incubation at 25°C when samples were packaged with 100 percent CO_2, regardless of water potential level. In general, most molds prefer high a_w values (> 0.8) while a few xerophilic molds prefer to grow at a_w values as low as 0.65.

3.2 Effect of temperature

Temperature plays a dominant role in mold growth and in the germination of spores. The majority of molds grow within a temperature range of 18.3–29.4°C. Chamberlain (1993) reported that the reduction in the storage temperature from 27°C to 21°C doubled the mold-free shelf life of cake and emphasized the need for care during distribution and storage.

3.3 Effect of pH

Guynot et al. (2005) studied the mold growth on fermented bakery product analogues (FBPA) of two different pH (4.5 and 5.5), different water activity (a_w) levels (0.80–0.90) and potassium sorbate concentrations (0–0.3 percent) by using seven molds commonly causing spoilage of bakery products (*Eurotium* sp., *Aspergillus* sp. and *Penicillium corylophilum*). For the description of fungal growth as a function of a_w, potassium sorbate concentration and pH, 10 terms polynomial models were developed. Modeling enables prediction of spoilage during storage as a function of the factors affecting fungal growth. At pH 4.5 the concentration of potassium sorbate could be reduced to some extent only at low levels of a_w, whereas at pH 5.5 fungal growths were observed even by adding 0.3 percent of potassium sorbate.

3.4 Effect of salt tolerance

The effect of NaCl and various NaCl replacers ($CaCl_2$, $MgCl_2$, KCl and $MgSO_4$) on the growth of *Penicillium roqueforti* and *Aspergillus niger* at 22°C have been evaluated by Samapundo et al. (2010). In addition, challenge tests were performed on white bread to determine the consequences of NaCl reduction with or without partial replacement on the growth of *Penicillium roqueforti*. The results obtained concluded that at equivalent water phase concentrations the isolates exhibited differing sensitivities to the salts evaluated with NaCl and $MgCl_2$ having the greatest inhibitory action on the growth of *Aspergillus niger* and *Penicillium roqueforti*, respectively. $MgSO_4$ had the least antifungal activity. At equivalent molalities, $CaCl_2$ had in general the largest antifungal activity. Although the water activity (a_w) lowering effects of the compounds studied play a large role in explaining the trends observed, at equivalent water phase concentrations $MgCl_2$ was found to have a smaller inhibitory effect on *Aspergillus niger* than that expected from its a_w depressing effect. The challenge tests revealed that no difference occurred in the growth of *Penicillium roqueforti* on standard white bread, bread with 30 percent less NaCl and bread in which 30 percent of the NaCl has been partially replaced by a mixture of KCl and Sub-salt.

4. Control of fungal contamination in bread

Several approaches can be used to control mold growth on bakery products including reformulation, freezing, and most commonly, the use of preservatives.

4.1 Reformulation to reduce bread A_w

Reformulation involves a reduction of available water, e.g., a_w in bakery products to obtain a longer shelf life. Reduction in product a_w can be achieved by dehydration, either through evaporation or freeze-drying or by high osmotically active additives, e.g., sugars and salts, incorporated directly into the food. The degree of a_w reduction is of practical significance in making a food non-perishable. The response to a given degree of a_w varies greatly among microorganisms in different environments (Gourama 1991). Water contained in solutions of sugars and salt becomes unavailable to microbes due to the increased concentration of crystalloid. Furthermore, microbes are directly damaged osmotically by concentrations of these substances. This effect may be due to the adverse influence of lowered water availability on all metabolic activities, since all chemical reaction of cells require an aqueous environment. Control of mold growth in bakery products normally relies on maintaining a sufficiently low a_w (Saranraj and Geetha 2012).

4.2 Freezing

It has been used for long term preservation of bakery products, particularly cream filled products. Quick freezing is important in controlling the formation of ice crystals. Large ice crystals are formed when the rate of freezing is slower; the large crystals can disrupt membranes and internal cellular structures (Banwart 2004).

Cakes, cookies, short cakes and pancakes are commonly frozen and marketed in the frozen form. Bread has been held fresh for many months by storage at –22°C (Desrosier and Desrosier 2006). In contrast to fresh bread, which stales in less than a week, frozen bread stales very slowly. Therefore, the lower the temperature, the more slowly it stales. Desrosier and Desrosier (2006) reported that bread frozen quickly after baking and held for one year at –18°C, was equivalent in softness to fresh bread held for two days at 20°C.

4.3 Preservatives

Preservatives are most commonly used to control mold growth in baked goods. The Code of Federal Regulations (CFR) defines preservatives "as an antimicrobial agent used to preserve food by preventing growth of microorganisms and subsequent spoilage". There are two classifications of preservatives: chemical and natural. Permitted chemical mold inhibitors in bread include acetic, sorbic, propionic acids and their salts. Natural food preservatives, such as cultured products, raisins and vinegar, are identified by their common name on the ingredient statement (Saranraj and Geetha 2012).

Effect of biopreservatives

In recent years, bio-preservative (the use of microorganisms and their metabolites to prevent spoilage and to extend the shelf life of foods) has gained increasing interest due to consumer's demands. Lactic acid bacteria (LAB) as bio-preservation organisms are of particular interest. The inclusion of antifungal LAB strains in the starter culture allowed a reduction in the calcium propionate concentration as a preservative (Hassan and Bullerman 2008).

5. Mycotoxins

Mycotoxins are low-molecular-weight natural products (i.e., small molecules) produced as secondary metabolites by filamentous fungi. These metabolites constitute a toxigenically and chemically heterogeneous assemblage that is grouped together only because the members can cause disease and death in human beings and other vertebrates. Mycotoxin from *Aspergillus flavus* known as aflatoxins. Mycotoxins sensitized scientists to the possibility that other occult mold metabolites might be deadly. Soon, the mycotoxin rubric was extended to include a number of previously known fungal toxins (e.g., the ergot alkaloids), some compounds that had originally been isolated as antibiotics (e.g., patulin), and a number of new secondary metabolites revealed in screens targeted at mycotoxin discovery (e.g., ochratoxin A). Other low-molecular-weight fungal metabolites such as ethanol that are toxic only in high concentrations are not considered mycotoxins (Turner et al. 2009; FDA 2013).

Currently, more than 400 mycotoxins are identified in the world. Considering their heat stability, these substances constitute a potential risk for human and animal health. Mycotoxins deteriorate the marketable quality of the contaminated products, causing heavy economic losses (Zinedine et al. 2007). Aflatoxins are often present in cereals (maize, sorghum, rice and wheat), oilseeds, spices and nuts. Aflatoxins were classified as group 1 carcinogen by the International Agency of Research on Cancer (IARC). Table 1 indicates the different types of mycotoxins produced by just two common fungal groups Asperglli and Penicilli (Tančinová et al. 2012) and there are many other types of mycotoxins produced by the rest of fungal groups.

Table 1. *In vitro* production of mycotoxins by aspergilli and penicilli isolated from breads.

Species	Number of tested isolates	Detection toxin	Evaluation +	Evaluation −
Aspergillus flavus	7	AFB1, AFG1		7
	7	CPA	7	
Aspergillus section *Nigri*	1	OTA		1
Penicillium chrysogenum	9	ROC	9	
Penicillium crustosum	8	ROC	8	
	9	PA	9	
Penicillium expansum	1	PAT		1
	1	ROC	1	
	1	CIT		1
Penicillium roqueforti	1	ROC	1	

AFB1—aflatoxin B1, AFG1—aflatoxin G1, CPA—cyklopiazonic acid, OTA—ochratoxin A, PA—penitrem A, PAT—patulin, ROC—roquefortin C, + production of mycotoxin confirmed, – production of mycotoxin was not detected
Source: Tančinová et al. 2012

According to the Food and Agriculture Organization of the United Nations (FAO 1997) over 25 percent of the agricultural commodities worldwide are significantly contaminated by mycotoxins. The best protection against mycotoxins is to monitor their presence in food.

Cell biologists put them into generic groups such as teratogens, mutagens, carcinogens and allergens. Organic chemists have attempted to classify them by their chemical structures (e.g., lactones, coumarins); biochemists according to their biosynthetic origins (polyketides, amino acid-derived, etc.); physicians by the illnesses they cause (e.g., St. Anthony's fire, stachybotryotoxicosis), and mycologists by the fungi that produce them (e.g., *Aspergillus* toxins, *Penicillium* toxins) (Zain 2011).

None of these classifications is entirely satisfactory. Moreover, as our anthropomorphic focus shifts attention, the same compound may get placed in different cognitive cubbyholes. Aflatoxin, for example, is a hepatotoxic, mutagenic, carcinogenic, difuran-containing, polyketide-derived *Aspergillus* toxin. Zearalenone is a *Fusarium* metabolite with potent estrogenic activity; hence, in addition to being called (probably erroneously) a mycotoxin, it also has been labeled a phytoestrogen, a mycoestrogen, and a growth promotant (Bennett and Klich 2003).

5.1 It is possible to decontaminate the mycotoxins

Several approaches have been developed for decontamination of mycotoxins in foods (Juodeikiene et al. 2012):

* Prevention of contamination;
* decontamination of mycotoxin-containing food and feed; and
* inhibition or absorption of mycotoxin content of consumed food into the digestive tract.

Additionally, knowledge of enzymes that take part in degradation of mycotoxins opens some new approaches (Halász et al. 2009):

* The production of genetically modified species of microorganisms commonly used in food production and their use for production of enzymes mentioned above; or
* the transfer of genes coding for these enzymes to transgenic plants and use the plants for production of mycotoxin degrading enzymes.

How to decontaminate the mycotoxins of the bread?

Prevention of mycotoxin formation is the best defense for protecting the consumer's health. However, prevention is not always possible, especially for those mycotoxins formed under field conditions. Introduction of further legislation for a wider range of mycotoxins in more food commodities means that there is a much greater need to determine how mycotoxins survive processing so that this can be taken into account when setting statutory or guideline limits. It is thus expected that there will be a trend towards further study of the fate of those mycotoxins that pose the greatest potential risk for humans. In some instances it may then be possible to introduce modifications to commercial processes that result in a significant reduction of mycotoxin content in the retail product. Gerez et al. (2009) have also investigated the ability of some LAB strains to inhibit *Aspergillus, Fusarium* and *Penicillium*, the main contaminants in bread. They assayed 95 strains of LAB and indicated that only four strains— *Lb. plantarum* CRL 778, *Lb. reuteri* CRL 1100, *Lb. brevis* CRL 772 and *Lb. brevis* CRL 796—displayed antifungal activity against tested molds. They observed that the inclusion of antifungal LAB strains in the starter culture allowed a reduction in the concentration of calcium propionate by 50 percent while still attaining the shelf life similar to that of traditional bread containing 0.4 percent calcium propionate.

Currently, in staple food such as bread and bakery products in the flour sector, yeast and lactobacilli now play an important role. It thus stands to reason that the same microbes and enzymes are the first to have been considered for use as detoxifying or decontaminating agents. This type of biodegradation could therefore prove a useful strategy for partially overcoming the problem of some mycotoxins. Indeed, this already takes place in bread and in sourdough processes (Bartkiene et al. 2008). This might offer new possibilities for reducing this mycotoxin in bread and bakery products and their raw materials (Patharajan et al. 2011).

6. Mycotoxins in bakery products: safety and regulations

The economic consequences of mycotoxin contamination are profound. Crops with large amounts of mycotoxins often have to be destroyed. Alternatively, contaminated crops are sometimes diverted into animal feed. Giving contaminated feeds to susceptible animals can lead to reduced growth rates, illness, and death. Moreover, animals consuming mycotoxin contaminated feeds can produce meat and milk that contain toxic residues and biotransformation products. Thus, aflatoxins in cattle feed can be metabolized by cows into aflatoxin M1, which is then secreted in milk (Van Egmond 1989). Ochratoxin in pig feed can accumulate in porcine tissues (Rutqvist et al. 1978). Court actions between grain farmers, livestock owners, and feed companies can involve considerable amounts of money. The ability to diagnose and verify mycotoxicoses is an important forensic aspect of the mycotoxin problem (Pier et al. 1980).

Many mycotoxins survive processing into flours and meals. When mold-damaged materials are processed into foods and feeds, they may not be detectable without special assay equipment. It is important to have policies in place that ensure that such "hidden" mycotoxins do not pose a significant hazard to human health.

The web sites for these commissions and organizations are excellent sources for the latest information. See, for example, the Council for Agricultural Science and Technology (www.cast-science.org), the Mycotoxicology Newsletter (www.mycotoxicology.org), the Society for Mycotoxin Research (www.mycotoxin.de), the American Oil Chemists Society Technical Committee on Mycotoxins (www.aocs.org), the Food and Agriculture Organization of the United Nations (www.fao.org), the International Union for Pure and Applied Chemistry Section on Mycotoxins and Phycotoxins (www.iupac.org), the Japanese Association of Mycotoxicology (www.chujo-u.ac.jp/myco/index.html), and the US Food and Drug Administration Committee on Additives and Contaminants (www.fda.gov).

Since it is normally impracticable to prevent the formation of mycotoxins, the food industry has established internal monitoring methods. Similarly, government regulatory agencies survey for the occurrence of mycotoxins in foods and feeds have established regulatory limits. Guidelines for establishing these limits are based on epidemiological data and extrapolations from animal models, taking into account the inherent uncertainties associated with both types of analysis. Estimations of an appropriate safe dose are usually stated as a tolerable daily intake (Smith et al. 1995; Kuiper-Goodman 1998).

Complete elimination of any natural toxicant from foods is an unattainable objective. Therefore, naturally occurring toxins such as mycotoxins are regulated quite differently from food additives (FAO 1997). The US Food and Drug Administration, the European Union, the Institute of Public Health in Japan, and many other governmental agencies around the world test products for aflatoxins and other mycotoxins and have established guidelines for safe doses, but there is a need for worldwide harmonization of mycotoxin regulations. The United States uses one set of guidelines, the European Union uses another, and Japan yet another, and many other guidelines have also been developed. Unfortunately, sometimes the regulatory community seems to be setting limits based more on current analytical capabilities than on realistic health factors (Wilson et al. 2002).

7. The molds contaminated bread must be identified...Why?

Many species of fungi are pathogenic and toxigenic. Thus, identification of potentially harmful microbes to species level is important for early diagnosis and environmental monitoring (Cornea et al. 2011).

Historically, the chief type of microbial spoilage of bakery industry has been moldiness. It is estimated that approximately 1–5 percent of the bread production goes wrong due to fungi activity. Referring to bread, mold contamination determines not only changes in color, taste, but also loss of the food quality as a result of possible formation of mycotoxins.

Moldiness is caused by external contamination of bread after baking, because the existing spores in flour during a normal technological process don't have any multiplication conditions, and during baking they are destroyed. Bread contamination with molds may occur in the following steps: the transportation of bread; during cooling and storage; and while cutting and packing (Vagelas et al. 2011).

7.1 Molecular approaches benefits

Generally, the traditional methods for identification of fungi species are based on the morphological characteristics of the colony and microscopic examination depend on the experience of the examiner are very time-consuming, laborious, and requires facilities and mycological expertise (Edwards et al. 2002). Moreover, these methods have low degree of sensitivity and do not allow the specification of mycotoxigenic species (Zhao et al. 2001). PCR-based methods that target DNA are considered a good alternative for rapid diagnosis because of their high specificity and sensitivity, and have been used for the detection of mycotoxigenic fungi (Somashekar et al. 2004).

Frisvad et al. (2006) detected specific spoilage molds of bread namely, *Penicillium roqueforti* and *P. carneum* based on the ribosomal gene sequences. One primer pair is group specific for *Penicillium* Subgenus *Penicillium*. The other primer set identified the two species *P. roqueforti* and *P. carneum*.

In the other study, Cornea et al. (2011) reported that the PCR method allowed identification of three species of potential toxigenic fungi: *Aspergillus flavus, A. niger* and *A. ochraceus* from bakeries. Moreover, molecular methods applied for the detection of some genes involved in aflatoxin biosynthesis led to the identification of aflatoxigenic strains of *A. flavus*.

8. Conclusions and future perspectives

Bakery products, like many processed foods especially bread, are subject to physical, chemical and microbiological spoilage. Filamentous microscopic fungi are the most frequent cause of bread decay. Although the bread is included in commodities with short durability, there is an effort to prolong it.

Mold spoilage is still a major problem limiting the shelf life of many high and intermediate moisture bakery products. Losses due to mold spoilage have been resulting in lost revenue to the baking industries. Therefore, methods to control mold growth and to extend the shelf life of bakery products is of great economic importance to the baking industry where an increased demand in global consumption exists. Other measures as good hygiene in the bakeries and if necessary complementary post packaging heat treatments or modified atmosphere packaging is the best alternatives.

Prevention of mycotoxin formation is the best defense for protecting the consumer's health. However, prevention is not always possible, especially for those mycotoxins formed under field conditions. There is a great need to determine how mycotoxins survive processing so that this can be taken into account when setting statutory or guideline limits. It is thus expected that there will be a trend towards further study of the fate of those mycotoxins that pose the greatest potential risk for humans. In some instances it may then be possible to introduce modifications to commercial processes that result in a significant reduction of mycotoxin content in the retail product. Introducing of further legislation for a wider range of mycotoxins in more food commodities in future. Also, the use of such methods could be of great interest to assess fungal contamination in bread as well as in food products.

Keywords: *Aspergillus*, bread moldiness, fungal control, molecular identification, mycotoxins, mycotoxins decontamination, *penicillium*, physical factors

References

Abellana, M., A.J. Ramos, V. Sanchis and P.V. Nielsen. 2000. Effect of modified atmosphere packaging and water activity on growth of *Eurotium amstelodami, E. chevalieri* and *E. herbariorum* on a sponge cake analogue. Journal of Applied Microbiology, 88: 606–616.

Abellana, M., X. Magri, V. Sanchis and A.J. Ramos. 1999. Water activity and temperature effects on growth of *Eurotium amstelodami, E. chevalier* and *E. herbaviorum* on a sponge cake analogue. International Journal of Microbiology, 52: 97–103.

Abellana, M., L. Torres, V. Sanchis and A.J. Ramos. 1997. Caracterización de diferentes productos de bollería industrial. II. Estudio de la micoflora. Alimentaria, 287: 51–56.

Banwart, G.J. 2004. Basic Food Microbiology, 2nd ed. Chapman & Hall Inc., New York.

Bartkiene, E., G. Juodeikiene and D. Vidmantiene. 2008. Evaluation of deoxynivalenol in wheat by acoustic method and impact of starter on its concentration during wheat bread baking process. Food Chemistry and Technology, 42: 5–12.

Bennett, J.W. and M. Klich. 2003. Mycotoxins. Clinical Microbiology Reviews, 16: 497–516.

Chamberlain, N. 1993. Mould growth on cake. Biscuit Maker and Plant Baker, 14: 961–964.

Chavan, J.K. and S.S. Kadam. 1993. Nutritional enrichment of bakery products by supplementation with nonwheat flours. Critical Review of Food Science Nutrition, 33: 189–226.

Coda, R., A. Cassone, C.G. Rizzello, L. Nionelli, G. Cardinali and M. Gobbetti. 2011. Antifungal activity of *Wickerhamomyces anomalous* and *Lactobacillus plantarum* during sourdough fermentation: identification of novel compounds and long-term effect during storage of wheat bread. Applied Environmental Microbiology, 77: 3484–3492.

Cornea, C.P., M. Ciucă, C. Voaides, V. Gagiu and A. Pop. 2011. Incidence of fungal contamination in a Romanian bakery: A molecular approach. Romanian Biotechnological Letters, 16: 5863–5871.

Desrosier, J.N. and N.W. Desrosier. 2006. The Technology of Food Preservation, 4th ed. CBS Publishers & Distributors Pvt. Ltd., New Delhi.

Edwards, S.G., J. O'Callaghan and A.D.W. Dobson. 2002. PCR-based detection and quantification of mycotoxigenic fungi. Mycological Research, 106: 1005–1025.

FAO. 1997. Worldwide Regulations for Mycotoxins 1995. A compendium. FAO Food and Nutrition Paper No. 64. Rome, Italy.

FDA. 2013. Food and Drug Administration. ORA Lab Manual, Volume IV, Section 7-Mycotoxin Analysis. pp. 1–23. Available online: http://www.fda.gov/downloads/ScienceResearch/FieldScience/UCM092245.pdf.

Frisvad, J.C., U. Thrane, R.A. Samson and J.I. Pitt. 2006. Important mycotoxins and the fungi which produce them. pp. 3–32. *In*: A.D. Hocking, J.I. Pitt, R.A. Samson and U. Thrane (eds.). Advances in Food Mycology, Vol. 571. Springer, New York.

Gerez, C.L., M.I. Torino, G. Rollan and G. Font de Valdez. 2009. Prevention of bread mould spoilage by using lactic acid bacteria with antifungal properties. Food Control, 20: 144–148.

Gourama, H. 1991. Growth and aflatoxin production of *Aspergillus flavus* in the presence *Lactobacillus* species. Ph.D. Thesis, University of Nebraska-Lincoln, Nebraska.

Guynot, M.E., S. Marin, V. Sanchis and A.J. Ramos. 2005. An attempt to optimize potassium sorbate use to preserve low pH (4.5–5.5) intermediate moisture bakery products by modelling *Eurotium* spp., *Aspergillus* spp. and *Penicillium corylophilum* growth. International Journal of Food Microbiology, 101: 169–177.

Halász, A., R. Lásztity, T. Abonyi and Á. Bata. 2009. Decontamination of mycotoxin-containing food and feed by biodegradation. Food Reviews International, 25: 284–298.

Hassan, Y.I. and L.B. Bullerman. 2008. Antifungal activity of *Lactobacillus paracasei* subsp. tolerans against *Fusarium proliferatum* and *Fusarium graminearum* in a liquid culture setting. Journal of Food Protection, 71: 2213–2216.

Hickey, C.S. 1998. Sorbate spray application for protecting yeast-raised bakery products. Baker's Digest, 54: 4–7.

Jarvis, B. 2001. Mould spoilage of food. Process Biochemistry, 7: 11–14.

Juodeikiene, G., L. Basinskiene, E. Bartkiene and P. Matusevicius. 2012. Mycotoxin decontamination aspects in food, feed and renewables using fermentation processes. pp. 171–204. *In*: A.A. Eissa (ed.). Structure and Function of Food Engineering. InTech., Rijeka.

Kuiper-Goodman, T. 1998. Food safety: Mycotoxins and phycotoxins in perspective. pp. 25–48. *In*: M. Miraglia, H. van Egmond, C. Brera and J. Gilbert (eds.). Mycotoxins and Phycotoxins—Developments in Chemistry, Toxicology and Food Safety. International Union of Pure and Applied Chemistry (IUPAC), Oxford U.K.

Malkki, Y. and O. Rauha. 2000. Mould inhibition by aerosols. Baker's Digest, 52: 47–50.

Membre, J.M., M. Kubaczka and C. Chene. 2001. Growth rate and growth-no-growth interface of *Penicillium brevicompactum* as functions of pH and preservative acids. Food Microbiology, 18: 531–538.

Moore, D., G.D. Robson and A.P.J. Trinci. 2011. 21st Century Guidebook to Fungi, 1st ed. Cambridge University Press, Cambridge.

Needham, R., J. William, N. Beales, P. Voysey and N. Magan. 2005. Early detection and differentiation of spoilage of bakery products. Sensors and Actuators B: Chemical, 106: 20–23.

Patharajan, S., K.R.N. Reddy, V. Karthikeyan, D. Spadaro, A. Lore, M.L. Gullino and A. Garibaldi. 2011. Potential of yeast antagonists on *in vitro* biodegradation of ochratoxin A. Food Control, 22: 290–296.

Pier, A.C., J.L. Richard and S.J. Cysewski. 1980. Implications of mycotoxins in animal disease. Journal of the American Veterinary Medical Association, 176: 719–724.

Ponte, J.G., J.D. Payne and M.E. Ingelin.1993. The shelf life of bakery foods. pp. 1143–1197. *In*: G. Charalambous (ed.). Shelf Life of Foods and Beverages. Elsevier Inc., Philadelphia.

Rutqvist, L., N.-E. Bjorklund, K. Hult, E. Hockby and B. Carlsson. 1978. Ochratoxin A as the cause of spontaneous nephropathy in fattening pigs. Applied and Environmental Microbiology, 36: 920–925.

Samapundo, S., N. Deschuyffeleer, D. Van Laere, I. De Leyn and F. Devlieghere. 2010. Effect of NaCl reduction and replacement on the growth of fungi important to the spoilage of bread. Food Microbiology, 27: 749–756.

Saranraj, P. and M. Geetha. 2012. Microbial spoilage of bakery products and its control by preservatives. International Journal of Pharmaceutical and Biological Archives, 3: 38–48.

Scott, P.M. 1991. Possibilities of reduction or elimination of mycotoxins in cereal grains. pp. 529–572. *In*: J. Chelkowski (ed.). Cereal Grain, Mycotoxins, Fungi and Quality in Drying and Storage. Elsevier, Amsterdam.

Smith, J.P., D.P. Daifas, W. EL-Khoury, J. Koukoutsis and A. EL-Khoury. 2004. Shelf life and safety concerns of bakery products—a review. Critical Review and Nutrition, 44: 19–55.

Smith, J.E., G. Solomons, C. Lewis and J.G. Anderson. 1995. Role of mycotoxins in human and animal nutrition and health. National Toxins, 3: 187–192.

Somashekar, D., E.R. Rati and A. Chandrashekar. 2004. PCR-restriction fragment length analysis of *aflR* gene for differentiation and detection of *Aspergillus flavus* and *Aspergillus parasiticus* in maize. International Journal of Food Microbiology, 93: 101–107.

Tančinová, D., Z. Barboráková, Z. Mašková, M. Císarová and T. Bojňanská. 2012. The occurrence of micromycetes in the bread samples and their potential ability to produce mycotoxins. Journal of Microbiology, Biotechnology and Food Science, 1: 813–818.

Turner, N.W., S. Subrahmanyam and S.A. Piletsky. 2009. Analytical methods for determination of mycotoxins: A review. Analytica Chimica Acta, 632: 168–180.

Vagelas, I., N. Gougoulias, E.-D. Nedesca and G. Liviu. 2011. Bread contamination with fungus. Carpathian Journal of Food Science and Technology, 3: 1–6.

Van Egmond, H.P. 1989. Aflatoxin M1: Occurrence, toxicity, regulation. pp. 11–55. *In*: H.P. Van Egmond (ed.). Mycotoxins in Dairy Products. Elsevier Applied Science, New York.

Vytřasová, J., P. Přibáňová and L. Marvanová. 2002. Occurrence of *Xerophilic* fungi in bakery production. International Journal of Food Microbiology, 72: 91–96.

Wareing, P. 2012. The fungal infection of agricultural produce and the production of mycotoxins. Available online: http://services.leatherheadfood.com/eman/FactSheet.aspx?ID=78.

Wilson, D.M., W. Mubatanhema and Z. Jurjevic. 2002. Biology and ecology of mycotoxigenic *Aspergillus* species as related to economic and health concerns. Advances in Experimental Medicine and Biology, 504: 3–17.

Zain, M.E. 2011. Impact of mycotoxins on humans and animals. Journal of Saudi Chemical Society, 15: 129–144.

Zhao, J., F. Kong, R. Li, X. Wang, Z. Wan and D. Wang. 2001. Identification of *Aspergillus fumigatus* and related species by nested PCR targeting Ribosomal DNA internal transcribed spacer regions. Journal of Clinical Microbiology, 39: 2261–2266.

Zinedine, A., C. Juan, J.M. Soriano, J.C. Moltó, L. Idrissiy and J. Mañes. 2007. Limited survey for the occurrence of aflatoxins in cereals and poultry feeds from Rabat, Morocco. International Journal of Food Microbiology, 115: 124–127.

9

Bread Fortification

Cristina M. Rosell

1. Introduction

Malnutrition, unbalanced diet, special nutrient requirement at specific life periods or some gastrointestinal diseases can cause nutrient deficiencies, which in turn could lead to different diseases. Nutrient deficiencies could have diverse origins and they are widespread through the world, resulting in important health and economic consequences in developing and industrialized countries. In fact, the World Health Organization (WHO) estimates that over two billion people are deficient in essential vitamins and minerals, and the worst situation is detected in infants, young children, pregnant and lactating due to their special physiological needs.

Food fortification programs developed through the last century allowed the eradication of diseases related to mineral or vitamin deficiencies like pellagra. Those food interventions have been voluntary or mandatory depending on the incidence of the nutrient deficiencies in each country. Nevertheless, through the fortification history successive supporters and opponents to this strategy have been declared (Kamien 2006).

It must be highlighted that although food fortification is a good strategy to solve nutritional deficiency in some population groups, there is a risk of over-nutrition in others. When defining a food fortification strategy it is necessary to define tolerable upper intake levels, also considered safe upper levels, which will allow evaluating the risk of excessive intakes of individual micronutrients (Fletcher et al. 2004). The EU Scientific Committee on Foods (2000) defines the upper intake levels (UL) as 'the maximum level of total chronic daily intake of a nutrient (from all sources, including foods, water, nutrient supplements and medicines) judged to be unlikely to pose a

Institute of Agrochemistry and Food Technology (IATA-CSIC). Avenida Agustín Escardino, 7. Paterna 46980. Valencia. Spain.
Email: crosell@iata.csic.es

risk of adverse health effects to almost all individuals in the general population'. In 2006, at the request of the European Commission by the Scientific Committee on Food (SCF) the Scientific Panel on Dietetic Products, Nutrition and Allergies (NDA) of European Food Safety Authority (EFSA) compiled scientific opinions up to April 2003 to support the implementation of impending harmonized EU legislation for food supplements and fortified foods with vitamins and minerals, and particularly to assist with the setting of maximum limits for micronutrients in these products (EFSA 2006). Therefore, in food fortification it is essential to define the correct balance of nutrient after an exhaustive evaluation of the benefits and risks at both ends of the intake scale (Fletcher et al. 2004).

Fortification can be defined as the addition of one or more vitamins and/or minerals to a food, regardless of its usual content in the food. Additions are carried out based on generally accepted scientific knowledge of the role of vitamins and minerals in attaining good health. Foods are fortified for the following reasons (Rosell 2007):

- to prevent or correct a demonstrated deficiency of one or more vitamins and/or minerals in the population or specific population groups; and
- to improve the nutritional status of the population and dietary intakes of vitamins or minerals due to changes in dietary habits.

Through the history, worldwide experience confirms that fortification is an effective strategy for mitigating nutrients deficiencies, although it is extremely important to select the adequate food target as vehicle and its consumption and also the deficiencies to alleviate. Numerous scientific studies have been conducted for verifying the utility of fortification (Allen et al. 2006). Fortification is perceived by consumers as beneficial to obtain healthy products and to tackle deficiencies. In fact, a consultation was carried out in UK to gather consumer preferences regarding folic acid (Tedstone et al. 2008). In that study, consumer must choose among to continue with women advice, take folic acid supplements, increase food enriched products, or to recommend the mandatory fortification of flour and cereal based products, and the mandatory fortification was the preferred option owing the outstanding concerns about spina bifida risk.

Enrichment is a term usually interchanged with fortification. If at all possible, enrichment should be equivalent to restoration. Therefore, the addition of vitamins and minerals, present in the edible portions of the food, should restore the levels lost during manufacturing, storage and handling.

The other relevant term in this subject is "nutritional equivalence," which means "being of similar nutritive value in terms of quantity and bioavailability of vitamins and minerals." Since fortification is a broader term, herein it will be used to refer to the addition of nutrients.

2. General considerations about food fortification

Minerals and vitamins may be added to foods only for the purpose of (1) restoration of nutrients lost during processing; (2) nutritional equivalence of substitute foods;

(3) fortification; and (4) ensuring the appropriate nutrient composition for a special purpose food.

Some considerations should be taken into account, prior to addition of any nutrient to foods (Baurenfiend and DeRitter 1991):

- The nutrient added should be present at a level that will not result in either an excessive or an insignificant intake, considering the amount provided from other dietary sources. The maximum safe amount to be added should be set considering the levels established by generally accepted scientific data and bearing in mind the diverse degree of sensitivity shown by different consumer groups.
- Nutrients should not be added to fresh products including meat, fish, fruits and vegetables, neither to beverages containing more than 1.2% by volume of alcohol.
- The nutrient added should be biologically available from the food and should not interfere in the metabolism of any other nutrient.
- The nutrient added should be sufficiently stable during packaging, storage, distribution, and end use, and should not affect both the sensory characteristics and the shelf life of the food.
- Technology and processing facilities should be available to permit the addition of the nutrient and also methods of measuring and controlling the levels of nutrient added.
- Fortification should not be used as a tool for providing nutrients in substitution of the natural nutrient sources, as this would lead to a change in the dietary patterns and thus jeopardize good dietary practices.

However, in any case fortification programs should include adequate Quality Assurance and Quality Control (QA/QC) at production level, regulatory monitoring of the nutrient content of fortified foods, as well as assessment methods to document the nutritional and health effectiveness when implementing fortification strategies. Policy for food fortification may vary from country to country.

Industrialized countries are facing social changes like industrialization, high per capita income, consumption of fast food outside the home that drive to increasing consumption of more highly processed foods, that often does not provide sufficient intake of recommended nutrients, mainly vitamins and minerals. In developed countries, like United States, children/adolescents have intakes of numerous micronutrients close to the recommended levels due to food fortification, without resulting in excessive intakes (Berner et al. 2014). However, no general consensus has been reached about fortification intervention. Advocators argue that manufacturers could use fortification as a promotional tool resulting in an excessive intake of certain nutrients that would represent a risk for consumer health. An uncontrolled food fortification program could result in excessive intakes of certain nutrients creating nutrient imbalances, and in consequence representing a health risk. It must have in mind that deficiencies provoke diseases but overdose of a vitamin or mineral also may cause health problems. For instance, excessive intake of vitamin A can cause birth defects, too much folate can hide symptoms of a vitamin B_{12} deficiency which can lead damage of the nervous system, and too much calcium can induce kidney problems.

In developing countries food fortification represents the best alternative to solve nutrient deficiencies, and so far the implementation of these programs has been very successful in correcting nutritional deficiencies of large segments of the population within a very short period. Although to reach that goal, a careful selection of the food vehicle is necessary. Target foods must be stable and routinely consumed by the population at risk and the amount of nutrient added must be sufficient to correct the possible deficiency.

Governments that mandate fortification should be able to ensure that the right concentrations of the needed nutrients are added to key foods and they should develop systems for assessment and monitoring. Food fortification is one of the most sustainable and cost-effective methods available to improve public health (Greiner 2007).

One of the most critical decisions when setting up a food fortification program is the selection of the appropriate food to act as a carrier of the nutrient. Basic criteria must include consumption at regular basis by the target population group, affordability, and availability all through the year.

Diets are different around the world and also deficiencies could be different. A study carried out to address at global level which foods to fortify, with which micronutrients, and in which countries, reported the most consumed foods in 48 countries (Fiedler and Macdonald 2009). In that study, from a household income and expenditure survey, which reflected the proportion of households purchasing any potential food fortification vehicles, wheat and maize flours and also those cereals based foods were identified as adequate carriers.

Cereals have been used as a basis of human diet from the ancient times and their implication in the human diet is still very significant. In addition, some populations with cereals as staple food have moved to eat increasingly available and affordable commercially processed cereals; thus those processed foods are also fundamental foods in the diet. Fortification of cereals and processed cereals can reach most vulnerable groups in countries where cereals are staple foods. In fact, flours were used as initial vehicles of fortification. Back, in the early 1900s, deficiencies of B vitamins were highly prevalent in the United States and despite the numerous deaths due to pellagra millers were really reticent to fortification. However, the decision of the British to sell only enriched flour had a great impact on Americans. The term "enriched flour" was coined during the Second World War when the American government decided to improve the soldiers' diet by purchasing only flour enriched with different nutrients. This campaign and the mandatory enrichment laws approved in different States encouraged flour and bread enrichment in US (Bishai and Nalubola 2002). Initially, the enrichment consisted of the addition of the three major B-vitamins (thiamine, riboflavin, and niacin) and iron, despite the scarce scientific information concerning the real nutritional improvement obtained with that proposal.

3. Cereals as food fortification vehicles and source of nutrients

Cereal grains have been used as a basis for the human diet from ancient times. Cereals and derivative foods provide the majority of the intake of these nutrients in low-income families. Today cereal production is estimated to be more than two million tons, of which around 20% of those are of wheat. In fact wheat consumption is around 66 kg per capita per year (FAOSTAT 2010), with the European continent having the highest consumption of wheat at 108 kg per capita per year. In Africa that value decreases to 45 kg per capita per year due to the high intake of other cereals such as oats, millet and sorghum. Globally, cereals account for 48% of total energy intake and they are also a cheap source of proteins, compared to the animal ones. Although, their relative contribution to human diet greatly depends on the production and the cultural differences, the popularity of cereals in the diet worldwide, mainly rice and wheat, make them the most appropriate vehicles for fortification strategies. Nevertheless, cereals are not directly consumed as grains; usually they undergo processing to transform the grain prior to its consumption with the subsequent reduction in nutrients and micronutrients that are mainly concentrated in the outer layers and germ. In the conversion of cereal grains to flour, twenty or more ingredients, such as thiamin, riboflavin, niacin, pyridoxine, folate, panthothenate, biotin, vitamin E, calcium, copper, iron, potassium, magnesium, manganese, phosphorus, zinc, chromium, fluorine, molybdenum and selenium are lost to the extent of 50 to 90% during the milling process (Rosell 2012). Cereal-fortification methods have been initially developed to restore the nutrients that have been removed during milling and to improve the nutrient intake level of specific population.

Cereals are an important source of energy and they supply different nutrients necessary for a healthy diet. Grains are rich of oligosaccharides, resistant starch and carbohydrates that function like dietary fiber, comprising cellulose, complex xylans, lignin and ß-glucans. The protein content of grains is also important, although the nutritional value of the cereal proteins is lower than that of the animal proteins owing to a deficiency in some essential amino acids, mainly lysine. The predominant amino acids are glutamic acid, proline, leucine and aspartic acid principally located in the germ. The fat content is low with absence of cholesterol. Grains also provide micronutrients like B vitamins, namely thiamine (B_1), riboflavin (B_2) and niacin (B_6), and minerals. Calcium, phosphorus, iron, sodium, magnesium and potassium are present in important amounts. Grains contain antioxidants, including vitamins and trace minerals, besides phenolic acids, lignans and phytic acid, which are thought to protect against cardiovascular disease and cancer. Phosphorus is mostly present as phytic acid or myo-inositol hexaphosphate that is not readily available and is considered an anti-nutritional compound because of its adverse effects on the bioavailability of minerals. In the gastrointestinal tract, the phytic acid or phytate forms insoluble complexes with multivalent cations, especially Zn^{2+}, Ca^{2+}, Mg^{2+} and Fe^{3+} (Davies and Nightingale 1975), decreasing the bioavailability of those minerals. Other health-promoting compounds, mainly concentrated in the germ and bran, are the phytoestrogens, which have the ability to protect against cancers such as breast and prostate (Slavin 2000).

The consumption of cereal grains by themselves is highly recommended due to their excellent nutritional profile. They are a source of: (i) complex carbohydrates, (ii) dietary fiber, (iii) minerals, especially calcium, phosphorus, iron and potassium, and (iv) B vitamins, and (v) have low fat content. This fact, besides their widespread consumption worldwide, supports the selection of cereal based product as one of the most effective food carriers in fortification strategies.

4. Bread fortification

There are different ways to fortify bread; among them are the use of flours from fortified crop varieties (agronomic fortification or biofortification), to blend flours with micronutrients at mills or at bakeries, or inducing enrichment during the breadmaking process.

4.1 Agronomic fortification

The term 'biofortification' refers to the increasing of micronutrients in the edible parts of the plants. Genetic variation in nutrient composition exists in cereals and can be exploited in conventional breeding programs and through gene technology. Cultural techniques, including fertilizer technology and organic farming, can impact the nutrient composition of cereals. By this strategy, human iron and zinc intake can be doubled. Some reports claim that this approach is potentially more sustainable than fortification and supplementation programs owing to its continuous intake. In the case of zinc it is especially important because it is needed almost daily (Graham et al. 2000).

Biofortification by mineral fertilization is a common practice in some countries that apply selenium-containing fertilizers as a short-term solution for improving the selenium content of wheat (Hawkesford and Zhao 2007). Selenium is an essential micronutrient for humans and may reduce the risk of degenerative diseases including cancer but it is deficient in at least a billion people worldwide. Further information about selenium enrichment can be found in the Chapter *Production of Selenium-enriched breads and their nutritional and nutraceutical properties.*

Biofortification through plant breeding consists of the development of micronutrient-enhanced crop varieties through conventional breeding. This method has potential to deliver a significant improvement in human micronutrient status. However further studies in the following areas are required: identification of genetic resources, determination of genotype x environment interactions in wheat, determination of the desired level of micronutrient increase, and establishment of the cost-effectiveness of biofortification programs (Ortiz-Monasterio et al. 2007). Genetic biofortification appears to be a sustainable and cost-effective approach to improve zinc and iron levels (Zhaoa and McGratha 2009).

In addition, Mendoza et al. (2001) reported the possible effect of reduced phytate content grains as an alternative for improving iron adsorption. When those maize flours were used for making cereal grain foods fortify with iron, no effect was observed due to the maize flour. Fortification of those maize based foods was only effective due to the supplementation with sodium iron EDTA. A more recent study shows that low phytic acid-containing maize varieties improved zinc bioavailability compared to wild-type counterparts (Moretti et al. 2014).

Further readings about agronomic fortification can be found in the Chapter *Agronomic Fortification and the Impact on Bread Fortification.*

4.2 Flour fortification

Different approaches to bring about a partial restoration of refined cereal flours to its initial nutritional value and to use cereal flours and related products as micronutrient vehicles have been reported. The simplest and most well recognized approach is the addition of compounds removed during milling by blending the flour in a direct process. At this point it must be stressed that the type of flour significantly affects the micronutrients bioavailability, particularly minerals. In fact, de-germination of maize flour improves bioavailability of iron and zinc due to the removal of phytic acid, a major inhibitor of both iron and zinc absorption (Moretti et al. 2014).

The term 'enriched flour' was firstly used during the World War II, when the American government, interested in winning the war, decided to improve soldiers' diet, by using bread as a carrier of different nutrients. In the beginning, enrichment consisted of the addition of the three major B vitamins (thiamine, riboflavin and niacin) and iron. At that time scarce scientific information was available about the nutritional improvement provided by this strategy. Currently, microencapsulation of micronutrients has been proposed to avoid the impact of fortifying agents on the sensory and technological properties of the food products (Majeed et al. 2013).

During the last decades, numerous studies related to fortification in different nutrients and the effectiveness of those measurements has been reported.

4.2.1 Iron fortification

The role of iron in the blood formation is well known and a deficiency of iron produces in its more extreme stage iron deficiency anemia. A recognized deficiency of iron has been detected in more than 20% of the world's population. The incidence of iron deficiency anemia is high among infants, teenagers, and women of child-bearing age, with no significant difference between developing and industrialized countries. Different studies confirmed that mineral and vitamins requirements varied with the life stages and extra supplementation is needed at some stages. For instance, iron requirements are greater in pregnancy, mainly during the last two trimesters, being the total requirement of a 55-kg woman is around 1000 mg, which corresponds to daily needs of 0.8 mg Fe in the first trimester, between 4 and 5 mg in the second trimester, and more than 6 mg in the third trimester (Bothwell 2000).

The iron supplementation is based mainly on non-hem iron which is absorbed to a lesser degree than hem iron and moreover it is subjected to much interference from inhibitors generally present in the diets, such as phenols, phytates, fibers, etc. Because of that some studies have been focused on the phytates reduction during processing. Hernandez et al. (2006) reported that baking of wheat dough improved the bioavailability of iron due to the decrease in the phytates content independently on the fortification. Conversely, tortilla preparation did not affect phytates content but in this type of bread fortification improved iron bioavailability, which was higher when fortification was carried out with ferrous sulfate and NaFeEDTA over reduced iron.

Food fortification with iron chemicals is one of the most efficient approaches for correcting the deficiency. Inorganic iron majorly used for iron supplementation has a very low bioavailability, because of that relatively high intakes of iron are required for reaching the required levels, but those levels may have detrimental effects on food quality. Numerous studies have been conducted to determine the levels of chemicals required to enrich the effects of processing and the effectiveness of those enrichment practices. Iron sources should be soluble and of high bioavailability even in the presence of inhibitors like phenols, phytates, fibers, etc. (MacPhail 2001). Hallberg et al. (1986) analyzed the bioavailability of commercial iron powders extensively used in flour enrichment. By specific labelling techniques, they found that the relative bioavailability of the iron was unexpectedly low and highly dependent on the meals in which they were incorporated; phytates, calcium and polyphenols decreased the bioavailability of iron. In addition, an inverse relationship has been found between the H-reduced iron (food grade $\leq$ 45 μm particle size) particle size and iron bioavailability; in fact if H-reduced iron is used in wheat flour fortification it should be added three times the level of ferrous sulphate to provide the same level of absorbed iron (Arredondo et al. 2006). Therefore, even particle size of the iron source affects bioavailability (Arredondo et al. 2006). This fact was pointed out when the bioavailability of two different particle size ($\geq$ 45 μm and 8 μm) hydrogen-reduced iron incorporated in iron fortified bread were compared. *In vitro* studies in Caco-2 cells indicated that ferritin and intracellular iron content were significantly higher when bread was fortified with 8 μm hydrogen-reduced iron. Nevertheless, the supplementation of wheat flour with iron is still a common practice adopted in some countries for solving hematological deficiencies.

$FeSO_4$ and NaFeEDTA have showed better effectiveness than electrolytic iron in improving iron storage in anemic students when consuming enriched wheat flour (Huang et al. 2009). Nevertheless, it must be taken into account that fortification might change flour proximate composition, decreasing protein content, dough rheology (increased water absorption) and also on the flour microbial stability during storage (Akhtar et al. 2009; Akhtar et al. 2008). Akhtar et al. (2008) reported that fortification with 40 ppm elemental iron and 30 ppm zinc oxide extends the microbial shelf life of whole wheat flours. Studies conducted by Nayak and Nair (2003) on iron-fortified chapattis indicated that the addition of ascorbic acid or disodium ethylenediaminetetraacetic acid (NaEDTA) to wheat flour can enhance the predicted bioavailability of both native and added iron. Iron fortified pocket-type flat breads obtained using $FeSO_4$, NaFeEDTA and elemental iron at levels of 52.1,133.2 and 228.7 mg iron/kg flour respectively were similar to unenriched flat breads in terms of sensory quality (Najm et al. 2010).

After initial fortification, the American Chemical Association (1972) analyzed the Food and Drug Administration's (FDA) proposal to increase the level of iron content in flours, due to the prevalence of iron-deficiency anemia in USA and concluded that the proposal was more beneficial than hazardous to human health. Since the 1950s, wheat flour has been fortified with iron and B vitamins by legislation in Chile, and in January 2000 it was mandatory the addition of 2.2 mg/kg of folic acid to wheat flour.

In 1996, the World Health Organization Eastern Mediterranean Region Office began recommending the use of ferrous sulfate at 30 ppm or reduced iron at 60 ppm along with 1.5 ppm folic acid in flour fortification in the Middle East without affecting the sensory characteristics of either the flour stored for up to three months at ambient hot (35°C) and humid (90%) conditions or foods made from fortified wheat flour. The level of iron should not reach the maximum iron requirement with a single fortified product to avoid over dosage. An advisable level of fortification is to provide the equivalent of 20–40% of the daily requirements with a single food item Huma et al. (2007).

From 1997, the Organización Panamericana de la Salud (OPS) has supported the supplementation of iron to the diet using wheat flour as the vehicle due to its low cost and extensive consumption. Different countries from South and Central America have implemented this measure for reducing the incidence of iron deficient anemia after the successful results obtained in Chile. In 1999, a multidisciplinary task force of international experts settled some guidelines on iron fortification. They recommended the use of ferrous sulfate or ferrous fumarate whenever possible, and that if that elemental iron powder was used, the electrolytic form was recommended at twice the level of iron present in iron salts (Ranum et al. 2001; Ranum 2006).

In South Africa, mandatory fortification of maize meal and wheat flour was launched in 2003 to combat the deficiencies in calcium, iron, zinc, riboflavin, niacin, vitamin B_6, folate, vitamin A, E and C found in children. Iron enrichment of flour is generally regulated in most countries by specifying a minimum iron level in the enriched flour, which includes both added and native iron, rather than by specifying the exact quantity of iron to be added. The minimum addition level recommended to restore the iron naturally present in the whole grain product is 25 ppm iron for white flour using ferrous sulfate or ferrous fumarate. This would give an iron level in the enriched flour of about 35 ppm, or equivalent to the original level found in a whole-wheat flour, although that value might be increased in countries where iron deficiency is prevalent (Ranum et al. 2001). In addition, iron bis-glycinate chelate (ferrochel) has been also tested as a chemical source of iron in sweet rolls (Wallace et al. 2000). The intervention carried out in pre-school children from families of low socioeconomic level in Brazil during six months with two fortified sweet rolls for a total daily iron intake of 4 mg confirmed the efficiency of the intervention, since the prevalence of iron deficiency anemia decay from 62 to 22%.

A complete study about the economic and health impact of iron fortification in Pakistan as well as the iron sources and levels for adding to flour was presented by Huma et al. (2007), stating the effectiveness of fortification in increasing the levels of iron in the population.

Albaldawi et al. (2005) proposed the use of slaughter blood haem encapsulated in lecithin: cholesterol liposomes as iron source to fortify wheat flour and in consequence bread. With the levels of fortification tested, 60 and 100 mg/100 g flour, the stability and rheological characteristics of the dough were improved, although the fat content of flours significantly increased.

4.2.2 Other minerals fortification

Other minerals that have been used to supplement wheat flour are zinc and calcium. Zinc is one of the essential trace elements needed by the human body owing its role as structural ion in transcription factors. It has a key role in reproductive physiology, immune modulation, growth and development. A zinc deficiency was recognized for the first time in 1961, and mainly affects infants, young children, pregnant and lactating women because at those physiological stages the zinc requirements are higher. Calcium intakes are critical during all life cycle stages; it contributes to bone mineral density and micro-architecture. Some subpopulation groups with special requirements of calcium and vitamin D have been identified, which include elderly persons, postmenopausal females, minorities, and individuals who have a low income level and/or are obese (Wallace et al. 2013).

Wang and Tang (1995) reported the effect of fortification with calcium and zinc lactate on the rheological and baking properties of wheat flour. They showed that the supplementation improved dough expansion without significant effects on the quality of the resulting bread and retaining 87–93% of the added calcium and zinc. A follow-up study to determine the impact of zinc fortification conducted with 771 participants confirmed a significant improvements in plasma zinc concentrations, indicator of zinc status (Das et al. 2013). Moreover, zinc fortification was associated with an increased serum concentration of the micronutrient, but large-scale studies will be needed to confirm the effectiveness of this approach.

Iron and zinc supplementation is still a topic of debate and a recent review compiled the information regarding food sources, dietary intakes, dietary recommendations, nutritional status, bioavailability and interactions, with a focus on adult population from economically developed countries (Lim et al. 2013).

Calcium has been added to breads to assist individuals with lactose intolerance and those who do not consume dairy products. Calcium-enriched bread can serve as a good source of bioavailable calcium, although diets with high fat content may interfere with calcium absorption. The intake of calcium-enriched bread with an elemental calcium content of 2.5% has been proposed as an effective treatment for ameliorating hyperphosphatemia without inducing hypercalcemia (Babarykin et al. 2004).

Iodine is an essential micronutrient that plays a crucial role in ensuring the normal development of most organs, especially brain. Iodine deficiency has been long detected in some areas of Australia. In October 2009, a mandatory iodine fortification program was launched in Australia, regulating that bread manufacturers must use iodized salt in the baking process at levels of 25–65 mg/kg flour, hence bread contained 48 μg of iodine/100 g. Iodine fortification has been effective increasing the iodine status of women (Charlton et al. 2013). Fortification of bread with iodized salt increased the urinary iodine concentrations of pregnant women from 68 μg/L to 84 μg/L, which is still far away from the recommended levels of the World Health Organization (150 μg/L) (Clifton et al. 2013), and also in school children (Skeaff et al. 2014), because of that recommendations are addressed to encourage to either consume iodine-rich foods or take appropriate iodine supplements (Rahman et al. 2011).

4.2.3 Vitamins fortification

Different vitamins have been added to flour to obtain fortified bread. Solon et al. (2000) studied the efficacy of bread fortification with vitamin A in 835 school age children in Philippines. Those authors added Vitamin A to wheat flour buns (fortified pandesal containing 133 µg retinol equivalents) and observed an increase in the initial serum retinol concentrations after a daily consumption of these buns for 30 weeks, improving in consequence the vitamin A status (Solon et al. 2000). However, the usefulness of vitamin A addition to wheat flour products is limited due to its low stability in the presence of oxygen or air. In fact, the loss of vitamin A during 1 h 10 min of baking at 202°C could be greater than 50% (Cakirer and Lachance 1975).

A deficiency in vitamin D has been encountered in America, Canada and other developed countries. Vitamin D is provided by sun exposure, but that is significantly reduced in winter times, which force to consume vitamin D containing foods for meeting recommended dietary allowances. Vitamin D fortification is not mandatory, and in some countries like United States and Canada fortification is made voluntarily in some foods, mainly dairy foods. Nevertheless, novel approaches for increasing vitamin D content in foods must be addressed (Calvo and Whiting 2013). The consumption of vitamin D_3 fortified bread or bread made with naturally vitamin D-rich yeast has been proposed to improve vitamin D status (Hohman and Weaver 2011).

Other vitamin that requires additional supplementation to meet daily intake levels is the vitamin E (200–800 IU). With the purpose of supplying additional vitamin E, Ranhotra et al. (2000) fortified breads with DL-alpha-tocopheryl acetate, and although no adverse effects were observed on bread quality, only around 66% of the added vitamin E was recovered in the breads. The study concluded that bread fortification with 1,600 IU vitamin E per loaf would provide 25% of the recommended daily intake.

Lately, B-vitamins supplementation has taken great consideration due to the reported folic acid deficiencies. Studies confirming the role of folates in congenital malformations and the development of chronic diseases in later life like Alzheimer disease (Czeizel and Dudas 1992) drove to encourage the supplementation of folic acid (vitamin B_9) in cereal-based foods (Rader et al. 2000). The main reason for that intervention was the association of periconceptional folate supplementation with the reduction in the incidence of neural tube defects (Shane 2003). Folate concentration in serum and erythrocytes is inversely associated with the plasma concentration of total homocysteine and moderate hyperhomocysteinemia is associated with an increased risk of chronic diseases, such as cardiovascular disease, dementia, and impaired cognition. Food fortification was chosen because folic acid supplementation failed in that prevention due to many women were unaware of their pregnancy during the initial period of gestation when the neural tube closes. In the European Union no mandatory fortification policy has been adopted in order to regulate the addition of folic acid. The US and Canada governments have passed the mandatory regulation for folic acid fortification of flour products to a level of 140–150 µg/100 g with the objective of increasing typical folate intakes around 100 µg/day. That level was selected because overdose of folic acid may mask the symptoms of vitamin B_{12} deficiency in elderly population. FDA regulations to have all flour fortified with folic acid (Food and Drug Administration 1996a,b,c) were published 5th March 1996, with the full compliance date 1st January 1998. To that date manufacturers have enough time to finish their suppliers of in-stock labels, set up processes and prepare new labels. In 2003, the analysis of the data regarding chronic folic acid intake and the levels of folate in plasma or serum indicated that typical intakes of folic acid from fortified foods were more than twice the level initially predicted. Later on, in 2005 Dietrich et al. (2005) explored the changes in serum and erythrocyte folate status of the adult U.S. population and in food sources and dietary total folate intake following fortification intervention. That study revealed that folic acid fortification resulted in significant increases in both serum (136%) and erythrocyte folate (57%) concentrations in all sex and age groups, but that enhancement was not enough for women of childbearing age, since less than 10% of women reached the recommended erythrocyte folate concentration to have a significant reduction in neural tube defect risk. The same study also revealed that bread, rolls, and crackers represented the largest contributor of total folate to the American diet (Dietrich et al. 2005).

Chile also regulated the fortification of wheat flour with 2.2 mg folic acid/kg flour since January 2000 to reduce the risk of neural tube defects in newborns. A follow-up study was carried out with 605 women of childbearing age in Santiago (Chile) to assess the effectiveness of the intervention (Hertrampf et al. 2003). The mean serum and red blood cell folate concentrations after fortification increased 4 and 2.4 times, respectively, compared to the values during pre-fortification period. That improvement in the levels of folic acid was reached by the consumption of approximately 219 g/day of bread obtained from fortified flour that contained 2020 ± 940 μg folic acid/kg bread (Hertrampf et al. 2003). Preliminary data from Chile revealed that the fortification of wheat flour with folic acid is a cost-effective intervention in that country, considering the cost of the fortification and the provision of medical care to children with spina bifida (Llanos et al. 2007). Nevertheless, some concerns about folic acid fortification arose due to the higher folic acid intake and possible unintended consequences (Crider et al. 2011). A study recently conducted in Spain revealed that an excessive intake of folic acid can occur in specific population groups, like children under six years old (Samaniego-Vaesken et al. 2013), and also in Chile later studies indicate that folic acid intake is higher than the estimated average requirement, and a revision of the regulated levels must be required (Castillo et al. 2010). Other uncertainty results from the later association of maternal exposure to folate in preconception and pregnancy with the development of early childhood asthma, allergy, and wheeze; although contradictory results were obtained with different cohort studies (Brown et al. 2014). Therefore, overall folic acid fortification has resulted in a marked reduction in the incidence of neural tube defects and also may reduce the occurrence of diseases related to folate deficiency and hyperhomocysteinemia (Ueland and Hustad 2008), but there is a potential risk for children and elderly, since preneoplastic lesions and cobalamin deficiency are common in elderly. This uncertainty stresses the need to continually monitor fortification programs and to revise recommendations regularly whenever additional information becomes available.

The supplementation of wheat flour with B-vitamins has to overcome the problem of the low stability of B-vitamins sources during storage. When enrichment is at the mill the vitamin content can decrease by 33.3–58.1%, while only 17.0–38.7% reduction is obtained when the same vitamins are added to the bread dough (Stepanova et al. 1988).

When fortifying with folic acid it is necessary to consider the impact of breadmaking process, flour type, and bread type (Anderson et al. 2010). Baking provokes a 22 to 32% reduction in the folic acid concentration and that decrease depends on the type of bread, being higher for wholemeal bread. Therefore, to meet authorities' recommendation for folic acid flour fortification should be 47% higher than the desired concentration in bread, concretely 225 µg folic acid/100 g flour to deliver 120 µg/100 g bread (Anderson et al. 2010). However, the contribution of the fortification program to the folic acid intake increase would depend on the amount of bread consumption. Nevertheless, known the masking effect of folic acid on vitamin B_{12}, different sources of folic have been searched. Calcium L-5-methyltetrahydrofolic acid, a synthetic form of reduced folate, has been proposed as safer source of folic acid that does not mask vitamin B_{12} deficiency (Green et al. 2013). Although a microencapsulated form of calcium L-5-methyltetrahydrofolic acid with sodium ascorbate and a modified starch must be used in breadmaking due to this form of folic acid is not stable in bread. The consumption of wheat rolls fortified with microencapsulated form of calcium L-5-methyltetrahydrofolic acid provides similar folic acid than rolls fortified with the molar equivalent of folic acid without the potential for masking the hematological symptoms of vitamin B_{12} deficiency (Green et al. 2013).

In United States, the FDA approves the supplementation of four B vitamins (thiamine, niacin, riboflavin and folic acid) and iron to the wheat flour, although this practice is not regulated by Federal law and depends on State law. In addition, in United Kingdom, it is regulated by law that the nutrients removed with the bran during the milling must be replaced in all types of flours except wholemeal. In this country, white and brown flours must have thiamine, niacin, iron and calcium, although the addition should not be done in amounts that might be harmful to people. There are some countries, such as Canada, where wheat flour fortification is mandatory, whereas others, such as New Zealand, Finland and Norway, where there are laws prohibiting the addition of micronutrients to wheat flour. Therefore, the enrichment of wheat flour with different nutrients is differently regulated by each country.

4.2.4 Fortification with other nutrients

Different ingredients, from different flour sources, have been proposed for fortifying breads, especially in dietary fiber and proteins. Those ingredients are usually blended with wheat flour during the breadmaking process. Some of those ingredients are discussed below to display the range of sources that have been proposed to nutritionally enhance cereal-based products.

When fortifying it is necessary to identify the nutritional patterns of the population and assess possible deficiencies associated to those patterns. For instance a basic food for the Latin American population and more specifically Mexican citizens is the maize tortilla, which constitutes the main source of proteins. However, as it was mentioned previously, cereals are deficient in essential amino acids such as lysine and tryptophan, because of that some attempts have been proposed for enriching tortillas with those amino acids (Waliszewski et al. 2000). Tortillas can be fortified using fortified nixtamalized maize flour containing 83% of suggested FAO recommendations for lysine (5.44 g/100 g protein) and tryptophan (0.96 g/100 g protein) without affecting the sensory characteristics. The level of fortification delivered with that supplementation will provide the appropriate amino acid intake to low income groups of Latin Americans that consume tortilla as their main daily source of proteins.

Graham et al. (1971) conducted studies to establish what amount of lysine it is adequate to add to make enriched flour in areas where wheat flour is the main source of proteins. They recommended at least 0.2% of lysine for wheat flour enrichment. Using fortified flour with up to 0.3% of lysine in breadmaking does not modify organoleptic evaluation of breads for appearance, texture, taste and overall acceptability (Yasoda-Devi and Geervani 1979). The nutritional improvement measured as the relative protein value was confirmed in adult rats, which showed better growth when fed with lysine enriched wheat flour (Mekhael et al. 1989). Defatted soybean flours have been frequently added to wheat flour for protein fortification of bread (Mashayekh et al. 2008). Adding up to 7% of defatted soybean flour to fortified wheat bread can increase 55% and 41% the content of ash and proteins, respectively, having similar characteristics than the wheat bread (Mashayekh et al. 2008).

Dried buttermilk and dried skim milk can be added up to 2% to nutritionally enriched bread without conferring strange flavors (Mostafa et al. 1982). Even fish protein obtained from cabrinha (*Prionotus punctatus*) has been used for bread enrichment replacing up to 50% of wheat flour (Centenaro et al. 2007). Sensory evaluation showed that bread containing 5% dry washed minced fish was not significantly different from the bread without added fish. With this approach it was possible to increase the protein content by 31, 45 and 48% when adding 3 and 5% of dry washed minced fish and 50% of wet washed minced fish, respectively.

Some nuts (almond, hazelnut, peanut and walnut) have been also proposed for enriching breads (Oliete et al. 2008). Nuts have high contents of unsaturated fatty acids that are beneficial with respect to chronic diseases such as hypertension and obesity, coronary heart disease, and diabetes. Nuts also contain important lipids, proteins, fiber and certain vitamins and minerals, together with other bioactive components, such as tocopherol and phytoestrogens. The addition of up to 15% nut paste to wheat flour leads to low bread volume and firm crumb. Breads containing 10 and 15% nut paste were most frequently and most persistently consumed and had the best texture (Oliete et al. 2008).

Chickpea flour (*Cicer arietinum*) has been added at levels of up to 15% of wheat flour, without seriously affecting bread quality and increasing by 3.5% the protein content of the breads (Figuerola et al. 1987). The supplementation of 5% edible grade cottonseed flour is recommended to increase the protein content of breads without any significant deleterious effect on their organoleptic qualities (El-Shaarawy and Mesallam 1987). Pumpkin seed products (raw, roasted, autoclaved, germinated, fermented, pumpkin protein concentrate and pumpkin protein isolate) are also proposed for protein fortification of wheat breads (El-Soukkary 2001). Loaf volume is not affected when up to 19% level for germinated, fermented and protein concentrate or 21% protein isolate is added, but a significant improvement in protein content and digestibility can be reached, besides an increase in the lysine and mineral content. Lentil protein concentrates and sweet lupin flour also have been added to enhance the nutritional value of wheat breads, although lentil protein concentrates decreased the overall acceptability. Different Andean crops like quinoa, amaranthus (kiwicha) and kañiwa have been blended at different levels with wheat flour to increase the nutritional value of the bakery products (Rosell et al. 2009). Replacement of wheat flour by 25% kañiwa, 50% kiwicha, or 50% quinua still produced breads with good sensory acceptability, but variable color.

Maize flour has been also fortified with amaranth flour to increase the protein supply through the enriched tortillas consumption. Vazquez-Rodriguez et al. (2013) reported nixtamalized maize flour fortified with common bean (*Phaseolus vulgaris*) and amaranth (*Amaranthus* spp.) flours in the proportion 90:3:7 to obtain bioavailable protein fortified tortillas. Bioassay of two generations with Wistar rats confirmed the enrichment in lysine (48%) and tryptophan (40%) content, and concerning the tortillas they showed similar rollability and tensile strength to commercial tortilla.

Nowadays, there is a growing interest for the valorization of food industry by-products (Collar and Rosell 2012) and one of the immediate applications of those products is to be used as food supplements for nutritional enrichment. In 1983, the Pan American Health Service developed bread enriched with cereal protein concentrates that were by-products of starch extraction. This bread was commercialized as 'Pan de Vida' in Honduras (Hammond 1983). The most common use of food industry by-products is feeding due to their nutrients content. Lately, those by-products are being incorporated in the human nutrition contributing to the nutrients recovery. For instance brewer's spent grain, the most important by-product of the brewing industry, contains 22.13% protein, 1.13% minerals, 131.0 mg/L polyphenols, 28.22% total fiber and 3.6% essential fatty acids (Waters et al. 2012). The brewer's spent grain has been added up to 10 % directly or after fermentation with lactic acid bacteria, *Lactobacillus plantarum* FST 1.7, to wheat flour yielding dough with good textural and handling technological properties and breads with softer crumbs than whole meal bread and moreover containing 13.9 g/day of dietary fiber (Waters et al. 2012).

In recent years, considerable scientific research has confirmed the beneficial role of the dietary fiber in the reduction of chronic ailments such as cardiovascular disease, certain forms of cancer and constipation (Lairon et al. 2005). The beneficial role of the dietary fiber intake has prompted the gaining in popularity of fiber-supplemented cereal-based foods (see chapter *The role of fibers in the nutrition and health benefits of bread*). Numerous fiber-enriched breads have been launched in recent years, although fibers negatively affect the technological quality of the bread, reducing loaf volume and increasing crumb hardness. Only non-conventional fibers used for bread enrichments will be mentioned in this chapter.

Either legume hulls or insoluble cotyledon fibers or soluble cotyledon fibers isolated from pea, lentil and chickpea flours have been incorporated at different levels (up to 7%) to fortified breads (Dalgetty and Baik 2006). Insoluble fibers reduce the volume of the bread and the opposite trend is observed when soluble fibers are used for fortification.

In some cases, past experience has revealed very interesting facts for improving health patterns. That is the case of incorporating phloem powder from the inner bark layer of the pine tree into rye bread in Finland (Vanharanta et al. 2002). Phloem powder is rich in fibers and polyphenols like flavonoids and lignans, useful as protective agents against acute coronary diseases. During the twentieth century this powder was used in Finland to cover the shortage of wheat flour for breadmaking. A randomized double-blind supplementation trial with rye bread enriched in phloem conducted by Vanharanta et al. (2002) confirmed its health benefits due to its lignans content, which enhanced the serum enterolactone levels that in turn reduce the risk of death from coronary heart disease.

Some cereal based products like flat bread has been used as fortification vehicle and different ingredients have been added to improve its nutritive value, among them milk, eggs, other cereals, legumes, dates or date syrup, dried fruits, leafy vegetables, cassava, green banana, flaxseed flour, sesame, black seeds, species, meat and dried or fresh herbs (Al-Dmoor 2012).

4.3 Fortification during breadmaking process

Breadmaking is a dynamic process accompanied by physico-chemical, microbiological and biochemical changes derived from the action of yeast, lactic acid bacteria and the endogenous enzymes of flours (Rosell 2011). Yeasts and lactic acid bacteria contain different enzymes responsible for the metabolism of microorganisms that modify dough characteristics and the technological and nutritional quality of bread. Amino acids are absorbed by yeast and lactic acid bacteria and metabolized as a nitrogen source for growth, and proteins can be hydrolyzed by the action of proteolytic enzymes from both flour and microorganisms as well as by yeast autolysis. As a result, the amino acid profile changes during breadmaking. The total amino acid content (and particularly the contents of ornithine and threonine) increases by 64% during mixing and decreases by 55% during baking, mostly affecting glutamine leucine, ornithine, arginine, lysine and histidine (Prieto et al. 1990). Additionally, the action of proteinases and peptidases from lactic acid bacteria on soluble polypeptides and proteins leads to an increase in small peptides. Jiang et al. (2008) also observed a decrease in 17 amino acids in steamed bread, mainly affecting alanine (17.1%), followed by tyrosine (12.5%) and leucine.

The vitamin content is also affected during the breadmaking process due to yeast metabolism. A 48% loss of thiamine and a 47% loss of pyridoxine in white bread has been reported, although those levels could be increased with longer fermentations (Batifoulier et al. 2005).

The use of different yeast strains have been also suggested for the production of enriched baked goods. Hjortmo et al. (2008) demonstrated that it is possible to increase the amount of folate in white wheat bread by using *Saccharomyces cerevisiae* CBS7764 cultured in a defined medium and harvested at a specific phase of growth. With this high folate producing strain it was possible to increase 3 to 5 fold the level of folate in white flour breads. A selenium-enriched yeast has been used to increase the selenium content of bread (Stabnikova et al. 2008). The wheat roll obtained with this yeast can provide 25% of the recommended daily allowance in the form of selenomethionine, which is the best form of selenium for humans. There is little knowledge on the role of selenium in the diet; however, consumers are favorable towards selenium enrichment of foods, particularly by biofortification.

Breadmaking process with wholemeal wheat flour yeast fermentation is beneficial for reducing the phytate content, which subsequently results in increases in magnesium and phosphorus bioavailability (Haros et al. 2001). The extent of phytase activity during breadmaking depends on the wheat flour extraction rate, the proofing temperature and time, dough pH, and the amount of yeast (Fernandez et al. 2002). Even the type of breadmaking process (frozen dough or bake-off technology) can lead to different impact on phytate content (Rosell et al. 2009). In consequence, it would be possible to modulate the phytate content by modifying the process conditions. In addition, specific strains of bifidobacteria species (*B. catenulatum, B. longum* and *B. breve*) with phytate degrading activity have been proposed as starters for the fermentation of wholemeal wheat bread to reduce the phytate content (Palacios et al. 2008). During fermentation in the presence of different bifidobacterial strains, the concentration of phytic acid showed a progressive decrease, leading to hydrolysis products without complexing activity.

5. Impact of enrichment or fortification on human health

While setting up a fortification program an important point is to have a follow up to evaluate the effectiveness of the measurement. In that assessment is necessary to establish the methodology for nutrient risk determination and to conduct the necessary test for setting 'tolerable upper levels of intake' for nutrients. It must be taken into account that fortification programs are set up for solving deficiencies but also they can lead to over-consumption in some population subgroups. Any intervention program must be monitored to assess the public health benefits of food fortification or supplement use while minimizing the risks that excessive intakes might cause. Therefore, evaluation and monitoring of the fortification programs are necessary to assess the effectiveness and modify if necessary the supplementation levels. After intervention, intermediate evaluations must be carried out to check the procedure. For instance, in 1999 it was detected that 33.4% of Iranian women were anemic according to hemoglobin levels, and 34.5% were iron deficient according to serum ferritin levels leading to a 16.6% prevalence of iron-deficiency anemia in Iranian women. After detecting the iron deficiency, a flour fortification program was initiated in 2001. A mid-term evaluation carried out in 2004 with 863 women of 15–49 years revealed an increase in the ferritin levels but to have an impact the hemoglobin levels and iron-deficiency anemia longer intervention were necessary (Sadighi et al. 2008). Nevertheless, it seems that iron fortification programs increase the ferritin levels (iron deficiency) but the prevalence of iron-deficiency anemia (low hemoglobin) might be not affected because in many developing countries anemia is not only due to iron deficiency but also to other nutritional deficiencies, malaria, helminthes and other inflammatory/infectious diseases (Sadighi et al. 2009).

In South Africa, a secondary data analysis was carried out in 2006 with 3229 adults to follow up the effectiveness of the intervention, showing that calcium, iron, folate and vitamin B$_6$ intakes were very low particularly in women (Steyn et al. 2008). In this country, fortification of maize meal and wheat flour (bread) augmented the levels of thiamine, riboflavin, niacin, vitamin B$_6$ and folate above the recommended nutrient intakes, although in women iron intakes remained below the recommended (Pandey et al. 2000).

An important point is the selection of the micronutrient source, for instance mineral sources for ensuring the bioavailability. That has been largely studied in the case of iron fortification using different salts. In fact, when different cereal foods were fortified with radiolabelled ferrous sulfate, ferrous fumarate, NaFeEDTA or ferric pyrophosphate, Hurrell et al. (2000) found that iron absorption from cereals fortified with ferrous sulfate and fumarate was similar. In infant cereals and bread rolls the iron absorption was higher when they were fortified with NaFeEDTA instead of ferrous sulfate. Those authors concluded that NaFeEDTA is the recommended iron source for cereal foods because iron absorption is higher when those products are fortified with it compared to ferrous sulfate or ferrous fumarate; besides, Na_2EDTA increases the iron bioavailability when added to cereal foods fortified with ferrous sulfate.

Bioavailability of calcium, iron and zinc as calcium carbonate, ferrous sulfate and zinc sulfate from fortified bread is different as revealed a study carried out with 64 female Sprague-Dawley Albino rats for a period of 28 days (Ahmad et al. 2012). Calcium levels in femur increased with fortification, whereas the iron and zinc levels were significantly higher in the plasma, liver and femur of rats. Multiple fortification of flour to address minerals malnutrition should be encouraged although it has been observed that multiple fortifications resulted in decreased bioavailability (Ahmed et al. 2012).

In the case of folic acid fortification of cereal foods, some reports have been published regarding the effectiveness of the intervention. In fact, Rader et al. (2000) surveyed 83 enriched cereal-grain products observing some divergences between the amount of folic acid declared in the label and the real values quantified in the enriched products. Same trend was observed when the iron and folate content was analyzed in grain foods observing significantly higher content than those declared in the label (Whittaker et al. 2001).

Nevertheless, a mixed longitudinal survey conducted within children and teenagers in Germany (Sichert-Hellert et al. 2000), to assess the nutrient intakes (protein, fat, carbohydrates, sugars, vitamins A, E, C, B_1, B_2, B_6, niacin, folate, calcium and iron) from fortified food, revealed that fortification was not always necessary. Specifically, the nutrient intake of that population was adequate regarding vitamins A, C, B_1, B_2, B_6, niacin and calcium; thus fortification was not necessary, but fortification with vitamin E and folate was effective improving the deficient intake.

Other group at risk of vitamin deficiencies is the elderly, particularly vitamin D deficiency, which increases the risk of falls and fractures. A study conducted among the nursing home residents (aged 58–89 years) identified that their requirements will be 125 µg of vitamin D_3 to achieve desirable levels of 25-hydroxyvitamin D to improve health (Costan et al. 2014). After one year consumption of one daily bun fortified with 125 µg vitamin D, serum 25-hydroxyvitamin D reached optimal status (> 75 nM) and bone health improved significantly, likewise the period time of the fortification was significantly related to pain perception, daily activities and locomotion.

6. Conclusions and future perspectives

As a foodstuff of great historical and contemporary importance, in many cultures worldwide, bread has significance beyond mere nutrition. Bread has ancient roots and is a staple of many diets throughout the world, from prosperous metropolises to developing nations. Bread comes in all shapes, flavors and forms, and is typically made from accessible and affordable ingredients. These ingredients are important because they help fill nutritional gaps in the diet as well as help you feel full and satisfied. The nearly ubiquitous consumption of bread all over the world gives bread an important position in international nutrition, due to either the nutrients provided with its consumption or as vehicle or carrier in food fortification.

Flour fortification is the most common way of introducing nutrients in the diet when a food intervention strategy is planned. Continuous follow-up or evaluation or monitoring of the population status is necessary because people could change their dietary habits and even life-style, besides the different requirements depending on gender, age, physiological status, and so on. Evaluation and monitoring results support the effectiveness of this strategy to ameliorate deficiencies detected in the minerals and vitamins intake.

Nevertheless, fortification strategies might not reach the targeted population. Population group in need of micronutrients should be clearly identify to increase effectiveness of the fortification strategies, which in consequence will lead to a reduction in the medical cost.

Acknowledgements

Authors acknowledge the financial support of the Spanish Ministry of Economy and Competitiveness (Project AGL2011-23802), the European Regional Development Fund (FEDER) and Generalitat Valenciana (Project Prometeo 2012/064).

Keywords: Bread, fortification, enrichment, vitamins, minerals, nutrients

References

Ahmad, Z., M.S. Butt, A. Ahmed, M. Riaz, S.M. Sabir, U. Farooq and F.U. Rehman. 2012. Effect of *Aspergillus niger* xylanase on dough characteristics and bread quality attributes. Journal of Food Science and Technology, 1–9. doi: 10.1007/s13197-012-0734-8.

Ahmed, A., F.M. Anjum, M.A. Randhawa, U. Farooq, S. Akhtar and M.T. Sultan. 2012. Effect of multiple fortification on the bioavailability of minerals in wheat meal bread. Journal of Food Science and Technology-Mysore, 49(6): 737–744. doi: 10.1007/s13197-010-0224-9.

Akhtar, S., F.M. Anjum, S.U. Rehman, M.A. Sheikh and K. Farzana. 2008. Effect of fortification on physico-chemical and microbiological stability of whole wheat flour. Food Chemistry, 110(1): 113–119. doi: 10.1016/j.foodchem.2008.01.065.

Akhtar, S., F. Anjum, R. Ur Saleem and M.A. Sheikh. 2009. Effect of mineral fortification on rhelogical properties of whole wheat flour. Journal of Texture Studies, 40(1): 51–65. doi: 10.1111/j.1745-4603.2008.00169.x.

Albaldawi, A., C.S. Brennan, K. Alobaidy, W. Alammar and D. Aljumaily. 2005. Effect of flour fortification with haem liposome on bread and bread doughs. International Journal of Food Science and Technology, 40(8): 825–828. doi: 10.1111/j.1365-2621.2005.00995.x.

Al-Dmoor, H.M. 2012. Flat bread: ingredients and fortification. Quality Assurance and Safety of Crops & Foods, 4(1): 2–8. doi: 10.1111/j.1757-837X.2011.00121.x.

Allen, L., B. Benoist, O. Dary and R. Hurrell. 2006. Guidelines on food fortification with micronutrients. World Health Organization and Food and Agriculture Organization of the United Nations. http://www.who.int/nutrition/publications/guide_food_fortification_micronutrients.pdf (accessed 10.12.13).

Anderson, W.A., D. Slaughter, C. Laffey and C. Lardner. 2010. Reduction of folic acid during baking and implications for mandatory fortification of bread. International Journal of Food Science and Technology, 45(6): 1104–1110. doi: 10.1111/j.1365-2621.2010.02226.x.

Arredondo, M., V. Salvat, F. Pizarro and M. Olivares. 2006. Smaller iron particle size improves bioavailability of hydrogen-reduced iron-fortified bread. Nutrition Research, 26(5): 235–239. doi: 10.1016/j. nutres.2006.05.009.

Babarykin, D., I. Adamsone, D. Amerika, A. Spudass, V. Moisejev, N. Berzina, L. Michule and R. Rozental. 2004. Calcium-enriched bread for treatment of uremic hyperphosphatemia. Journal Renal Nutrition, 14: 149–156.

Batifoulier, F., M.A. Verny, E. Chanliaud, C. Rémésy and C. Demigné. 2005. Effect of different breadmaking methods on thiamine, riboflavin and pyridoxine contents of wheat bread. Journal of Cereal Science, 42: 101–108.

Baurenfiend, J.C. and E. DeRitter. 1991. Foods considered for nutrient addition: Cereal grain products. pp. 143–209. *In*: J.C. Baurenfiend and P.A. LaChance (eds.). Nutrient additions to Food, Connecticut, Food and Nutrition Press.

Berner, L.A., D.R. Keast, R.L. Bailey and J.T. Dwyer. 2014. Fortified Foods Are Major Contributors to Nutrient Intakes in Diets of US Children and Adolescents. Journal of the Academy of Nutrition and Dietetics, 114(7): 1009–1022. doi: 10.1016/j.jand.2013.10.012.

Bishai, D. and R. Nalubola. 2002. The history of food fortification in the United States: Its relevance for current fortification efforts in developing countries. Economic Development and Cultural Change, 51(1): 37–53. doi: 10.1086/345361.

Bothwell, T.H. 2000. Iron requirements in pregnancy and strategies to meet them. American Journal of Clinical Nutrition, 72(1): 257S–263S.

Brown, S.B., K.W. Reeves and E.R. Bertone-Johnson. 2014. Maternal folate exposure in pregnancy and childhood asthma and allergy: a systematic review. Nutrition Reviews, 72(1): 55–64. doi: 10.1111/nure.12080.

Cakirer, O.M. and P.A. Lachance. 1975. Added micronutrients: their stability in wheat flour during storage and the baking process. Bakers' Digest, 49(1): 53–57.

Calvo, M.S. and S.J. Whiting. 2013. Survey of current vitamin D food fortification practices in the United States and Canada. Journal of Steroid Biochemistry and Molecular Biology, 136: 211–213. doi: 10.1016/j.jsbmb.2012.09.034.

Castillo, C., J.A. Tur and R. Uauy. 2010. Flour fortification with folic acid in Chile. Unintended consequences. Rev. Med. Chil., 138(7): 832–840.

Centenaro, G.S., V. Feddern, E.T. Bonow and M. Salas-Mellado. 2007. Bread enrichment with fish protein. Ciencia e Tecnologia de Alimentos, 27: 663–668.

Charlton, K.E., H. Yeatman, E. Brock, C. Lucas, L. Gemming, A. Goodfellow and G. Ma. 2013. Improvement in iodine status of pregnant Australian women 3 years after introduction of a mandatory iodine fortification programme. Preventive Medicine, 57(1): 26–30. doi: 10.1016/j.ypmed.2013.03.007.

Clifton, V.L., N.A. Hodyl, P.A. Fogarty, D.J. Torpy, R. Roberts, T. Nettelbeck and B. Hetzel. 2013. The impact of iodine supplementation and bread fortification on urinary iodine concentrations in a mildly iodine deficient population of pregnant women in South Australia. Nutrition Journal, 12. doi: 10.1186/1475-2891-12-32.

Collar, C. and C.M. Rosell. 2012. Bakery and confectionary. pp. 554–582. *In*: M. Chandrasekaran (ed.). CRC Book on Valorization of food processing by products. CRC.

Costan, A.R., C. Vulpoi and V. Mocanu. 2014. Vitamin D fortified bread improves pain and physical function domains of quality of life in nursing home residents. Journal of Medicinal Food, 17(5): 625–631. doi: 10.1089/jmf.2012.0210.

Crider, K.S., L.B. Bailey and R.J. Berry. 2011. Folic acid food fortification-its history, effect, concerns, and future directions. Nutrients, 3(3): 370–384. doi: 10.3390/nu3030370.

Czeizel, A.E. and I. Dudas. 1992. Prevention of first occurrence of neural tube defects by periconceptional vitamin supplementation. New England Journal of Medicine, 327: 1832–1835.

Dalgetty, D.D. and B.K. Baik. 2006. Fortification of bread with hulls and cotyledon fibers isolated from peas, lentils, and chickpeas. Cereal Chemistry, 83(3): 269–274. doi: 10.1094/cc-83-0269.

Das, J.K., R. Kumar, R.A. Salam and Z.A. Bhutta. 2013. Systematic review of zinc fortification trials. Annals of Nutrition and Metabolism, 62: 44–56. doi: 10.1159/000348262.

Davies, N.T. and R. Nightingale. 1975. The effect of phytate on intestinal absorption and secretion of zinc and wholebody retention of zinc, copper, iron and manganese in rats. Journal of Nutrition, 34: 243–247.

Dietrich, M., C.J.P. Brown and G. Block. 2005. The effect of folate fortification of cereal-grain products on blood folate status, dietary folate intake, and dietary folate sources among adult non-supplement users in the United States. Journal of the American College of Nutrition, 24(4): 266–274.

EFSA. 2006. http://www.efsa.europa.eu/en/ndatopics/docs/ndatolerableuil.pdf (last access 28th October 2014).

El-Shaarawy, M.I. and A.S. Mesallam.1987. Feasibility of Saudi wheat flour enriched with cottonseed flour for bread making. Zeitschrift fuer Ernaehrungswissenschaft, 26(2): 100–106.

El-Soukkary, F.A.H. 2001. Evaluation of pumpkin seed products for bread fortification. Plant Foods for Human Nutrition, 56(4): 365–384. doi: 10.1023/a:1011802014770.

FAOSTAT. 2010. Food Balance Sheet, 2007, Food Agric Org, U.N. FAO Statistic Division.

FAO (2002). Economic and Social Department. http://www.fao.org/WAICENT/FAOINFO/ECONOMIC/ESN/fortify/reguls.htm.

Fernandez, A., M. Haros and C.M. Rosell. 2002. Nutritional improvement of whole wheat bread through the phytases activity during breadmaking. Proceedings of the European Symposium on Enzymes in Grain Processing 3 (ESEGP-3), Belgium.

Fiedler, J.L. and B. Macdonald. 2009. A strategic approach to the unfinished fortification agenda: Feasibility, costs, and cost-effectiveness analysis of fortification programs in 48 countries. Food and Nutrition Bulletin, 30(4): 283–316.

Figuerola, R.F., A.A. Estevez and V.E. Castillo. 1987. Supplementation of wheat flour with chickpea (Cicer arietinum) flour. I. Preparation of flours and their breadmaking properties. Archivos Latinoamericanos Nutricion, 37(2): 378–387.

Fletcher, R.J., I.P. Bell and J.P. Lambert. 2004. Public health aspects of food fortification: a question of balance. Proceedings of the Nutrition Society, 63(4): 605–614. doi: 10.1079/pns2004391.

Food and Drug Administration, USA. 1996a. Food standards: amendment of standards of identity for enriched grain products to require addition of folic acid: final rule, (21 CFR Parts 136, 137 and 139). Federal Register, 61: 8781–8797.

Food and Drug Administration, USA. 1996b. Food standards: food labelling: health claims and label statements: folate and neural tube defects: final rule, (21 CFR Part 101). Federal Register, 61: 8752–8781.

Food and Drug Administration, USA. 1996c. Food additives permitted for direct addition to food for human consumption; folic acid (folacin); final rule, (21 CFR Part 172). Federal Register, 61: 8797–8807.

Graham, G.G., E. Morales, A. Cordano and R.P. Placko. 1971. Lysine enrichment of wheat flour: prolonged feeding of infants. American Journal Clinical Nutrition, 24: 200–206.

Graham, R.D., J.M. Humphries and J.L. Kitchen. 2000. Nutritionally enhanced cereals: A sustainable foundation for a balanced diet. Asia Pacific Journal of Clinical Nutrition, 9: S91–S96. doi: 10.1046/j.1440-6047.2000.00185.x.

Green, T.J., Y.Z. Liu, S. Dadgar, W.Y. Li, R. Bohni and D.D. Kitts. 2013. Wheat rolls fortified with microencapsulated L-5-methyltetrahydrofolic acid or equimolar folic acid increase blood folate concentrations to a similar extent in healthy men and women. Journal of Nutrition, 143(6): 867–871. doi: 10.3945/jn.113.174268.

Greiner, T. 2007. Fortification of processed cereals should be mandatory. Lancet, 369(9575): 1766–1768. doi: 10.1016/s0140-6736(07)60791-0.

Hallberg, L., M. Brune and L. Rossander. 1986. Low bioavailability of carbonyl iron in man: studies on iron fortification of wheat flour. American Journal of Clinical Nutrition, 43(1): 59–67.

Hammond, N. 1983. Utilization of wheat protein concentrates in baked products in Central America. Developments in Food Science, 5B: 1069–1074.

Haros, M., C.M. Rosell and C. Benedito. 2001. Use of fungal phytase to improve breadmaking performance of wholewheat bread. J. Agric. Food Chem., 49(11): 5450–5454. doi: 10.1021/jf0106421.

Hawkesford, M.J. and F.J. Zhao. 2007. Strategies for increasing the selenium content of wheat. Journal of Cereal Science, 46: 282–292.

Hernandez, M., V. Sousa, S. Villalpando, A. Moreno, I. Montalvo and M. Lopez-Alarcon. 2006. Cooking and Fe fortification have different effects on Fe bioavailability of bread and tortillas. Journal of the American College of Nutrition, 25(1): 20–25.

Hertrampf, E., F. Cortes, J.D. Erickson, M. Cayazzo, W. Freire, L.B. Bailey and C. Pfeiffer. 2003. Consumption of folic acid-fortified bread improves folate status in women of reproductive age in Chile. Journal of Nutrition, 133(10): 3166–3169.

Hjortmo, S., J. Patring, J. Jastrebova and T. Andlid. 2008. Biofortification of folates in white wheat bread by selection of yeast strain and process. International Journal of Food Microbiology, 127: 32–36.

Hohman, E.E. and C.M. Weaver. 2011. Vitamin D bread could help solve insufficiency problem. Agro Food Industry Hi-Tech, 22(5): 24–25.

Huang, J., J. Sun, W.X. Li, L.J. Wang, J.S. Huo, J.S. Chen, C.M. Chen and A.X. Wang. 2009. Efficacy of different iron fortificants in wheat flour in controlling iron deficiency, Biomedical Environmental Science, 22: 118–121.

Huma, N., R. Ur Salim, F.M. Anjum, M.A. Murtaza and M.A. Sheikh. 2007. Food fortification strategy—Preventing iron deficiency anemia: A review. Critical Reviews in Food Science and Nutrition, 47(3): 259–265. doi: 10.1080/10408390600698262.

Hurrell, R.F., M.B. Reddy, J. Burri and J.D. Cook. 2000. An evaluation of EDTA compounds for iron fortification of cereal-based foods. British Journal of Nutrition, 84(6): 903–910.

Jiang, X.L., Z. Hao and J.C. Tian. 2008. Variations in amino acid and protein contents of wheat during milling and norther-style steamed breadmaking. Cereal Chemistry, 85: 504–508.

Kamien, M. 2006. The repeating history of objections to the fortification of bread and alcohol: from iron filings to folic acid. Medical Journal of Australia, 184(12): 638–640.

Lairon, D., N. Arnault, S. Bertrais, R. Planells, E. Clero, S. Hercberg and M.C. Boutron-Ruault. 2005. Dietary fibre intake and risk factors for cardiovascular disease in French adults. American Journal of Clinical Nutrition, 82: 1185–1194.

Lim, K.H.C., L.J. Riddell, C.A. Nowson, A.O. Booth and E.A. Szymlek-Gay. 2013. Iron and zinc nutrition in the economically-developed world: a review. Nutrients, 5(8): 3184–3211. doi: 10.3390/nu5083184.

Llanos, A., E. Hertrampf, F. Cortes, A. Pardo, S.D. Grosse and R. Uauy. 2007. Cost-effectiveness of a folic acid fortification program in Chile. Health Policy, 83: 295–303.

MacPhail, A.P. 2001. Iron deficiency and the developing world. Archivos Latinoamericanos De Nutricion, 51(1): 2–6.

Majeed, H., H.J. Qazi, W. Safdar and Z. Fang. 2013. Microencapsulation can be a novel tool in wheat flour with micronutrients fortification: Current Trends and Future Applications—a Review. Czech Journal of Food Sciences, 31(6): 527–540.

Mashayekh, M., M.R. Mahmoodi and M.H. Entezari. 2008. Effect of fortification of defatted soy flour on sensory and rheological properties of wheat bread. International Journal of Food Science and Technology, 43(9): 1693–1698. doi: 10.1111/j.1365-2621.2008.01755.x.

Mendoza, C., F.E. Viteri, B. Lonnerdal, V. Raboy, K.A. Young and K.H. Brown. 2001. Absorption of iron from unmodified maize and genetically altered, low-phytate maize fortified with ferrous sulfate or sodium iron EDTA. American Journal of Clinical Nutrition, 73(1): 80–85.

Moretti, D., R. Biebinger, M.J. Bruins, B. Hoeft and K. Kraemer. 2014. Bioavailability of iron, zinc, folic acid, and vitamin A from fortified maize. Technical Considerations for Maize Flour and Corn Meal Fortification in Public Health, 1312: 54–65. doi: 10.1111/nyas.12297.

Mostafa, M.K., A.S. Hamed and Y.H. Foda. 1982. Enrichment of wheat flour with dry skim-milk and dry buttermilk and its effect on the baking quality. Egyptian Journal Food Science, 8: 33–39.

Najm, N.E.O., A. Olabi, S. Kreyydieh and I. Toufeili. 2010. Determination of visual detection thresholds of selected iron fortificants and formulation of iron-fortified pocket-type flat bread. Journal of Cereal Science, 51: 271–276.

Nayak, B. and K.M. Nair. 2003. *In vitro* bioavailability of iron from wheat flour fortified with ascorbic acid, EDTA and sodium hexametaphosphate, with or without iron. Food Chemistry, 80: 545–550.

Oliete, B., M. Gomez, V. Pando, E. Fernandez-Fernandez, P.A. Caballero and F. Ronda. 2008. Effect of nut paste enrichment on physical characteristics and onsumer acceptability of bread. Food Science Technology International, 14: 259–269.

Ortiz-Monasterio, J.I., N. Palacios-Rojas, E. Meng, K. Pixley, R. Trethowan and R.J. Pena. 2007. Enhancing the mineral and vitamin content of wheat and maize through plant breeding. Journal of Cereal Science, 46: 293–307.

Pandey, A., P. Nigam, C.R. Soccol, V.T. Soccol, D. Singh and R. Mohan. 2000. Advances in microbial amylases. Biotechnol. Appl. Biochem., 31(2): 135–152.

Palacios, C., M. Haros, Y. Sanz and C.M. Rosell. 2008. Phytate degradation during whole wheat dough fermentation: effect of different Bifidobacterium strains. European Food Research and Technology, 226: 825–831.

Prieto, J.A., C. Collar and C. Benedito. 1990. Reversed phase high performance liquid chromatographic determination of biochemical changes in free amino acids during wheat flour mixing and bread baking. Journal of Chromatography Science, 28: 572–577.

Rader, J.I., C.M. Weaver and G. Angyal. 2000. Total folate in enriched cereal-grain products in the United States following fortification. Food Chemistry, 70(3): 275–289. doi: 10.1016/s0308-8146(00)00116-3.

Rahman, A., G.S. Savige, N.J. Deacon, J.E. Chesters and B.C. Panther. 2011. Urinary iodine deficiency in Gippsland pregnant women: the failure of bread fortification? Medical Journal of Australia, 194(5): 240–243.

Ranhotra, G.S., J.A. Gelroth and B.M. Okot-Kotber. 2000. Stability and dietary contribution of vitamin E added to bread. Cereal Chemistry, 77(2): 159–162. doi: 10.1094/cchem.2000.77.2.159.

Ranum, P. 2006. Update on iron fortification of milled cereals. Cereal Foods World, 51: 87–88.

Ranum, P., S. Lynch, T. Bothwell, L. Hallberg, R. Hurrell, P. Whittaker, J.L. Rosado, L. Davidsson, V. Mannar, T. Walter, S. Fairweather-Tait, O. Dary, J. Rivera, L. Bravo, M. Reddy, M.N. Garcia-Casal, E. Hertrampf and I. Parvanta. 2001. Guidelines for iron fortification of cereal food staples. Published online at www.sustaintech.org/publications/pubm7.pdf. SUSTAIN, Washington, DC.

Rosell, C.M., E. Santos, J.M. Sanz Penella and M. Haros. 2009. Wholemeal wheat bread: A comparison of different breadmaking processes and fungal phytase addition. Journal of Cereal Science, 50(2): 272–277. doi: 10.1016/j.jcs.2009.06.007.

Rosell, C.M. 2012. The nutritional enhancement of wheat flour. pp. 687–710. *In:* S. Cauvain (ed.). Breadmaking: Improving quality. 2nd edn. Woodhead Publishing, UK.

Rosell, C.M. 2011. The science of doughs and bread quality. pp. 3–14. *In:* V.R. Preedy, R.R. Watson and V.B. Patel (eds.). Flour and breads and their fortification in health and disease prevention. Academic Press, Elsevier, London, Burlington, San Diego.

Rosell,C.M. 2007. Vitamin and mineral fortification of bread. pp. 336–361. *In:* B. Hamaker (ed.). Technology of Functional Cereal Products. Woodhead Publishing Ltd., Cambridge, UK.

Rosell, C.M., G. Cortez and R. Repo-Carrasco. 2009. Breadmaking use of the Andean crops quinoa (*Chenopodium quinoa*), kañiwa (*Chenopodium pallidicaule*), kiwicha (*Amaranthus caudatus*), and tarwi (*Lupinus mutabilis*). Cereal Chemistry, 86: 386–392.

Sadighi, J., K. Mohammad, R. Sheikholeslam, M.A. Amirkhani, P. Torabi, F. Salehi and Z. Abdolahi. 2009. Anaemia control: Lessons from the flour fortification programme. Public Health, 123(12): 794–799. doi: 10.1016/j.puhe.2009.09.024.

Sadighi, J., R. Sheikholeslam, K. Mohammad, H. Pouraram, Z. Abdollahi, K. Samadpour and M. Naghavi. 2008. Flour fortification with iron: a mid-term evaluation. Public Health, 122(3): 313–321. doi: 10.1016/j.puhe.2007.05.002.

Samaniego-Vaesken, M.L., E. Alonso-Aperte and G. Varela-Moreiras. 2013. Voluntary food fortification with folic acid in Spain: Predicted contribution to children's dietary intakes as assessed with new food folate composition data. Food Chemistry, 140(3): 526–532. doi: 10.1016/j.foodchem.2013.01.092.

Shane, B. 2003. Folate fortification: enough already? American Journal of Clinical Nutrition, 77(1): 8–9.

Sichert-Hellert, W., M. Kersting, U. Alexy and F. Manz. 2000. Ten-year trends in vitamin and mineral intake from fortified food in German children and adolescents. Eur. J. Clin. Nutr., 54(1): 81–86. doi: 10.1038/sj.ejcn.1600897.

Skeaff, S., Y. Zhao, R. Gibson, M. Makrides and S.J. Zhou. 2014. Iodine status in pre-school children prior to mandatory iodine fortification in Australia. Maternal and Child Nutrition, 10(2): 304–312. doi: 10.1111/j.1740-8709.2012.00419.x.

Slavin, J.L. 2000. Whole grains, refined grains and fortified refined grains: What's the difference? Asia Pacific Journal of Clinical Nutrition, 9: S23–S27. doi: 10.1046/j.1440-6047.2000.00171.x.

Solon, F.S., R.D.W. Klemm, L. Sanchez, I. Darnton-Hill, N.E. Craft, P. Christian and K.P. West. 2000. Efficacy of a vitamin A-fortified wheat-flour bun on the vitamin A status of Filipino schoolchildren. American Journal of Clinical Nutrition, 72(3): 738–744.

Stabnikova, O., V. Ivanov, I. Larionova, V. Stabnikov, M.A. Bryszewska and J. Lewis. 2008. Ukrainian dietary bakery product with selenium-enriched yeast. LWT—Food Science Technology, 41: 890–895.

Stepanova, E.N., L.N. Shatnyuk, M.F. Verzhinskaya, M.G. Kostyleva, N.A. Bukina, V.B. Spirichev, A.F. Shukhnov, N.N. Kosteltseva, A.I. Bistrova and I.B. Emtseva. 1988. Effect of method of vitaminization of high grade wheat flour bread on its content on thiamine, riboflavin and niacin. Voprosy-Pitaniya, 2: 67–71.

Steyn, N.P., P. Wolmarans, J.H. Nel and L.T. Bourne. 2008. National fortification of staple foods can make a significant contribution to micronutrient intake of South African adults. Public Health Nutr., 11(3): 307–313. doi: 10.1017/s136898000700033x.

Tedstone, A., M. Browne, L. Harrop, C. Vernon, V. Page, J. Swindells and L. Stockley. 2008. Fortification of selected foodstuffs with folic acid in the UK: consumer research carried out to inform policy recommendations. Journal of Public Health, 30(1): 23–29. doi: 10.1093/pubmed/fdm073.

Ueland, P.M. and S. Hustad. 2008. Homocysteine and folate status in an era of folic acid fortification: Balancing benefits, risks, and B-vitamins. Clinical Chemistry, 54(5): 779–781. doi: 10.1373/clinchem.2008.103218.

Vanharanta, M., J. Mursu, T. Nurmi, S. Voutilainen, T. Rissanen, R. Salonen and J.T. Salonen. 2002. Phloem fortification in rye bread elevates serum enterolactone level. Eur. J. Clin. Nutr., 56(10): 952–957. doi: 10.1038/sj.ejcn.1601510.

Vazquez-Rodriguez, J.A., C.A. Amaya-Guerra, J.G. Baez-Gonzalez, M.A. Nunez-Gonzalez and J.D. Figueroa-Cardenas. 2013. Study of the fortification with bean and amaranth flours in nixtamalized maize tortilla. Cyta-Journal of Food, 11: 62–66. doi: 10.1080/19476337.2012.753644.

Waliszewski, K.N., Y. Estrada and V. Pardio. 2000. Lysine and tryptophan fortification of nixtamalized corn flour. International Journal of Food Science and Technology, 35(5): 523–527. doi: 10.1046/j.1365-2621.2000.00415.x.

Wallace, J.M.W., A.J. McCabe, P.J. Robson, M.K. Keogh, C.A. Murray, P.M. Kelly and J.J. Strain. 2000. Bioavailability of n-3 polyunsaturated fatty acids (PUFA) in foods enriched with microencapsulated fish oil. Annals of Nutrition and Metabolism, 44(4): 157–162. doi: 10.1159/000012839.

Wallace, T.C., C. Reider and V.L. Fulgoni. 2013. Calcium and vitamin D disparities are related to gender, age, race, household income level, and weight classification but not vegetarian status in the United States: Analysis of the NHANES 2001-2008 Data Set. Journal of the American College of Nutrition, 32(5): 321-330. doi: 10.1080/07315724.2013.839905.

Wang, S. and Y.R. Tang. 1995. Fortification of Ca and Zn in wheat flour. Journal Zhengzhou Grain College, 16(1): 26–34.

Waters, D.M., F. Jacob, J. Titze, E.K. Arendt and E. Zannini. 2012. Fibre, protein and mineral fortification of wheat bread through milled and fermented brewer's spent grain enrichment. European Food Research and Technology, 235(5): 767–778. doi: 10.1007/s00217-012-1805-9.

Whittaker, P., P.R. Tufaro and J.I. Rader. 2001. Iron and folate in fortified cereals. Journal of the American College of Nutrition, 20(3): 247–254.

Yasoda-Devi, M. and P. Geervani. 1979. Acceptability of fortified wheat products. Indian Journal Nutrition Dietetics, 16(2): 49–51.

Zhaoa, F. and S.P. McGratha. 2009. Biofortification and phytoremediation. Current Opinion in Plant Biology, 12: 373–380.

10

Agronomic Fortification and the Impact on Bread Fortification

Aly F. El Sheikha[1,2]

1. Introduction

Through the years, grain millers found removing bran led to more desirable flour. Taste became milder and less susceptible to oxidation as rancidity-prone oils were no longer present. Removal of the grain's bran and germ, however, left the flour short on naturally occurring vitamins, minerals and phytonutrients.

Bread's relatively low cost and commonality to countless diet plans made it an excellent vehicle for nutrients missing from many consumers' diets. Shortly after issuing its Recommended Daily Allowances (RDAs) in 1941, FDA was joined by bread manufacturer Continental Baking Co. in developing a bread-enrichment, adding niacin, riboflavin (B_2), thiamin (B_1), calcium and iron to bread to help stop the spread of nutritional-deficiency-related diseases, including beriberi, pellagra and severe nutritional anemia, in the United States. More recently, folic acid has become a common enrichment ingredient, helping prevent neural tube birth defects like spina bifida (Fig. 1) (Wesley and Ranum 2004).

Because enriched bread is typically consumed as part of a greater meal item, its added vitamins and minerals are better absorbed. Calcium, for example, is more effectively absorbed in the presence of protein. Consuming calcium-fortified bread as a peanut butter or meat-and-cheese sandwich, therefore, improves the absorption of the added calcium (Ahmed et al. 2008; Ahmed et al. 2012).

[1] Minufiya University, Faculty of Agriculture, Department of Food Science and Technology, 32511 Shibin El Kom, Minufiya Government, Egypt.
[2] Al-Baha University, Faculty of Sciences, Department of Biology, P.O. Box 1988, Al-Baha, Saudi Arabia. Email: elsheikha_aly@yahoo.com

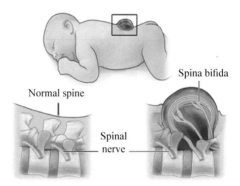

Figure 1. Illustrated drawing of infant with defect of spina bifida.

Consumers have discovered that bread provides nutrients but their fast-paced diets fall short on health-conscious. Unlike "enrichments" where vitamins and minerals are added to enhance or replace naturally occurring elements, "fortification" programs add nutritive elements normally not present. Consumers are turning for help in their quest for better health to these fortified products.[1]

This chapter highlights the application strategies and importance of agronomic fortification and proved that micronutrient fortification of nutrient-deficient soils can not only help boost crop yields but can also improve the content and bioavailability of these nutrients in plants when consumed by humans. Also, explain how the agronomic fortification reflected positively for countries' economies especially of the developing countries.

This chapter also answered several important questions, including:

- Is agronomic fortification of tools combating the hidden hunger?
- Is agronomic fortification a sufficient tool for fortification?
- What are the complementary relationship between agronomic fortification and the flour fortification?
- What is the role of bio-fortification in sustainable development?

2. Why we need the agronomic fortification?

Billions of people, mostly in developing countries, suffer from micronutrient deficiencies, sometimes called "hidden hunger". The problem of hidden hunger—micronutrient deficiency—affects far more people than hunger. It can be difficult to count those affected. About 1 in 3 people affected, according to the Micronutrient Initiative. Figure 2 shows the areas suffering from deficiencies of the most common micronutrients worldwide at three severity levels (low, medium and high).

The micronutrients most commonly associated with human health problems on a global scale include those to deal with iron, zinc and selenium deficiencies. In contrast to food security, nutrition security has been traditionally viewed as being within the

---

[1] http://www.foodproductdesign.com/articles/2008/06/bread-fortification-on-the-rise.aspx

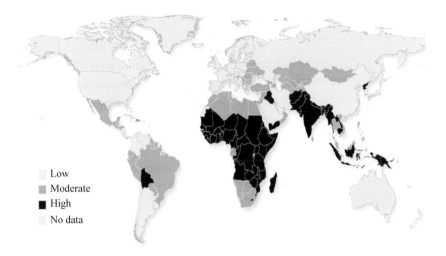

Figure 2. Severity levels deficiencies of the most common micronutrient worldwide (Source: http://www.harvestplus.org/content/nutrients).

realm of health professionals. Yet the entire agri-food chain has a vital role to play in addressing this problem. Producing more nutritious food and feed, or "farming for health", should therefore be a central objective. This means increasing micronutrient content through fertilization "agronomic fortification", which holds out the promise of fighting deficiencies in soils, plants, animals and people (IFA 2010).

The costs of these deficiencies in terms of lives lost and poor quality of life are staggering (Table 1).

Table 1. Extent and consequences of micronutrient deficiencies.

Micronutrient	Prevalence in the world	Groups most affected	Consequences
Iron (Fe)	60 percent of the world population	All, but especially women and children	Reduced cognitive ability; childbirth complications; reduced physical capacity and productivity
Zinc (Zn)	30 percent of the world population	Women and children	Illness from infectious diseases, poor child growth; pregnancy and childbirth complications; reduced birth weight
Selenium (Se)	15 percent of the world population	All, but especially men	Increased risk of thyroid and immune dysfunction, viral infections, cancer and inflammatory conditions

Source: Adapted from ACC/SCN 2000; Whitney et al. 2002; Rolfes et al. 2011; Bilski et al. 2012; Das et al. 2013

2.1 Basic definitions related to bread fortification

Fortification: Addition of lost or missing minerals to a massively consumed or targeted bread vehicle that is consumed regularly in predictable amounts, without affecting the vehicle's organoleptic characteristics.

Bio-fortification: Enhancement of iron or zinc in edible portion of a staple food crop through traditional plant breeding without sacrificing agronomic qualities (i.e., yield). No additional cost to consumer.[2] In another definition **Bio-fortification**: Plant breeding, genetic engineering and agronomic techniques to increase Fe, Zn, I and Se in plant foods. **Plant Breeding**: Select for high micronutrient content or bioavailability and cross breed. **Genetic Engineering**: Use molecular methods to transfer across species genes that will improve micronutrient content or bioavailability. **Agronomic**: Application of fertilizers.[3]

Agronomic bio-fortification: Determine how to use agronomic means, particularly fertilization and crop management, to increase micronutrient levels in the edible parts of plants (IFA 2010).

Bio-fortification differs from ordinary fortification because it focuses on making plant foods more nutritious as the plants are growing, rather than having nutrients added to the foods when they are processed.[4] This is an improvement on ordinary fortification when it comes to providing nutrients for the rural poor, who rarely have access to commercially fortified foods (Islam 2007). As such, bio-fortification is seen as an upcoming strategy for dealing with deficiencies of micronutrients in the developing world. In the case of iron, WHO estimated that bio-fortification could help curing the two billion people suffering from iron deficiency-induced anemia (de Benoist et al. 2008).

Bioavailability "in nutritional sciences": Covers the intake of nutrients and non-drug dietary ingredients. The concept of bioavailability lacks the well-defined standards associated with the pharmaceutical industry. The pharmacological definition cannot apply to these substances because utilization and absorption is a function of the nutritional status and physiological state of the subject (Heaney 2001), resulting in even greater differences from individual to individual (inter-individual variation). Therefore, bioavailability for dietary supplements can be defined as the proportion of the administered substance capable of being absorbed and available for use or storage (Srinivasan 2001).

The Food Fortification Initiative (FFI): Formerly the Flour Fortification Initiative is an international partnership working to improve health by advocating for fortification in industrial grain mills. It specializes in wheat and maize flour and rice.

The FFI global network of partners provides advocacy support and technical assistance to help you plan, implement, and monitor high-quality fortification practices (FFI 2014).

---

[2] http://www.umb.no/statisk/costaction/final_eboy_mineral_fortification_of_foods.pdf
[3] http://www.umb.no/statisk/costaction/120514_cost_action_fa0905_june_2012.pdf
[4] http://www.dartmouth.edu/~news/releases/2007/11/19a.html

The WHO e-Library of Evidence for Nutrition Actions (eLENA): An online library of evidence-informed guidance for nutrition interventions. It is a single point of reference for the latest nutrition guidelines, recommendations and related information including supporting materials such as scientific evidence, background materials and commentaries from invited experts.

eLENA aims to help countries successfully implement and scale-up nutrition interventions by informing as well as guiding policy development and program design.

2.2 Why agronomic fortify?

When vitamins and minerals are added to wheat and maize flour, commonly eaten foods become more nutritious. Consequently, consumers improve their health without changing their habits. The extra nutrition helps people become smarter, stronger and healthier.

The three main benefits of agronomic fortification are:

1. Improved health
2. Increased productivity
3. Economic progress

Improved nutrition prevents diseases, strengthens immune systems, and improves productivity and cognitive development. Cereals—especially rice, wheat, and maize—provide nutrition to the populations of many developing countries. Most of the population in such countries depends on a low-protein and low-mineral diet comprising these staple foods. Meanwhile, according to an estimate, over 60 percent of the world's people are iron deficient, over 30 percent are deficient in zinc, and about 15 percent lack sufficient selenium in their systems.[5]

Agronomic fortification as part of a country's nutrition strategy is supported by global organizations such as UNICEF, the World Health Organization (WHO), the U.S. Centers for Disease Control and Prevention (CDC), the Global Alliance for Improved Nutrition (GAIN), and the Micronutrient Initiative (MI). For the latest evidence and guidance on nutrition interventions, eLENA provides important information on nutrition interventions which is organized in an intuitive manner (FFI 2014).

3. Agronomic fortification...improved health?

The agronomic fortification strategy seeks to take advantage of the consistent daily consumption of large amounts of food staples by all family members, including women and children who are most at risk for micronutrient malnutrition. Soils poor in micronutrients may cause crop and food deficiencies, resulting in deficiencies in animals and people. Increasing the micronutrient density of food crops for human health reasons could require higher application rates than those needed to achieve optimal crop yields (IFA 2010).

---

[5] http://tribune.com.pk/story/451650/crop-bio-fortification-can-combat-hidden-hunger/

Bio-fortified crops "especially cereals", which have been bred to have higher amounts of micronutrients, can help provide these needed vitamins and minerals. They can be effective in reducing hidden hunger as part of a strategy that includes dietary diversification, supplementation, and commercial fortification, among others.[6]

Iron (Fe), zinc (Zn) and selenium (Se) deficiencies are serious public health issues and important soil constraints to crop production, particularly in the developing world (Lyons et al. 2004; Cakmak 2010).

Various physiological diseases, such as anemia and some neurodegenerative diseases are triggered by Fe deficiency (Andreini et al. 2006). Human health problems caused by Fe deficiency can be prevented by specific attention to food composition and by choosing a balanced diet with sufficient Fe concentration.

This potential is shown schematically in Fig. 3, in which a high percentage of the iron-deficient population is shown to be relatively mildly deficient. For those who are severely deficient, supplements (the highest-cost intervention) are required.

Zinc is one of the most important micronutrients in biological systems, and plays a critical role in protein synthesis and metabolism. Several of Zn-binding proteins are transcription factors necessary for gene regulation and necessary for more than a half of enzymes and proteins involved in ion transport (Black 2003). Any decrease in Zn concentration in human body may result in number of cellular dis-functions, including a high susceptibility to infectious diseases, retardation of mental development, and stunted growth of children. Zinc deficiency is considered one of major causes of children death in the world. It is responsible for more than four percent of the deaths of children less than five years of age (Rayman 2000). High consumption of cereal-based foods with low concentration of Zn is the major reason of Zn deficiency in human populations, especially in developing world (Eichler et al. 2012). This problem

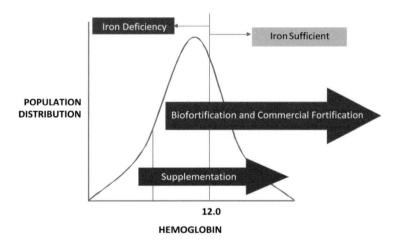

Figure 3. Biofortification improves status for those less deficient and maintains status for all at low coast. Iron adequacy for a population is indicated as 12.0 mg.dL^{-1} on the plot. Biofortification will shift the population into a more Fe-sufficient range (Source: Bouis and Welch 2010).

---

[6] http://www.harvestplus.org/content/nutrients

is aggravated by growing cereal crops on potentially Zn deficient soils. A widespread deficiency of Zn in humans occurs mainly in the regions where soils have Zn deficiency problem and cereals are major source of daily calorie intake (Cakmak 2010).

Selenium (Se) is an essential micronutrient for normal mammalian cell function, with antioxidant, anti-cancer and anti-viral properties, and cereal crops are major dietary sources of Se (Lyons et al. 2004; Kabata-Pendias and Mukherjee 2010).

Selenium deficiency is widespread and likely manifested in populations as increased risk of thyroid and immune dysfunction, viral infections, cancer and inflammatory conditions (Lyons et al. 2004). There is strong evidence suggesting that supranutritional Se intake provides protection against cancer (Combs 2001; Cakmak 2009). In many soils Se is poorly available to plants, and of concern is a trend toward a reduction of Se in a global food chain, possibly caused by fossil fuel burning (with release of sulphur, a Se antagonist), acid rain, soil acidification and use of high-S fertilizers. As cereal crops are major dietary sources of Se, it is important to modify agronomic practices, mainly through plant fertilization, that may influence Se concentration in these crops in order to maintain, if not increase, the concentration of selenium in plants (Lyons et al. 2004).

Impacts of micronutrient deficiencies on human health could be summarized as follow (IFA 2010):

- Premature deaths;
- Impairment of mental and cognitive development;
- Reduced productivity, with higher rates of chronic disease and disabilities; and
- Increased sensitivity to disease.

It is important to highlight that the use of agronomical bio-fortification might be especially desirable in various developing countries. Most of farmers in such countries (e.g., in Africa) cannot afford application of mineral fertilizers, and it would be desirable to find a solution through the application of some cheap materials which would serve as potential fertilizers, would contain a variety of micronutrients, and would be considered as non-toxic from environmental health point of view (Bilski et al. 2012).

Table 2 provides conservative estimates of the amounts of iron and β-carotene that may add through bio-fortification to diets for wheat as one of the important staple crops for the indicated sub regions.

4. Agronomic fortification...increased productivity?

In the field of crop nutrient management, an emerging concern is how to ensure that micronutrient levels in harvested products are adequate for human nutrition. Much of the relevant research focuses on the bioavailability of zinc, selenium, iron and possibly boron and iodine in staple cereal grains, wheat and rice. The use of iron for agronomic bio-fortification is not viable since this essential nutrient is not mobile. Nevertheless, increasing micronutrient density and bioavailability warrant consideration in a greater number of crops. In human and animal diets the range of essential micronutrients

Table 2. Estimated increments in iron and β-carotene intakes due to bio-fortification of wheat.

Region/subregion	Iron increment (mg/day)	Increment in beta-carotene (mg/day)
Latin America	1.7	0.6
Central America	1.3	0.4
Caribbean	1.5	0.5
South America	1.8	0.6
Africa/Near East Asia	2.7	0.9
North, Northwest Africa	5.2	1.7
Near East Asia	5.7	1.9
Western Africa	0.3	0.1
Central Africa	0.4	0.1
Eastern Africa	0.4	0.1
Southern Africa	2.1	0.7
Asia	2.1	0.7
South Asia	2.4	0.8
Southeast Asia	0.5	0.2

Source: Adapted from CIAT and IFPRI 2002

is broader than in the case of plants, extending to a number of organic compounds including vitamin A. The importance of adequate micronutrient levels of chromium (Cr), cobalt (Co), iodine (I), selenium (Se), silicon (Si) and fluorine (F) should also be considered.

Lastly, micronutrient fertilization can also be an effective treatment against plant diseases. For instance, the addition of copper to fertilizers has been shown to be effective in soils prone to ergot, a fungal disease that grows on cereal crops and can cause hallucinations in humans and other illnesses if ingested.[7]

Impacts of micronutrient deficiencies on crop production could be summarized as follow (IFA 2010):

- Reduced yields;
- Poor quality produces, e.g., low oil content, poor fiber quality, deformed fruits;
- Decreased N fixation by leguminous crops;
- Reduced crop vigour;
- Low germination rates;
- Shorter storage life; and
- Reduced efficiency of macronutrients.

5. Agronomic fortification...economic progress?

The economic benefits a country experiences because of investing in fortification are tremendous. The fertilizer industry has a significant role to play in those parts of

---

[7] http://www.foodsecurity.ac.uk/blog/index.php/2013/10/fortifying-fertilizers-can-fortify-food/

the world where large numbers of people suffer from deficiencies of micronutrients such as zinc, selenium, boron and iodine. These four micronutrients can be supplied through fertilization. Strong market development opportunities constitute a powerful business case for the fertilizer industry to contribute to human well-being by making micronutrient products available (FFI 2014).

The cost-effectiveness of an intervention is expressed in terms of the cost of achieving a specified outcome. Analyses of cost-effectiveness are particularly useful for comparing different interventions that share the same outcome. In assessments of health interventions, the two most widely used effectiveness measures are "cost per death averted" and the "cost per disability adjusted life-year saved" (cost per DALY saved). Both measures can apply to micronutrient interventions. Although the latter measure combines mortality and morbidity outcomes into a single indicator, its calculation is generally more demanding in terms of data needs and assumptions (Allen et al. 2006).

Cost-effectiveness and cost-benefit analyses have shown that:

- Both iodine and iron fortification have the potential to achieve high cost–benefit ratios, given the prevailing levels of micronutrient deficiency and the economic situation of many low-income countries;
- Bio-fortification with iron and zinc is highly cost-effective in children and pregnant women; and
- Agronomic fortification becomes increasingly cost-effective the higher the proportion of the population in need of the intervention. Because of the predominance of food staples in the diets of the poor, this strategy implicitly targets low-income households.

6. Application strategies for agronomic fortification

Generally, the micronutrient requirements of crops met by adding micronutrient fertilizers either directly to soils or as foliar spray. Low concentrations of micronutrients (typically a few kilograms per hectare) are sufficient for optimum crop production.

Several application strategies exist for agronomic fortification (IFA 2010):

- *Blended fertilizers*: Bulk blending of granular macronutrient and micronutrient fertilizers is widely practiced. A large number of blends of different grades can produce regionally to meet specifications for different soils, crops, or even particular fields.
- *Fluid fertilizers*: Micronutrient compounds can add to fluid N, NP or NPK carrier fertilizers for soil or foliar application.
- *Compound fertilizers*: In compound fertilizers, the micronutrients are incorporated during manufacture. They are either added during the production of fertilizer granules or sprayed onto the granule surface.
- *Controlled-release fertilizers*: These are polymer-coated granules or prills designed to allow a slow dispersal of the nutrient content in the soil. Wide ranges of such products contain micronutrients.

- *Foliar spray*: Foliar application of micronutrients is the method of choice for some field crops in Europe and North America, as well as for many fruit, vegetable and flower crops around the world. Its importance for field crops is increasing, especially in developing countries. Micronutrients can apply to crops in liquid form or as a suspension.
- *Fertigation*: Micronutrients can apply in water-soluble solutions through irrigation systems, particularly trickle or drip irrigation.
- *Hydroponics*: Micronutrients apply in water-soluble solutions in systems that use inert material such as gravel, sand, perlite or rockwood instead of soil.

7. Agronomic fortification fights "hidden hunger"...but how?

Agronomic fortification with micronutrients can be used as an effective and quick agricultural tool to improve the nutrition and health of people in developing economies (Bell and Dell 2008).

The International Fertilizer Industry Association (IFA) recently launched an initiative to assess linkages between fertilizer applications and human health, with the ultimate objective of developing practical fertilizer recommendations that combine crop productivity, environmental protection and human health considerations.

The fertilizer industry works with farming communities worldwide to teach farmers the best way to use their products. Best practices need to evolve constantly. Unless supply increases at the same rate as crop removal, deficiencies may emerge where they did not previously limit crop growth. However the continued use of micronutrients may lead, over time, to excessive levels that could threaten food safety or environmental quality, particularly in the case of micronutrients such as selenium where there is a narrow margin between deficiency and toxicity (IFA 2010).

8. Agronomic fortification...is it enough?

Fortification of a staple food is a highly effective tool to improve public health. Wheat flour fortification offers a tremendous opportunity toward improving the micronutrient status of populations because more than 400 million tons of wheat is eaten each year, most of which is milled by large roller mills. In its natural state, wheat is an excellent source of many vitamins. But because most of them are concentrated in the outer layers of the wheat grain, a significant proportion is lost during the milling process (FFI 2014).

8.1 Need of flour fortification

Bread and flour-based foods are an important part of the diet for millions of people worldwide. Their complex nature provides energy, protein, minerals and many other macro- and micronutrients. However, consideration must be given to three major aspects related to flour and bread. The first is that not all cultures consume bread made from wheat flour. There are literally dozens of flour types, each with their distinctive heritage, cultural roles and nutritive contents. Second, not all flours are used to make leavened bread in the traditional (i.e., Western) loaf form. Flours are used in many different ways in the production of staple foods. Third, flour and breads provide a suitable means for fortification: either to add components that are removed in the milling and purification process or to add components that will increase palatability or promote health and reduce disease per se (Preedy et al. 2011; Preedy et al. 2013). All details under this title are discussed earlier in chapter titled "Bread Fortification".

8.2 Enriching flour...enriching lives

Wheat, the "Staff of Life", has been an essential commodity to human existence through the centuries and is currently the most widely consumed staple food (Bagriansky 2003). As versatile as they are nutritious, wheat products have graced tables in all continents. The range of forms this staple food takes correspondingly varied: crusty French bread, soft Mexican tortillas and spicy Indonesian noodles being a few examples. Fortunately, for wheat eaters, wheat flour naturally contains many nutrients essential to human growth and development (Wesley and Ranum 2004).

Wheat is important not only to stimulate appetite; it also plays an important role in ending "hidden hunger". "Hidden hunger" is caused by subtle vitamin and mineral inadequacies, which show themselves over time in the reduced productive capacity of individuals and nations (Gautam 2003). Vitamin and mineral deficiencies cause "hunger" because the body will wither and die without the necessary levels of these nutrients. This hunger is "hidden" because vitamin and mineral deficiencies do not stimulate the appetite.

Approximately two billion people throughout the world are affected by "hidden hunger". Two of the chief nutrient deficiencies causing "hidden hunger" are those of iron and folic acid. These nutrients are essential for mothers to give birth to healthy babies and for children to reach their full intellectual and physical capabilities. Flour processing reduces the natural level of iron and folic acids, and people's inability to consume balanced diets. People in many countries who consume large amounts of flour suffer from iron and folic acid deficiencies. These deficiencies cause paralyzing birth defects and reduce the ability of children to learn and of adults to work hard (Gautam 2003).

9. Bio-fortification: challenge program scope and objectives

The ultimate goal of the bio-fortification strategy is to reduce mortality and morbidity rates related to micronutrient malnutrition and to increase food security, productivity, and the quality of life for poor populations of developing countries by breeding staple crops that provide, at low cost, improved levels of bioavailable micronutrients in a fashion sustainable over time. Developing plant breeding tools, crossing, testing various lines for nutritional effects, eventual dissemination of nutritionally improved varieties, and measuring their effectiveness in reducing malnutrition, indeed putting in place a new paradigm for agriculture and nutrition is a process that will take a decade. Some intermediate outputs, however, can be made available in a 3- to 5-yr period.

Funding is sought for a 4-yr project that is part of a 10-yr plan. At the end of four years, it will be possible to evaluate progress and the viability of further investments in the 10-yr plan. The 10-yr plan is described below, and outputs of the first 4-yr project are identified within that plan (CIAT and IFPRI 2002).

The primary objectives of the 10-yr plan are to:

- Select and breed nutritionally improved varieties of six major staple food crops with superior agronomic properties that make them attractive to farmers to grow.
- Demonstrate convincingly in the short to medium term the nutritional efficacy of the bio-fortification strategy.
- Develop efficient, accelerated mechanisms for testing materials on farms, including in areas among the most nutritionally disadvantaged, in order to identify varieties with superior agronomic, socioeconomic, and farmer-acceptable traits.
- Undertake activities to promote the adoption and dissemination of these varieties efficiently and rapidly in selected developing countries in Africa, Asia, and Latin America among the nutritionally disadvantaged.
- Measure the nutritional and other impacts of these nutritionally improved varieties in community based studies where these varieties have adopted.

Complementary objectives are to:

- Initiate pre-breeding studies to determine the feasibility of undertaking full-scale breeding programs for an additional 11 food staple crops.
- Understand better how dietary factors determine the bioavailability of micronutrients in malnourished populations in developing countries, especially interactions among micronutrients, anti-nutrients such as phytates, promoter compounds, and physiological status.
- Inform decision-makers in developing countries about cost-effective strategies to reduce micronutrient malnutrition through food-based approaches and policies to improve dietary quality among the poor.

Staple food crops under the project classified into two groups:

- Phase 1 crops, for which the knowledge base already exists to breed for improved micronutritional quality: wheat, maize, rice, sweet potatoes, common beans and cassava; and
- Phase 2 crops, for which the knowledge base must be established: sorghum, millet, groundnuts, pigeon peas, lentils, barley, cowpeas, yams, potatoes, bananas and plantains.

The primary target micronutrient deficiencies are iron, zinc and vitamin A. Delivery of improved, biofortified varieties to end-users will assure through an alliance of international centers, NARES, ARIs, NGOs, and farmers' organizations and the use of participatory breeding techniques. As already stated, the bio-fortification breeding strategy is envisioned as a complement to other successful ongoing approaches, including supplementation and fortification (CIAT and IFPRI 2002).

9.1 Why a challenge program?

The Bio-fortification Challenge Program pushes the boundaries of agricultural research beyond the traditional limits of food security and sustainability and makes direct linkages with the human health and nutrition sectors. By making a formal connection between what people grow and consume and how healthy they are as a result, the program marries the often separate agendas of the international nutrition and agricultural research communities in the context of working concertedly to address a specific problem of global concern: micronutrient malnutrition.

This linkage of agricultural research and human health goals raises the profile of the international agricultural research system and gives new relevance to the often-unheralded work done throughout the CGIAR-supported Future Harvest Centers and our partners in the developing and developed world (CIAT and IFPRI 2002).

Building on a solid foundation of research results, the program will develop, deploy and measure the nutritional impact of micronutrient-improved varieties of staple crops consumed by the poorest of the poor in Africa, Asia, and Latin America. Activities will be undertaken by an international alliance of Future Harvest Centers, national agricultural research and extension systems (NARES), departments of human nutrition and plant science at universities in developing and developed countries, advanced research institutes (ARIs) with expertise in micronutrients in plants and animals, and genomics, nongovernmental organizations (NGOs), farmers' organizations in developing countries, and private-sector partnerships. The Future Harvest Centers involved in the Bio-fortification Challenge Program are world renowned for their plant breeding expertise and extensive germplasm banks, strong ties to national agricultural extension programs, and links to the human nutrition community. Thus, they are well placed to coordinate the proposed activities. However, close collaboration with institutions that offer complementary scientific expertise, skills and experience not found within the Future Harvest Centers is critical to a successful outcome. To achieve the goals and objectives of the Program, new ways of working together, both within the CGIAR system and with external partners, are needed. Such arrangements are possible under the Challenge Program framework but not under a Systemwide Initiative (CIAT and IFPRI 2002).

There are significant advantages to working together in a coordinated fashion, under the rubric of a challenge program:

- Program success depends critically on the alignment of objectives and the coordinated efforts of institutions with diverse disciplinary perspectives, experience and skills.
- These multiple partnerships, many formed with nontraditional collaborators of the CGIAR system, require strong central coordination to avoid loss of program focus.
- Interdisciplinary communication within single crop activities and common experiences across these crop activities will stimulate fresh insights and discovery of novel solutions.

- Standardization of methodologies (such as sample analyses) will lead to greater acceptance and applicability of results.
- Program-coordinated work in nutritional genomics, identification of breeding objectives, and other core research applicable across crops or nutrients will avoid duplication of efforts and result in cost savings.
- Consolidation of the main advocacy, fund-raising, communications, and other administrative burdens will permit the individual partners to focus on the core research, development, deployment, and impact analysis activities.
- Attraction of new sources of funding is best handled through centralized coordination.

The program will heighten the profile of the CGIAR system as an important world body addressing pressing global concerns.

Table 3 shows that how the bio-fortification could contribute to the millennium development goals.

10. Comparative advantages of bio-fortification

Eliminating micronutrient malnutrition in any one country will require bringing to bear an array of interventions including supplementation, commercial fortification, and greater dietary diversity through nutrition education and higher incomes. Bio-fortification must have some comparative advantages relative to existing interventions to justify investments in this approach. These comparative advantages are discussed below.

10.1 Reaching the malnourished in rural areas

The biofortification strategy seeks to put the micronutrient-dense seed trait in the most profitable, highest yielding varieties being released to farmers. This will be feasible by agricultural research systems—as many released lines as future research and experience. Thus, nutritionally improved varieties would reach into relatively remote rural areas not presently well covered by commercial fortification and supplementation programs. Moreover, marketed surpluses of these crops would make their way into retail outlets, reaching consumers in both rural and urban areas. The direction of the flow, as it were, is from rural to urban. Often commercial fortification works best for imported foods (such as wheat flour) that are processed at a few central industrial establishments. These foods flow from urban to rural locations. This situation clearly shows the complementarity of biofortification and commercial fortification (CIAT and IFPRI 2002).

10.2 Cost-effectiveness and low cost

Unlike the continual financial outlays required for supplementation and fortification programs, a one-time investment in breeding-based solutions can yield micronutrient-

Table 3. How biofortification can contribute to the millennium development goals?

Goals and indicators	How biofortification can contribute?
Goal 1: Eradicate extreme poverty and hunger • Proportion of population below $1 a day • Poverty gap ratio (*incidence × depth of poverty*) • Share of poorest quintile in national consumption • Prevalence of underweight in children (under five years of age) • Proportion of population below minimum level of dietary energy consumption	Improved micronutrient status has shown to improve work productivity, mental and psychomotor performance, and appetite, and to promote faster growth. Biofortification targets the rural poor, in particular, who consume large amounts of food staples and little else.
Goal 2: Achieve universal primary education • Net enrolment ratio in primary education • Proportion of pupils starting grade 1 who reach grade 5 • Literacy rate of 15- to 24-yr-olds	Improved micronutrient status has shown to improve cognitive and psychomotor abilities. Children who do well in school are more likely to want to stay in school and their parents are more likely to support their education.
Goal 3: Reduce child mortality • Under-five mortality rate • Infant mortality rate	Improved micronutrient status has shown to reduce under-five mortality and morbidity; infant mortality rates may be benefited from improved micronutrient status of mothers during pregnancy.
Goal 4: Improve maternal health • Maternal mortality ratio	Improved micronutrient status has shown to reduce mortality and morbidity.
Goal 5: Combat HIV/AIDS, malaria and other diseases • HIV prevalence among 15- to 24-yr-old pregnant women • Number of children orphaned by HIV/AIDS • Prevalence and death rates associated with malaria • Prevalence and death rates associated with tuberculosis	The severity, mortality from, and perhaps incidence of HIV-AIDS, malaria, tuberculosis and other diseases are exacerbated by poor micronutrient status.
Goal 6: Ensure environmental sustainability • Change in land area covered by forest • Proportion of population with access to secure tenure [rural areas]	When topsoil dries, roots in the dry soil zone (which are easiest to fertilize) largely deactivate and the plant must rely on deep roots for further nutrition. Roots of plant genotypes are efficient in mobilizing surrounding; external trace minerals are not only more disease-resistant but also better able to penetrate deficient subsoils and so make use of moisture and minerals contained in subsoils. This reduces need for fertilizers and improves drought tolerance. Also, fewer herbicides and pesticides would have to be used because micronutrient-efficient genotypes should have greater resistance to plant pathogens.

rich plants for farmers to grow around the world for years to come. It is this multiplier aspect of bio-fortification across time and distance that makes it so cost-effective (Table 4).

High-iron and high-zinc traits appeared to be genetically linked. Thus, it should be relatively easy to breed high-iron and high-zinc varieties simultaneously. The

Table 4. How much nutrition an US$80 million investment can buy, by intervention?

Supplementation	Plant breeding/Biofortification
Provides vitamin A supplementation to 80 million women and children in South Asia for two yr, 1 in 15 persons in the total population, at a cost of 25 cents for delivery of each pill, each effective for six months.	Develops six nutrient-dense staple crops for dissemination to the entire world's people for consumption year after year. This includes dissemination and evaluation of nutritional impact in selected countries.

Source: Adapted from Horton and Ross 2003

calculations above count no benefit to human nutrition of increased zinc intakes or to improved productivity due to higher loading of zinc into seeds. Moreover, of course, the calculations do not count any benefits prior to year 16 or after year 25, even though bio-fortified varieties would be available before and after these years (Horton and Ross 2003).

10.3 Sustainability of bio-fortification

Once in place, the system described in the previous section is highly sustainable. The major, fixed costs of developing the varieties and convincing the nutrition and plant science to communities of their importance and effectiveness will have already been borne. Government attention to micronutrient issues may fade. International funding for micronutrient interventions may substantially reduce. Nevertheless, the nutritionally improved varieties will continue to grow and consumed year after year. To be sure, recurrent expenditures are required for monitoring and maintaining these traits in crops. However, these recurrent costs are low compared with the cost of the initial development of the nutritionally improved crops and the establishment, institutionally speaking, of nutrient content as a bona fide breeding objective (CIAT and IFPRI 2002).

10.4 Behavioral change

Mineral micronutrients make up a tiny fraction of the physical mass of a seed, 5–10 parts per million in milled rice. Dense bean seeds may contain as many as 100 parts per million. Whether such small amounts will alter the appearance, taste, texture, or cooking quality of foods need to be investigated. If increased densities in iron and zinc are not noticeable by consumers, the dissemination strategy for trace minerals, then, could rely on existing producer and consumer behavior. Analogous to the addition of fluoride to drinking water in some developed countries, successful implementation would not require that farmers and consumers know that they are producing and eating more nutritious varieties, although this information would be publicly advertised and publicly available.

In contrast, higher levels of beta-carotene will turn varieties from white or light colors of yellow to dark yellow and orange. Often, consumers much prefer white varieties of, for example, milled rice, wheat flour, maize, and cassava. Major nutrition education programs will have to mount to encourage consumers to switch to varieties that are more nutritious (and incorporated in benefit-cost calculations such as in the previous section). If these nutrition education programs are successful, however, the yellow-orange color will distinguish the more nutritious varieties from the less nutritious and a disadvantage will have turned into an advantage (Hagenimana and Low 2000).

11. Conclusions and perspectives

The production of high-quality, nutritious food through increased agricultural productivity—focusing on more efficient, effective and sustainable use of all available nutrient resources—will help restore the food supply and demand balance, making food affordable, increasing farmers' incomes and reducing the number of those who are food-deprived, hungry, malnourished and undernourished. Fighting micronutrient deficiencies is crucial to the health and economic development of millions of people worldwide. Iron deficiency in adults is so widespread that it is lowering the energies of nations and the productivity of work forces with estimated losses of up to two percent of GDP in the worst affected countries. As an example, when calculated as a proportion of the gross domestic product, productivity losses in South Asia alone are estimated at close to $5 billion annually.

Economically marginalized households may not have access to such foods and other vulnerable population groups, particularly children under 5 yr of age, may not be able to consume large enough quantities of the fortified food to satisfy an adequate level of their daily requirements. All these issues need to be assessed carefully and discussed in detail.

As we strive as a species to eliminate hunger and poverty, we must take steps to eliminate suffering to. Even small efforts to improve micronutrient status have a snowball effect as well-nourished children grow up to be stronger adults and can help pull their communities out of poverty. It will take a combination of efforts, including gardens, supplements, food preparation methods, fortification, bio-fortification, and more to reach all people in need. It makes no sense to reject any of the possible solutions in favor of one or the other. There is no silver bullet, but we have silver buckshot.

Keywords: Advantages of bio-fortification, agronomic fortification, application strategies, bio-fortification, economic benefits, hidden hunger, increased productivity, need of agronomic fortification, sustainability of bio-fortification

References

ACC/SCN. 2000. United Nations Administrative Committee on Coordination Sub-Committee on Nutrition. Fourth Report on the World Nutrition Situation. Geneva: ACC/SCN in collaboration with International Food Policy Research Institute (IFPRI). Available online: http://www.ifpri.org/sites/default/files/publications/4threport.pdf.

Ahmed. A., F.M. Anjum, M.A. Randhawa, U. Farooq, S. Akhtar and M.T. Sultan. 2012. Effect of multiple fortification on the bioavailability of minerals in wheat meal bread. Journal of Food Science and Technology, 49: 737–744.

Ahmed, A., F.M. Anjum, S. Ur Rehman, M.A. Randhawa and U. Farooq. 2008. Bioavailability of calcium, iron and zinc fortified whole wheat flour Chapatti. Plant Foods for Human Nutrition, 63: 7–13.

Allen, L., B. de Benoist, O. Dary and R. Hurrell. 2006. Guidelines on Food Fortification with Micronutrients. WHO Press, Geneva.

Andreini, C., L. Banci and A. Rosato. 2006. Zinc through the three domains of life. Journal of Proteome Research, 5: 3173–3178.

Bagriansky, J. 2003. Experience with flour fortification in South Africa. *In*: G. Maberly (ed.). Enriching Lives through Flour Fortification. Available online: www.sph.emory.edu/wheatflour/Main.htm.

Bell, R.W. and B. Dell. 2008. Micronutrients for sustainable food, feed, fibre and bioenergy production. International Fertilizer Industry Association (IFA), Paris, France. Available online: www.fertilizer. org/ifa/Home-Page/LIBRARY/Our-selection/Fertilizer-use.html.

Bilski, J., D. Jacob, F. Soumaila, C. Kraft and A. Farnsworth. 2012. Agronomic biofortification of cereal crop plants with Fe, Zn, and Se, by the utilization of coal fly ash as plant growth media. Advances in Bioresearch, 3: 130–136.

Black, R.E. 2003. Zinc deficiency, infectious disease and mortality in the developing world. The Journal of Nutrition, 133: 1485–1489.

Bouis, H.E. and R.M. Welch. 2010. Biofortification—a sustainable agricultural strategy for reducing micronutrient malnutrition in the global South. Crop Science, 50: S20–S32.

Cakmak, I. 2009. Enrichment of cereal grains with zinc: Agronomic or genetic biofortification? Plant and Soil, 302: 1–17.

Cakmak, I. 2010. Biofortification of cereals with zinc and iron through fertilization strategy. 19th World Congress of Soil Science, 1–6 August, Brisbane, Australia, 4–6.

CIAT and IFPRI. 2002. International Center for Tropical Agriculture and International Food Policy Research Institute. Biofortified Crops for Improved Human Nutrition. Available online: http://www.cgiar.org/ www-archive/www.cgiar.org/pdf/biofortification.pdf.

Combs, G. 2001. Selenium in global food systems. British Journal of Nutrition, 85: 517–547.

Das, J.K., R.A. Salam, R. Kumar and Z.A. Bhutta. 2013. Micronutrient fortification of food and its impact on woman and child health: A systematic review. Systematic Reviews, 2: 1–24.

de Benoist, B., E. McLean, I. Egli and M. Cogswell. 2008. Worldwide Prevalence of Anaemia 1993–2005: WHO Global Database on Anaemia. WHO Press, Geneva.

Eichler, K., S. Wieser, I. Rüthemann and U. Brügge. 2012. Effects of micronutrient fortified milk and cereal food for infants and children: A systematic review. BMC Public Health, 2: 1–13.

FFI. 2014. Flour Fortification Initiative. Flour Fortification. Online Database. Available online: http://www. unicef.org/eapro/fact_sheet_06.pdf.

Gautam, K.C. 2003. A global partnership to end hidden hunger. International Grains Conference, London, England.

Hagenimana, V. and J. Low. 2000. Potential of orange-fleshed sweet potatoes for raising vitamin A intake in Africa. Food Nutrition Bulletin, 21: 414–418.

Heaney, R.P. 2001. Factors influencing the measurement of bioavailability, taking calcium as a model. The Journal of Nutrition, 131: 1344S–1348S.

Horton, S. and J. Ross. 2003. The economics of iron deficiency. Food Policy, 28: 51–75.

IFA. 2010. International Fertilizer Industry Association. Feeding the Earth: Micronutrients for Macro Impacts "Fighting Malnutrition through Micronutrient Fertilization". International Fertilizer Industry Association (IFA), Paris, France. Available online: http://www.atpnutrition.ca/_uploads/ documents/2010_ifa_micronutrients_brief.pdf.

Islam, Y. 2007. Growing goodness. Developments, 38: 36–37.

Kabata-Pendias, A. and A.B. Mukherjee. 2010. Trace Elements from Soil to Humans. Springer Verlag, Belrin, Heidelberg.

Lyons, G., J. Lewis, M. Lorimer, R. Holloway, D. Brace, J. Stangoulis and R. Graham. 2004. High-selenium wheat: agronomic biofortification strategies to improve human nutrition. Food, Agriculture and Environment, 2: 171–174.

Preedy, V.R., R. Srirajaskanthan and V.B. Patel. 2013. Handbook of Food Fortification and Health: From Concepts to Public Health Application (Vol. 1). Humana Press, Springer, New York.

Preedy, V.R., R.R. Watson and V.B. Patel. 2011. Flour and Breads and their Fortification in Health and Disease Prevention. Academic Press, London.

Rayman, M. 2000. The importance of selenium in human health. The Lancet, 356: 233–241.

Rolfes, S.R., K. Pinna and E.N. Whitney. 2011. Understanding Normal and Clinical Nutrition (9th Ed.). Wadsworth/Cengage Learning, Belmont, California.

Srinivasan, V.S. 2001. Bioavailability of nutrients: A practical approach to *in vitro* demonstration of the availability of nutrients in multivitamin-mineral combination products. The Journal of Nutrition, 131: 1349S–1350S.

Wesley, A. and P. Ranum. 2004. Fortification Handbook: Vitamin and Mineral Fortification of Wheat Flour and Maize Meal "Micronutrient Initiative". Ottawa. Available online: http://www.micronutrient.org/resources/publications/Fort_handbook.pdf.

Whitney, E.N., D.B. Cataldo and S.R. Rolfes. 2002. Understanding Normal and Clinical Nutrition (6th Ed.). Wadsworth/Thomson Learning, Belmont, California.

11

Physical Processing of Grains and Flours Leading Nutritious Breads

Ioanna Mandala[1],* and *Cristina M. Rosell*[2]

1. Introduction

Physical treatment of the raw materials and particularly flours, is gaining interest in recent years due to consumer's rejection of chemicals and the trend of food technologists to look for green label foods. In this scenario, diverse physical modifications of the raw materials have been lately reported, which are focused on reducing particle size distribution or in changing by non-thermal treatments the functional properties of the constituents. However, besides the different functionality, those certain physical treatments are also affecting the nutritional properties of the foods. Because of that, this chapter will give an overview of the physical transformation of the raw materials and their impact on both the technological quality and nutritional aspects of foods, namely bread.

2. Impact of particle size reduction of flours on bread

Technologies such as micron- or nano-technology in food research and product development have gained much attention in recent years. They lead in new applications and products with improved characteristics. In addition to the technological benefits,

[1] Laboratory of Food Engineering, Department of Food Science & Human Nutrition, Agricultural University of Athens, Greece.
Email: imandala@aua.gr
[2] Institute of Agrochemistry and Food Technology (IATA/CSIC), Avenida Agustin Escardino 7, Paterna, 46980 Valencia, Spain.
Email: crosell@iata.csic.es
* Corresponding author

widening the raw materials applications, particle size has an important impact in nutrition, particularly in the glycaemic-insulin response and the satiety rating (Holt and Miller 1994). That fact was confirmed when comparing the effect of whole grains, cracked grains, coarse and fine wholemeal flour on plasma glucose response and satiety after ingesting equal carbohydrate portions of four test meals based on four different grades of wheat. Fine flour meal elicited the highest insulin response followed by the coarse flour, cracked grain and wholegrain meal; and satiety responses showed the opposite trend. Conversely, Behall et al. (1999) when compared the effect of consumption of conventional wholegrain wheat or ultra-fine wholegrain wheat on glucose and insulin responses observed similar responses.

2.1 Technologies for reducing particle size

To understand the different characteristics of flours associated to particle size distribution it is necessary to briefly describe the processing systems used to reduce the particle size of the flours. Jet milling is one of the processes for ultragrinding. It is a fluid energy impact-milling technique which is commonly used to produce particle sizes less than 40 microns (Chamayou and Dodds 2007). The final particle size depends on the feedstock size, the nozzles' number, the grinding pressure, the feed rate and the passes. Improved final products can be formulated by adding fine powders of specific properties and controllable particle size. Thus, reverse food engineering is applied in food containing fine powders. Jet milling has a noticeable effect on the characteristics of the wheat flour (Protonotariou et al. 2014a,b). It allows the micronisations of the flour to the level of starch granules size and different milling conditions give different particle sizes. Jet milling belongs to macromolecular fractionation processes, which aim not only at tissue separation (e.g., bran tissue) but also at sub-cellular constituents' isolation. Sub-cellular constituents should be liberated in such a way that they can be separated and that is only achieved in superfine grinding, where cells are broken (Hemery et al. 2007). Fractionation and separation methods need to be improved to achieve a complete macromolecular fractionation. However, these processes present interesting prospects to produce isolated, novel food ingredients.

2.2 Particle size reduction effect in flour

Functionality and chemical composition of the flours are affected by the particle size distribution. Sapirstein et al. (2007) proposed the reduction of particle size to improve breadmaking performance of different genotypes of durum wheat. Particle size reduction of the semolina by gradual reduction shortened the development time during mixing and increased the amount of starch damage. Flour fractions of different particle sizes sieved from the same flour result in chemical composition differences (Toth et al. 2006). Flours with particle size ranged from 125–63 μm had better baking performance and much higher nutritional value. Specifically, their macroelement contents (carbon, calcium, potassium, magnesium, nitrogen, phosphorous and sulphur) and essential microelements (iron, zinc, copper, chromium, lithium and manganese) contents, with the exception of calcium and manganese, are higher in the fraction with smaller particle size (< 63 μm). Protein and ash content increase with the reduction of the particle size (Toth et al. 2006).

Recently, Brewer et al. (2014) even found differences in the phytochemicals extractability and antioxidant capacity when comparing wheat bran fractions with differing particle size distributions (whole coarse bran, medium and fine). Particle size of bran affected the phytochemicals extractability. The coarse fraction displayed significantly higher total antioxidant capacity (426.72 mg ascorbic acid eq./g) and ferric reducing/antioxidant power value (53.04 lmol $FeSO_4$/g) than fine bran fraction (314.55 ascorbic acid eq./g and 40.84 lmol $FeSO_4$/g, respectively). With particle size reduction (greater for 200 μm than unmilled bran), there was a significant increase in extracted anthocyanins, carotenoids, phenolic acid and flavonoids and oxygen radical absorbance capacity (ORAC) value increased by over 80% (Brewer et al. 2014).

Fractionation using sieving and air classification can result in enriched fractions of flour. Beta-glucans' enriched barley fractions can be obtained (Ferrari et al. 2009), or effective separation of hull from the grain in barley, that further promotes its use, can be achieved (Srinivasan et al. 2012).

Particle size distribution greatly affects the functionality of gluten free flours. In fact, rice flour fractionation has been proposed as an alternative physical method for modulating the technological functionality of rice flour and also its digestibility (de la Hera et al. 2013a). Particle size heterogeneity on rice flour significantly affects functional properties and starch features. De la Hera et al. (2013a) found that rice flour hydration properties increase with the reduction of particle size, but particle size reduction beyond < 80 μm showed much greater effect attributable to molecular and structural changes of grain components. Hence, particle size distribution significantly affected water holding capacity, water binding capacity and oil absorption capacity, which might be related to the greater surface area exposed to water molecules binding in fine particles. Regarding enzymatic digestibility, it increased with the reduction of the particle size (de la Hera et al. 2013a).

The combination of soaking and particle size reduction has been also proposed for improving the properties of the flours; such is the case of rice flour to obtain gluten-free bread (Song and Shin 2007). Soaking of rice grains affected the particle size distribution of flour and the pasting properties of the flours, particularly a decrease in the pasting temperature and setback was observed when decreasing the particle size; and what was more important is that flours with particle size lower than 150 μm had the best breadmaking performance.

By reducing the particle size distribution of the flours it is possible to modify the susceptibility of the starch granules to undergo enzymatic hydrolysis by amylases, as has been reported for barley and sorghum (Al-Rabadi et al. 2009). Hydrolysis rate of the starches decreases with increasing particle size due to the effect on enzyme diffusion through the particles.

Other flours that has been also subjected to particle reduction are the pulses flours like dehulled yellow pea flour (*Pisum sativum* L.) of fine particle size and other pulse flours including dehulled green lentils (*Lens esculenta*), navy beans (*Phaseolus vulgaris*) with the hull, and pinto beans (*P. vulgaris*) with the hull (Borsuk et al. 2011). Coarse pulse flours blended with wheat flour have higher water absorption and require higher water amount for mixing. When pulse flours were incorporated in wheat pita bread, specific loaf volumes of pitas containing 25% coarse lentil and 25% coarse navy bean flours were similar to the control, despite pulse flours decreased it (Borsuk et al. 2011; Borsuk et al. 2012). Therefore, it could increase the protein, fiber, antioxidants, minerals and vitamins of the pitas breads adding pulse flours; although the substitution level is limited to 25% (Borsuk et al. 2012). Similarly, when those pulse (green lentil, navy and pinto bean) flours with different particle size were tested on wheat cookies for increasing the nutritional value, namely protein content and antioxidant capacity, incorporation of fine flours increased cookies' hardness (Zucco et al. 2011). Coarse navy beans flour was the best alternative to be blended with wheat flour for production of cookies (Zucco et al. 2011).

2.3 Particle size reduction on baked products

Particle size distribution of wheat flour has attracted increasing attention in the last decade due to the different functionality observed in the fractions. Wheat flour with high proportion of small particles (< 55 µm) shows increasing starch damage which might be responsible for the higher water retention ability. Wheat flours with intermediate (55–88 µm) particle size led to produce larger volume of sponge cake (Choi and Baik 2013).

Given the importance of fiber enrichment of cereal based products and the technological drawbacks promoted by fiber particles on fermented products, the particle size reduction of the wholegrains has been proposed as an alternative for modifying the functional properties of the flours. Micro-particulated flour, using a jet milling process, can be used in products of high wholemeal flour amount. Fine powders could be used to substitute white flour in greater amounts than commonly found in the market without altering the physical and sensorial attributes of the final product (Fig. 1).

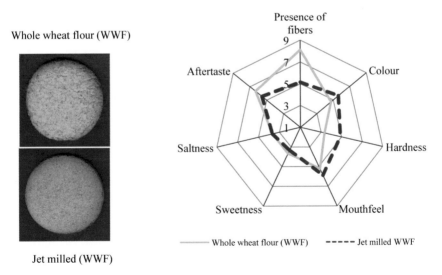

Figure 1. Sensory evaluation of biscuits with whole wheat flour (WWF) and jet milled WWF (Protonotariou et al. 2014a).

In the bread industry, specifically, the addition of micronized wheat brans in bread increased the concentration of free amino acids, total phenols and dietary fiber as well as the phytase and antioxidant activities of doughs. Moreover, fine bran fractions are considered good sources of vitamin E and might be used in breadmaking (Engelsen and Hansen 2009).

Wheat bran fiber particles isolated from wheat bran can be pulverized to submicron scale. Then, they can be used in several foodstuffs, as ultra-fine grinding can change their physical structure. A ball mill was used in cryogenic conditions and different bran fractions were received with increased surface area and decreased particle size to values smaller than 50 µm. Breads enriched with micronized bran and fermented with sourdough exhibited increased concentration of functional compounds and decreased value of hydrolysis index (HI) (Rizzello et al. 2012). However, ultrafine bran incorporation in bread can have negative effects on its quality such as lower specific volume and denser crumb texture as shown by Noort et al. (2010). However, those authors indicated that gluten dilution, gas cells breakage and gluten network interference cannot explain the negative effects of fibers. Conversely, it seems that particle reduction of fiber affects the physical properties of gluten because smaller fiber particles have large surface to interact with gluten impairing the gluten network, and also released components (conjugated ferulic acid monomers, reducing components as thiols like glutathione and phytate) from the cell breakage may interact with gluten also interfering in its formation (Noort et al. 2010). Bran fractions antioxidant capacity was linearly correlated with the specific surface and with the D50 values (Rossa et al. 2013). Similarly, aleurone micronization increases its antioxidant activity (Zhou et al. 2004).

Three pin milling steps and air classification were used for aleurone cells separation, in order to reduce bran particle size. The dissociation of aleurone cell walls (rich in fiber) and aleurone cell contents (rich in vitamins and minerals) was achieved. A very fine fraction of D50 at 7 µm was received, which mainly contained aleurone cells, although micronisation needs further improvements in order to achieve a complete fractionation of the bran (Antoine et al. 2004).

Whole barley flour has been reported as an interesting source of fibers and particularly beta-glucans approved as soluble fiber. Nevertheless, like the rest of wholemeal flours, they impair gluten structure affecting bread volume and other sensory characteristics of bakery products. A reduction in the particle size of the wholebarley flour was proposed by Prasopsunwattana et al. (2009) for enriching wheat tortillas. With that objective authors compared the effect of regular (237 µm), intermediate (131 µm) and microground (68 µm) particle size when added at 9 and 15% (flour basis) to wheat flour for producing wheat tortillas. Wholebarley enriched tortillas were darker than the wheat tortillas, but the color was lighter as particle size decreased. Regarding the chemical composition, protein and moisture content decreased when decreasing the particle size but beta-glucan content was constant. The sensory analysis carried out with 95 untrained panelists to evaluate tortilla appearance, color, flavor, texture, and overall acceptability revealed that no flavor differences were detected and tortillas made with the largest particle size were more similar in texture and flavor to those tortillas made with refined bread flour (Prasopsunwattana et al. 2009).

Hemery et al. (2011) applied a cryogenic grinding process in order to make the wheat bran brittle and to achieve a more efficient particle size reduction. Grinding at such low temperature (i.e., at glass transition temperature) presents the advantage of no heat generation that result in the preservation of the activity of heat-sensitive compounds, such as B and E vitamins. Cryogenic and grinding at ambient conditions can be combined, as grinding at low temperature favors fragmentation, whereas at ambient temperature dissociation takes place that leads to the production of different fractions' compositions. However, cost issues should be taken into account.

As mentioned before, in gluten-free products development, the particle size of the flours is crucial for obtaining good bakery products. de la Hera et al. (2013b) reported that the finest rice flours (< 80 μm) had low gas retention capacity for holding the carbon dioxide produced during fermentation and led to rice gluten-free breads with lower specific volume. Those changes in functionality resulted in rice gluten-free breads with high content of slowly digestible starch and resistant starch when made with coarse rice flours (de la Hera et al. 2014). Therefore, the coarse fraction rice flour besides high dough hydration (90–110%) was the most advisable combination for developing rice bread with adequate bread volume and crumb texture, but for lowering starch digestibility the lowest dough hydration might be recommended to limit starch gelatinization and in consequence to hinder the *in vitro* starch digestibility (de la Hera et al. 2014). Similarly, maize flours with fine particle size have low development during fermentation and only flours with compact particles (> 130 μm) yielded high specific bread volume, besides lower values of hardness and resilience in gluten-free maize bread (de la Hera et al. 2013c).

Odonnell et al. (1989) reported that flour particle size had a significant effect on postprandial glucose absorption, when coarse and fine flour made breads were ingested by middle age people, non-insulin diabetics and young people.

Bread made with coarse flours induced less insulin response, thus it might decrease the risk of hypertension, atherosclerosis and obesity if consumed on a regular basis. In addition, coarse bread led to reduced amount of bioavailable starch for bowel adsorption, in consequence reducing the implantation of colonic diseases like cancer. Therefore, authors recommended the ingestion of bread made from coarse wheat flour to control diabetes (Odonnell et al. 1989).

2.4 Functionalities of fibers under grinding

Fibers can be an interesting case of fine powders with improved characteristics. Research in the field of insoluble fibers from fruits, seeds or vegetables, demonstrated the improved functionality of the latter by the application of grinding.

Intense grinding can change the properties of wheat bran, such as water holding or water retention capacity, that are decreased, but additionally, a redistribution of fiber components from insoluble to soluble fractions occurs (Rossa et al. 2013).

In fact, wheat bran of different particle sizes (170, 280, 425 and 750 μm) act differently when added to Barbari bread, a type of flat bread highly consumed in Asian countries, for its enrichment in fibers (Majzoobi et al. 2013). Those authors reported that coarse bran required higher amount of water for mixing and led to darker flat breads. Simultaneously, the sensory analysis indicated that for obtaining fiber enriched flat breads it would be advisable up to 15% bran with particle sizes shorter than 280 μm (Majzoobi et al. 2013). Same research group (Majzoobi et al. 2013) tested the applicability of those brans in sponge cake making. The particle size reduction of the brans decreased the content of the crude fiber and phytic acid. Coarse particle size bran led to cakes with lighter crust and crumb color and low density. Sensory analysis indicated that it would be advisable to incorporate no more than 10% bran with particle size smaller than 170 μm, which gave a total dietary fiber and phytic acid content of 5.95% and 2.90 (mg/g), respectively (Majzoobi et al. 2013).

Similar observation was also observed in case of rye bran. Decreasing the particle size of rye bran from 440 μm to 28 μm using extrusion processing resulted in higher amounts of SDF (soluble dietary fiber) compared to coarse-particle sized rye bran. These extrudates also had improved structural and mechanical properties, i.e., they were crispier, softer and more expanded than their coarse counterparts (Alam et al. 2014).

A redistribution of fibers can be also observed in other kind of fibers as well. As an example, sweet potato dietary fiber (DF) treated by micronization can be referred. The particle size of sweet potato DF was 18 μm and fibers presented a porous structure (Mei et al. 2014). Furthermore, improved functional properties, in terms of water holding capacity, release of antioxidant compounds and *in vitro* hypoglycemic potential, were observed for carrot insoluble fiber (Chau et al. 2007). Micronization treatments give an opportunity to improve the functionality of insoluble fibers for further exploitation in food enrichment applications (Chau et al. 2007).

Moreover, ultrafine grinding can enhance the antioxidant properties of DF, as found for wheat bran DF and buckwheat DF without any prior extraction (Rossa et al. 2013; Zhu et al. 2010; Zhu et al. 2014). Micronized insoluble dietary fibers showed increased chelating activity, reducing power and total phenolic content (TPC). The intense grinding process using a ball milling can damage or change the fiber matrix resulting in the release or greater exposure of some phenolic compounds that are embedded or linked to that matrix. They also present a decreased 1,1-diphenyl-2-picrylhydrazyl (DPPH) radical scavenging activity (Zhu et al. 2010). The bioaccessibility and/or bioavailability of phenolic acids can then increase, because an increase in particle surface area can result in a higher release of bioactive compounds from the material matrix due to the higher solvent-compounds interactions (Hemery et al. 2011). However, the enhanced antioxidant properties of micronized bran should be preserved, as the small particle size could accelerate their loss during storage due to chemical reactions such as oxidation. Thus, storage conditions as also processing conditions of selected cultivars might influence the antioxidant compounds maintenance (Cheng et al. 2006).

Ellis et al. (1991) even analyzed the possible impact of particle size distribution of the fibers, specifically guar gum on the post-prandial blood glucose and plasma insulin levels in human subjects. In doing so, they investigated the effects of wheat breads containing guar gum samples varying in molecular weight and particle size (characteristics that strongly influence the rheological properties of guar gum) on post-prandial blood glucose and plasma insulin levels in healthy subjects but no significant differences in the post-prandial blood glucose responses were found between the control and guar breads due to the diverse particle size.

Finally, grape skin powders—comprised essentially of fibers and antioxidants—of different particle size can be used on gel structure formation such as that of fruit candies, developing innovative confectionery product (Cappa et al. 2014). Red grape skins (GS) of Barbera cultivar (*Vitis vinifera* L.), were sieved to separate the skins from the seeds and the powders were collected: small (S 125 mm), medium (125 < M < 250 mm) and large (250 < L 500 mm). The ratio of SDF/IDF increased as the particle size decreased. The antioxidant activity was not reduced after heating, whereas their texture was stronger; thus candy products can be successfully developed.

2.5 Potential of dry fractionation for protein isolates production

Protein isolates are widely used in food industry applications, in order to improve the texture and the nutritional quality of end-products, or as replacers of the gluten protein in the development of high quality gluten-free breads and products. However simple replacement of gluten from other proteins did not lead to gluten-free products of high quality (Hüttner and Arendt 2010). The latter experience evidences that a variety of food products benefit from the complex composition of different proteins (and other components) with their (native) functionality (Schutyser et al. 2011). The production of protein isolates and concentrates is conventionally carried out with wet fractionation techniques. Those methods were considered high energy and water consuming and cause partial loss of the native functionality of the proteins (denaturation) due to the pH shifts and drying. Moreover, milling of vegetable sources with high starch content is easy to perform as starch granules can be removed after milling by means of air-classification. However, when the starch amount of the source is low, protein isolation is much more difficult and new techniques should be applied (Dijkink and Willemsen 2006). Jet milling and air classification methods are considered a more sustainable alternative to wet fractionation, since they use no or less water and less energy for heating or drying. Furthermore end product can be easily controlled in terms of functionality and of purity. In the end, jet milling equipment can be easily scaled up and be located close to the potential application.

An example of the above-mentioned use of jet milling is the production of pea protein concentrates. A good knowledge and control of the air flow and the classifier wheel speed in the air classification process leads to protein concentration of desired particle size, and therefore of desired protein content (Pelgrom et al. 2013).

Lupin protein concentrates from lupin seeds can be also produced by jet milling and an ultra-rotor as described in a patent, which imply a protein enrichment of 150% (Dijkink and Willemsen 2006).

Fine powders of proteins can be also used as fat substitutes. A jet mill can produce powders from egg white, casein and soybean hull. Casein powders had increased hydrophobicity (Hayakawa et al. 1993).

These examples indicate the potential of utilizing ultra-grinding or size fractionation for improving functionality and structure of raw materials creating new aspects for micronization.

3. Understanding high hydrostatic pressure

Food safety has been a continuous goal in research and different technologies have been developed with the aim of obtaining safe foods with extended shelf life. At the end of the last century, high hydrostatic pressure (HHP) was developed and applied to foods for reducing the microorganism's population working within the pressure range (100–1000 MPa). High hydrostatic pressure is a physical non-thermal process that allows inactivating microorganisms and enzymes affecting minimally to food quality and constituents. Numerous studies have been carried out on the effect of high hydrostatic pressure on microbial physiology and sterilization, control of enzymatic reaction and food processing (Estrada-Giron et al. 2005).

3.1 Effect of HHP on proteins

HHP can irreversibly change the structural and functional properties of proteins (Winter 2003). The effects of HHP on proteins are primarily due to disruption of non-covalent interactions within proteins, and secondly the formation of intra- and intermolecular bonds within or between proteins (Messens et al. 1997).

Kato et al. (2000) even used the HHP for reducing the allergenic level of proteins in rice grains. Those authors observed that HHP treatment (100–400 MPa) of rice grains allowed releasing the 16-kDa albumin, R-globulin and 33-kDa globulin—major rice allergens. Likely, the partial destruction of endosperm cells favors the accessibility of the surrounding solution and the subsequent solubilization of the rice proteins, preferentially the allergen ones. Therefore, pressurization of rice grains could be an alternative processing for obtaining hypoallergenic rice.

The same effect has been observed in buckwheat flour, in which the treatment at high pressure reduced the content of 24-kDa allergenic as indicated the enzyme-linked immunosorbent assay using a monoclonal antibody specific for buckwheat 24-kDa protein (Tomotake et al. 2012).

Even the allergenicity of the soybean isolate proteins has been decreased by 49% when treated with HHP at 300 MPa and 15 min (Li et al. 2012). The HHP effect on the proteins differed depending on the pressure and time duration of the treatment. In the ranges of 200–300 MPa a treatment for 5–15 min resulted in an increase of the free SH content and hydrophobicity of the soybean protein isolate, but with more intense conditions those interactions decreased. Those changes affected the secondary structure of the proteins and in consequence the epitopes of soybean protein isolate allergens reducing its allergenicity.

High hydrostatic pressure has been applied to different bakery ingredients. For instance, dairy proteins treated with high hydrostatic pressure were incorporated in breadmaking (Kadharmestan et al. 1998). HHP (586 MPa during 30 min) was applied to modify the functionality of the proteins, namely to decrease their emulsifying and foaming ability. Those conditions decreased the solubility of the proteins from 91% to 16% due to denaturation. At wheat flour replacement of 5% or 10%, HHP proteins reduced bread volume and increase crumb hardness. However, protein content of the bread increased up to 20% and increased the proportion of essential amino acids, including lysine, threonine, isoleucine, leucine, methionine and valine.

3.2 Effect of HHP on starch

HPP also has great impact on starch granules, with an action similar to the heat gelatinization process (Rubens et al. 1999). Initially the hydration of the amorphous regions of the starch granules led to swelling and an alteration of crystalline regions. Then, the crystalline regions become more accessible to water. Conversely to heat induced gelatinization, pressure-gelatinized starches undergo limited swelling (up to twofold in diameter) and they keep their granular character (Stute et al. 1996). Nevertheless, the range of pressure necessary for promoting starch gelatinization is dependent on the starch origin (Stute et al. 1996).

Gomes et al. (1998) applied HHP ranging 400–600 MPa to increase the total soluble carbohydrate and reduce sugar content of wheat samples. Under those conditions a significant increase of the activity of starch degrading enzymes (alfa and beta amylases) was detected due to non-thermal starch gelatinization that starts at around 400 MPa. Treatments at pressure above 600 MPa induced the inactivation of the enzymes likely due to either the modification of the active site or partial or total unfolding of the enzyme.

HHP has been also applied to improve technological characteristics of glutinous rice (or sticky rice), which required extended soaking for improving starch gelatinization during cooking (Ahromrit et al. 2006). Rice treatment at high pressures up to 600 MPa accelerated water uptake kinetics during soaking, temperature affecting the effective diffusion coefficient below 300 MPa, but without a significant effect at higher pressures. Therefore, the effective combination of high pressure and temperatures allow increasing the quantity and the rate of water absorption by rice (Ahromrit et al. 2006). Rice starch gelatinization only started when pressure exceeded 200 MPa at ambient temperature and it could be completed at 500 and 600 MPa at 70°C when the rice was soaked in water during 120 min (Ahromrit et al. 2007). Huang et al. (2009) investigated the combination effects of pressure (200 to 500 MPa) and temperature (20, 40 and 50°C) on the water uptake and gelatinization characteristics of *Japonica* rice grains. These authors observed that no gelatinization of starch in *Japonica* rice grains occurred at pressures below 300 MPa and temperatures of 20 and 40°C; and the highest degree of gelatinization was obtained at 500 MPa and 50°C for 120 min. Therefore, an appropriate combination of pressure and temperature is necessary to facilitate water uptake and gelatinization.

This strategy was also proposed by Nguyen et al. (2007) to prepare starch-based high energy density gruels as feeding supplements for young child. In this case, pre-heating of the slurry combined with HHP treatment was applied, which facilitated the starch hydrolysis by amylolytic lactic acid bacteria.

3.3 Effect of HHP on cereal flours

HHP has been applied to grains and flours, in the former to modify flours functionality, but the effects on the health components have been barely investigated. Only some studies have been carried out in flours, mainly gluten-free flours, but scarce information exists on the possible health effect of breads obtained from HHP treated flours. HHP has been used as a processing technique for improving the functionality of gluten-free flours, based on the possibility of inducing a matrix creation. HHP has been also applied to other cereal flours like oats. Huttner et al. (2009) analyzed the effect of HHP (200, 300, 350, 400 or 500 MPa for 10 min) on oat batters and confirmed a significant impact on starch and proteins. At a pressure of 350 MPa, a significant reduction of the water and salt-soluble proteins was observed due to the formation of new non-covalent bonds. Nevertheless, pressures of 300 MPa were sufficient to induce the formation of urea-insoluble complexes and/or disulfide bonds owing to denaturation, aggregation, gelation or possible interactions with other proteins or flour components. The starch gelatinization of oat flour started at 300 MPa and 500 MPa was necessary to complete it. When those HHP treated oat flours were used for replacing untreated oat flour at 10, 20 or 40% levels, a significant improved bread volume was obtained with the addition of 10% oat batter treated at 200 MPa (Huttner et al. 2010). In addition, the bread staling was reduced when containing oat batter was treated at 200 MPa. On the other hand, the supplementation with oat batters treated at pressure higher than 350 MPa led to bread quality deterioration.

Similarly, sorghum flour was treated at pressures from 200 to 600 MPa at 20°C for obtaining sorghum breads (Vallons et al. 2010). The treatment at 300 MPa pressure resulted in the weakening of the batter structure owing to the protein depolymerization and a simultaneous increase of the batter consistency due to pressure-induced gelatinization of starch. A delay in the staling was observed when 2% of those treated batters at 600 MPa were added into a sorghum bread recipe although a decrease in the specific volume and low quality was obtained (Vallons et al. 2010). Nevertheless, with the addition of 200 MPa treated flour a similar quality to the reference breads were obtained.

Angioloni and Collar (2012) compared the quality of breads obtained from different cereal blends (wheat, oat, millet and sorghum) after treating the flours with HHP (350 MPa, 10 min). The ratio between wheat and the other cereals was kept at 60:40 or 40:60 and HHP treated flours were replacing the non-gluten cereals for making breads. Breads containing HHP treated flours were sensory scored better than their non-treated counterparts, although reduced specific volume was observed in wheat and oat breads and faster staling kinetics in millet and sorghum containing breads. In wheat breads HHP induced an increase in starch digestibility and antiradical activity, and a decrease in the free, bound and bio-accessible phenols, also in the flavonoids content. Protein digestibility of breads decreased as consequence of HHP likely the formation of agglomerates and the intra and inter-linkage between proteins chains is responsible for that effect. In all the blended breads with other cereals the HPP affected negatively the total and bio-accessible polyphenol contents but their antiradical activity was enhanced. These authors did not find any significant difference regarding starch hydrolysis and expected glycaemic index between non-treated and their HHP treated counterparts (Angioloni and Collar 2012).

3.4 Effect on the microorganisms

As was previously mentioned, HHP was initially conceived as a non-thermal treatment for inactivating microorganisms. However, the use of HHP for food processing leads to identify the range of pressure required for modifying food ingredients without inducing microorganisms' inactivation. In fact, Barcenas et al. (2010) proposed the use of HHP combined with breadmaking process for obtaining wheat breads with different technological properties. Treatment of wheat dough with high hydrostatic pressure induced rapid reduction of the microbial population but sufficient yeast survival, for ensuring bread dough fermentation, was obtained using mild pressure conditions (50–250 MPa, for 2 min at 20°C). This treatment resulted in increased dough hardness and adhesiveness but decreased dough stickiness. Microstructure analysis revealed that proteins were affected at pressure range from 50 to 150 MPa, but starch modification required higher pressure levels. HPP treated yeast doughs allowed obtaining wheat breads with brownish crumb color and uneven gas cells distribution with increased hardness due to new crumb structure. This study suggests that HHP in the range 50–200 MPa could be an alternative technique for obtaining novel textured cereal based products.

4. Concluding remarks or future trends

Specific physical treatments can affect the functional and the nutritional properties of the foods giving them new characteristics. In this chapter an overview about two processes—superfine grinding and high pressure—is presented. Their influence on the physical characteristics of the raw materials and their further impact on the technological quality and nutrition aspects of final products, namely bread, are analyzed.

Superfine grinding aims at the production of very fine particles of improved functionalities. For example, fine powders of pulse flours or bran can be used to substitute white flour in great amounts without altering the physical and sensorial attributes of the final product. Moreover, a sub-cellular constituents' isolation can be achieved, as in case of bran grinding. Sub-cellular constituents can be then separated and further used in many foods, giving new functional and nutritional attributes in the baked end products. Finally, protein powders as fat substitutes produced by a dry fractionation can be achieved.

However, the particle size of milled grains influences the baking performance. According to Turner (2003) there would appear to be an optimal granulation for whole-wheat functionality. Fine flours have increased water binding capacity. The susceptibility of the starch granules to undergo enzymatic hydrolysis by amylases is also modified and the hydrolysis rate of the starches often increases with decreasing the particle size. Moreover, fine bran powders have large surface to interact with gluten impairing the gluten network, although the large surface can result in a higher release of bioactive compounds from the material matrix due to the higher solvent-compounds interactions. All these issues should be taken into consideration in further development of particle micronization process for the improvement of ultra-fine powders' characteristics.

On the other hand, pressurization of grains or of individual components presents another alternative proposition for obtaining new functionalities in foods. Specifically, high hydrostatic pressure of grains could be an alternative processing for obtaining hypoallergenic flours, namely rice flour. Starch and proteins can be also modified under high pressure application. Pressure-induced gelatinization of starch or denaturation of proteins is achieved. This leads to the decrease in emulsifying and foaming ability of proteins or the decrease in their solubility, or to the enhancement of water uptake and starch gelatinization. However, it is necessary to combine in an appropriate way the pressure and the temperature to find the optimal conditions for desired functionality of the treated samples. By choosing the appropriate pressure-temperature combination, possible drawbacks such as the weakening of the batter structure owing to the protein depolymerization and an increase of the batter consistency due to pressure-induced gelatinization of starch, can be avoided.

To conclude, the processes presented offer many possibilities in powders or flours treatment. They can offer raw material with enhanced nutritional characteristics and functionalities that can be used in a successful development of many foods or substitute other materials. More studies are needed in this area to better understand the findings presented. In the future such alternative processes would be further developed for the benefit of manufacturing, balancing added value and cost issues.

Acknowledgements

Authors acknowledge the financial support of the Spanish Ministry of Economy and Competitiveness (Project AGL2011-23802), the European Regional Development Fund (FEDER) and Generalitat Valenciana (Project Prometeo 2012/064).

Keywords: particle size, jet milling, high pressure, flours, proteins, fibers

References

Ahromrit, A., D.A. Ledward and K. Niranjan. 2006. High pressure induced water uptake characteristics of Thai glutinous rice. Journal of Food Engineering, 72(3): 225–233.

Ahromrit, A., D.A. Ledward and K. Niranjan. 2007. Kinetics of high pressure facilitated starch gelatinisation in Thai glutinous rice. Journal of Food Engineering, 79(3): 834–841.

Alam, S.A., J. Järvinen, S. Kirjoranta, K. Jouppila, K. Poutanen and N. Sozer. 2014. Influence of particle size reduction on structural and mechanical properties of extruded rye bran. Food and Bioprocess Technology, 7(7): 2121–2133.

Al-Rabadi, G.J.S., R.G. Gilbert and M.J. Gidley. 2009. Effect of particle size on kinetics of starch digestion in milled barley and sorghum grains by porcine alpha-amylase. Journal of Cereal Science, 50(2): 198–204.

Angioloni, A. and C. Collar. 2012. Effects of pressure treatment of hydrated oat, finger millet and sorghum flours on the quality and nutritional properties of composite wheat breads. Journal of Cereal Science, 56(3): 713–719.

Antoine, C., S. Peyron, V. Lullien-Pellerin, J. Abecassis and X. Rouau. 2004. Wheat bran tissue fractionation using biochemical markers. Journal of Cereal Science, 39: 387–393.

Barcenas, M.E., R. Altamirano-Fortoul and C.M. Rosell. 2010. Effect of high pressure processing on wheat dough and bread characteristics. LWT-Food Science and Technology, 43(1): 12–19.

Behall, K.M., D.J. Scholfield and J. Hallfrisch. 1999. The effect of particle size of whole-grain flour on plasma glucose, insulin, glucagon and thyroid-stimulating hormone in humans. Journal of the American College of Nutrition, 18(6): 591–597.

Borsuk, Y., S. Arntfield and O. Lukow. 2011. Incorporation of pulse flours (green lentils, navy beans, yellow peas, and pinto beans) of different particle sizes into pita bread. Canadian Journal of Plant Science, 91(2): 373–373.

Borsuk, Y., S. Arntfield, O.M. Lukow, K. Swallow and L. Malcolmson. 2012. Incorporation of pulse flours of different particle size in relation to pita bread quality. J. Sci. Food Agric., 92(10): 2055–2061.

Brewer, L.R., J. Kubola, S. Siriamornpun, T.J. Herald and Y.-C. Shi. 2014. Wheat bran particle size influence on phytochemical extractability and antioxidant properties. Food Chemistry, 152(1): 483–490.

Cappa, C., V. Lavelli and M. Mariotti. 2014. Fruit candies enriched with grape skin powders: physicochemical properties. LWT-Food Science and Technology (in press).

Chamayou, A. and J.A. Dodds. 2007. Chapter 8: Air Jet Milling. Handbook of Powder Technology, 12: 421–435.

Chau, C.-F., Y.-T. Wang and Y.-L. Wen. 2007. Different micronization methods significantly improve the functionality of carrot insoluble fibre. Food Chemistry, 100(4): 1402–1408.

Cheng, Z.H., I. Su, J. Moore, K.Q. Zhou, M. Luther, J.J. Yin and L.L. Yu. 2006. Effects of post-harvest treatment and heat stress on availability of wheat antioxidants. Journal of Agricultural and Food Chemistry, 54: 5623–5629.

Choi, H.W. and B.K. Baik. 2013. Significance of wheat flour particle size on sponge cake baking quality. Cereal Chemistry, 90(2): 150–156.

de la Hera, E., M. Gomez and C.M. Rosell. 2013a. Particle size distribution of rice flour affecting the starch enzymatic hydrolysis and hydration properties. Carbohydrate Polymers, 98(1): 421–427.

de la Hera, E., M. Martinez and M. Gomez. 2013b. Influence of flour particle size on quality of gluten-free rice bread. LWt-Food Science and Technology, 54(1): 199–206.

de la Hera, E., M. Talegon, P. Caballero and M. Gomez. 2013c. Influence of maize flour particle size on gluten-free breadmaking. J. Sci. Food Agric., 93(4): 924–932.

de la Hera, E., C.M. Rosell and M. Gomez. 2014. Effect of water content and flour particle size on gluten-free bread quality and digestibility. Food Chemistry, 151: 526–531.

Dijkink, B.H. and J.H.A. Willemsen. 2006. WO2006006845 A1, access 25/9/2014.

Ellis, P.R., F.M. Dawoud and E.R. Morris. 1991. Blood-glucose, plasma-insulin and sensory responses to guar-containing wheat breads—effects of molecular-weight and particle-size of guar gum. British Journal of Nutrition, 66(3): 363–379.

Engelsen, M.M. and Å. Hansen. 2009. Tocopherol and tocotrienol content in commercial wheat mill streams. Cereal Chemistry, 86(5): 499–502.

Estrada-Giron, Y., B.G. Swanson and G.V. Barbosa-Canovas. 2005. Advances in the use of high hydrostatic pressure for processing cereal grains and legumes. Trends in Food Science & Technology, 16(5): 194–203. doi: 10.1016/j.tifs.2004.10.005.

Ferrari, B., F. Finocchiaro, A. Gianinetti and A.M. Stanca. 2009. Optimization of air classification for the production of β-glucan-enriched barley flours. Journal of Cereal Science, 50(2): 152–158.

Gomes, M.R.A., R. Clark and D.A. Ledward. 1998. Effects of high pressure on amylases and starch in wheat and barley flours. Food Chemistry, 63(3): 363–372.

Hayakawa, I., Y. Yamad and Y. Fujio. 1993. Microparticulation by jet mill grinding of protein powders and effects on hydrophobicity. Journal of Food Science, 58(5): 1026–1029.

Hemery, Y., M. Chaurand, U. Holopainen, A.-M. Lampi, P. Lehtinen, V. Piironen, A. Sadoudi and X. Rouau. 2011. Potential of dry fractionation of wheat bran for the development of food ingredients, part I: Influence of ultra-fine grinding. Journal of Cereal Science, 53: 1–8.

Hemery, Y., X. Rouau, V. Lullien-Pellerin, C. Barron and J. Abecassis. 2007. Dry processes to develop wheat fractions and products with enhanced nutritional quality. Journal of Cereal Science, 46(3): 327–347.

Holt, S.H.A. and J.B. Miller. 1994. Particle-size, satiety and the glycemic response. European Journal of Clinical Nutrition, 48(7): 496–502.

Huang, S.L., C.L. Jao and K.C. Hsu. 2009. Effects of hydrostatic pressure/heat combinations on water uptake and gelatinization characteristics of japonica rice grains: A kinetic study. Journal of Food Science, 74(8): E442–E448.

Hüttner, E.K. and E.K. Arendt. 2010. Recent advances in gluten-free baking and the current status of oats. Trends in Food Science & Technology, 21: 303–312.

Huttner, E.K., F. Dal Bello and E.K. Arendt. 2010. Fundamental study on the effect of hydrostatic pressure treatment on the bread-making performance of oat flour. European Food Research and Technology, 230(6): 827–835.

Huttner, E.K., F. Dal Bello, K. Poutanen and E.K. Arendt. 2009. Fundamental evaluation of the impact of high hydrostatic pressure on oat batters. Journal of Cereal Science, 49(3): 363–370.

Kadharmestan, C., B.K. Baik and Z. Czuchajowska. 1998. Whey protein concentrate treated with heat or high hydrostatic pressure in wheat-based products. Cereal Chemistry, 75(5): 762–766.

Kato, T., E. Katayama, S. Matsubara, Y. Omi and T. Matsuda. 2000. Release of allergenic proteins from rice grains induced by high hydrostatic pressure. J. Agric. Food Chem., 48(8): 3124–3129.

Li, H.J., K.X. Zhu, H.M. Zhou and W. Peng. 2012. Effects of high hydrostatic pressure treatment on allergenicity and structural properties of soybean protein isolate for infant formula. Food Chemistry, 132(2): 808–814.

Majzoobi, M., A. Farahnaky, Z. Nematolahi, M.M. Hashemi and M.J.T. Ardakani. 2013. Effect of Different Levels and Particle Sizes of Wheat Bran on the Quality of Flat Bread. Journal of Agricultural Science and Technology, 15(1): 115–123.

Mei, X., T. Mu, X. Chen, J. Guan and J. He. 2014. Effect of micronization on composition and physicochemical properties of sweet potato dietary fiber. Journal of the Chinese Cereals and Oils Association, 29(2): 76–81.

Messens, W., J. Van Camp and A. Huyghebaert. 1997. The use of high pressure to modify the functionality of food proteins. Trends in Food Science and Technology, 8(4): 107–112.

Nguyen, T.T.T., J.P. Guyot, C. Icard-Verniere, I. Rochette and G. Loiseau. 2007. Effect of high pressure homogenisation on the capacity of *Lactobacillus plantarum* A6 to ferment rice/soybean slurries to prepare high energy density complementary food. Food Chemistry, 102(4): 1288–1295.

Noort, M.W.J., D. van Haaster, Y. Hemery, H.A. Schols and R.J. Hamer. 2010. The effect of particle size of wheat bran fractions on bread quality—Evidence for fibre protein interactions. Journal of Cereal Science, 52(1): 59–64.

Odonnell, L.J.D., P.M. Emmett and K.W. Heaton. 1989. Size of flour particles and its relation to glycemia, insulinemia, and colonic disease. British Medical Journal, 298(6688): 1616–1617.

Pelgrom, P.J.M., A.M. Vissers, R.M. Boom and M.A.I. Schutyser. 2013. Dry fractionation for production of functional pea protein concentrates. Food Research International, 53: 232–239.

Prasopsunwattana, N., M.B. Omary, E.A. Arndt, P.H. Cooke, R.A. Flores, W. Yokoyama and S.P. Lee. 2009. Particle size effects on the quality of flour tortillas enriched with whole grain waxy barley. Cereal Chemistry, 86(4): 439–451.

Protonotariou, S., A. Drakos, V. Evageliou, C. Ritzoulis and I. Mandala. 2014b. Sieving fractionation and jet mill micronization affect the functional properties of wheat flour. Journal of Food Engineering, 134(1): 24–29.

Protonotariou, S., C. Batzaki and I. Mandala. 2014a. Increasing the amount of whole wheat flour in biscuits using jet milling. 12th International Hydrocoloids Conference (IHC). Taipei, Taiwan, 5-9/5/2014.

Rizzello, C.G., R. Coda, F. Mazzacane, D. Minervini and M. Gobbetti. 2012. Micronized by-products from debranned durum wheat and sourdough fermentation enhanced the nutritional, textural and sensory features of bread. Food Research International, 46: 304–313.

Rossa, N.N., C. Barron, C. Gaiani, C. Dufour and V. Micard. 2013. Ultra-fine grinding increase the antioxidant capacity of wheat bran. Journal of Cereal Science, 57: 84–90.

Rubens, P., J. Snauwaert, K. Heremans and R. Stute. 1999. *In situ* observation of pressure-induced gelation of starches studied with FTIR in the diamond anvil cell. Carbohydrate Polymers, 39(3): 231–235.

Sapirstein, H.D., P. David, K.R. Preston and J.E. Dexter. 2007. Durum wheat breadmaking quality: Effects of gluten strength, protein composition, semolina particle size and fermentation time. Journal of Cereal Science, 45(2): 150–161.

Schutyser, M.A.I. and A.J. van der Goot. 2011. The potential of dry fractionation processes for sustainable plant protein production. Trends in Food Science & Technology, 22: 154–164.

Song, J.Y. and M. Shin. 2007. Effects of soaking and particle sizes on the properties of rice flour and gluten-free rice bread. Food Science and Biotechnology, 16(5): 759–764.

Srinivasan, R., K.B. Hicks, J. Wilson and R.K. Challa. 2012. Effect of barley roller milling on fractionation of flour using sieving and air classification. Applied Engineering in Agriculture, 28(2): 225–230.

Stute, R., R.W. Klingler, S. Boguslawski, M.N. Eshtiaghi and D. Knorr. 1996. Effects of high pressures treatment on starches. Starch-Starke, 48(11-12): 399–408.

Tomotake, H., R. Yamazaki and M. Yamato. 2012. An autoclave treatment reduces the solubility and antigenicity of an allergenic protein found in buckwheat flour. J. Food Prot., 75(6): 1172–1175.

Toth, A., J. Prokisch, P. Sipos, E. Szeles, E. Mars and Z. Gyori. 2006. Effects of particle size on the quality of winter wheat flour, with a special focus on macro- and microelement concentration. Communications in Soil Science and Plant Analysis, 37(15-20): 2659–2672.

Turner, J.B. 2003. Whole wheat flour milling: effects of variety and particle size. Kansas State University. Master Thesis.

Vallons, K.J.R., L.A.M. Ryan, P. Koehler and E.K. Arendt. 2010. High pressure-treated sorghum flour as a functional ingredient in the production of sorghum bread. European Food Research and Technology, 231(5): 711–717.

Winter, R. 2003. Proteins in lipid nanocontainers—Effects of hydration, temperature, pressure and confinement. Biophysical Journal, 84: 198A–198A.

Zhou, K., L. Su and L.L. Yu. 2004. Phytochemicals and antioxidant properties in wheat bran. Journal of Agricultural and Food Chemistry, 52: 6108–6114.

Zhu, F., B. Du, R. Li and J. Li. 2014. Effect of micronization technology on physicochemical and antioxidant properties of dietary fiber from buckwheat hulls. Biocatalysis and Agricultural Biotechnology, 3(3): 30–34.

Zhu, K.X., S. Huang, W. Peng, H.F. Qian and H.M. Zhou. 2010. Effect of ultrafine grinding on hydration and antioxidant properties of wheat bran dietary fiber. Food Research International, 43(4): 943–948.

Zucco, F., Y. Borsuk and S.D. Arntfield. 2011. Physical and nutritional evaluation of wheat cookies supplemented with pulse flours of different particle sizes. LWT-Food Science and Technology, 44(10): 2070–2076.

12

Raw Material Characteristics for Healthy Breadmaking

Marina Carcea,* Francesca Melini and *Valentina Narducci*

1. Introduction

Plain leavened bread is originally produced from four ingredients: cereal flour, water, yeast or other leavening agent and salt (Dewettinck et al. 2008). Wheat flour is particularly suitable for baking leavened loaves because it contains large amounts of gluten-forming proteins, which makes the dough soft, elastic and resistant, capable to rise and produce bread with soft, elastic and open crumb (Cauvain and Young 2007).

Some other cereal flours can form gluten to a lesser extent, e.g., rye and barley, and traditions of leavened bread made from other cereals than wheat exist in many countries. Minor cereals (that is, barley, rye, oats, hulled wheat) were rather used in the past and have been dropped over the years to the advantage of the more productive, easily processed and technologically superior wheat. However, in recent years, they are attracting interest again because they have been found rich in nutrients and substances which are beneficial for human health, such as fibres and phytochemicals, and they are interesting for wholemeal products which are attracting again the interest of health authorities and consumers (Rui 2007).

Cereals not containing gluten proteins (like maize, rice, sorghum, millet) are used for breadmaking in certain parts of the world and their flour is generally mixed with wheat flour to obtain better results. However, in recent years, they are increasingly used in combination with other ingredients to make gluten-free bread for people suffering celiac disease.

Council for Agricultural Research and Economics - Research Center on Food and Nutrition - CRA NUT (formerly INRAN). Via Ardeatina 546, I-00178 Rome, Italy.

Emails: marina.carcea@entecra.it; francesca.melini@entecra.it; valentina.narducci@entecra.it

* Corresponding author

Flours obtained from vegetable species other than cereals can also be used in breadmaking. It is the case of the so-called *pseudocereals* such as buckwheat, quinoa and amaranth; of legumes like soy or pulses; of tubers like cassava; or of oily seeds like sunflower. The use of some of these flours is traditional in certain parts of the world. However, thanks to the recent rediscovery of their nutritional properties, they are receiving attention as healthy ingredients for breadmaking in combination with wheat flour or to increase the nutritional quality of gluten-free bread. Economic reasons might also be important in some cases when there is a need for reducing expensive wheat import and for increasing the value of local crops by enhancing their use.

The absence of gluten poses significant technological challenges that can be overcome by using additives and by adopting suitable fermentation procedures. Emulsifiers, hydrocolloids, enzymes and sourdough fermentation have been shown to improve the technological and nutritional quality of non-wheat bread (Mettler and Seibel 1993; Collar et al. 1999; Rosell et al. 2001; Shittu et al. 2009; Sciarini et al. 2012).

In the following paragraphs, the technological and nutritional characteristics of vegetable flours will be discussed in general, whereas specific information on raw materials, coming from different plant species but wheat and widely used in breadmaking, will be given in greater detail.

2. Cereals

From a technological point of view, cereal grains at maturity can be hulled or free threshing. Hulled grains possess strong hulls, i.e., toughened glumes that tightly enclose the grains and that have to be removed by specific processing before the grains can be consumed. Examples are einkorn, emmer, spelt, rice and barley. In free threshing (or naked) forms such as durum wheat and soft wheat, the glumes are fragile and they break up on threshing releasing the grain.

As far as nutrition is concerned, cereals are a major source of carbohydrates, proteins, vitamins (especially of the B group) and minerals. They also contain dietary fibre and a number of phytochemicals that contribute to good health (McKevith 2004).

Cereals contain about 50–80 percent carbohydrates, mainly starch, whereas up to about 10 percent are non-starch polysaccharides contained in the outer layers (bran) and constituting dietary fibre (McKevith 2004; Dewettinck et al. 2008). According to the rate of glucose release and absorption in the gastrointestinal tract, starch is classified into rapidly digestible starch (RDS), digested in about 20 min; slowly digestible starch (SDS), digested between 20 and 120 min, which leads to a lower glycaemic response; and resistant starch (RS), not digested and included in soluble fibre (Gil et al. 2011). Bread contains all starch fractions, with SDS being the most represented and RS increasing with staling. However, the relative amounts of the starch fractions vary according to the cereal used. Wholegrain bread has a lower glycaemic response with respect to white bread, since fibre slows the absorption of nutrients. It is generally recommended that 45–65 percent of caloric intake derive from carbohydrate-based foods assumed in a number of servings per day and that half of them be wholegrain (Aisbitt et al. 2008; EFSA 2010; USDA 2010). A wide range of benefits for human health are consistently reported in association with consumption of carbohydrate-based equilibrated diets including an important whole grain quota. These effects include a reduced risk of cardiovascular diseases, cancer, diabetes, improved control of glycaemia and weight (FAO-WHO 2007; Aisbitt et al. 2008; Gil et al. 2011).

Cereals are a fundamental source of proteins for humans worldwide. Proteins typically range 6–15 percent (McKevith 2004), though they can approach 20 percent in certain species, like einkorn (Hidalgo and Brandolini 2014). Proteins are concentrated in the grain endosperm and in some cereals, up to 80 percent of them can be gluten-forming proteins belonging to the classes of prolamins and glutelins, rich in the amino acids proline and glutamine, but generally containing limited quantities of the essential amino acid lysine and, to a lesser extent, threonine (Dewettinck et al. 2008). The remaining 20 percent proteins are soluble proteins instead, belonging to the class of albumins and globulins, which are concentrated in the outer layers. Soluble proteins contain higher levels of essential amino acids than the gluten ones; however they are scarcely present in refined flours. Cereal proteins generally have a lower percentage of postprandial utilization than legume proteins and animal proteins (Dewettinck et al. 2008).

Lipids in cereals are concentrated in the germ (which is generally removed during milling except for wholemeal flour) and their quantity ranges 1–10 percent (dry weight) (McKevith 2004). They are valuable especially for their composition, being rich in unsaturated fatty acids: particularly linoleic acid (C18:2, essential), but also oleic acid (C18:1) and linolenic acid (C18:3, essential). In addition, the cereal lipid fraction can contain fat-soluble vitamins E, D, K, carotenoids (with or without A vitamin activity) and phytosterols (Dewettinck et al. 2008).

Whole cereals in general are considered an important source of the B group vitamins, especially thiamine, riboflavin, niacin and pyridoxine (McKevith 2004; Dewettinck et al. 2008). Wheat, barley and oats also provide biotin and, together with rye, folic acid (Dewettinck et al. 2008). Cereals are not sources of pantothenic acid or C vitamin instead. As regards lipid soluble vitamins, they are present in small quantity in cereals because of the small quantity of the lipid fraction; however, wheat germ oil is rich in vitamin E and various cereal oils can contain D and K vitamins and carotenoids with A vitamin activity.

Cereals contain about 1.5–2.5 percent of minerals: phosphorus, potassium, magnesium, calcium, iron, zinc, copper and selenium (McKevith 2004; Dewettinck et al. 2008; Nuss and Tanumihardjo 2010; Sullivan et al. 2013). All cereals are good source of potassium whereas they have low levels of sodium. Other minerals are mostly present in the outer layers of the grains and their content is reduced in refined flours. Phosphorus is present in the largest amounts, especially in the form of calcium and magnesium phytates. The presence of phytates (mioinositol-hexakisphosphates) is a characteristic of cereals, but phytates are considered to be anti-nutritional factors since they form stable complexes with cations thus reducing their absorption. Phytate content is reduced (and phosphorus made available as well) in bread produced by means of sourdough fermentation (Buddrick et al. 2014).

Traditionally, dietary fibre is classified as insoluble and soluble. Insoluble fibre in cereals is composed by cellulose, hemicelluloses (e.g., arabinoxylanes and arabinogalactanes) and lignin. Soluble fibre (gel-forming fraction) in cereals includes soluble hemicelluloses, β-glucans, pentosans, inulin and resistant starch. Phytic acid, tannins and phytosterols are also associated with it.

Cereals contain a number of bioactive substances that can help in preventing oxidative stress and related diseases. These are generally more concentrated in the outer layers of grains, so that their actual amount in flours depends on the degree of milling. The most represented antioxidants in cereals are phenolic acids (ferulic in highest amounts, vanillic, caffeic, p-coumaric, etc.). Other bioactive substances are present in different amounts depending on the cereal species: phenolic substances like flavonoids, carotenoids with or without vitamin A activity, lignans, phytoestrogens and phytosterols (Rui 2007).

Cereals also contain antinutrients, which include chelating agents, inhibitors of digestive enzymes, anti-vitamins, goitrogens and lathyrogens. They are generally contained in the outer layers of grains and their presence in flours increases with the extraction rate. The most common antinutrient in cereals is phytate (inositol hexakisphosphate), a chelating agent capable of binding cations like iron, calcium and zinc thus decreasing their availability for absorption (McKevith 2004). Apart from debranning, fermentations, e.g., sourdough technology, were shown to reduce phytate content (Buddrick et al. 2014). Other examples of anti-nutrients are tannins in sorghum that bind and precipitate proteins, and goitrogen flavonoids in pearl millet. Dehulling, germination, fermentation and soaking followed by thermal processing can reduce the amount of both kinds of substances (Taylor and Duodu 2014).

2.1 Barley

Barley (*Hordeum vulgare* L.) generally contains 65–68 percent starch, 10–17 percent proteins, 2–3 percent free lipids, 1.5–2.5 percent minerals, 11–34 percent total dietary fibre of which 3–20 percent is soluble (Baik and Ullrich 2008; Sullivan et al. 2013).

Hulled and hulless varieties, normal starch vs. waxy or high amylose starch varieties can be found. Hulless or dehulled barley, which is minimally debranned, has 11–20 percent total dietary fibre, 11–14 percent insoluble and 3–10 percent soluble.

Barley endosperm contains a high percentage of prolamin storage proteins capable to form gluten (about 80 percent of total protein), named hordeins, that are rich in proline and glutamine and are lacking lysine. High lysine mutants have been selected, but are scarcely marketed for human consumption (Baik and Ullrich 2008).

Barley is a very good source of dietary fibre and, particularly, it contains 5–10 percent of β-glucans, which are components of the soluble fraction (Sullivan et al. 2013). β-glucans are attracting interest since they are extensively reported to be hypocholesterolaemic and hypoglycaemic (Baik and Ullrich 2008; Sullivan et al. 2013). Barley soluble fibre also contains inulin, a fructose polymer, which is reported to have prebiotic activity (Rui 2007).

Barley contains various classes of bioactive substances, particularly phenolics, tocols and carotenoids (Goupy et al. 1999; Peterson 2001; Baik and Ullrich 2008).

2.2 Maize

A very large number of maize (*Zea Mais* L.) varieties exist, that show differences in kernel shape, colour and chemical composition and have different end uses (Nuss and Tanumihardjo 2010). Whole common yellow maize has a mean content of 9.4 percent proteins, 74.3 percent carbohydrates, 4.7 percent lipids, 1.2 percent ash, 7.3 percent dietary fibre and contains B group, E and A vitamins (USDA 2014).

Maize proteins generally range 7–11 percent, they are not able to form a gluten network and their amino acid profile lacks lysine and tryptophan like most cereals (Brites et al. 2010; Nuss and Tanumihardjo 2010; Saturni et al. 2010).

Maize starch is about 72 percent of kernel weight. Together with normal starch varieties, waxy and high amylose varieties exist. Dietary fibre is concentrated in the pericarp and it is mainly insoluble, whereas soluble fibre is generally less than two percent. Maize fibre as a dietary supplement has been reported to have a hypocholesterolaemic effect (Nuss and Tanumihardjo 2010).

Lipids in whole maize range 3.5–6 percent of the total kernel weight (Nuss and Tanumihardjo 2010). The most represented fatty acids in maize oil are the unsaturated essential linoleic (C18:2, 60 percent) and the unsaturated oleic (C18:1, 24 percent) acid, then the saturated palmitic acid follows (C16:0, 11 percent).

Maize contains vitamins of the B group. However, niacin is not bioavailable unless maize is treated by alkali processing (Nuss and Tanumihardjo 2010). The oil fraction contains lipophilic carotenoid pigments and E vitamin as tocopherols. Maize carotenoids include beta carotene, alpha carotene and beta cryptoxanthin, all having A vitamin activity, together with lutein and zeaxantin. Carotenoids are not contained in white varieties (Nuss and Tanumihardjo 2010).

According to the variety, maize can also contain various other phenolic substances with antioxidant activity, like flavonoids and anthocyanins that are associated with kernel colour (Nuss and Tanumihardjo 2010).

Traditional alkali processing, like nixtamalization, increase the availability of niacin and essential amino acids and raise the amount of calcium, but decrease the availability of other B vitamins. The flour obtained is also more capable to absorb water and form a dough, due to carbohydrate polymer modification (Nuss and Tanumihardjo 2010).

2.3 Oats

The nutritional value of oats (*Avena sativa* L.), a hulled species, as a food for humans has recently been re-discovered (Lásztity 1998; Butt et al. 2008; Mäkinen et al. 2013). Whole oat flour typically contains 15–17 percent proteins, 59–70 percent starch and sugars, 4–9 percent lipids, 5–13 percent fibre (Sontag-Strohm et al. 2008).

Oat proteins are richer in lysine than wheat proteins (Lásztity 1998; Mäkinen et al. 2013) but they are unable to form gluten, hence they are unsuitable for baking unless they are used in addition to wheat flour (Butt et al. 2008). Recent studies indicated that oats can be tolerated by celiac people, hence their use to enrich the nutritional quality of gluten-free bread formulas (Hüttner and Arendt 2010).

Lipids are present in oats in higher quantity than in wheat and are more distributed throughout the kernel with respect to wheat (Butt et al. 2008). Oat lipids are mostly unsaturated and the more represented fatty acids are oleic acid (C18:1) and linoleic acid (C18:2) (Sontag-Strohm et al. 2008).

Whole oats are rich in insoluble and soluble dietary fibre. They generally contain high levels of ß-glucan (2–6 percent), which is distributed in the endosperm and in aleurone cell walls (Butt et al. 2008; Wood 2010). Oats are also rich in antioxidants, which include tocols (20–30 mg/kg), phenolic acids, avenantramides, flavonoids and sterols.

2.4 Rice

A large number of rice (*Oryza sativa* L.) cultivars exist with noticeable differences in kernel shape, flavour, composition and end-use. Whole-grain rice (brown rice) is reported to have a mean protein content of 7.3 percent, fat 2.2 percent, available carbohydrates 64.3 percent, dietary fibre 0.8 percent, ash 1.4 percent (14 percent wet basis). Polished rice has a highly reduced content of proteins, fat, fibre, minerals, vitamin and bioactive substances (Zhou et al. 2002).

Brown rice is regarded as the cereal having the lowest protein content; however, the net protein utilization and digestible energy of rice are the highest amongst those of the common cereal grains (Zhou et al. 2002; Chandi and Sogi 2007). Rice does not form gluten and it is allowed in gluten-free diets (Saturni et al. 2010).

Rice has a high lipids content compared to other grains, especially wheat (Zhou et al. 2002; Dipti et al. 2012). The most represented fatty acids in rice are linoleic acid (C18:2, unsaturated), palmitic acid (C16:0, saturated) and oleic acid (C18:1, unsaturated).

Rice starch can be normal or waxy according to the cultivar. Rice has the smallest starch granules amongst cereals and has a higher glycaemic index with respect to wheat (Zhou et al. 2002). Rice endosperm contains virtually no soluble fibre and insoluble fibre is concentrated in the outer layers (Slavin 2004). High levels of tocotrienols and tocopherols with E vitamin activity are found in brown rice, together with B-group vitamins (Dipti et al. 2012). Phytochemicals reported to be present in rice are phytosterols, gamma-oryzanol, policosanols, saponins, phenolic acids and several classes of phenolic compounds that vary with the cultivar (e.g., flavonoids and antocyanidins related to grain colour) (Dipti et al. 2012) even if rice has less total phenolics and total antioxidant activity than corn, wheat and oats (Adom and Liu 2002; Rui 2007).

2.5 Rye

Rye (*Secale cereale* L.) is a traditional staple food in German-speaking regions and Scandinavian countries in Europe and in the former USSR (Vinkx and Delcour 1996). Rye grains are reported to have a mean protein content of 8.9 percent, a lipid content of 2.4 percent, starch and sugars 57.7 percent, ash 1.6 percent and dietary fibre 14.4 percent (Frølich et al. 2013).

Vinkx and Delcour (1996) report a protein content range from 6 to 15 percent, a mean total dietary fibre content of 18 percent of which 3–4 percent is soluble. Rye proteins are similar to those of wheat and barley and show the same lack in lysine (Tatham and Shewry 2012).

Rye is a very good source of dietary fibre (Nyman et al. 1984; Åman et al. 1997) and the main components are arabinoxylans which are present in higher quantity than in any other cereal and are partly insoluble, partly soluble (Vinkx and Delcour 1996). Arabinoxylans influence the technological properties of rye (Vinkx and Delcour 1996). Rye also contains ß-glucans (Wood 2010) and it is a source of the B-group vitamins and of the E vitamin (Clydesdale 1994; Åman et al. 1997; Adlercreutz 2010).

Rye is also rich in bioactive compounds, particularly phenolic acids, alkylresorcinols and lignans; these latter ones are present in the highest amount compared to other cereals (Adlercreutz 2007; Bondia-Pons et al. 2009; Adlercreuz 2010).

2.6 Sorghum and millets

The most cultivated species of sorghum is *Sorghum bicolor* L., of which many varieties are grown (white and red, low-tannin and high-tannin), whereas millet is a generic name indicating several small grained cereal crops, that belong to different genera and species: Pearl millet (*Pennisetum glaucum* L. and other species of the *Pennisetum* genus), Finger millet (*Eleusine coracana* L. Gaertn.), Proso or common millet (*Panicum miliaceum* L.), Foxtail millet (*Setaria italica* (L.) P. Beauvois), Teff (*Eragrostis teff* Zucc. Trotter), Fonio (white fonio *Digitaria exilis* Stapf., black fonio *Digitaria iburua* Stapf.), Guinea millet (*Brachiaria deflexa* (Schumach.) Robyns) and even others (FAO and ICRISAT 1996; Belton and Taylor 2004).

From a nutritional point of view, sorghum and millets are comparable to other cereal grains (Belton and Taylor 2004; Shahidi and Chandrasekara 2013).

Sorghum and millets have an elevated content in bioactive substances, particularly phenolic compounds. Sorghum phenolics include phenolic acids, a variety of flavonoids and particularly anthocyanins, and tannins (Awika and Rooney 2004). These latter components are known to reduce proteins and other nutrients absorption, but don't cause toxicity problems and are also known as potent antioxidants (Dykes and Rooney 2006). Moreover, high tannin sorghum varieties are even preferred by certain African populations because they produce a long-lasting sense of satiety compared to other cereals and to low-tannin sorghum (Awika and Rooney 2004). Sorghum also contains phytosterols and policosanols.

Millets are also reported to be rich in phenolic substances, especially phenolic acids and several classes of flavonoids (Shahidi and Chandrasekara 2013). Besides *in vitro* studies on the antioxidant properties and potential health benefits of bioactive compounds, studies on human consumption of sorghum and millets indicate health benefits (Awika and Rooney 2004; Dykes and Rooney 2006; Shahidi and Chandrasekara 2013).

Millet and sorghum flour have been successfully used to partially replace wheat in breadmaking (Angioloni and Collar 2013).

2.7 Hulled wheat (Einkorn, Emmer, Spelt)

Einkorn (*Triticum monococcum* L. sp. *monococcum*), emmer (*Triticum dicoccum* Schrank ex Scübl) and spelt (*Triticum spelta* L.) are hulled species of the genus *Triticum*, often referred to as "ancient wheats" (Shewry 2009; Hammed and Simsek 2014; Hidalgo and Brandolini 2014). As domestication of cereals developed, they were slowly abandoned in favour of more productive and free-threshing modern wheat, which also showed a better performance in breadmaking (Shewry 2009).

Hulled wheat are partly similar to modern bread wheat in composition, but they also show some distinctive traits. Generally, they are richer in proteins (17–19 percent) and ash (a measure of mineral content), whereas they are lower in dietary fibre (below 10 percent), with respect to modern wheat (Hammed and Simsek 2014; Hidalgo and Brandolini 2014).

Hulled wheat have a lipid content similar to that of modern wheat, but einkorn and spelt are reported to be richer in unsaturated fatty acids.

A similar or more elevated content of thiamine, tocols, carotenoids, phenolic compounds (notably phenolic acids, flavonoids, alkylresorcinols) and phytosterols is also reported in hulled wheats with respect to modern wheat (Hammed and Simsek 2014; Hidalgo and Brandolini 2014).

Einkorn has been particularly studied also because there had been evidences that it could be tolerated by celiac people. However, more recent studies don't support this hypothesis (Hidalgo and Brandolini 2014).

3. Pseudocereals

This term refers to not-true cereals, that is, plants that share some similarities with cereals, such as, starchy fractions, edible and non-starchy aleurone layer, and fruits and seeds that can be processed into flour for bread and other staples, but do not belong to the cereal family *Poaceae* and are classified in a number of different genera. Moreover, they are dicotyledonous plants and as such contain no endosperm but an embryo enclosing perisperm.

Amaranth, buckwheat and quinoa are by far the most used pseudo-cereals in breadmaking, and they have attracted a renewed interest for their excellent nutrient profile and their potential health benefits.

Pseudocereals are, in fact, important energy sources due to their starch content; they provide good quality protein, dietary fibre and lipids rich in unsaturated fats (Alvarez-Jubete et al. 2010). Moreover, they contain adequate levels of important micronutrients, such as minerals and vitamins, and significant amounts of bioactive components, i.e., saponins, phytosterols, squalene, fagopyritols and polyphenols (Alvarez-Jubete et al. 2010).

The proteins in amaranth, quinoa and buckwheat are mainly composed of globulins and albumins and their amino acid composition is well balanced, with a high content of essential amino acids, and is thus superior to that of common cereals. Moreover, protein bioavailability in pseudo-cereals is high, and has shown to be superior to that of common cereals, and close to the quality of animal proteins (Alvarez-Jubete et al. 2010). Amaranth, quinoa and buckwheat seeds, being naturally gluten-free, are increasingly emerging as healthy alternatives to gluten-containing grains in gluten-free diets (Alvarez-Jubete et al. 2010).

Pseudocereals also represent good sources of dietary fibre. Buckwheat seeds are significantly richer in dietary fibre than amaranth and quinoa, which have fibre levels comparable to those found in common cereals (Alvarez-Jubete et al. 2010).

Another important characteristic of pseudocereals composition is their lipid content that is two-fold higher in amaranth and quinoa than in buckwheat and in common cereals (Alvarez-Jubete et al. 2010). Lipids are, moreover, characterized by a high degree of unsaturation, which is desirable from a nutritional point of view: linoleic acid is the most abundant fatty acid, followed by oleic acid and palmitic acid (Alvarez-Jubete et al. 2010). The high α-linolenic acid (C18:3 n-3) content found in quinoa (3.8–8.3 percent) is particularly beneficial from a nutritional point, as an increased intake of n-3 fatty acids reportedly reduces biological markers associated with many degenerative diseases, such as CVDs, cancer, osteoporosis, and inflammatory and autoimmune diseases.

Pseudocereals are also rich in bioactive components with outstanding health benefits, e.g., fagopyritols, polyphenol compounds and phytosterols. In the last decades, the reason of interest in pseudo-cereals is, nevertheless, to be identified not only in their nutritional profile but also in the need to identify raw materials suitable for gluten-free breadmaking.

Pseudocereals also contain in the pericarp of their seeds anti-nutritional factors, such as saponins and tannins. Quinoa is reportedly the richest pseudo-cereal in saponins, that is, strongly bitter tasting, surface active compounds present in its seeds at significant levels, and ranging in different varieties between 0.01 and 4.65 percent with a mean value of 0.65 percent (Alvarez-Jubete et al. 2010). In amaranth, saponins are on the other hand present in low amount and are relatively toxic for consumers. Pseudo-cereal hulls are rich in tannins, like legumes, and these polyphenolic secondary plant metabolites range 80–420 mg/100 g in amaranth and 0–500 mg/100 g in quinoa (Valcárcel-Yamani and Caetano da Silva Lannes 2012). Buckwheat seeds are also rich in thermally resistant trypsin inhibitors and tannins and their abundance partly explains, for instance, the low protein digestibility of buckwheat protein (Wijngaard and Arendt 2006).

However, processing such as grain abrasive dehulling, water extraction (either running or alkaline water), cooking and/or roasting, have become increasingly required to allow bread formulation with raw materials having reported health benefits (Alvarez-Jubete et al. 2010).

3.1 Amaranth

Amaranth (*Amaranthus* sp. family *Amaranthaceae*) shares from a nutritional point of view characteristics of both a cereal and a leguminous seed, because its protein content and amino acid composition are somewhat in between those of a cereal and a bean. It has high soluble fibre content (4.2 percent) and a protein content (12.5–18.19 percent) with high lysine and methionine concentration. Lipid content ranges between

1.9 and 9.7 percent. Fatty acids, palmitic (19 percent), oleic (26 percent) and linoleic (47 percent) are the most characterizing for amaranth. It is also rich in vitamin and mineral content, e.g., riboflavin, niacin, ascorbic acid, calcium and magnesium (Caselato-Sousa and Amaya-Farfán 2012).

Admixtures of amaranth and wheat flours increase bread nutritive value, and the composite bread, depending on the percentage added, shows a high content of proteins, lipids, dietary fibre and ash. The replacement ratio and the production technology affect the technological parameters of dough and the quality characteristics of the final product. An increase of the amaranth replacement ratio from 10 percent to 30 percent, determines an increase of water absorption, gelatinization temperature, development time and stability as for pulse flours. When replacement ranges around 30 percent, some adverse effects on sensory characteristics can appear, and at 40 percent substitution crumb hardness and elasticity increases (Venskutonis and Kraujalis 2013). Dough formulations with pure amaranth flour also show high water absorption during dough making due to the presence of larger amounts of crude fibre in the amaranth flour than wheat flour (Caselato-Sousa and Amaya-Farfán 2012).

So, in general, wheat-amaranth composite flour, compared to wheat flour, produces dough with weaker viscoelastic properties and the composite bread has smaller, darker-coloured and denser-textured slices than the pure wheat bread (Venskutonis and Kraujalis 2013) and hardness increases (Sanz-Penella et al. 2013). In addition, the composite bread shows a slightly bitter after-taste sensation.

Amaranth flour has also been used in sourdough breadmaking processes, but evidence (Venskutonis and Kraujalis 2013) shows that sourdough has no effect on the product volume and moisture.

3.2 Buckwheat

Common buckwheat (*Fagopyrum esculentum* Moench, family Polygonaceae) contains proteins of high nutritional value, a high percentage of total carbohydrates (67.8–70.1 percent), thereof starch (54.5 percent), resistant starch (33.5 percent) and dietary fibre (7.0 percent) are the most important components, a high content of flavonoids and polyphenols, but also minerals and vitamins (Wijngaard and Arendt 2006).

Buckwheat starch is similar to cereals in content, shape and composition, but other properties, such as high viscosity values, correspond more to tuber starches. Moreover, the high amount (33.5 percent) of resistant starch in raw buckwheat groats suggests that buckwheat is also suitable for low GI foods, which are very important for diabetic control (Wijngaard and Arendt 2006). Incorporating buckwheat in bread blends also implies a high intake of dietary fibre, buckwheat being an interesting source of it (27.4 percent in seeds or 7.0 percent in groats).

However, the interest in buckwheat relies on its protein profile and on the amino acid composition that is well-balanced and nutritionally superior to that of cereal proteins. Globulins are the major storage proteins found in buckwheat and there are only a small percentage of prolamins (Wijngaard and Arendt 2006). This is why celiac sufferers can consume bread formulated with this raw material. The optimization of bread formulations has allowed to observe that when dehulled buckwheat flour is added up to 40 percent, dough development is good because of increased viscosity, due to high dietary fibre content, but also because of the swelling and gelling properties of starch, and the emulsion-forming and stabilizing properties of the globulin protein fraction (Mariotti et al. 2013).

The addition of buckwheat flour to wheat flour can also influence the ratio of total unsaturated to saturated fatty acids content that becomes higher in wheat-buckwheat flour admixtures; mono-, di- and triacylglycerols composition also influences dough extensibility (Nikolić et al. 2011).

Antioxidant properties and sensory value of bread are also influenced (Alvarez-Jubete et al. 2010; Chlopicka et al. 2012). In general, the phenolic content is lower in bread than in flours, being the antioxidant active compounds in flours damaged or degraded during baking. Bread formulated with buckwheat flour shows significantly higher antioxidant capacity and total phenol content than wheat bread and maintains polyphenols in significant quantities.

Buckwheat flour also confers to bread a more positive sensory profile than amaranth and quinoa bread in terms of colour, odour and taste (Chlopicka et al. 2012).

3.3 Quinoa

Quinoa (*Chenopodium quinoa* Willd, family Chenopodiaceae) like amaranth and buckwheat is recognized as an important source of nutrients. The protein content ranges between 12.9 and 16.5 percent (Valcárcel-Yamani and Caetano da Silva Lannes 2012). Globulins and albumins are the main proteins. However, quinoa, more than any other pseudo-cereal, shows the best amino acid profile, as there is no deficiency of any essential amino acid. It shows, in particular, high levels of histidine, isoleucine and aromatic amino acids, e.g., phenylalanine and tyrosine, but also leucine and tryptophan (Valcárcel-Yamani and Caetano da Silva Lannes 2012).

Due to gluten absence, quinoa flour can only partially substitute wheat flour in breadmaking and other baked products. Moreover, the sensory evaluation of flavour, texture and appearance shows products to be moderately acceptable, despite a crunchy texture and a nutty or wheat flavour in baking products are sometimes reported (Stikic et al. 2012).

Blends containing 5 or 10 percent quinoa flour exhibit good breadmaking properties and have been reported to be acceptable based on dough stability, loaf volume, weight, structure, texture, taste and colour. Blends from 15 percent up to 30 percent quinoa flour do not meet consumer acceptance because of the high breakdown number and low dough stability. Moreover, a bitter aftertaste is reported at such high quinoa flour levels (Stikic et al. 2012), maybe due also to a deficient seed processing. Quinoa also has a low glycaemic index, and its incorporation in flour admixtures allows bread formulations with potential hypocholesterolemic and hypoglycaemic effects.

Dietary fibre content ranges between 12.88 and 14.20 percent and is present especially in the embryo. Fat concentration is high (5.2–9.7 percent) with elevated levels of unsaturated fatty acids and phospholipids which, due to the presence of vitamin E, remain stable during storage (Collar and Angioloni 2014). Quinoa chemical composition reveals, therefore, the potential as a valuable ingredient in the preparation of bread and other cereal foods with improved nutritional characteristics.

Besides flour, seeds and leaves have been taken into consideration for breadmaking. The addition of quinoa to wheat flour in the form of seeds do not reportedly reflect on dough development and stability and allows, therefore, the manufacturing of nutritionally valuable products with good sensory acceptance (Stikic et al. 2012). As regards addition of quinoa under the form of dried leaves, enrichment of wheat bread with quinoa leaves is an effective technique to improve the antioxidant potential of the final product. However, the addition of quinoa leaves to bread results in decreased loaf volume, as well as increased hardness, cohesiveness and gumminess of the bread with no significant influence on bread elasticity (Świeca et al. 2014).

4. Legumes

The terms 'legumes' and 'pulses' are often used interchangeably but actually refer to two different groups of raw materials. The term "legumes" refers generally to the plants of the family *Leguminosae*, alternatively known *Fabaceae*, whose fruit is enclosed in a pod (FAO 1994). The term "pulses" is limited to crops harvested solely for dry grain, thereby excluding crops harvested green for food (green peas, green beans, etc.) which are classified as vegetable crops, and also excluding those crops used mainly for oil extraction (e.g., soybean and groundnuts) and leguminous crops (e.g., seeds of clover and alfalfa) that are used exclusively for sowing purposes (FAO 1994).

Pulses are an important source of nutrients. In particular, they are rich in proteins (18.5–30.0 percent), dietary fibre (14.6–26.3 percent on dw) and complex carbohydrates, e.g., starch (35–52 percent), that make them an important part of any healthy diet, including gluten-free diet (Boye et al. 2010; Wang and Toews 2011). In breadmaking, the reason of interest in pulses is the nutritional quality of their proteins, in particular their composition of essential amino acids. Pulses are, in fact, generally high in lysine, leucine, aspartic acid, glutamic acid and arginine, while are deficient in methionine, cysteine and tryptophan (Boye et al. 2010). This composition is complemented in daily diets by cereal proteins that, on the contrary, are short of lysine and rich in methionine and cysteine (Boye et al. 2010). As a consequence, pulses flours have been extensively used in bread formulations as part of composite flours.

Carbohydrates constitute the main fraction in pulses, accounting for up to 55–65 percent (dw) (Boye et al. 2010). Starch accounts for 22–45 percent (Maaran et al. 2014) and amylose is in general the main fraction.

In addition to starch, pulses are also very rich in dietary fibre, both soluble and insoluble, whose beneficial role in health and nutrition has been extensively demonstrated (Tosh and Yada 2010; Wang and Toews 2011). Pulses are also an important source of minerals and contain plant secondary metabolites that are being increasingly recognized for their potential benefits for human health: isoflavones, phytosterols, bioactive carbohydrates, alkaloids and saponins. In the last decades, interest has also grown in separating pulse crops into protein, starch and fibre that are therefore increasingly used as single ingredients in food systems for their enhanced nutritional quality. Protein concentrates and isolates contain 65–90 percent protein and more than 90 percent protein on a dry matter basis (Toews and Wang 2013).

The benefits of wheat-legume composite flours are therefore largely centered on the above nutritional properties and on the possibility to formulate low glycaemic index (GI) bread. It is known that conventional bakery products belong to medium-to-high GI categories due to their richness in sugar and white flour; white wheat bread, in particular, is the main contributor to the GI of the human diet, as its starch is rapidly digested and absorbed, eliciting high glucose and insulin responses (GI > 70) (Ferrer-Mairal et al. 2012).

Therefore, in the last decades, pulses and other legumes have been increasingly processed into flours for formulation of wheat bread with increased protein content, protein digestibility, dietary fibre and resistant starch. However, challenges in terms of dough functional properties, bread sensory characteristics, presence of anti-nutritional compounds (Ma et al. 2011), and diluted gluten network have generally hampered so far an extensive development of bread with wheat-legume composite flours.

Researchers have therefore increasingly tried to identify optimal formulations of legume-wheat bread by studying the influence of legume/pulses supplementation on dough rheological properties and on the organoleptic and glycaemic response of composite bread (Fenn et al. 2010).

Considering that different legume species might have different nutritional and technological characteristics, the peculiarities of each group are reported in dedicated paragraphs.

4.1 Beans

Common bean (*Phaseolus vulgaris* L.) seeds can be round, elliptical, somewhat flattened or rounded elongate in shape, with a rich assortment of coat colours and patterns. Several *Phaseolus* sp. exist: kidney, haricot bean (*Ph. vulgaris*); lima, butter bean (*Ph. lunatus*); adzuki bean (*Ph. angularis*); mungo bean, golden, green gram (*Ph. aureus*); black gram, urd (*Ph. mungo*); scarlet runner bean (*Ph. coccineus*); rice bean (*Ph. calcaratus*); moth bean (*Ph. aconitifolius*); and tepary bean (*Ph. acutifolius*) (FAO 1994).

The common bean presents high protein content (22.5 percent), carbohydrates (38.5 percent starch and 2.7 percent sugars), fibre (18.8 percent with insoluble fibre being the main component), some minerals and vitamins (Alonso et al. 2001; Ruiz-Ruiz et al. 2008; Batista et al. 2011; The Bean Institute 2014).

Fortification of bread with beans allows, therefore, an important increase of both total protein and fibre content (Bhol and Don Bosco 2014; Viswanathan and Ho 2014). In spite of its excellent nutritional profile, the common bean presents, nevertheless, some disadvantages related to the anti-nutritional factors present in it, including, e.g., saponins, phytic acid, plant sterols, phenolic compounds, enzyme inhibitors, and lectins, that reduce the activity of some enzymes, the biological action of several chemical compounds and the absorption of metabolites (Batista et al. 2010).

However, in the last decades reduction in activity of anti-nutritional factors, concomitantly with an improvement of the digestibility of proteins and starch, has become possible, thanks to the use of alternative technologies, such as dry and wet fractionating, alkaline thermal treatment and extrusion (Batista et al. 2010). Extrusion-cooking, in particular, has become the method of choice for food industry also to deal with the disadvantages of the so-called Hard-To-Cook (HTC) effect: a phenomenon caused by storage duration and conditions that makes grains hard, alters biochemical and physical properties and reduces starch and protein availability, by lowering the nutritional contribution of these seeds (Batista et al. 2011).

Even though bean flour addition alters bread specific volume that decreases with the increasing of the substitution degree, some studies show that bread produced with bean flours addition has very good sensory characteristics and consumers acceptance (Batista et al. 2010; Batista et al. 2011).

4.2 Carob

The carob tree (*Ceratonia siliqua* L.), called also locust bean, is a leguminous shrub native to the Mediterranean area (Dakia et al. 2007) which is cultivated for its edible pods which can be dried and processed. Seeds are also interesting for the food industry that produces from them carob bean gum and carob germ flour (Gharnit et al. 2006).

Carob bean gum, carob germ flour and carob fibres are certainly the most utilized fractions in breadmaking because of their specific nutritional and functional properties. Germ flour has a high protein content, almost 50 percent, with a high content of lysine and arginine (Bengoechea et al. 2008) and it is particularly used for protein supplementation in food (Dakia et al. 2007) or as an ingredient in cereal-derived foods for celiac people. It also has high amounts of dietary fibre and micronutrients.

Addition of carob germ proteins to wheat flour is also very interesting from a technological point of view because they have been shown to possess functional properties similar to wheat gluten thanks to the presence of the caroubin, the water-insoluble protein isolated from carob bean germ, that is a mixture of polymerized and disulfide bonded high molecular weight proteins of different size able to form a wheat-like dough (Bengoechea et al. 2008; Smith et al. 2012; Tsatsaragkou et al. 2014a; Tsatsaragkou et al. 2014b). Moreover, in the last decades, gluten-free bread containing carob germ flour has been successfully and increasingly produced (Smith et al. 2012).

Locust bean gum incorporation in bread results in a significantly increased elastic character, structure strength, stability during mixing and decreased starch retrogradation. Purified gum at 2 percent level might also be recommended as an improvement in the breadmaking performance owing to its good rheological and crumb softening effects (Blibech et al. 2013).

Addition of carob fibre in wheat breadmaking affects dough rheological properties but allows an increase of the daily intake of fibre without promoting negative effects on the overall acceptability of the resulting breads (Wang et al. 2002; Miś 2011; Miś et al. 2012).

4.3 Chickpea

Chickpeas (*Cicer arietinum* L.) are largely classified in two different varieties: Kabuli and Desi. Kabuli variety, also known as white chickpea, is large, cream-coloured and has a thin seed coat; whereas Desi variety, also known as black chickpea, has small, wrinkled at beak, thicker coated and brown coloured seeds, with generally higher amounts of protein than the Kabuli varieties. They contain moderately high amount of proteins (17–22 percent); low fat (6.48 percent), high available carbohydrate (50 percent) and crude fibre content (3.82 percent) (Asif et al. 2013).

Chickpea protein content is higher than in other pulses (Idriss et al. 2012) and their largest fraction is represented by globulins that range between 53 and 60 percent (Asif et al. 2013). Bread with improved nutritional value can be therefore potentially obtained when using wheat-chickpea composite flour.

Chickpea flours are also considered a promising ingredient for the improvement of bread quality in terms of better glycaemic response. Chickpeas are, in fact, considered a low GI food because of the slow digestibility of its starch and high proportion of resistant starch (Idriss et al. 2012; Zafar et al. 2013). Chickpea flour is also rich in dietary fibre (16.4 percent) (Zafar et al. 2013).

At technological level, the more chickpea flour is added, the more water absorption increase is observed due to the significant levels of soluble non-starch polysaccharides, about ten times higher than bread wheat flour. Substitution of wheat flour with chickpea flour at level of 10 to < 20 percent produces dough with very good properties, almost similar to the wheat flour dough whereas with an addition > 20 percent, the dough becomes sticky and difficult to process (Idriss et al. 2011; Idriss et al. 2012). Pure chickpea flour dough is not possible, because no homogeneous network dough is formed (Idriss et al. 2012).

Chickpea bread is judged very soft bread and, together with soya bread, is in general the best evaluated in terms of acceptance (Miñarro et al. 2012). The interest in wheat flour supplementation with chickpea flours, due to bread enhanced quality and protein nutritional value, is therefore counteracted by the challenge of formulating bread with good physical and sensory properties.

Emulsifiers showed to be of interest since they could improve crumb structure, porosity and gas retention, resulting in increased loaf volume, softer crumb and finer pore structure (Yamsaengsung et al. 2010). Monoglycerides, in particular, are used as dough strengtheners and crumb softeners, because of anti-firming properties related to the ability to affect the amylose structure after baking and retard retrogradation.

4.4 Cowpea

Cowpea (*Vigna unguiculata* L. Walpers) proteins are rich in essential amino acids, isoleucine, lysine, and phenylalanine (Asif et al. 2013) and, when it is blended with cereals, cowpea produces mixtures with complementary amino acid profiles and improves nutritional quality (Mcwatter et al. 2004). It is also a good source of B-vitamins and a promising source of many minerals such as calcium, potassium, phosphorus, zinc and iron (Asif et al. 2013).

It can be easily processed into flour and blended with wheat flour (Mcwatter et al. 2004); its use in bread formulation is nevertheless limited because it lacks gluten (Asif et al. 2013). Cowpeas also contain non-digestible oligosaccharides, i.e., raffinose, stachyose and verbascose, and anti-nutritional compounds such as trypsin inhibitors (Asif et al. 2013). They can nevertheless be removed by appropriate processing methods so as to improve nutritional value and sensory acceptability (Mcwatter et al. 2004).

Condensed tannins are also found bound to cowpea proteins, but heat treatments such as boiling to an eating-soft condition (atmospheric boiling), pressure cooking, steaming, frying, and roasting allow to consume cowpeas without contraindications (Asif et al. 2013). Extrusion, in particular, destroys the anti-nutritional factors and inactivates through heat the lipoxygenase enzymes responsible for the beany flavour development, thus, allowing overcoming the drawbacks to cowpea utilization in foods.

Extensive literature on the use of cowpea in breadmaking is lacking. However available experimental studies show that when extruded cowpea flour is added at a 15 percent level, no significant difference from wheat-bread are found as to sensory quality and acceptability. This range of replacement neither adversely affects baking performance nor eating quality. Higher levels of cowpea substitution (raw or extruded) adversely affect, on the other hand, baking performance and sensory acceptability of bread (Mcwatter et al. 2004).

Cowpea protein isolates can be improved for their functionality to be utilized for product development after enzymatic or chemical modifications.

4.5 Lentil

Lentils (*Lens culinaris* Medikus) are composed of about two-thirds carbohydrates and 24–30 percent proteins and are a good source of dietary fibre (Longnecker et al. 2002; Lee et al. 2007; Asif et al. 2013). When processed into flours, they contribute to making bread with low GI, probably one of the lowest amongst pulses (Gharnit et al. 2006).

Lentils also contain anti-nutritional components, e.g., trypsin inhibitors, phytic acid and tannins that, to some extent, limit their utilization. However, germination and fermentation and heat-treatment can remove or significantly decrease the content of non-desirable components, thus improving nutritional quality and enhancing sensory characteristics of products (Sadowska et al. 1999).

Lentils are found in different colours, ranging from yellow and red-orange to green, black and brown and this characteristic can influence bread colour (Aider et al. 2012; Asif et al. 2013).

Lentil protein isolates are also used in breadmaking and possess good foaming, emulsifying and fat absorption properties (Asif et al. 2013). Fermented and non-fermented lentil flours are also used with different influences on dough rheological properties. At comparable level of supplementation, dough with non-fermented lentil flour addition generally shows a more advantageous rheological behaviour for breadmaking (Sadowska et al. 1999).

4.6 Lupin

Lupin (*Lupinus* sp.) is a leguminous seed with high protein content (about 35 percent dw), very similar to that of soybean, but with lower oil content. Globulins represent about 90 percent of the total protein content (Paraskevopoulou et al. 2010).

The development of bread enriched in lupin proteins has been quite extensively studied and substitution of wheat flour by full fat lupin flour, concentrated lupin flour and defatted concentrated lupin flour within a certain range (5 percent substitution), reportedly increases the stability and the tolerance index of the dough (Paraskevopoulou et al. 2010). When the supplementation rate increases (15 percent) a marked decrease in bread volume is observed, as for any other legume/pulse.

The addition of lupin isolates, obtained by isoelectric precipitation and ultrafiltration and enriched in proteins belonging to the lupin protein globulin and albumin fractions, has further demonstrated the real effect of different protein fractions on dough and bread characteristics (Paraskevopoulou et al. 2010; Paraskevopoulou et al. 2012).

4.7 Soybean

Soybean (*Glycine max* L.) is the most important legume in relation to total world grain production. Due to the high protein content and quality, it is widely used by the food industry. In breadmaking, in particular, soybean is used under the form of soy flours (full fat soy- and defatted soy-flour) and soy protein isolates. Thus protein content in soy products ranges from 40 to over 90 percent (Ribotta et al. 2005) and their addition to wheat flour significantly increases flour protein content and nutritional quality (Dhingra and Jood 2001).

Soybean is also rich in fat (18–20 percent), dietary fibre and other biologically active components, including saponins, lunasin and isoflavones. Fat content is higher in full fat soy flour than any other flour, whereas dietary fibre shows different values in full and defatted soy flour depending on soybean being dehulled or otherwise. Insoluble fibres are, in fact, mainly present in hulls and soluble fibres in cotyledons (Dhingra and Jood 2001).

The use of soy flours in breadmaking follows an increased consumption of soy foods because of their reported beneficial health effects (Ribotta et al. 2005). Isoflavones, in particular, have been studied because they are found in physiologically relevant amounts only in soybeans and foods derived from this legume and they were effective in reducing the risk of coronary heart diseases and several cancers (Sabanis and Tzia 2009; Messina 2010; Toews and Wang 2013). However, isoflavones content depends on processing, and apparently changes from soybean to soy flours in terms of both content and profile occur (Shao et al. 2009).

Processing is very important for the use of soy flours in breadmaking also because of anti-nutritional factors. Soybean must be, in fact, heat-processed to destroy and/or partially inactivate anti-nutritional factors, such as protease inhibitors, haemagglutinins, antivitamins and phytates.

As regards technology, soy ingredients have been traditionally added to white bread in low amounts (1–3 percent) to whiten the crumb colour and lower the staling rate (Nilufer-Erdil et al. 2012). Defatted soy flour, in particular, is the primary soy product used as a partial replacement (up to 3 percent) for non-fat dry milk, since it provides improved water absorption, dough handling properties and a tenderizing effect (Nilufer-Erdil et al. 2012).

Despite some attractive functional properties, the challenge of formulating bread with soybean hinges on incorporation at levels sufficient to induce health benefits, while guaranteeing optimal functional properties and maintaining organoleptic quality (Ribotta et al. 2005). In fact, incorporating high levels of soy protein (up to 50 percent) depresses loaf volume, gives poor crumb characteristics and decreases acceptability (Sabanis and Tzia 2009; Asif et al. 2013). A complete replacement of wheat flour by 100 percent of soy flour is, moreover, difficult to achieve due to the resulting extremely sticky dough (Sabanis and Tzia 2009), dense texture, but also a characteristic beany flavour due to the lipoxygenase-catalysed oxidation of unsaturated fatty acid in soybean oil to volatile compounds (Shin et al. 2013).

Recently, soybean germination and heat-treatments such as steaming, roasting and baking showed to be potentially able to remove the beany aroma. Germinated soy flour gives optimal soy bread quality, highest loaf volume and softest texture (Shin et al. 2013). Improved loaf volume and soft texture can also be attained by adding, for instance, hydroxypropyl-methylcellulose (HPMC) to roasted flour that also offers an extra source of dietary fibre (Shin et al. 2013).

Flour mixtures with soy products containing denatured proteins are also generally able to form gluten: it is possible, in fact, that the unfolding of soy proteins enhances the interaction with wheat proteins. Finally, when enzyme-active defatted soy flour is added, better performance on specific loaf volume is shown than other supplemented breads. Enzyme-active soy flours have, in fact, high protein solubility and high protein denaturation enthalpy (Ribotta et al. 2005).

In conclusion, bread up to 20 percent level of full fat and defatted soy flour can be baked with satisfactory performance (Dhingra and Jood 2001; Sabanis and Tzia 2009).

5. Roots and tubers

They are plants yielding roots, tubers, rhizomes, corms and stems rich in starch, and they are used as such or in processed form. In breadmaking, potatoes, sweet potatoes and cassava are the raw materials of choice for wheat flour supplementation.

5.1 Cassava

Cassava (*Manihot esculenta* Crantz), also called manioc, is primarily a source of carbohydrates and is relatively rich in calcium and ascorbic acid, but contains very little fat or protein. Both bitter and sweet varieties contain antinutritional factors and toxins and must be properly prepared before consumption. The use of cassava flour fortified with legume/cereal flours and/or bran sources has recently made cassava an interesting raw material in breadmaking and its functionality and nutritional attributes can be favourably modified also through pre-treatment with amylases and pre-gelatinization (Jisha et al. 2008).

According to a study by Shittu et al. (2008), not only the level of supplementation but also the cassava genotype and fertilizer application are important in breadmaking. In particular, the greatest effect of genotype can be identified in crumb moisture, while fertilizer application has the greatest effect on the bread crumb texture (Shittu et al. 2008).

Among the several attempts to identify the best fortifications, addition of xanthan gum to composite cassava-wheat bread (Shittu et al. 2009) has shown interesting effects on dough handling properties. For instance, a maximum of one percent xanthan gum is reportedly sufficient to retard moisture loss and firming of the bread crumb.

5.2 Potato

Potatoes (*Solanum tuberosum* L.) have been processed into flour since ancient times. When added in small quantities, potato flour provides a distinctive flavour, helps retain the freshness of bread, improves toasting qualities, reduces product firming and staling, and assists in the leavening of the product.

Potato flour has a high viscosity compared to other flours, and its addition to wheat flour increases water absorption and consistency, and decreases dough development time. The addition of 2–4 percent potato flour does not affect the exterior quality of the bread, but improves interior qualities such as texture, aroma and flavour. Potato flour has been found to be useful also in preparation of gluten-free bread (Rajarathnam and Narpinder 2011).

5.3 Sweet potato

Sweet potato (*Ipomoea batatas* Lam) is high in potassium and its phytochemicals (e.g., carotenoids and anthocyanins), especially in coloured-flesh cultivars, makes it interesting from the nutritional point of view. Evidence widely showed that sweet potato can be considered an excellent novel source of natural health-promoting compounds, such as β-carotene and anthocyanins, present in high concentration (Hathorn et al. 2008).

Transformation of this tuber into sweet potato flour has thus allowed increasing the intake of its nutrients in specialty breads. However, as a consequence of sweet potato lack of proteins, dough formulated with wheat and sweet potato needs additional ingredients, e.g., dough enhancers or dough conditioners (such as hydrocolloids, phospholipids, spices, vitamins, gluten) to improve loaf volume, texture, flavour, shelf-life, and overall quality (Grosh and Wieser 1999; Azizi et al. 2003; Gallagher et al. 2003).

6. Oilseeds

Flour mixtures of wheat and whole oilseeds (i.e., sunflower, sesame and flaxseeds) or flour remaining after oil extraction are also used in breadmaking. This interest relates to their high content of polyunsaturated fatty acids, vegetable proteins, phosphorous, iron, vitamin E, niacin, folates, phytochemicals and fibre.

6.1 Flaxseeds

Flaxseeds (*Linum usitatissimum*) have recently gained a lot of attention as functional foods because of their unique nutrient profile, and are often processed into either raw or roasted ground flaxseed flour to develop enriched functional bread.

The incorporation of flaxseed influences bread dough rheology parameters, e.g., dough stickiness and water absorption and the more flaxseed amount is added, the more water absorption and dough stickiness increase. However, crumb softness also increases with increase in flaxseed level (Marpalle et al. 2014).

6.2 Sunflower seeds

Sunflower seeds (*Helianthus annuus* L.) are excellent source of vegetable proteins with high nutritional value and functional properties. They contain around 20 percent protein, high level of potassium (710 mg/100 g) and magnesium (390 mg/100 g) and are especially rich in polyunsaturated fatty acids (approximately 31.0 percent) in comparison with other oilseeds (Škrbić and Filipčev 2008).

Supplementation of wheat bread with high-oleic sunflower seeds contribute to meeting dietary reference intakes for various nutrients (mineral, tocopherols, fatty acids, proteins). Sunflower seeds can be added to bread up to levels of 16 percent (flour basis) without significant adverse effects regarding the crust colour, crumb grain structure and uniformity (Škrbić and Filipčev 2008). Addition significantly decreases crumb elasticity but not to the level that would disqualify the product. Bread containing sunflower seeds at all levels has rather scored high for flavour, thus showing a potential consumer acceptance.

Besides sensory properties, sunflower seed supplemented bread also has important nutritional aspects as it maintains the significant amount of tocopherols, essential fatty acids, copper, zinc, fat, and crude fibre possessed by the raw material (Škrbić and Filipčev 2008). In particular, supplementation might contribute to meeting up to 10 percent of DRIs for zinc with white breads and 20 percent of DRIs for zinc with wholegrain bread (Škrbić and Filipčev 2008). Improvement of wheat flour is also made by addition of sunflower concentrates and isolates.

6.3 Sesame seeds

Sesame seeds (*Sesamum indicus*) are incorporated in wheat flour under different forms: sesame meal, roasted sesame meal, autoclaved sesame meal, sesame protein isolate and sesame protein concentrates (El-Adawy 1995). That influences the rheological, physical, sensory, chemical and nutritional properties of bread.

Analysis of bread made with wheat flour and sesame products shows that, in case of protein isolates, protein content is significantly higher ($p < 0.05$); in case of protein concentrates and autoclaved sesame meal, level of crude fibre is significantly higher ($p < 0.05$). So, in general, addition of sesame products to wheat flour can increase both protein and ash content in bread. No significant increase/decrease is observed in fat content, with the exception of sesame protein isolate bread which shows a low fat content.

As to bread baking properties, loaf volume is decreased with increasing levels of sesame product proteins, though no significant depression is observed up to 18 percent level of protein supplementation. In this case, crust colour is not significantly different. Crust colour and texture, flavour and overall quality change only when protein supplementation is higher than 16 percent (El-Adawy 1995).

7. Conclusions

Vegetable flours coming from different species belonging to the cereals, legumes, roots and tubers and oilseeds groups can be conveniently used for breadmaking in combination with wheat flour and in different proportions to produce conventional bread with higher protein, dietary fibre, minerals, bioactive substances content and/or with different and attractive textures and tastes. Also the protein quality and in particular the amino acidic profile of bread can be improved by combining complementary species, i.e., wheat and legumes. The same vegetable flours without wheat flour addition are used to formulate gluten-free bread that is becoming more and more popular amongst people suffering from the coeliac disease.

Formulating bread with or without wheat and other vegetable flours poses the challenge of incorporating raw materials at levels sufficient to induce health benefits, while guaranteeing optimal functional properties and maintaining organoleptic quality. For example the incorporation of high levels of fibre and proteins has often detrimental effect on dough rheological and viscoelastic properties, on bread functional properties, as well as on its organoleptic ones.

However, traditional as well as modern processing of raw materials (decortication, water extraction, heat treatments, extrusion, spray drying, etc.) and the use of additives such as enzymes, hydrocolloids and emulsifiers can be used to improve dough performance and bread technological, nutritional and sensory quality to the advantage of both consumers and breadmaking industry.

Acknowledgements

The authors wish to acknowledge the secretarial help of Mr. Francesco Martiri in the preparation of this chapter.

Keywords: Barley, hulled wheat, legumes, maize, millets, oats, oilseeds, pseudocereals, rice, roots, rye, sorghum, tubers

References

Adlercreutz, H. 2007. Lignans and human health. Critical Reviews in Clinical Laboratory Sciences, 44(5-6): 483–525.
Adlercreutz, H. 2010. Can rye intake decrease risk of human breast cancer? Food and Nutrition Research, 54: 5231 - DOI: 10.3402/fnr.v54i0.5231 (accessed September 2014).

Adom, K.K. and R.H. Liu. 2002. Antioxidant activity of grains. Journal of Agriculture and Food Chemistry, 50: 6182–6187.

Aider, M., M. Sirois-Gosselin and J.I. Boye. 2012. Lentil and chickpea protein application in breadmaking. Journal of Food Research, 1(4): 160–173.

Aisbitt, B., H. Caswell and J. Lunn. 2008. Cereals—Current and emerging nutritional issues. Nutrition Bulletin, 33(3): 169–185.

Alonso, R., L.A. Rubio, M. Muzquiz and F. Marzo. 2001. The effect of extrusion cooking on mineral bioavailability in pea and kidney bean seed meals. Animal Feed Science Technology, 94: 1–13.

Alvarez-Jubete, L., E.K. Arendt and E. Gallagher. 2010. Nutritive value of pseudocereals and their increasing use as functional gluten free ingredients. Trends in Food Science and Technology, 21: 106–113.

Alvarez-Jubete, L., H. Wijngaard, E.K. Arendt and E. Gallagher. 2010. Polyphenol composition and *in vitro* antioxidant activity of amaranth, quinoa buckwheat and wheat as affected by sprouting and baking. Food Chemistry, 119: 770–778.

Åman, P., M. Nilsson and R. Andersson. 1997. Positive health effects of rye. Cereal Foods World, 42: 684–688.

Angioloni, A. and C. Collar. 2013. Suitability of oat, millet and sorghum in breadmaking. Food Bioprocess Technology, 6: 1486–1493.

Asif, M., L.W. Rooney, R. Ali and M.N. Riaz. 2013. Application and opportunities of pulses in food system: a review. Critical Reviews in Food Science and Nutrition, 53: 1168–1179.

Awika, J.M. and L.W. Rooney. 2004. Sorghum phytochemicals and their potential impact on human health. Phytochemistry, 65: 1199–1221.

Azizi, M.H., N. Rajabzadeh and E. Riahi. 2003. Effect of monodiglyceride and lecithin on dough rheological characteristics and quality of flat bread. LWT-Food Science and Technology, 36: 189–193.

Baik, B.K. and S.E. Ullrich. 2008. Barley for food: characteristics, improvement, and renewed interest. Journal of Cereal Science, 48(2): 233–242.

Batista, K.A., S.H. Prudêncio and K.F. Fernandes. 2010. Changes in the functional properties and antinutritional factors of extruded hard-to-cook common beans (*Phaseolus vulgaris* L.). Journal of Food Science, 75(3): C286–C290.

Batista, K.A., S.H. Prudêncio and K.F. Fernandes. 2011. Wheat bread enrichment with hard-to-cook bean extruded flours: nutritional and acceptance evaluation. Journal of Food Science, 76(1): S108–S113.

Belton, P.S. and J.R.N. Taylor. 2004. Sorghum and millets: protein sources for Africa. Trends in Food Science and Technology, 15: 94–98.

Bengoechea, C., A. Romero, A. Villanueva, G. Moreno, M. Alaiz, F. Millán, A. Guerrero and M.C. Puppo. 2008. Composition and structure of carob (*Ceratonia siliqua* L.) germ proteins. Food Chemistry, 107: 675–683.

Bhol, S. and S.J. Don Bosco. 2014. Influence of malted finger millet and red kidney bean flour on quality characteristics of developed bread. LWT-Food Science and Technology, 55: 294–300.

Blibech, M., S. Maktouf, F. Chaari, S. Zouari, M. Neifar, S. Besbes and R. Ellouze-Ghorbel. 2013. Functionality of galactomannan extracted from Tunisian carob seed in bread dough. Journal of Food Science and Technology, 50(2): 1–7.

Bondia-Pons, I., A.M. Aura, S. Vuorela, M. Kolehmainen, H. Mykkänen and K. Poutanen. 2009. Rye phenolics in nutrition and health. Journal of Cereal Science, 49: 323–336.

Boye, J., Z. Fatemeh and P. Alison. 2010. Pulse proteins: Processing, characterization, functional properties and applications in food and feed. Food Research International, 43: 414–431.

Brites, C., M.J. Trigo, C. Santos, C. Collar and C.M. Rosell. 2010. Maize-based gluten-free bread: influence of processing parameters on sensory and instrumental quality. Food and Bioprocess Technology, 3(5): 707–715.

Buddrick, O., O.A.H. Jones, H.J. Cornell and D.M. Small. 2014. The influence of fermentation processes and cereal grains in wholegrain bread on reducing phytate content. Journal of Cereal Science, 59: 3–8.

Butt, M.S., M. Tahir-Nadeem, M.K.I. Khan, R. Shabir and M.S. Butt. 2008. Oat: unique among the cereals. European Journal of Nutrition, 47(2): 68–79.

Caselato-Sousa, V.M and J. Amaya-Farfán. 2012. State of knowledge on amaranth grain: a comprehensive review. Journal of Food Science, 77(4): R93–R104.

Cauvain, S.P. and L.S. Young. 2007. Technology of Breadmaking. Springer Science and Business Media, New York (USA).

Chandi, G.K. and D.S. Sogi. 2007. Biochemical characterisation of rice protein fractions. International Journal of Food Science and Technology, 42: 1357–1362.

Chlopicka, J., P. Pasko, S. Gorinstein, A. Jedryas and P. Zagrodzki. 2012. Total phenolic and total flavonoid content, antioxidant activity and sensory evaluation of pseudocereal breads. LWT-Food Science and Technology, 46: 548–555.

Clydesdale, F.M. 1994. Optimizing the diet with whole grains. Critical Reviews in Food Science and Nutrition, 34: 453–471.

Collar, C. and A. Angioloni. 2014. Pseudocereals and teff in complex breadmaking matrices: Impact on lipid dynamics. Journal of Cereal Science, 59: 145–154.

Dakia, P.A., B. Wathelet and M. Paquot. 2007. Isolation and chemical evaluation of carob (*Ceratonia siliqua* L.) seed germ. Food Chemistry, 102: 1368–1374.

Dewettinck, K., F. Van Bockstaele, B. Kühne, D. Van de Walle, T.M. Courtens and X. Gellynck. 2008. Nutritional value of bread: Influence of processing, food interaction and consumer perception. Journal of Cereal Science, 48(2): 243–257.

Dhingra, S. and S. Jood. 2001. Organoleptic and nutritional evaluation of wheat breads supplemented with soybean and barley flour. Food Chemistry, 77: 479–488.

Dipti, S.S., C. Bergman, S.D. Indrasari, T. Herath, R. Hall, H. Lee, F. Habibi, P. Zaczuk Bassinello, E. Gratero, J.P. Ferraz and M. Fitzgerald. 2012. The potential of rice to offer solutions for malnutrition and chronic diseases. Rice, 5:16 http://www.thericejournal.com/content/5/1/16 (accessed june 2015).

Dykes, L. and L.W. Rooney. 2006. Sorghum and millet phenols and antioxidants. Journal of Cereal Science, 44: 236–251.

EFSA (European Food Safety Authority). Panel on Dietetic Products, Nutrition and Allergies (NDA) 2010. Scientific Opinion on Dietary Reference Values for carbohydrates and dietary fibre. EFSA Journal, 2010 8(3): 1462 [77 pp.].

El-Adawy, T.A. 1995. Effect of sesame seed proteins supplementation on the nutritional, physical, chemical and sensory properties of wheat flour bread. Plant Foods for Human Nutrition, 48: 311–326.

FAO (Food and Agriculture Organization of the United Nations). Cereals. 1994. Definition and classification of commodities, last accessed 25 July 2014, Available online: http://www.fao.org/waicent/faoinfo/economic/faodef/faodefe.htm

FAO and ICRISAT (Food and Agriculture Organization of the United Nations and International Crops Research Institute for the Semi-Arid Tropics). 1996. The World Sorghum and Millet Economies: Facts, Trends and Outlook. A joint study by the Basic Foodstuffs Service of FAO Commodities and Trade Division, FAO Headquarters, Rome, Italy and the Socioeconomics and Policy Division of the International Crops Research Institute for the Semi-Arid Tropics, Patancheru, Andhra Pradesh, India. ISBN 92-5-103861-9.

FAO/WHO (Food and Agriculture Organization of the United Nations/World Health Organization). 2007. Scientific update on carbohydrates in human nutrition. Guest Editors: C. Nishida, F. Martinez Nocito and J. Mann. European Journal of Clinical Nutrition, 61(Supplement 1): S1–S137.

Fenn, D., O.M. Lukow, G. Humphreys, P.G. Fields and J.I. Boye. 2010. Wheat-legume composite flour quality. International Journal of Food Properties, 13: 381–393.

Ferrer-Mairal, A., C. Peñalva-Lapuente, I. Iglesia, L. Urtasun, P. De Miguel-Etayo, S. Remón, E. Cortés and L.A. Moreno. 2012. *In vitro* and *in vivo* assessment of the glycaemic index of bakery products: influence of the reformulation of ingredients. European Journal of Nutrition, 51: 947–954.

Frølich, W., P. Åman and I. Tetens. 2013. Whole grain foods and health—a Scandinavian perspective. Food and Nutrition Research, 57: 18503 – DOI: 10.3402/fnr.v57i0.18503 (accessed September 2014).

Gallagher, E., T.R. Gormley and E.K. Arendt. 2003. Crust and crumb characteristics of gluten free breads. Journal Food Engineering, 56: 156–161.

Gharnit, N., N. El Mtili, A. Ennabili and F. Sayah. 2006. Pomological characterization of carob tree (*Ceratonia siliqua* L.) from the province of Chefchaouen (NW of Marocco). Moroccan Journal of Biology, 2-3: 1–11.

Gil, A., R.M. Ortega and J. Maldonaldo. 2011. Wholegrain cereals and bread: a duet of the Mediterranean diet for the prevention of chronic disease. Public Heath Nutrition, 14(12A): 2316–2322.

Goupy, P., M. Hugues, P. Boivin and M.J. Amiot. 1999. Antioxidant composition and activity of barley (*Hordeum vulgare*) and malt extracts and of isolated phenolic compounds. Journal of the Science of Food and Agriculture, 79: 1625–1634.

Grosh, W. and H. Wieser. 1999. Redox reactions in wheat dough as affected by ascorbic acid. Journal of Cereal Science, 29: 1–16.

Hammed, A.M. and S. Simsek. 2014. Hulled wheats: a review of nutritional properties and processing methods. Cereal Chemistry, 91(2): 97–104.

Hathorn, C.S., M.A. Biswas, P.N. Gichuhi and A.C. Bovell-Benjamin. 2008. Comparison of chemical, physical, micro-structural, and microbial properties of breads supplemented with sweetpotato flour and high-gluten dough enhancers. LWT-Food Science and Technology, 41: 803–815.

Hidalgo, A. and A. Brandolini. 2014. Nutritional properties of einkorn wheat (*Triticum monococcum* L.). Journal of the Science of Food and Agriculture, 94(4): 601–612.

Hüttner, E.K. and E.K. Arendt. 2010. Recent advances in gluten-free baking and the current status of oats. Trends in Food Science and Technology, 21(6): 303–312.

Idriss, M., R.A. Abdelrahman and B. Senge. 2011. Dynamic rheological properties of chickpea and wheat flour dough's. Journal of Applied Sciences, 11: 3405–3412.

Idriss, M., A.R. Ahmed and B. Senge. 2012. Dough rheology and bread quality of wheat-chickpea flour blends. Industrial Crops and Products, 36: 196–202.

Jisha, S., G. Padmaja, S.N. Moorthy and K. Rajeshkumar. 2008. Pre-treatment effect on the nutritional and functional properties of selected cassava-based composite flours. Innovative Food Science and Emerging Technologies, 9: 587–592.

Lásztity, R. 1998. Oat grain—A wonderful reservoir of natural nutrients and biologically active substances. Food Review International, 14: 99–119.

Lee, H.C., A.K. Htoon, S. Uthayakumaran and J.L. Paterson. 2007. Chemical and functional quality of protein isolated from alkaline extraction of Australian lentil cultivars: Matilda and Digger. Food Chemistry, 102: 1199–1207.

Longnecker, N., R. Kelly and S. Huang. 2002. The lentil lifestyle-Health benefits of lentils and their use in diets. Proceedings of Lentil Focus 2002: National Conference, Horsham, Victoria, pp. 58–59.

Ma, Z., J.I. Boye, B.K. Simpson, S.O. Prasher, D. Monpetit and L. Malcolmson. 2011. Thermal processing effects on the functional properties and microstructure of lentil, chickpea, and pea flours. Food Research International, 44: 2534–2544.

Maaran, S., R. Hoover, E. Donner and Q. Liu. 2014. Composition, structure, morphology and physicochemical properties of lablab bean, navy bean, rice bean, tepary bean and velvet bean starches. Food Chemistry, 152: 491–499.

Mäkinen, O.E., E. Zannini and E.K. Arendt. 2013. Germination of oat and quinoa and evaluation of the malts as gluten free baking ingredients. Plant Foods for Human Nutrition, 68: 90–95.

Mariotti, M., M.A. Pagani and M. Lucisano. 2013. The role of buckwheat and HPMC on the breadmaking properties of some commercial gluten-free bread mixture. Food Hydrocolloids, 30: 393–400.

Marpalle, P.N., S.K. Sonawane and S.S. Arya. 2014. Effect of flaxseed flour addition on physicochemical and sensory properties of functional bread. LWT—Food Science and Technology, 58(2): 614–619.

McKevith, B. 2004. Nutritional aspects of cereals. Nutrition Bulletin, 29(2): 111–142.

Mcwatter, K.H., R.D. Phillips, S.L. Walker, S.E. Mccullough, Y. Mensa-Wilmot, F.K. Saalia, Y.C. Hung and S.P. Patterson. 2004. Baking performance and consumer acceptability of raw and extruded cowpea flour breads. Journal of Food Quality, 27(5): 337–351.

Messina, M. 2010. A brief historical overview of the past two decades of soy and isoflavones research. The Journal of Nutrition, 140: 1350S–1354S.

Mettler, E. and W. Seibel. 1993. Effects of emulsifiers and hydrocolloids on whole wheat bread quality: response surface methodology study. Cereal Chemistry, 70(3): 373–376.

Miñarro, B., E. Albanell, N. Aguilar, B. Guamis and M. Capellas. 2012. Effect of legume flours on baking characteristics of gluten-free bread. Journal of Cereal Science, 56: 476–481.

Miś, A. 2011. Interpretation of mechanical spectra of carob fibre and oat wholemeal-enriched wheat dough using non-linear regression models. Journal of Food Engineering, 102: 369–379.

Miś, A., S. Grundas, D. Dziki and J. Laskowski. 2012. Use of farinograph measurements for predicting extensograph traits of bread dough enriched with carob fibre and oat wholemeal. Journal of Food Engineering, 108: 1–12.

Nikolić, N., M. Sakač and J. Mastilović. 2011. Effect of buckwheat flour addition to wheat flour on acylglycerols and fatty acids composition and rheology properties. LWT—Food Science and Technology, 44: 650–655.

Nilufer-Erdil, D., L. Serventi, D. Boyacioglu and Y. Vodovotz. 2012. Effect of soy milk powder addition on staling of soy bread. Food Chemistry, 131: 1132–1139.

Nuss, E.T. and S.A. Tanumihardjo. 2010. Maize: a paramount staple crop in the context of global nutrition. Comprehensive Reviews in Food Science and Food Safety, 9: 417–436.

Nyman, M., M. Siljeström, B. Pedersen, K.E. Bach Knudsen, N.-G. Asp, C.-G. Johansson and B.O. Eggum. 1984. Dietary fibre content and composition in six cereals at different extraction rates. Cereal Chemistry, 61(1): 14–19.

Paraskevopoulou, A., E. Provatidou, D. Tsotsiou and V. Kiosseoglou. 2010. Dough rheology and baking performance of wheat flour-lupin protein isolate blends. Food Research International, 43: 1009–1016.

Paraskevopoulou, A., A. Chrysanthou and M. Koutidou. 2012. Characterisation of volatile compounds of lupin protein isolate-enriched wheat flour bread. Food Research International, 48: 568–577.

Peterson, D.M. 2001. Oat antioxidants. Journal of Cereal Science, 33: 115–129.

Rajarathnam, E. and S. Narpinder. 2011. Use of potato flour in bread and flat bread. pp. 247–259. *In:* V.R. Preedy, R.R. Watson and V.B. Patel (eds.). Flour and Breads and their Fortification in Health and Disease Prevention. Elsevier, UK.

Ribotta, P.D., S.A. Arnulphi, A.E. León and M.C. Añón. 2005. Effect of soybean addition on the rheological properties and breadmaking quality of wheat flour. Journal of the Science of Food and Agriculture, 85: 1889–1896.

Rosell, C.M., J.A. Rojas and C. Benedito de Barber. 2001. Influence of hydrocolloids on dough rheology and bread quality. Food Hydrocolloids, 15(1): 75–81.

Rui, H.L. 2007. Whole grain phytochemicals and health. Journal of Cereal Science, 46: 207–219.

Ruiz-Ruiz, J., A. Martinez-Ayala, S. Drago, R. Gonzalez, D. Batancur-Ancona and L. Chel-Guerrero. 2008. Extrusion of a hard-to-cook bean (*Phaseolus vulgaris* L.) and quality protein maize (*Zea mays* L.) flour blend. Food Science and Technology, 41: 1799–1807.

Sabanis, D. and C. Tzia. 2009. Effect of rice, corn and soy flour addition on characteristics of bread produced from different wheat cultivars. Food Bioprocess Technology, 2: 68–79.

Sadowska, J., J. Fornal, C. Vidal-Valverde and J. Frias. 1999. Natural fermentation of lentils. Functional properties and potential in breadmaking of fermented lentil flour. Nahrung, 43(6): 396–401.

Sanz-Penella, J.M., M. Wronkowska, M. Soral-Smietana and M. Haros. 2013. Effect of whole amaranth flour on bread properties and nutritive value. LWT-Food Science and Technology, 50: 679–685.

Saturni, L., G. Ferretti and T. Bacchetti. 2010. The gluten-free diet: safety and nutritional quality. Nutrients, 2: 16–34.

Sciarini, L.S., P.D. Ribotta, A.E. León and G.T. Pérez. 2012. Incorporation of several additives into gluten free breads: effect on dough properties and bread quality. Journal of Food Engineering, 111: 590–597.

Shahidi, F. and A. Chandrasekara. 2013. Millet grain phenolics and their role in disease risk reduction and health promotion: a review. Journal of Functional Foods, 5: 570–581.

Shao, S., A.M. Duncan, R. Yang, M.F. Marcone, I. Rajcan and R. Tsao. 2009. Tracking isoflavones: from soybean to soy flour, soy protein isolates to functional soy bread. Journal of Functional Foods, 1: 119–127.

Shewry, P.R. 2009. Wheat. Journal of Experimental Botany, 60(6): 1537–1553.

Shin, D.-J., W. Kim and Y. Kim. 2013. Physicochemical and sensory properties of soy bread made with germinated, steamed and roasted soy flour. Food Chemistry, 141: 517–523.

Shittu, T.A., A. Dixon, S.O. Awonorin, L.O. Sanni and B. Maziya-Dixon. 2008. Bread from composite cassava–wheat flour. II: Effect of cassava genotype and nitrogen fertilizer on bread quality. Food Research International, 41: 569–578.

Shittu, T.A., A.A. Rashidat and O.A. Evelyn. 2009. Functional effects of xanthan gum on composite cassava-wheat dough and bread. Food Hydrocolloids, 23: 2254–2260.

Škrbić, B. and B. Filipčev. 2008. Nutritional and sensory evaluation of wheat breads supplemented with oleic-rich sunflower seed. Food Chemistry, 108: 119–129.

Slavin, J. 2004. Whole grains and human health. Nutrition Research Reviews, 17: 99–110.

Smith, B.M., S.R. Bean, T.J. Herald and F.M. Aramouni. 2012. Effect of HPMC on the quality of wheat-free bread made from carob germ flour-starch mixtures. Journal of Food Science, 77(6): C684–C689.

Sontag-Strohm, T., P. Lehtinen and A. Kaukovirta-Norja. 2008. Oat products and their current status in the celiac diet. pp. 191–202. *In:* E.K. Arendt and F. Dal Bello (eds.). Gluten-Free Cereal Products and Beverages. Academic Press, MN, USA.

Stikic, R., D. Glamoclija, M. Demin, B. Vucelic-Radovic, Z. Jovanovic, D. Milojkovic-Opsenica, S.E. Jacobsen and M. Milovanovic. 2012. Agronomical and nutritional evaluation of quinoa seeds (*Chenopodium quinoa* Willd.) as an ingredient in bread formulations. Journal of Cereal Science, 55: 132–138.

Sullivan, P., E. Arendt and E. Gallagher. 2013. The increasing use of barley and barley by-products in the production of healthier baked goods. Trends in Food Science and Technology, 29(2): 124–134.

Świeca, M., L. Sęczyk, U. Gawlik-Dziki and D. Dziki. 2014. Bread enriched with quinoa leaves—The influence of protein-phenolics interactions on the nutritional and antioxidant quality. Food Chemistry, 162: 54–62.

Tatham, A.S. and P.R. Shewry. 2012. The S-poor prolamins of wheat, barley and rye: revisited. Journal of Cereal Science, 55: 79–99.

Taylor, J.R. and K.G. Duodu. 2014. Effects of processing sorghum and millets on their phenolic phytochemicals and the implications of this to the health-enhancing properties of sorghum and millet food and beverage products. Journal of the Science of Food and Agriculture (in press). DOI 10.1002/jsfa.6713 (accessed September 2014).

The Bean Institute, Composition of Beans (2014). Available online: http://beaninstitute.com/beans-101/nutrients/

Toews, R. and N. Wang. 2013. Physicochemical and functional properties of protein concentrates from pulses. Food Research International, 52: 445–451.

Tosh, S.M. and S. Yada. 2010. Dietary fibres in pulse seeds and fractions: characterization, functional attributes and applications. Food Research International, 43: 450–460.

Tsatsaragkou, K., G. Gounaropoulos and I. Mandala. 2014a. Development of gluten free bread containing carob flour and resistant starch. LWT-Food Science and Technology, 58: 124–129.

Tsatsaragkou, K., S. Yiannopoulos, A. Kontogiorgi, E. Poulli, M. Krokida and I. Mandala. 2014b. Effect of carob flour addition on the rheological properties of gluten-free breads. Food and Bioprocess Technology, 7(3): 868–876.

USDA (United States Department of Agriculture). 2014. National Nutrient Database for Standard Reference Release 27. Basic Report 2014 Corn, Yellow.

USDA-HHS (United States Department of Agriculture-U.S. Department of Health and Human Services). 2010. Dietary Guidelines for Americans, 2010, 7th Edition. U.S. Government Printing Office, Washington, DC: 95 pp.

Valcárcel-Yamani, B. and S. Caetano da Silva Lannes. 2012. Applications of Quinoa (*Chenopodium Quinoa* Willd.) and Amaranth (*Amaranthus* sp.) and their influence in the nutritional value of cereal based foods. Food and Public Health, 2(6): 265–275.

Venskutonis, P.R. and P. Kraujalis. 2013. Nutritional components of amaranth seeds and vegetables: A review on composition, properties, and uses. Comprehensive Reviews in Food Science and Food Safety, 12: 381–412.

Vinkx, C.J.A. and J.A. Delcour. 1996. Rye (*Secale cereale* L.) arabinoxylans: a critical review. Journal of Cereal Science, 24: 1–14.

Viswanathan, K. and P. Ho. 2014. Fortification of white flat bread with sprouted red kidney bean (*Phaseolus vulgaris*). Acta Scientiarum Polonorum Technologia Alimentaria, 13(1): 27–34.

Wang, J., C.M. Rosell and C. Benedito de Barber. 2002. Effect of the addition of different fibres on wheat dough performance and bread quality. Food Chemistry, 79(2): 221–226.

Wang, N. and R. Toews. 2011. Certain physicochemical and functional properties of fibre fractions from pulses. Food Research International, 44: 2515–2523.

Wijngaard, H.H. and E.K. Arendt. 2006. Buckwheat. Cereal Chemistry, 83(4): 391–401.

Wood, P. 2010. Oat and rye beta-glucan: properties and function. Cereal Chemistry, 87(4): 315–330.

Yamsaengsung, R., R. Scoenlechner and E. Berghofer. 2010. The effects of chickpea on the functional properties of white and whole wheat bread. International Journal of Food Science and Technology, 45: 610–620.

Zafar, T.A., F. Al-Hassawi, F. Al-Khulaifi, G. Al-Rayyes, C. Waslien and F.G. Huffman. 2013. Organoleptic and glycaemic properties of chickpea-wheat composite breads. Journal of Food Science and Technology (in press). DOI 10.1007/s13197-013-1192-7 (accessed September 2014).

Zhou, Z., K. Robards, S. Helliwell and C. Blanchard. 2002. Composition and functional properties of rice. International Journal of Food Science and Technology, 37: 849–868.

13

Non-conventional Raw Materials for Nutritional Improvement of Breads

Georgia Ane Raquel Sehn, Amanda de Cássia Nogueira and
*Caroline Joy Steel**

1. Introduction

Bread is a staple food consumed all over the world in different forms. Its basic
formulation includes wheat flour, water, yeast and salt, but many optional ingredients
are also used. As bread reaches a great part of the population and is greatly accepted,
it can be used as a carrier for bioactive compounds or other nutritionally important
components. Fruit, legume and root and tuber flours (or the flours produced from the
residues of their processing to obtain juice, refined flours or starch) can be considered
non-conventional raw materials in breadmaking. This chapter proposes reviewing
the literature that involves the application of these non-conventional raw materials in
bread, with a focus on improving nutritional value, but also taking into account all the
technological and sensory changes that these incorporations may cause. For this, the
chapter is divided in three sections: (1) Fruit flours, (2) Root and tuber flours, and (3)
Legume flours. Special emphasis is made on flours origin, if they are residues, their
major nutritional contribution, proportions to be applied in breads and what effect
they have on technological and sensory characteristics; also, when possible, reference
is made to the maintenance of nutritional benefits after processing.

Department of Food Technology – School of Food Engineering – University of Campinas (UNICAMP)
– Campinas, SP, Brazil.
* Corresponding author

2. Fruit flours

Fruit flours, when used in partial substitution of wheat flour, can improve the nutritional quality of breads, by adding fibers, vitamins and minerals, resistant starch and phenolic compounds. Some of these compounds can also contribute with flavor, aroma and color different to those observed in white breads, produced solely with wheat flour. Furthermore, the use of fruit flours is an alternative to reduce the production of solid organic residues from the fruit juice extraction industry. A great part of these residues generated during processing—peels, albedo and seeds—are sources of dietary fiber and other functional compounds, having economic and nutritional potential (Dall'Asta et al. 2013; Ho et al. 2013; Nascimento et al. 2013). Next sections describe diverse studies involving the incorporation of banana, apple, orange and chestnut flours in bread, also mentioning the rheological and sensory alteration caused by these incorporations to evaluate their viability.

2.1 Banana (*Musa* spp.)

Banana is a climacteric and low value fruit, originated in Asia, specifically in India. It is grown mainly in tropical and subtropical developing countries, and has a prominent place in world agricultural production, once its cultivation is developed in approximately 130 countries. Banana is consumed in the mature state and, therefore, about one-fifth of all harvested fruit is discarded. To minimize losses, the fruit is often converted to more stable forms, such as flour and chips (Noor Aziah et al. 2012; Shittu et al. 2013; FAO 2014).

Plantain (*Musa paradisiaca* L.), a variety of banana, is rich in iron (Aremu and Udoessien 1990), as well as other micronutrients including carotenoids, ascorbic acid, and minerals such as calcium, phosphorus and potassium (Adeniji et al. 2006). When bananas are harvested while still unripe, they are a source of indigestible carbohydrates, which are composed of cellulose, hemicellulose, lignin, starch, dietary fiber, and especially high resistant starch content (about 40.9 to 58.5%) (Juarez-Garcia et al. 2006; Tribess et al. 2009).

The resistant starch found in unripe green bananas is the sum of starch and products of starch degradation not absorbed in the small intestine of healthy individuals. The undigested starches are fermented by bacterial microflora in the large intestine, affecting physiological functions and causing beneficial health effects, such as reduction of blood glucose and insulinaemic responses to food, hypocholesterolemic action, and reduced risk of colorectal cancer (Asp et al. 1996; Juarez-Garcia et al. 2006). During fruit ripening, this starch reserve decreases, mainly due to the action of enzymes; therefore, the flour should be produced from unripe bananas (Zhang et al. 2005).

Juarez-Garcia et al. (2006) studied the total replacement of wheat flour by unripe plantain flour, with levels of 17.5% resistant starch and 14.5% dietary fiber, in breadmaking. After the manufacturing process, the bread with unripe plantain flour presented resistant starch content of 6.7%, while the control bread containing 100% wheat flour exhibited 1% resistant starch. Similar behavior was observed for dietary fiber content, since the value found for the bread with unripe banana flour was 5.1%, higher than the value found for the control bread (2.3%). According to these authors, bakery products prepared with unripe plantain flour can be an alternative for people with special caloric requirements.

According to Ho et al. (2013), banana production generates large amounts of agricultural waste such as the leaves and the pseudo-stem or trunk, which may reach up to 88% by weight of the plant, causing serious environmental problems. The stem of this plant has been studied since it contains fibrous components rich in cellulosic material, minerals, dietary fibers, low molecular weight sugars and antioxidant compounds. These authors have replaced 10% of wheat flour by banana pseudo-stem flour (*Musa acuminata* x *balbisiana* cv. Awak) in bread, aimed at improving the nutritional value of this product. The replacement of wheat flour by banana pseudo-stem flour (BPSF) increased, from 2.9 to 3.1 times, the insoluble dietary fiber content as compared to the control bread with wheat flour. The insoluble fraction is represented by lignin, hemicellulose and cellulose, the latter present in greater quantity. The same behavior was observed for soluble dietary fiber (1.31 and 1.71% in the control bread and bread with BPSF, respectively), and consequently for total dietary fiber content, which varied from 3.68% (control bread) to 8.51% (bread with BPSF). Also, according to these authors, the replacement of 10% wheat flour by this alternative flour in bread formulation resulted in an increase in total phenolics content from 139.24 mg GAE/100 g in the control bread to 204.16 mg GAE/100 g in bread with BPSF, and a higher DPPH and FRAP scavenging activity was also found in bread with banana pseudo-stem flour. With regard to the technological characteristics of breads, the addition of 10% BPSF resulted in a decrease of both bread specific volume (from 5.11 cm^3/g to 4.38 cm^3/g) and the color parameter L* of the crust. In contrast, an increase was observed for the parameters a* and b*.

Shittu et al. (2013) studied the technological changes caused by flour replacements of 0, 10 and 20% flour made from unripe green bananas harvested at 7, 8, 9 and 10 weeks. For specific volume, the samples showed no significant difference ($P < 0.05$) when compared to the control, except for the bread produced with 20% flour from bananas harvested at nine weeks, which showed lower specific volume (4.3 cm^3/g) as compared to the control (5.1 cm^3/g). For the color parameter L*, lower values were observed in the crust with increasing degree of ripeness. The authors attributed this change to the higher sugar content in the flour, which increases as the bananas ripen. The color parameter L* of the crumb was greater at eight weeks of maturation, with 10% unripe banana flour (70.1). In addition, all formulations were significantly ($P < 0.05$) darker than the control (91.5), with lower L* values. Unripe green bananas are rich in polyphenols, thus the darkening effect can be due to polyphenol oxidase activity that is present in the fruit ground into flour. Authors concluded that the degree of ripeness of the bananas was less significant than the percent replacement of the flour, and the bread samples made with bananas harvested in the eighth week of maturation were most acceptable by consumers.

2.2 Apple (*Malus domestica*)

Apple juice is the main product of apple processing. Fruit is usually cold pressed to extract the juice, resulting in great volumes of waste or by-products, called apple pomace. Apple pomace contains 94.5% peels and pulp, 4.4% seeds and 1.1% of the center of the fruit. It is composed mainly of carbohydrates and dietary fiber, small amounts of protein, fat and ash, and high total sugar contents, about 40% on a dry basis. The apple pomace is also a good source of phytochemicals, mainly phenolic acids and flavonoids (Wang and Thomas 1989; Coelho and Wosiacki 2010; Reis et al. 2014). Phytochemicals in apples have been associated with many health benefits, for example, decreases in cancer cells proliferation, lipid oxidation and cholesterol (O'Shea et al. 2012).

Masoodi and Chauhan (1998) investigated water absorption, volume, weight, firmness and sensory changes caused by the incorporation of 0, 2, 5, 8 and 11% apple pomace flour into bread. The study was performed with the alkali neutralization of the dough to pH 5.4 to neutralize excess acid from the pomace, as compared with the unneutralized dough. The water absorption increased with higher apple pomace flour contents, from 62% (control) to 72.4 and 73% (11% flour from apple pomace) for unneutralized and neutralized doughs, respectively. Greater flour addition caused a reduction in bread volume, and the unneutralized breads presented a lower volume than those made with the neutralized dough, evidencing that the acidity of apple pomace flour may have a negative effect on the gluten network, reducing bread volume. On the other hand, greater flour additions resulted in heavier breads because of higher water absorption. Breads containing higher contents of apple pomace flour exhibited higher firmness (3 N in control, and 12 N and 10 N in unneutralized and neutralized doughs with 11% pomace, respectively), evidencing that bread firmness was reduced with dough neutralization. Sensory scores decreased with increasing concentrations of apple pomace flour in breads; however, the sensory texture of the neutralized dough presented no significant difference ($P > 0.05$) up to 5% pomace. With respect to aroma and flavor, the bread with 5% pomace was considered better than the breads containing 2%, probably due to the critical level of enhanced apple aroma that was appreciated by consumers. Authors also concluded that apple pomace flour can be incorporated in breads up to 5% without changing the quality of the final product.

2.3 Orange (*Citrus sinensis* L.)

Orange is a citrus fruit consumed in large quantities throughout the world in its natural form, either peeled or as juice. Brazil is the largest grower, producing about 18 million tons in 2012, followed by the United States and China (FAO 2014). Orange juice accounts for nearly 50% of the weight of fresh oranges; generating large amounts of waste (peel, pulp and seeds) (Braddock 1995; Rezzadori et al. 2012).

The fruit contains many nutrients, including vitamins C, A and B, minerals (calcium, phosphorous, potassium), dietary fiber and many phytochemicals, including flavonoids, amino acids, triterpenes, phenolic acids and carotenoids (Roussos 2011;

Rezzadori et al. 2012). The orange residue contains 16.9% soluble solids, 9.21% cellulose, 10.5% hemicellulose and 42.5% pectin, which is the most important component (Rivas et al. 2008; Rezzadori et al. 2012).

Ocen and Xu (2013) evaluated the effect of 0, 1, 2, 3, 4 and 5% citrus fiber incorporation in breads made from frozen dough, on specific volume, firmness, crumb color, and total dietary fiber. The specific volume of the breads ranged from 1.82 to 3.15 cm^3/g as compared to the control sample without fiber addition (3.41 cm^3/g), and decreased with increasing amounts of orange fiber. This decrease may be due to the effect of the addition of fibers in frozen dough, which may have affected the formation of the gluten network. The incorporation of orange fiber resulted in an increase in the bread firmness, ranging from 360.31 N (control) to 366.83–804.52 N (breads containing citrus fiber). The increase in firmness was attributed to the effect of the fiber on the gluten network. With respect to the color parameters, L* value was 75.97 for the control, ranging from 72.21 to 76.69 for the breads with 5% and 1% citrus fiber, respectively. The control sample presented the lowest a* value (0.91), which ranged from 1.28 to 3.03 in the samples with citrus fiber. For the b* value, the control was 18.39 and differed ($P < 0.05$) only from the sample with 5% fiber (20.93). The results showed that the addition of orange fiber caused an increase in total dietary fiber, and the highest content was found with 5% incorporation, which explains the lower specific volume and the higher firmness observed for this percentage. This study demonstrated the significant potential of producing fiber-rich breads from frozen dough with a citrus by-product constituting an alternative fiber source.

2.4 Chestnut (Castanea sp.)

Chestnuts are a traditional product in several countries such as the Republic of Korea, Japan, Italy, Spain and China, the latter being the main grower of this fruit, producing nearly 1.6 million tons in 2012 (FAO 2014).

These seeds or fruits have a long history of health benefits related to their composition (excellent source of energy due to their high starch content) and the presence of effective nutritional compounds such as omega-3 fatty acids, vitamins E and C, as well as antioxidant compounds such as phenolics and tannins (De Vasconcelos et al. 2010; Dall'Asta et al. 2013).

The feasibility of bread supplementation with chestnut flour from Italian cultivars was evaluated by Dall'Asta et al. (2013). These authors investigated the effect of chestnut flour addition at 0, 20 and 50% levels to wheat flour on the antioxidant capacity, volatile profile, specific volume, texture and color of the breads. The antioxidant capacity of bread samples were 0.73, 1.00 and 1.04 μmolTroloxeq/g for 0, 20 and 50% supplementation, respectively. Breads with higher chestnut flour contents showed significantly higher TEAC values (Trolox Equivalent Antioxidant Capacity; μmolTroloxeq/g), when compared to the bread samples produced with refined wheat flour. The compounds that contributed to the volatile fraction of the breads were alcohols, followed by aldehydes, ketones and furans. A total of 38 volatiles were detected and identified by gas chromatography in the bread samples, most of them already detected in the chestnut flour.

The specific volume decreased with increasing chestnut flour, probably due to the high fiber content of the flour interacting with gluten, thus decreasing gas retention capacity. Crumb hardness was significantly lower ($P < 0.05$) when 20% chestnut flour was incorporated (2.0 N) as compared to 0 and 50% supplementation (3.0 and 3.3 N, respectively), which had similar values, even with different specific volumes. Significant differences were observed for the L* parameter of the crumb in all samples, indicating that the color of chestnut flour had a darkening effect on the breads. Breads supplemented with 50% chestnut flour had the lowest lightness (49.4), whereas breads without chestnut flour presented the highest value (66.4). Similar differences were observed for the parameter a*, once the highest value (4.9) was found for the sample with 50% chestnut flour, while the samples without chestnut flour (0%) showed the lowest a* value (1.0). For the parameter b*, a significant difference was observed only for 20% chestnut flour (9.2). Crust color analysis showed that all bread samples containing chestnut flour exhibited a dark crust or lower L* values, which may be due to the browning effect of the chestnut flour, as well as the Maillard and caramelization reactions, since these samples have a high sugar content. No significant differences were observed for the parameters a* and b* of the crust. These results show that supplementation of breads with chestnut flour could be an interesting approach, in the nutritional and technological point of view, for the formulation of functional breads, mainly the supplementation with 20% chestnut flour.

Demirkesen et al. (2010) studied the effect of chestnut/rice flour in gluten-free breads at different proportions (0/100, 10/90, 20/80, 30/70, 40/60, 50/50 and 100/0 flour) on volume characteristics, hardness and color. When larger amounts of chestnut flour were added, the breads exhibited harder texture and lower volume due to the compact and rigid structure of chestnut flour fibers. According to the authors, the relatively high sugar content in chestnut flour may have prevented or reduced starch gelatinization during cooking, leading to lower volume and firmer texture. The L* values of the breads decreased with increasing chestnut flour content and an opposite effect was observed for parameter a*, since higher values were found with higher proportions of chestnut flour. However, for the color parameter b*, almost no variation was observed. According to the results, the ratio of 30/70 chestnut/rice flour was the most effective formulation in terms of quality parameters.

3. Roots and tubers

For their use in bakery products, most roots and tubers are transformed into flour and then incorporated to wheat flour, as a partial substitute in the production of breads. The main justifications for this incorporation are the nutritional enrichment proportioned by the addition of these ingredients, the use of residues from other processes (environmental impact and low cost) and the deficit of wheat in some developing countries, which have their commercial balances impacted by their need to import wheat. Apart from this, the processing to flour and/or starch is also one of the best means to preserve these raw materials (Perez et al. 2005), once they have a short shelf life due to their high water content.

The flours can be obtained from the roots and tubers themselves, or from their agro-industrial residues, as for example, potato and cassava peelings, often alternative sources of nutrients and dietary fibers. These flours, as the roots and tubers from which they come, are known and appreciated for their high starch contents, as well as proteins, fibers, vitamins, minerals and compounds with antioxidant properties. However, their maintenance in the flour depends greatly on the process used, as they can be degraded by various factors, such as light, heat, enzymes, among others. Thus, there is a need to optimize flour processing and storage conditions to minimize losses. Another important factor is the variation of the contents of these compounds in the raw material itself, that makes standardization of their quantities in the flours, and consequently in the final products in which they are applied, more difficult.

The higher the level of substitution of wheat flour by root and tuber flours, the greater the contents of these nutrients and compounds in the final product, but the rheological, technological and sensory characteristics are affected at levels above 15–20%. These levels can vary depending on the process and also on the quality of the wheat flour used. Taking all this into account, studies are necessary to improve the use of these flours to obtain good quality products. Some studies involving the incorporation of potato, sweet potato, cassava, yam and ginger are mentioned below.

3.1 Potato (*Solanum tuberosum* L.)

Potatoes (*Solanum tuberosum* L.) are a good source of carbohydrates, contain high quality proteins, good amounts of vitamin C and some B vitamins such as niacin, thiamine and vitamin B_6, and are also a good source of minerals like iron, phosphorus, magnesium and potassium (ABBA 2005). Additionally, it is high in dietary fiber, especially when eaten with the peel, and rich in antioxidants including polyphenols, carotenoids and tocopherols (Storey 2007). Potato is consumed fresh or as a raw material for the production of starch, ethanol, chips, among others. However, a great portion of the product is discarded during the industrialization process without use of the peel, which contains many of the nutrients mentioned above, especially iron, calcium, potassium, phosphorus, zinc, vitamin B and high fiber content (Fukelmann 2004).

The potato peel flour process is based on cleaning and sanitizing the peels, removing excess moisture, followed by drying and grinding (Orr et al. 1982; Fernandes et al. 2008; Garmus et al. 2009). Potato peel flour provides good levels of fiber and minerals, including phosphorus, calcium and magnesium. Fernandes et al. (2008) found values of 500 mg/100 g, 140 mg/100 g and 80 mg/100 g of these minerals, respectively, and 1.46% crude fiber, which was different from the 4.6% value found by Garmus et al. (2009). These differences can be explained by differences in cultivars, cultural practices, climate, soil, maturation and storage, as well as the conditions of peeling potatoes. According to Orr et al. (1982), potato peel flour also has a good water retention capacity, minor amounts of starch-rich components and no phytate.

Fernandes et al. (2008) studied the rheological properties of wheat flour with the addition of potato peel flour, and obtained higher water absorption capacity, as expected, due to the increased amount of damaged starch in the product, the high fiber content compared to white flour and low initial moisture content of the potato peel flour. A higher stability was observed with substitution levels of 3 and 6%, demonstrating that tolerance to mixing was not affected by these substitutions. However, replacements from 9 to 12% promoted a decrease in stability due to dilution of gluten and consequent weakening of the dough. In the alveographic parameters, these authors observed an increase in W and in the P/L ratio with increasing replacement of wheat flour by potato peel flour, due to the higher tenacity of the dough.

Regarding technological characteristics, Fernandes (2006) used the potato peel flour in breads at levels of 3% and 6%, without affecting bread volume and crumb firmness. Good scores were obtained in the sensory evaluation of the breads containing potato peel flour. However, replacement levels of 9 and 12% led to greater firmness and compact structure due to weakening of the gluten, which is also one of the main reasons for the decrease in bread volume. Orr et al. (1982) added 5, 10 and 15% potato peel flour in breads and obtained acceptable and good quality breads. Therefore potato peel may be used to increase dietary fiber, although at high flour concentrations could confer moldy odor, as well as an influence on flavor.

3.2 Sweet Potato (*Ipomoea batatas* L.)

Sweet potato (*Ipomoea batatas* L.) is one of the most important root crops in the world, being cultivated in more than 110 countries, with a production of 104 million tons. It is a traditional staple food in tropical countries, although it is widely cultivated in subtropical and temperate regions (FAO 2014). It is typically consumed cooked and may be used in domestic preparations or as raw material for industrial processes to obtain sweets, flour, flakes and potato starch (Silva et al. 2006; Roesler et al. 2008).

When compared to other starch-containing plants, sweet potato (*Ipomoea batatas* L.) has higher content of dry matter, carbohydrates, lipids, calcium and fibers than potatoes, more lipids and carbohydrates than yam, and more proteins than cassava (Clark and Moyer 1988; Woolfe 1992). Besides being rich in fiber, minerals and vitamins, it presents high levels of antioxidants, such as phenolics, anthocyanins, tocopherol and ß-carotene (Woolfe 1992). Antioxidants, carotenoids and phenolic compounds also provide sweet potatoes with their distinctive colors (cream, deep yellow, orange and purple) (Teow et al. 2007). These compounds, which are important for human health, have attracted attention by their antioxidant (Teow et al. 2007; Rumbaoa et al. 2009), anticarcinogenic (Hagiwara et al. 2002), antimutagenic (Yoshimoto et al. 1999) and antihyperglycemic properties (Kusano et al. 2001). Other studies indicate that these phytochemicals, especially polyphenols, can also eliminate free radical activity, which helps to reduce the risk of chronic diseases such as cardiovascular disease, cancer, cataracts and macular degeneration (Ames et al. 1993; Rodriguez-Amaya 2001; van Jaarsveld et al. 2006; Rodriguez-Amaya et al. 2008).

The carotenoids content may vary according to the cultivar. For example, different cultivars in Africa ranged from 7.780 to 19.400 µg of β-carotene per 100 g fresh weight (van Jaarsveld et al. 2006; Faber et al. 2007). Varieties of purple skinned white potato showed carotenoids and phenolics levels of 35.67 µg/100 g and 59.39 µg/100 g, respectively, while the purple skinned potato presented 18.84 µg/100 g and

90.25 µg/100 g (Amaro et al. 2013). Given the content of carotenoids and other compounds present in sweet potatoes, they may be a natural, plentiful and inexpensive source of beta-carotene (Rodriguez-Amaya 2004).

Sweet potato flour, if prepared from roots with high β-carotene content, is an alternative for food enrichment to combat hypovitaminosis A. Once it is a source of pro-vitamin A and has the same benefits already mentioned. Vitamin A deficiency has been considered a health problem in 118 countries. Some studies have shown a high prevalence of this deficiency in rural areas of southern Africa, northwestern Ethiopia, Brazil, Nepal and Vietnam (Al-Mekhlafi et al. 2010), often in regions with high poverty rates. According to Rodriguez-Amaya et al. (2011), the production of flour from sweet potatoes increases product shelf life and facilitates their incorporation into various products, including the partial substitution of wheat flour in various bakery products (Rodriguez-Amaya et al. 2011; Alves et al. 2012), since the high consumption and the scope of these products, especially breads, enables the enrichment to guarantee the nutrient supply. In addition, sweet potato flour becomes an alternative for farmers as a possible sales market (van Hal 2000).

Various levels of substitution of wheat flour by sweet potato flour were studied. In general, the degree of substitution ranges from 10 to 15% (Woolfe 1992), but other levels were also investigated. Gattas et al. (1983) obtained viable breads by incorporating only 6–8% of sweet potato flour.

Dansby and Bovell-Benjamin (2003) and Greene and Bovell-Benjamin (2004) produced sweet potato flour according to the following steps: washing, drying and weighing of sweet potatoes, manual peeling, further washing, slicing, drying at 70°C for 12 hours, grinding and storage at 14°C until use. Greene and Bovell-Benjamin (2004) replaced wheat flour by 50, 55, 60 and 65% orange-fleshed sweet potato flour and found beta-carotene contents of 6.480 and 5.748 g/100 g on days 0 and 4, respectively, for the 65% replacement level, which were significantly higher than the values found for the other levels. Dansby and Bovell-Benjamin (2003) also found a reduction of ß-carotene in sweet potato flour over time. With respect to vitamin C content, breads showed 1.0 to 1.6 mg/100 g (without significant changes in the formulations and during the storage period). The bread volumes varied widely (from 825 to 1,405 mL), decreasing as the level of sweet potato flour was increased. There was no difference in color parameters (L, a, b) among the levels of substitution or during storage. In the descriptive analysis, the sensory attributes wheat flavor and aroma, cell size, denseness and grittiness of the breads containing sweet potato flour were different from the commercial bread (100% wheat flour).

Low and van Jaarsveld (2008) investigated the replacement of 38% wheat flour (by weight) by different varieties of orange-fleshed sweet potato puree. The potato varieties were prepared by two methods, as follows: (1) the potatoes were cut into chips of 1 to 3 mm and dried in an electric dryer for eight hours at 60°C and rehydrated to form a puree before being added to the formulation; and (2) the potatoes were boiled for 25 minutes, peeled and crushed to the consistency of a puree. The total β-carotene of the medium intensity sweet potato varieties ranged from 18 to 21 µg/g in bread, of which 13–16 µg/g were *trans*-β-carotene, which represented from 65 to 81 µg vitamin A (µg retinol activity equivalent RAE/60 g bread). In conclusion, authors emphasized that breads made from medium intensity orange-fleshed sweet potato puree showed higher carotenoid levels than the lighter intensity varieties, being a viable alternative.

3.3 Cassava (Manihot esculenta Crantz)

Cassava (*Manihot esculenta* Crantz) is one of the most important tropical crops amongst roots and tubers (Silva et al. 2003), and is among the most important sources of energy in many countries. Again, the most popular form of consumption is the cooked form.

Freitas et al. (1997) added cassava flour (from 5 to 40%) to wheat flour, and found a lower specific volume only at 30% substitution, which affected tenderness (more compact crumb) and consumer acceptability. Breads containing up to 30% cassava flour showed no significant difference for the parameters symmetry, shape, size and cell distribution, taste and flavor, when compared to the control, being well accepted by the panelists. According to Ciacco and Appolonia (1978), replacing part of the wheat flour by tuber flour in bakery products is possible at levels from 5 to 15% without affecting the quality of the final product, and breads made with 10% cassava flour had good acceptability.

Cassava processing industries generate large amounts of waste, particularly solid waste, like the peels (periderm and inner bark) and the fibrous mass or bagasse (cortex and starch parenchyma) (Souza and Fialho 2003). These residues, besides having a high starch content, are good sources of dietary fiber (Cereda 1996). However, there are some limitations to the use of cassava peels and bagasse, including their high moisture content, which makes these products rapidly fermentable by microorganisms coming from the ground. Thus, it is necessary to process them immediately after harvest to reduce this risk (Vilhalva et al. 2011). Furthermore, the presence of hydrocyanic acid content, a toxic compound in some varieties, is also a concern. Some varieties, called "mandiocabrava" have a bitter taste and a high hydrocyanic acid content (above 100 mg HCN/kg peeled root), and can only be consumed after processing as flour, starch and other products. Vilhalva et al. (2011) mention that during the drying process and in the stage of bread baking this compound is volatilized and eliminated. However, other studies indicate that the industrial processing normally used does not remove all the cyanide present in cassava roots (Yeoh and Sun 2001).

The flour from cassava peel is obtained through the following operations: collection, transportation, drying, grinding and packaging. Regarding its physicochemical characteristics, the flour stands out for high levels of fiber (around 50 g/100 g, with 96.4% of insoluble dietary fiber and 3.6% of soluble dietary fiber), demonstrating that cassava by-products represent excellent sources of fiber that can enrich food products (Vilhalva et al. 2011).

Several studies are found in the literature on the substitution of wheat flour by cassava peel flour at levels ranging from 5 to 30%. The concentration of cassava peel flour influences dough expansion and bread color, since it has similar color to whole wheat flour. Thus increasing the degree of substitution may cause darkening of the bread. A lower bread volume is also observed with increasing substitution levels, but with higher fiber contents. Breads with up to 15% substitution of wheat flour by cassava peel flour can be a viable alternative for inclusion of a good source of fiber on the market (Vilhalva et al. 2011).

3.4 Yam (*Dioscorea* spp.)

The culture of yam is present in various parts of the world, but the vast majority of cultivated species is originally from tropical areas of Asia and West Africa (Monteiro 2002). Aside from its relatively high content of proteins and starch, some nutritional and functional properties are attributed to yam, due to its mineral content (chlorine, silicium, phosphorus, aluminum, iron, manganese, potassium and sodium) and vitamins (A, B_1, B_2, B_5 and C), as well as its content of phytochemicals such as anthocyanins, polyphenols and saponins, in addition to the fiber content (Araújo 1982; Miamoto 2008).

The most popular form of consuming yam is cooked, or macerated after cooking to form purees, which can be used directly or added to soups and solid foods (Miamoto 2008). The production of flour is an alternative for use in breadmaking. There is also the yam mucilage, which is a natural additive that has emulsifying activity and can be used by industries in the bakery segment (Fonseca 2006).

Yam flour can be used to replace part of the wheat flour in breadmaking. To improve its beneficial effects, yam flour is produced through lyophilization or freeze-drying (selection, cleaning, peeling, cutting, freezing, lyophilization and packaging), in order to preserve its antioxidant properties (Hsu et al. 2004), and to provide vitamins, minerals, fiber and protein (Zarate et al. 2002). Miamoto (2008) found 3.19 mg vitamin A and 2.49 mg of β-carotene per 100 g of whole yam flour, and 15 and 22.5 mg/kg of manganese and zinc, respectively. In adults, the zinc and manganese content represents 25% and 3.74% of the RDI, respectively. The flour may also be obtained by conventional drying, however, with further loss of these nutrients. Batista et al. (2008) used the following procedure to produce yam flour: pre-selection of yam, peeling, cutting, drying (70°C/7 h), grinding, sieving and packing. Replacement levels from 0 to 25% of wheat flour by lyophilized yam flour were tested by Hsu et al. (2004). No change in the specific volume was observed with 5% replacement, but increasing replacement levels resulted in a decrease of the specific volume, reaching a 45% reduction. According to the authors, up to 20% yam flour can be included in bread formulations without interfering with the sensory acceptance, significantly increasing the antioxidant capacity.

3.5 Ginger (*Zingiber officinale* Roscoe)

Ginger is widely used around the world as a spice in foods. Products of ginger rhizome are available as fresh ginger, in syrup or brine, dried, powder, oils and oleoresin (Vasala 2001). Most production is concentrated in Asia, and the main producers are India and China (FAO 2014).

Currently, there is interest in ginger mainly due to its pharmacological properties and its isolated compounds. Among some properties, anti-tumorigenic, anti-inflammatory, and anti-hyperglycemic stand out. Furthermore, it is known to be a potent antioxidant ingredient which can mitigate or prevent the generation of free radicals (Ali et al. 2008). The constituents of ginger are numerous and vary depending on the place of origin, and if the rhizomes are fresh or dried. The pungency of fresh ginger is mainly due to the gingerols, which are a homologous series of phenols. In contrast, the pungency of dried ginger is mainly the result of shogaols, which are formed during thermal processing (Wohlmuth et al. 2005; Ali et al. 2008).

Balestra et al. (2011) incorporated 3, 4, 5 and 6% of ginger powder into wheat flour, and observed higher values of modulus of elasticity in dough containing higher ginger powder (6%). This level also decreased brightness and hue angle, and increased chroma of the crumb, with characteristics similar to whole wheat bread (Rosell et al. 2009). The addition of ginger powder did not affect the characteristics of the crust, but the Maillard reaction was much more notable. The phenolics content increased proportionally with the increase in ginger powder levels, which was observed in both the crumb and the crust, and was higher in the crust. The same behavior was observed for the radical scavenging activity. In conclusion, among the samples studied, the bread with 3% ginger powder showed good rheological characteristics, doubled the antioxidant content compared to the control bread and obtained higher sensory acceptability. The sensory disagreement in some studies may be associated with differences in eating habits between populations, as well as the spicy flavor, which may vary depending on the content of the active components of the ginger (Ali et al. 2008; Balestra et al. 2011).

4. Legumes

Legumes or pulses are considered good sources of proteins, starch, fibers, vitamins and minerals. They are usually consumed cooked in water, salt and other seasonings and in many countries, together with a cereal, constitute the basic diet. Rice and beans consumed almost every day by most of the population in Brazil have a good amino acid balance because beans supply lysine that is limiting in rice, and rice supplies methionine that is limiting in beans. This same rationale can be used when thinking of the supplementation of wheat (cereal) flour by legume flours in breads.

The total production of pulses in the world in 2013 was just over 73 million tons, with India, Canada, Myanmar and China being the top producers (FAO 2014). The main legumes and pulses produced in the world are common beans (*Phaseolus vulgaris* L.) (red kidney, black and navy beans, string beans), chickpeas or Bengal grams (*Cicer arietinum* L.), peas (*Pisum sativum* L.), cowpeas (*Vigna unguiculata* L. Walp.), lentils or red dahls (*Lens culinaris* Medic.), pigeon peas or red grams or dahls (*Cajanus cajan* L. Millsp.) and broad beans or faba beans (*Vicia faba* L.) with world productions of approximately 23, 13, 11, 5.7, 5, 4.7 and 3.4 million tons, respectively, in 2013 (FAO 2014). Other minor legumes include lupines (*Lupinus* spp.), bambara beans or groundnuts (*Vigna subterranea* L. Verdc.), red beans or rice beans (*Vigna umbellate* Thunb. Ohwi and Ohashi), mung beans or black grams (*Vigna mungo* L. Hepper), mung beans or green grams (*Vigna radiata* L. R. Wilczek), moth beans (*Vigna aconitifolia* Jacq. Marechal), fenugreek (*Trigonella foenumgraecum* L.) and lablab or Egyptian bean (*Dolochos lablab*). Many of these minor pulses are important in developing countries.

Apart from the use of low commercial value products, such as hard-to-cook beans, to produce flours that can be applied in bakery products, or the fiber and protein-rich residues from the legume starch extraction process, novelty products can be obtained by malting, popping and roller drying, conventional or extrusion cooking of wheat-legume based mixtures or even germinating and/or fermenting legumes to produce high nutritive value products.

Studies carried out all over the world including some of the above-mentioned legumes and processing technologies for application in breads are included in this section. The nutritional benefits of legume incorporation are highlighted, as well as strategies to inactivate or eliminate anti-nutritional factors in some of these seeds. As legume flours contain no gluten, the amounts added to bread may affect dough rheological properties and, consequently, technological quality characteristics of the final products, as well as sensory acceptability. These aspects will also be mentioned, as no nutritional advantage can be brought if products are not acceptable to be consumed.

Chavan and Kadam (1993) mention the air classification of flours to obtain protein-rich non-wheat flours and their products among the strategies suggested to improve the nutritional composition of bakery products. The flours and protein products of legumes (as well as from other sources such as oilseeds, other cereals, tubers, corn gluten and germ and rice bran) can be used effectively as vegetable protein sources for nutritional enrichment of the bakery products.

Duodu and Minnaar (2011) reviewed the nutritional, functional, sensory and phytochemical qualities of legume-cereal composite flours and baked goods, concluding that compositing results in improved nutritional quality because of an overall increase in the protein content and a better amino acid balance. Also, simpler technologies than that used for leguminous oilseed flours can be used for processing flours from grain legumes because of their low fat content. However, the extent of compositing is directly influenced by the sensory quality of the final product. They also conclude that little information is available on phytochemical properties of legume composite flours and baked goods.

Scazzina et al. (2013) justify that bread is the most relevant source of available carbohydrates in the diet and describe numerous studies carried out to lower its dietary glycaemic index (GI), mostly through the addition of fiber-rich flours or pure dietary fiber. The reviewed literature suggests that the presence of intact structures not accessible to human amylases, as well as a reduced pH that may delay gastric emptying or create a barrier to starch digestion, seems to be more effective than dietary fiber itself in improving glucose metabolism. Amongst the studies, the addition of fractions from legumes also appears as an effective strategy. And the need to review the manufacturing protocol, reconsidering several technological parameters in order to obtain high-quality and consumer-acceptable breads is highlighted.

Ballesteros et al. (1984) used linear programing to define least cost formulations based on cereals and legumes, taking into account the amino acid profile and the technological feasibility. From a mixture based on wheat, chick-pea, sorghum and soybean flours, they developed bread, tortillas and cookies. Bread was further evaluated and obtained a protein efficiency ratio (PER) of 1.69, as compared to 0.68 for the control. Sensory evaluation also showed that there were no significant differences in taste, texture, color or overall acceptability of the developed bread product as compared to the control.

4.1 Beans

Beans or common beans (*Phaseolus vulgaris* L.) constitute the largest group amongst legumes and pulses and can be of different varieties (red kidney, black and navy beans, string beans). Wulf et al. (1989) and Yanez et al. (1989), from Chile, studied the use of bean (*Phaseolus vulgaris* L.) flour for bread fortification, evaluating technological aspects and nutritive value.

Vásquez Carrillo et al. (1991) proposed the use of hardened beans to prepare bean flours for incorporation in bread formulations. Different soaking temperatures (22, 30, 40 and 50°C) and testa removal methods (under moist and dry conditions) were tested in laboratory and pilot-plant levels to prepare the flours, giving different yields and protein contents. These flours were added to wheat flour at 5, 10 and 15% for bread making. The addition of 5.0% gave breads with similar protein content and sensory characteristics to those of the wheat flour control. A diet based on bean-flour bread resulted in greater weight gain than that with casein for gold hamsters. The study also demonstrated the importance of heat-treating bean flours, because when flour without previous heat treatment was administered, the animals lost weight and died. This effect was overcome by the process of baking the flours at 140°C for 4 hours.

Batista et al. (2011) describe the enrichment of wheat bread with hard-to-cook black bean (*Phaseolus vulgaris*) (BBEF) and cowpea (*Vigna unguiculata*) (CEF) extruded flours. Breads containing 10% BBEF and 10% CEF presented increases of 9% and 10% in protein content, respectively. Fiber content was also 2.6% higher in 10% BBEF bread and 2.2% higher in 10% CEF bread in comparison to the standard bread. Despite protein and fiber increasing, the energetic value of substituted breads remained unchanged. An increase in the substitution to 15% resulted in a decrease of specific volume of the breads. Sensory analysis results for 10% BBEF bread and 10% CEF bread were positive.

Viswanathan and Ho (2014), concerned with protein quantity and quality in food products to eradicate undernutrition in developing countries, studied the fortification of flat bread with legumes in order to increase the total protein content of the product to 13–15%, necessary to meet at least 1/3 of protein requirement of an adult recommended daily allowance. They added sprouted red kidney bean (*Phaseolus vulgaris*) flour at 5, 15 and 25% to white flour and analyzed the composite bread for crude protein and *in vitro* protein digestibility using the Kjeldahl and pepsin-pancreatin method. The protein content of raw beans increased slightly on soaking for 17 h and sprouting for three days, but a remarkable increase was observed in protein digestibility. However, protein digestibility in breads decreased by 12% from control, due to the presence of dietary fibers which bind with protein and inhibit its digestibility. Breads made using 15% legume flour had overall acceptable quality.

4.2 Peas, Lentils and Chickpeas

Chickpeas, peas and lentils are three other important legumes or pulses which we decided to group together, as they are well known to us in Western societies. Many studies were found incorporating chickpea flour to bread, highlighting its slowly digestible carbohydrates and lowering glycaemic response properties.

Figuerola et al. (1987) assessed the feasibility of adding chickpea flour to substitute part of the wheat flour in yeast-leavened breads in order to increase their protein value. A 70% extraction chickpea flour of commercial particle size (150 µm) was prepared. Wheat flours of 74% and 78% extraction were then blended with 5%, 10% and 15% chickpea flour. Addition of chickpea flour increased protein, fiber, ash and fat contents in the blends, not causing a severe effect on quality, even at the 15% level of substitution. Blends showed an increase in maltose content, W alveographic value and bread specific volume.

Utrilla-Coello et al. (2007) prepared chickpea flour (CF) and used it as an ingredient for the elaboration of bread with different levels of wheat (80:20 and 60:40, wheat flour:chickpea flour). Available starch (AS), resistant starch (RS), dietary fibre (DF), the *in vitro* starch hydrolysis indices (HIs), using a chewing/dialysis digestion protocol, and the acceptability of the experimental breads were compared with those of a control bread prepared only with wheat flour. HIs were used to predict glyceamic indices (pGI). CF-bread had higher protein, RS and DF amounts than the control bread. HI-based pGI for the CF-breads were 46.92 and 34.67% for 20 and 40% CF breads, respectively, which were significantly lower than control bread (65.31%), suggesting a 'slow carbohydrate' characteristic for the CF-based products. The slow digestion characteristics of chickpea were largely retained in the experimental breads, indicating that CF might be used as a potential ingredient for bakery products with slowly digestible carbohydrates.

Mohammeda et al. (2012) studied the partial substitution of wheat flour with chickpea flour at the levels of 10, 20 and 30%, evaluating rheological properties and baking performance. Chickpea flour addition increased water absorption and dough development time, while dough extensibility and resistance to extension were reduced. Regarding dough stability, 10% chickpea exhibited higher stability and resistance to mechanical mixing than the control, while they decreased as the substitution level increased from 20% to 30%. Blends with 20% and 30% chickpea also produced "sticky" dough surfaces. The presence of chickpea flour in dough affected bread quality in terms of volume, internal structure and texture. The color of crust and crumb got progressively darker as the level of chickpea flour substitution increased. The substitution of wheat flour with 10% chickpea flour gave loaves similar to the control.

Hefnawy et al. (2012) highlight the importance of legume flours to improve the nutritional value of bread and bakery products, due to their amino acid composition and fiber content. They analyzed the influence of total or partial replacement of wheat flour by chickpea flour on the quality characteristics of toast bread. Chickpea flour was added to medium strength wheat flour to replace 15 and 30% w/w of wheat flour. The effects of chickpea flour supplementation on dough physical properties, such as water absorption capacity, dough development time, dough stability, crumb porosity and toast bread structure and other bread quality parameters were studied. Chickpea flour at 15 and 30% substitution levels increased water absorption, arrival time, dough development time, stability and also the weakening of the dough. The volumes of the breads decreased as the level of chickpea flour increased due to the dilution of the gluten present in wheat flour. Nevertheless, substitutions at

15 and 30% produced acceptable toast breads, in terms of weight, volume, texture and crumb structure.

Zafar et al. (2013) mention that the prevalence of obesity and type-2-diabetes requires dietary manipulation. They hypothesized that wheat-legume composite breads can reduce the spike of blood glucose and increase satiety. Four pan bread samples were prepared: white bread (WB) as standard, whole-wheat bread (WWB), WWB supplemented with chickpea flour at 25% (25%ChB) and 35% (35%ChB) levels. These breads were tested in healthy female subjects for acceptability and for effect on appetite, blood glucose, and physical discomfort in digestion. The breads were rated > 5.6 on a 9-point hedonic scale with WB significantly higher than all other breads. No difference in the area under the curve (AUC) for appetite was found, but blood glucose AUC was reduced as follows: 35%ChB < WB and WWB, WB > 25%ChB = WWB or 35%ChB. They concluded that the addition of chickpea flour at 35% to whole wheat produces bread that is acceptable to eat, causing no physical discomfort and lowers the glycemic response.

Fenn et al. (2010) produced wheat-legume composite flours by blending Canada Western Extra Strong (CWES) and Canada Western Red Spring (CWRS) wheat with varying amounts (0, 2, 5 and 8%) of three legume proteins (yellow pea, chickpea and soybean). Legume protein addition produced breads with lower specific loaf volume, coarser crumb and firmer texture. The CWES wheat compensated for the negative baking effects of the legume proteins as much as the CWRS wheat. Yellow pea protein produced the greatest quality changes, followed by chickpea and soybean protein.

Miñarro et al. (2012) studied the characteristics of four gluten-free bread formulations and the possibility of substituting soya protein with other legume proteins. Four bread recipes were prepared with chickpea flour, pea isolate, carob germ flour or soya flour. Carob germ flour batter structure was thicker compared with the other batters, probably due to the different protein behavior and the residual gums present in carob germ flour. However, carob germ flour bread obtained the lowest specific volume values (2.51 cm³/g), while chickpea bread obtained the highest (3.26 cm³/g). Chickpea bread also showed the softest crumb. Confocal scanning-laser microscopy results showed a more compact microstructure in carob germ flour bread compared with soya and chickpea formulations. Chickpea bread exhibited the best physicochemical characteristics and, in general, good sensory attributes, indicating that it could be a promising alternative to soya protein.

Baik and Han (2012) studied the effects of cooking, roasting and fermentation on the composition and protein properties of grain legumes and evaluated the characteristics of dough and bread incorporated with these legume flours to determine the most appropriate pretreatment. Oligosaccharide content of legumes was reduced by 76.2–96.9% by fermentation, 44.0–64.0% by roasting, and 28.4–70.1% by cooking. Cooking and roasting decreased protein solubility but improved *in vitro* protein digestibility. Mixograph absorption of wheat and legume flour blends increased from 50–52% for raw legumes to 68–76, 62–64 and 74–80% for cooked, roasted and fermented legumes, respectively. Bread dough with cooked or roasted legume flours was less sticky than that with raw or fermented legume flour. Loaf volume of bread baked from wheat and raw or roasted legume flour blends with or without gluten addition was consistently higher for chickpeas, lower for peas and lentils, and lowest for soybeans. Roasted legume flour exhibited more appealing aroma and greater loaf volume of bread than cooked legume flour, and it appears to be the most appropriate preprocessing method for incorporation into bread.

Sadowska et al. (1999) prepared good quality breads with 2.5 to 10% non-fermented lentil flour (NFLF) and fermented lentil flour (FLF) supplementation (except for bread with 10% FLF addition which had medium quality). Fermentation of lentil flour improved water hydration capacity and fat binding capacity, irrespective of fermentation temperature (28–42°C) and flour concentration (79–221 g/L). In contrast, the emulsion capacity and stability of FLF were very low and flours fermented at 42°C did not even form an emulsion.

Dalgetty and Baik (2006) prepared bread from wheat flour and wheat flour fortified with either 3, 5 and 7% legume hulls or insoluble cotyledon fibers, or with 1, 3 and 5% soluble cotyledon fibers isolated from pea, lentil, and chickpea flours. Incorporation of hulls or insoluble fibers resulted in increases in dough water absorption by 2–16% and mixing time of dough by 22–147 s. Addition of soluble fiber resulted in decreases in water absorption as the substitution rate increased and similar mixing times to the control dough. Loaf weights of breads containing hulls or insoluble fibers were generally higher than that of control bread. However, the loaf volume of breads fortified with legume hulls and fibers was lower than that of the control bread. Breads containing soluble fibers were more attractive in terms of crumb uniformity and color than breads containing either hulls or insoluble fibers. Breads fortified with legume hulls and fibers were higher in moisture content than control bread regardless of the type, source, or fortification rate. Bread fortified with up to 7% hulls or insoluble cotyledon fibers or up to 3% soluble cotyledon fibers, with the exception of 7% insoluble pea fiber, exhibited similar firmness after seven days of storage compared with the control bread, despite their smaller loaf volume. Breads containing hull fibers exhibited the lowest starch transition enthalpies as determined by DSC after seven days of storage, while the starch transition enthalpies of breads containing added soluble or insoluble fibers were not significantly different from the control bread.

4.3 Broadbeans or Fababeans

Abdel-Aal et al. (1993) formulated composite flour blends containing wheat (W), fababean (F), cottonseed and sesame flours to provide the FAO/WHO/UNU protein requirements for 2- to 5-year old children, and evaluated them in pan and flat bread applications. Water absorption of composite flour doughs was up to 35% greater than the control but gluten strength and slurry viscosities were markedly reduced. Loaf volume and specific volume of pan breads prepared from composite flours were 25–60% lower than that of the control bread but flat breads tolerated the protein supplements very well. The W/F flat bread, containing 27% of fababean flour, received acceptable taste, texture and color scores and was only slightly inferior to the control in puffing and layer separation. Additions of cottonseed or sesame flours to the W/F blend failed to improve sensory properties of the flat breads.

Abdel-Kader (2000) studied the physical, rheological and baking properties of decorticated cracked broadbeans-wheat composite flours and the acceptability of the Egyptian "Balady" bread by sensory tests. Decorticated cracked broadbeans flour (DCBF) was used to replace 5%, 10%, 15% and 20% of the wheat flour (WF) in bread. Farinographic studies showed that water absorption, arrival time and dough development time increased as the amount of DCBF increased, while dough stability increased at 5% and 10% of DCBF substitution and decreased at 15% and 20% substitution. Also, the extensographic energy of the dough decreased as DCBF substitution increased, while the ratio between resistance and extensibility increased. There was a decrease in peak viscosity with increased amounts of DCBF. A reduction of the diameter and weight of the bread loaf was observed as the amount of DCBF increased. It was concluded that the replacement of wheat flour (WF) with up to 10% decorticated cracked broadbeans flour produced acceptable Egyptian "Balady" bread.

Abdel-Kader (2001) also studied the nutritional improvement of the Egyptian "Balady" breads made with decorticated cracked broadbeans flour (DCBF) replacing 5%, 10%, 15% and 20% of the wheat flour (WF). The nutrient composition of DCBF, WF, wheat bread and DCBF-fortified bread was studied. When DCBF fortification was increased from 0 to 20%, there was an increase of 36% in protein, 18% in fat, 123% in calcium, 52% in phosphorus and 40% in iron contents. DCBF contained greater amounts of lysine and histidine compared to WF. All essential amino acids increased when DCBF substituted WF from 0 to 20%, except methionine, which decreased. The biological quality of the breads was investigated. The protein efficiency ratio (PER) was 10%. DCBF bread (1.60) was found to be significantly greater ($P < 0.05$) than that of 5%-DCBF bread (1.48) and wheat bread (1.17).

However, Mur Gimeno et al. (2007) considering hidden foods or ingredients as those that are not specified in the labels or are referred to with an unknown name for the consumer, showed concern with broad bean flour. They mention that there are different kinds of presliced breads that include legumes (broad bean or *Vicia faba* flour) as an additive, in some cases not specified on the label. They demonstrated the existence of allergens from broad beans in a slice of bread that caused a type-I reaction in a legume-allergic patient and recommend an extensive labelling of commercial foods to avoid unexpected reactions in susceptible allergic patients.

4.4 Lupines

Zacarías et al. (1985), from Chile, determined the effect of incorporating 3, 6, 9 and 12% sweet lupine flour (SLF) to bread, on the organoleptic characteristics and acceptability of the product, evaluated by 25 trained judges using a 9-point hedonic scale. At the 9 and 12% SLF levels external color ($P < 0.05$) was significantly different. Regarding the internal characteristics, a significant difference for color was found at the 3% SLF; and at 6, 9 and 12% SLF, for appearance. The general acceptability was good at all the levels tested, with no significant differences among them. An acceptability study at the consumer level for 9% lupine flour bread was carried out in a group of 90 girls, aged 10–12 years, during a 10-day period. The results showed a very good acceptability of the product.

Pollard et al. (2002) support that the nutritional quality of various food products could be improved by supplementation with grain legumes to increase protein content and to improve the balance of essential amino acids. The lupin grain is a good candidate for this role, given its yield potential in a range of climatic environments and soil types. To establish the practicality of extending the use of lupins as food additives, the functional properties of various species and cultivars of lupin were studied for their effect as additives to baked products and their ability to provide foaming and emulsifying properties. Of the two lupin species that are commonly cultivated commercially, *Lupinus albus* showed the greater potential as a bread additive; loaf height and structure were maintained when wheat flour was substituted by lupin flour at levels up to 5%. This level of substitution offered the advantage of reducing mixing time. The detrimental effects at higher substitution levels appeared to be associated with the nonprotein components of the lupin flour. *L. albus* showed better functionality than *L. angustifolius* in emulsifying attributes, although *L. angustifolius* showed greater potential as a foaming agent. Defatting the lupin flour may be necessary to show these properties to best advantage.

Hall et al. (2005) mention that the addition of some legume ingredients to bread has been associated with effects on glycaemic, insulinaemic and satiety responses that may be beneficial in controlling type 2 diabetes, cardiovascular disease and obesity. However, the effect of Australian sweet lupin (*Lupinus angustifolius*) flour (ASLF) was unknown. Thus, their investigation examined the effect of adding ASLF to standard white bread on post-meal glycaemic, insulinaemic and satiety responses and palatability in healthy subjects. ASLF addition to the breakfast reduced its glycaemic index (mean ± SEM; ASLF bread breakfast = 74.0 ± 9.6. Standard white bread breakfast = 100, $P = 0.022$), raised its insulinaemic index (ASLF bread breakfast = 127.7 ± 12.0. Standard white bread breakfast = 100, $P = 0.046$), but did not affect palatability, satiety or food intake. ASLF addition resulted in a palatable breakfast; however, the potential benefits of the lowered glycaemic index may be eclipsed by the increased insulinaemic index.

Güémes-Vera et al. (2008) developed procedures for detoxifying *Lupinus mutabilis* seeds, decreasing or eliminating the yellow color in their derivatives. An evaluation was done of the effect of replacement of wheat flour with the detoxified and decolorized *L. mutabilis* derivatives on the quality properties of three types of bread products (loaf, bun and sweet). Physicochemical and nutritional analyses coincided with previous reports. The *Lupinus* protein concentrate and isolate had lower phenolic compound and oligosaccharide concentrations than the untreated seeds. Amino acid composition was determined for wheat flour (WF), *L. mutabilis* defatted and detoxified flour (LF), *L. mutabilis* protein concentrate (LPC) and *L. mutabilis* protein isolate (LPI). The resulting values were used to calculate the replacement levels at which lysine content would be increased significantly in WF–lupin blends. Replacement levels were: LF (5%, 10%, 15% and 20%); LPC (2.5%, 5%, 7.5% and 10%); LPI (0.5%, 1%, 2%, 3% and 4%). The detoxifying treatments employed decreased non-nutritional and toxic compounds present in original lupin seed. The use of citric acid (1%) reduced yellow coloration in lupin flour (LF) and lupin protein concentrate (LPC).

Guillamón et al. (2010) report that there has been increased interest in using lupine for human nutrition in recent years due to its nutritional properties and health benefits. Moreover, lupine is used as an ingredient in breadmaking because of its functional and technological properties. However, a higher number of allergic reactions to this legume have recently been reported as a consequence of a more widespread consumption of lupine-based foods. In a previous study, several thermal treatments were applied to lupine seeds and flours resulting in reduced allergenicity. In order to study how this thermal processing (autoclaving and boiling) affects the breadmaking properties, raw and thermally processed lupine flours were used to replace 10% of wheat flour. The effect of supplementing wheat flour with lupine flour on physical dough properties, bread structure and sensory characteristics were analyzed. The results indicated that thermally-treated lupine flours had similar breadmaking and sensorial properties as untreated lupine flour. These thermal treatments could increase the potential use of lupine flour as a food ingredient while reducing the risk to provoke allergic reactions.

Paraskevopoulou et al. (2010) studied the impact of the addition of two lupin protein isolates (LPI), enriched either in proteins belonging to globulin (LPI G) or to albumin (LPI A) fractions, on wheat flour dough and bread characteristics. LPI addition increased dough development time and stability, resistance to deformation and extensibility of the dough. The presence of LPI proteins in dough affected bread quality in terms of volume, internal structure and texture, while extra gluten addition to the blends to compensate for wheat gluten dilution, resulting from LPI addition, led to an improvement of bread quality characteristics. Generally, the incorporation of LP isolates to wheat flour delayed bread firming. The authors suggest a possible action of LPI particles as a filler of the gluten network and possible interactions between the gluten protein constituents and those of lupin.

5. Conclusions and future trends

There are many alternative raw materials from a great number of different sources (fruits, roots, tubers and legumes) that can be applied in bread making with different health benefits. Increases in fiber, protein, vitamin, mineral and antioxidant contents and reduction in glycaemic index are some of the benefits mentioned in the studies reviewed. Future trends include formulation and process optimization to overcome some of the drawbacks observed, such as reductions in volume and sensory acceptance in some cases; physical or bio-processing of the alternative raw materials (especially residues) for the same objective and further treatment (such as germination or fermentation) to produce other physiologically functional compounds, such as bioactive peptides, that may also be applied in bread. It would also be interesting to have more information on the effect of the different stages of the bread making process (mixing, proofing and baking) on the nutritionally important compounds added.

Keywords: bread, by-products, fruit, roots and tubers, legumes

References

ABBA (Associação Brasileira da Batata). 2005. Batata. Available at: <http://www.abbabatatabrasileira. com.br>. Access in: May 2014.

Abdel-Aal, E.-S.M., F.W. Sosulski, I.M.M. Youssef, A. Adel and Y. Shehata. 1993. Selected nutritional, physical and sensory characteristics of pan and fiat breads prepared from composite flours containing fababean. Plant Foods for Human Nutrition, 44: 227–239.

Abdel-Kader, Z.M. 2000. Enrichment of Egyptian 'Balady' bread. Part 1. Baking studies, physical and sensory evaluation of enrichment with decorticated cracked broadbeans flour (*Vicia faba* L.). Die Nahrung, 44: 418–421.

Abdel-Kader, Z.M. 2001. Enrichment of Egyptian 'Balady' bread. Part 2. Nutritional values and biological evaluation of enrichment with decorticated cracked broadbeans flour (*Vicia faba* L.). Die Nahrung, 45: 31–34.

Adeniji, T.A., L.O. Sanni, I.S. Barimalaa and A.D. Hart. 2006. Determination of micronutrients and colour variability among new plantain and banana hybrids flour. World Journal of Chemistry, 1: 23–27.

Ali, B.H., G. Blunden, M.O. Tanira and A. Nemmar. 2008. Some phytochemical, pharmacological and toxicological properties of ginger (*Zingiber officinale* Roscoe): a review of recent research. Food and Chemical Toxicology, 46: 409–420.

Al-Mekhlafi, M.S.H., J. Surin, A.A. Sallam, A.W. Abdullah and M.A.K. Mahdy. 2010. Giardiasis and poor vitamin a status among aboriginal school children in rural Malaysia. American Journal Tropical Medicine and Hygiene, 83: 523–527.

Alves, R.M.V., D. Ito, J.L.V. Carvalho, W.F. Melo and R.L.O. Godoy. 2012. Stability of biofortified sweet potato flour. Brazilian Journal of Food Technology, 15: 59–71.

Amaro, F.S., L.F. Souza, I.B.I. Barros, E.M.P. Facco, B. Monego, J. Parisotto and S.R. Silva. 2013. Experiência da construção do Grupo de Agroecologia KAIWOÀ na Universidade Federal de Santa Maria. Cadernos de Agroecologia 8(2). *In*: Resumos do VIII Congresso Brasileiro de Agroecologia, Porto Alegre/Rio Grande do Sul.

Ames, B.M., M.K. Shigena and T.M. Hagen. 1993. Oxidants, antioxidant and the degenerative diseases of aging. Proceedings of the National Academy of Sciences, 90: 7915–7922.

Araújo, F.C. 1982. Aspectos sobre o cultivo do inhame-da-costa. Recife: EMATER-PE, 4 p.

Aremu, C.Y. and E.I. Udoessien. 1990. Chemical estimation of some inorganic elements in selected tropical fruits and vegetables. Food Chemistry, 37: 229–240.

Asp, N.G., J.M.M. Van Amelsvoort and J.G.A.J. Hautvast. 1996. Nutritional implications of resistant starch. Nutrition Research, 9: 1–31.

Balestra, F., E. Cocci, G. Pinnavaia and S. Romani. 2011. Evaluation of antioxidant, rheological and sensorial properties of wheat flour dough and bread containing ginger powder. LWT—Food Science and Technology, 44: 700–705.

Ballesteros, M.N., G.M. Yépiz, M.I. Grijalva, E. Ramos and M.E. Valencia. 1984. Elaboration, by linear programming, of new products from cereals and legumes. Archivos Latinoamericanos de Nutrición, 34: 130–145.

Batista, K.A., S.H. Prudêncio and K.F. Fernandes. 2011. Wheat bread enrichment with hard-to-cook bean extruded flours: nutritional and acceptance evaluation. Journal of Food Science, 76: S108–S113.

Batista, V., C.S.S. Ramos, W.F. Silva, M.R.V. Cardoso and F.G. Carlos. 2008. Farinha de inhame: uma alternativa para celíacos. *In*: I Jornada Científica e VI FIPA do CEFET Bambuí/ Minas Gerais.

Braddock, R.J. 1995. By-products of citrus fruit. Food Technology, 49: 74–77.

Baik, B.-K. and I.H. Han. 2012. Cooking, roasting, and fermentation of chickpeas, lentils, peas, and soybeans for fortification of leavened bread. Cereal Chemistry, 89: 269–275.

Cereda, M.P. 1996. Caracterização, usos e tratamentos de resíduos da industrialização da mandioca. Botucatu: Centro de Raízes Tropicais.

Chavan, J.K. and S.S. Kadam. 1993. Nutritional enrichment of bakery products by supplementation with nonwheat flours. Critical Reviews in Food Science and Nutrition, 33: 189–226.

Ciacco, C.T. and B.L. D'Appolonia. 1978. Baking studies with cassava and yam flour. II. Rheological and baking studies of tuber wheat flour blends. Cereal Chemistry, 55: 423–435.

Clark, C.A. and J.W. Moyer. 1988. Compendium of sweet potato diseases. Saint Paul: APS, 74 p.

Coelho, L.M. and G. Wosiacki. 2010. Avaliação sensorial de produtos panificados com adição de farinha de bagaço de maçã. Ciência e Tecnologia de Alimentos, 30: 582–588.

Dalgetty, D.D. and B.-K. Baik. 2006. Fortification of bread with hulls and cotyledon fibers isolated from peas, lentils, and chickpeas. Cereal Chemistry, 83: 269–274.

Dall'Asta, C., M. Cirlini, E. Morini, M. Rinaldi, T. Ganino and E. Chiavaro. 2013. Effect of chestnut flour supplementation on physico-chemical properties and volatiles in bread making. LWT—Food Science and Technology, 53: 233–239.

Dansby, M.Y. and A.C. Bovell-Benjamin. 2003. Production and proximate composition of a hydroponic sweet potato flour during extended storage. Journal of Food Processing and Preservation, 27: 153–64.

De Vasconcelos, M., R. Bennett, E. Rosa and J. Ferreira-Cardoso. 2010. Composition of European chestnut (*Castanea sativa* Mill.) and association with health effects: fresh and processed products. Journal of the Science of Food and Agriculture, 90: 1578–1589.

Demirkesen, I., B. Mert, G. Sumnu and S. Sahin. 2010. Utilization of chestnut flour in gluten-free bread formulations. Journal of Food Engineering, 101: 329–336.

Duodu, K.G. and A. Minnaar. 2011. Legume composite flours and baked goods: nutritional, functional, sensory, and phytochemical qualities. pp. 193–203. *In*: V. Preedy, R. Watson and V. Patel (eds.). Flour and Breads and their Fortification in Health and Disease Prevention. Academic Press.

Faber, M. and P.J. van Jaarsveld. 2007. Review: The production of provitamin A—rich vegetables in home-gardens as a means of addressing vitamin A deficiency in rural African communities. Journal of the Science of Food and Agriculture, 87: 366–377.

Freitas, R.E., S.C. Stertz and N. Waszczynskyj. 1997. Viabilidade da produção de pão, utilizando farinha mista de trigo e mandioca em diferentes proporções. Boletim do Centro de Pesquisa de Processamento de Alimentos, 15: 197–208.

FAO (Food and Agriculture Organization of the United Nations—Statistics Division). 2014. Available at: <http://www.faostat.fao.org/>. Access in: May 2014.

Fenn, D., O.M. Lukow, G. Humphreys, P.G. Fields and J.I. Boye. 2010. Wheat-legume composite flour quality. International Journal of Food Properties, 13: 381–393.

Fernandes, A.F. 2006. Utilização da farinha de casca de batata inglesa (*Solanum tuberosum* L.) na elaboração de pão integral. Dissertação de mestrado, Universidade Federal de Lavras, Lavras, Minas Gerais.

Fernandes, A.F., J. Pereira, R. Germani and J. Oiano-Neto. 2008. Efeito da substituição parcial da farinha de trigo por farinha de casca de batata (*Solanum tuberosum* Lineu). Food Science and Technology, 28: 56–65.

Figuerola, F.E., A.M. Estévez and E. Castillo. 1987. Supplementation of wheat flour with chickpea (*Cicer arietinum*) flour. I. Preparation of flours and their properties for bread making. Archivos Latinoamericanos de Nutrición, 37: 378–387.

Fonseca, E.W.N. 2006. Utilização da mucilagem de inhame (*Dioscorea* spp.) como melhorador na produção de pão de forma. Dissertação de Mestrado, Universidade Federal de Lavras, Lavras, Minas Gerais.

Fukelmann, M. 2004. É batata. Available at: <http://www.folhaonline.com.br./pensata>. Access in: May 2014.

Garmus, T.T., J.R.M.V. Bezerra, M. Rigo and K.R.V. Córdova. 2009. Elaboração de biscoitos com adição de farinha de casca de batata (*Solanum tuberosum* L.). Revista Brasileira de Tecnologia Agroindustrial, 3: 56–65.

Gattas, V.E., D. Ballester and E. Yanez. 1983. Sensory evaluation of bread with potato flour. Archivos Latinoamericanos de Nutrición, 33: 56–66.

Greene, J.L. and A.C. Bovell-Benjamin. 2004. Macroscopic and sensory evaluation of bread supplemented with sweet-potato flour. Journal of Food Science: Sensory and Nutritive Qualities of Food, 69: 167–173.

Güémes-Vera, N., R.J. Peña-Bautista, C. Jiménez-Martínez, G. Dávila-Ortiz and G. Calderón-Domínguez. 2008. Effective detoxification and decoloration of *Lupinus mutabilis* seed derivatives, and effect of these derivatives on bread quality and acceptance. Journal of the Science of Food and Agriculture, 88: 1135–1143.

Guillamón, E., C. Cuadrado, M.M. Pedrosa, A. Varela, B. Cabellos, M. Muzquiz and C. Burbano. 2010. Breadmaking properties of wheat flour supplemented with thermally processed hypoallergenic lupine flour. Spanish Journal of Agricultural Research, 8: 100–108.

Hagiwara, A., H. Yoshino, T. Ichihara, M. Kawabe, S. Tamano, H. Aoki, T. Koda, M. Nakamura, K. Imaida, N. Ito and T. Shirai. 2002. Prevention by natural food anthocyanins, purple sweet potato color and red cabbage color, of 2-amino-1-methyl-6-phenylimidazo[4,5-b]-pyridine (PhIP)-associated colorectal carcinogenesis in rats initiated with 1,2-dimethylhydrazine. The Journal of Toxicological Sciences, 27: 57–68.

Hall, R.S., S.J. Thomas and S.K. Johnson. 2005. Australian sweet lupin flour addition reduces the glycaemic index of a white bread breakfast without affecting palatability in healthy human volunteers. Asia Pacific Journal of Clinical Nutrition, 14: 91–97.

Hefnawy, T.M.H., G.A. El-Shourbagy and M.F. Ramadan. 2012. Impact of adding chickpea (*Cicer arietinum* L.) flour to wheat flour on the rheological properties of toast bread. International Food Research Journal, 19: 521–525.

Ho, L.H., N.A.A. Aziz and B. Azahari. 2013. Physico-chemical characteristics and sensory evaluation of wheat bread partially substituted with banana (*Musa acuminata* x *balbisiana* cv. Awak) pseudo-stem flour. Food Chemistry, 139: 532–539.

Hsu, C., S. Hurang, W. Chen, Y. Weng and C. Tseng. 2004. Qualities and antioxidant properties of bread as affected by the incorporation of yam flour in the formulation. International Journal of Food Science and Technology, 39: 231–238.

Juarez-Garcia, E., E. Agama-Acevedo, S.G. Sáyago-Ayerdi, S.L. Rodríguez-Ambriz and L.A. Bello-Pérez. 2006. Composition, Digestibility and Application in Breadmaking of Banana Flour. Plant Foods for Human Nutrition, 61: 131–137.

Kusano, S., H. Abe and H. Tamura. 2001. Isolation of antidiabetic components from white-skinned sweet potato (*Ipomoea batatas* L.). Bioscience, Biotechnology and Biochemistry, 65: 109–114.

Low, J.W. and P.J. van Jaarsveld. 2008. The potential contribution of bread buns fortified with β-carotene–rich sweet potato in Central Mozambique. Food and Nutrition Bulletin, 29: 98–107.

Masoodi, F.A. and G.S. Chauhan. 1998. Use of apple pomace as a source of dietary fiber in wheat bread. Journal of Food Processing and Preservation, 22: 255–263.

Miamoto, J.B.M. 2008. Obtenção e caracterização de biscoito tipo cookie elaborado com farinha de inhame (*Colocasia esculenta* L.) Dissertação de mestrado, Universidade Federal de Lavras, Lavras, Minas Gerais.

Miñarro, B., E. Albanell, N. Aguilar, B. Guamis and M. Capellas. 2012. Effect of legume flours on baking characteristics of gluten-free bread. Journal of Cereal Science, 56: 476–481.

Mohammeda, I., A.R. Ahmeda and B. Sengea. 2012. Dough rheology and bread quality of wheat-chickpea flour blends. Industrial Crops and Products, 36: 196–202.

Monteiro, D.A. 2002. Situação atual e perspectiva da cultura do taro no estado de São Paulo. pp. 77–84. *In*: C.A.S. do Carmo (ed.). Inhame e taro: sistemas de produção familiar. Vitória, Incaper.

Mur Gimeno, P., F. Feo Brito, A. Martín Iglesias, M. Lombardero Vega and P. Bautista Martínez. 2007. Allergic reaction caused by a new hidden food, broad bean flour. Allergy, 62: 1340–1341.

Nascimento, E.M.G.C., J.L.R. Ascheri, C.W.P. Carvalho and M.C. Galdeano. 2013. Benefits and risks of using passion fruit peel (*Passiflora edulis*) as an ingredient in food production. Revista do Instituto Adolfo Lutz, 72: 1–11.

Noor Aziah, A.A., L.H. Ho, A.A. Noor Shazliana and R. Bhat. 2012. Quality evaluation of steamed wheat bread substituted with unripe banana flour. International Food Research Journal, 19: 869–876.

O'Shea, N., E.K. Arendt and E. Gallagher. 2012. Dietary fibre and phytochemical characteristics of fruit and vegetable byproducts and their recent applications as novel ingredients in food products. Innovative Food Science and Emerging Technologies, 16: 1–10.

Ocen, D. and X. Xu. 2013. Effect of citrus orange (*Citrus sinensis*) by-product dietary fiber preparations on the quality characteristics of frozen dough bread. American Journal of Food Technology, 8: 43–53.

Orr, P.H., R.B. Toma, S.T. Munson and B. D'appolonia. 1982. Sensory evaluation of breads containing various levels of potato peel. American Potato Journal, 59: 605–611.

Paraskevopoulou, A., E. Provatidou, D. Tsotsiou and V. Kiosseoglou. 2010. Dough rheology and baking performance of wheat flour-lupin protein isolate blends. Food Research International, 43: 1009–1016.

Perez, E., F.S. Schultzb and E. Pacheco de Delahaye. 2005. Characterization of some properties of starches isolated from Xanthosoma *Saggitifolium* (tannia) and *Colocasia esculenta* (taro). Carbohydrate Polymers, 60: 139–145.

Pollard, N.J., F.L. Stoddard, Y. Popineau, C.W. Wrigley and F. MacRitchie. 2002. Lupin flours as additives: dough mixing, breadmaking, emulsifying, and foaming. Cereal Chemistry, 79: 662–669.

Reis, S.F., D.K. Rai and N. Abu-Ghannam. 2014. Apple pomace as a potential ingredient for the development of new functional foods. International Journal of Food Science and Technology, doi:10.1111/ijfs.12477.

Rezzadori, K., S. Benedettia and E.R. Amante. 2012. Proposals for the residues recovery: orange waste as raw material for new products. Food and Bioproducts Processing, 90: 606–614.

Rivas, B., A. Torrado, P. Torre, A. Converti and J.M. Domínguez. 2008. Submerged citric acid fermentation on orange peel autohydrolysate. Journal Agriculture Food Chemistry, 56: 2380–2387.

Rodriguez-Amaya, D.B. 2001. A guide to carotenoid analysis in foods. Washington: ILSI—International Life Sciences Institute, 64 p.

Rodriguez-Amaya, D. and M. Kimura. 2004. HarvestPlus Handbook for Carotenoid Analysis. HarvestPlus Technical Monograph 2. Washington, DC and Cali: International Food Policy Research Institute (IFPRI) and International Center for Tropical Agriculture (CIAT). Copyright HarvestPlus.

Rodriguez-Amaya, D.B., M. Kimura, H.T. Godoy and J. Amaya-Farfan. 2008. Updated Brazilian database on food carotenoids: factors affecting carotenoid composition. Journal of Food Composition and Analysis, 21: 445–463.

Rodriguez-Amaya, D.B., M.R. Nutti and J.L.V. Carvalho. 2011. Carotenoids of sweet potato, cassava, and maize and their use in bread and flour fortification. pp. 301–311. *In*: R.R. Preedy, R.R. Watson and V.B. Patel. (eds.). Flour and Breads and their Fortification in Health and Disease Prevention. Burlington, London. Academic Press, San Diego.

Roesler, P.V.S.O., S.D. Gomes, A.C.B. Kummer and M.P. Cereda. 2008. Produção e qualidade de raiz tuberosa de cultivares de batata doce no oeste do Paraná. Acta Scientiarum Agronnomy, 30: 117–122.

Rosell, C.M., E. Santos, J.M. Sanz-Penella and M. Haros. 2009. Wholemeal wheat bread: a comparison of different breadmaking processes and fungal phytase addition. Journal of Cereal Science, 50: 272–277.

Roussos, P.A. 2011. Phytochemicals and antioxidant capacity of orange (*Citrus sinensis* (l.) Osbeck cv. Salustiana) juice produced under organic and integrated farming system in Greece. Scientia Horticulturae, 129: 253–258.

Rumbaoa, R.G.O., D.F. Cornago and I.M. Geronimo. 2009. Phenolic content and antioxidant capacity of Philippine sweet potato (*Ipomoea batatas*) varieties. Food Chemistry, 113: 1133–1138.

Sadowska, J., J. Fornal, C. Vidal-Valverde and J. Frias. 1999. Natural fermentation of lentils. Functional properties and potential in breadmaking of fermented lentil flour. Nahrung-Food, 43: 396–401.

Scazzina, F., S. Siebenhandl-Ehn and N. Pellegrini. 2013. The effect of dietary fibre on reducing the glycaemic index of bread. British Journal of Nutrition, 109: 1163–1174.

Shittu, T.A., R.I. Egwunyenga, L.O. Sanni and L. Abayomi. 2013. Bread from composite plantain-wheat flour: I. Effect of plantain fruit maturity and flour mixture on dough rheology and fresh loaf qualities. Journal of Food Processing and Preservation. doi:10.1111/jfpp.12153.

Silva, J.B.C., C.A. Lopes and J.S. Magalhães. 2006. Cultura da batata-doce. Available at: <http://www.cnph.embrapa.br/>. Access in: May 2014.

Silva, R.M., G. Bandel and P.S. Martins. 2003. Mating system in an experimental garden composed of cassava (*Manihot esculenta* Crantz) ethnovarieties. Euphytica, 134: 127–135.

Souza, L.S. and J.F. Fialho. 2003. Cultivo da Mandioca para a Região do Cerrado. Embrapa Mandioca e Fruticultura, sistemas de produção. Available at: <http://sistemasdeproducao.cnptia.embrapa.br/>. Access in: May 2014.

Storey, M. 2007. The harvested crop. pp. 441–470. *In*: D. Vreugdenhil. (ed.). Potato biology and biotechnology advances and perspectives. Elsevier, Oxford.

Teow, C.C., V. Truong, R.F. McFeeters, R.L. Thompson, K.V. Pecota and G.C. Yencho. 2007. Antioxidant activities, phenolic and ß-carotene contents of sweet potato genotypes with varying flesh colours. Food Chemistry, 103: 829–838.

Tribess, T.B., J.P. Hernandez, M.G.C. Montealvo, E.W. Menezes, L.A. Bello-Perez and C.C. Tadini. 2009. Thermal properties and resistance starch content of unripe banana flour (*Musa cavendishii*) produced at different drying conditions. LWT—Food Science and Technology, 42: 1022–1025.

Utrilla-Coello, R.G., P. Osorio-Díaz and L.A. Bello-Pérez. 2007. Alternative use of chickpea flour in breadmaking: chemical composition and starch digestibility of bread. Food Science and Technology International, 13: 323–327.

van Hal, M.V. 2000. Quality of sweet potato flour during processing and storage. Food Reviews International, 16: 1–37.

van Jaarsveld, P.J., D.W. Marais, E. Harmse, P. Nestel and D.B. Rodriguez-Amaya. 2006. Retention of β-carotene in boiled, mashed orange-fleshed sweet potato. Journal of Food Composition and Analysis, 19: 321–329.

Vasala, P.A. 2001. Ginger. pp. 195–206. *In*: K.V. Peter. (ed.). Handbook of herbs and spice. DC: Peter CRC Press, Boca Raton Boston, New York, Washington.

Vásquez Carrillo, M.G., M.L. Ortega Delgado and E. Estrada Lugo. 1991. Flour of hard bean (*Phaseolus vulgaris*) in the preparation of bread. Archivos Latinoamericanos de Nutrición, 41: 620–630.

Vilhalva, D.A.A., M.S.S. Júnior, C.M.A. Moura, M. Caliari, T.A.C. Souza and F.A. Silva. 2011. Utilization of cassava peel flour for preparing loaf bread. Revista Instituto Adolfo Lutz, 70: 514–521.

Viswanathan, K. and P. Ho. 2014. Fortification of white flat bread with sprouted red kidney bean (*Phaseolus vulgaris*). Acta Scientiarum Polonorum Technologia Alimentaria, 13: 27–34.

Wang, H.J. and R.L. Thomas. 1989. Direct Use of Apple Pomace in Bakery Products. Journal of Food Science, 54: 618–620, 639.

Wohlmuth, H., D.N. Leach, M.K. Smith and S.P. Myers. 2005. Gingerol content of diploid and tetraploid clones of ginger (*Zingiber officinale* Roscoe). Journal of Agricultural and Food Chemistry, 53: 5772–5778.

Woolfe, J.A. 1992. Sweet potato: an untapped food resource. Cambridge: Cambridge University, 188 p.

Wulf, H., C. Cafati and E. Yanez. 1989. Bread fortification with bean (*Phaseolus vulgaris* L.) flour. I. Farinological and panification aspects. Archivos Latinoamericanos de Nutrición, 39: 613–619.

Yanez, E., H. Wulf, C. Cafati, G. Acevedo and V. Reveco. 1989. Bread fortification with bean (*Phaseolus vulgaris* L.) flour. II. Nutritive value of bread fortified with bean flour. Archivos Latinoamericanos de Nutrición, 39: 620–630.

Yeoh, H.H. and F. Sun. 2001. Assessing cyanogen content in cassava-based food using the enzyme-dipstick method. Food and Chemical Toxicology, 39: 649–653.

Yoshimoto, M., S. Okuno, M. Yoshinaga, O. Yamakawa, M. Yamaguchi and J. Yamada. 1999. Antimutagenicity of sweetpotato (*Ipomoea batatas*) roots. Bioscience, Biotechnology and Biochemistry, 63: 537–541.

Zacarías, I., E. Yáñez, E. Araya and D. Ballester. 1985. Sensory evaluation and acceptability study, at the consumer level, of bread supplemented with sweet lupine flour. Archivos Latinoamericanos de Nutrición, 35: 119–129.

Zafar, T.A., F. Al-Hassawi, F. Al-Khulaifi, G. Al-Rayyes, C. Waslien and F.G. Huffman. 2013. Organoleptic and glycemic properties of chickpea-wheat composite breads. Journal of Food Science and Technology. Published online: 20 Oct. 2013.

Zarate, N.A.H., M.C. Vieira and A. Minuzzi. 2002. Produtividade de cinco clones de inhame, custos e uso na panificação caseira. Ciência e Agrotecnologia, 26: 1236–1242.

Zhang, R.L., J.N. Whistler, B.R. BeMiller and B.R. Hanaker. 2005. Banana starch: production, physicochemical properties and digestibility—a review. Carbohydrate Polymers, 59: 443–458.

14

Effect of Fibre in Enriched Breads

*Manuel Gómez** and *Bonastre Oliete*

1. Introduction

Dietary fibre encompasses a heterogeneous group of compounds that are not digested in the small bowel. Despite difficulties in the definition and classification, fibres have been promoted for their nutritional properties. Research is on-going into the effect of dietary fibre on cardiovascular health and its use in the control of diabetes, obesity, constipation, other gastrointestinal disorders and certain types of cancer, although results are sometimes controversial. Despite their positive effects on health, in general, fibre intake in Western countries does not reach the minimum recommended levels. The addition of fibre to bakery products would therefore favour compliance with recommendations on the type and amount of fibre intake, and would produce nutritional benefits for consumers. However, the addition of fibre can modify the behaviour of ingredients in the formula, the process and the quality of each product. Not only do these modifications depend on the characteristics of the fibre—type, percentage used, size and shape of the fibres, previous treatments applied, interaction between fibres and presence of other components added with the fibre (when using by-products from the food industry, for example)—but they also vary with process conditions during kneading, handling and fermentation, and these conditions should be adjusted to minimise changes in rheology and texture.

Finally, it is important to consider the type of product being prepared. Bread, cookies and cakes use different formulations and processes of elaboration. These will modify the behaviour of fibres in the product in different ways, and the final quality of each product will depend on distinct properties. It is important to realise that it may not be possible to obtain the desired characteristics with a single type of fibre,

Food Technology. E.T.S. Ingenierías Agrarias. Valladolid University. Campus La Yutera. Avda. de Madrid, 44. 34004 Palencia.
  Email: pallares@iaf.uva.es
* Corresponding author

and mixtures of fibres may be required. All these factors must be taken into account in order to improve the final quality of fibre-enriched products. Apart from these practical aspects, the production of fibre-enriched bakery products must also comply with legislation on health and nutrition claims and the price must be appropriate. Only meticulous consideration of all these conditions will enable us to achieve high-quality, fibre-enriched bakery products.

2. Types of fibre

The definition of dietary fibre is still controversial. A common feature of most definitions is non-digestibility in the small bowel. In general, we could say that there are two distinct schools of thought on the definition and method of analysis of dietary fibre: those who define dietary fibre as only non-starch polysaccharides, and those who prefer a wider definition of fibre as measured by the method of the Association of Official Analytical Chemists (AOAC). Taking into account the broader point of view, Thebaudin et al. (1997) stated that dietary fibres are oligosaccharides, polysaccharides and the (hydrophilic) derivates that cannot be digested by human digestive enzymes to absorbable components in the upper alimentary tract. The European Food Safety Authority (EFSA) Panel recommends that dietary fibre should include all non-digestible carbohydrates because of the key importance of digestibility in the small bowel for the nutritional effects of carbohydrates in humans. On this basis, dietary fibre comprises the following substances (Gray 2006):

- Non-starch polysaccharides (NSP), including cellulose, hemicelluloses, pectins and hydrocolloids (β-glucans, gums, mucilages)
  - Cellulose is a polysaccharide comprising up to 10,000 closely packed glucose units, arranged linearly, making it highly insoluble and resistant to digestion by human enzymes. It is the main component of the cell walls of most plants and it accounts for about 25% of the fibre in grains and fruit and about a third in vegetable and nuts.
  - Hemicelluloses are polysaccharides formed of sugars other than glucose. These substances are associated with cellulose in cell walls and include both water-soluble and water-insoluble forms. Hemicelluloses account for about a third of the fibre in vegetables, fruits, legumes and nuts. The main dietary sources are cereal grains.
  - Pectins are polysaccharides composed of galacturonic acid and a variety of sugars. They are soluble in hot water and form a gel on cooling. They are found in the cell walls and intracellular tissue of fruits and vegetables and represent 15% to 20% of the fibre in vegetables, legumes and nuts.
  - β-glucans are glucose polymers that, unlike cellulose, have a branched structure enabling them to form viscous solutions. They are the major components of the cell wall in oats and barley.
  - Gums and mucilages: Gums are hydrocolloids derived from plant exudates. Mucilages are present in the cells of the outer layers of seeds of the plantain family, for example, psyllium.

- Resistant oligosaccharides or non-digestible oligosaccharides (NDOs) formed of three to ten sugar units occur naturally in plants consumed as foods, mainly vegetables, cereals and nuts. They can also be obtained chemically or enzymatically from mono- and disaccharides and by enzymatic hydrolysis of polysaccharides. Examples include fructo-oligosaccharides (FOS) and galacto-oligosaccharides (GOS).
- Resistant starch refers to starch and starch degradation products that are not absorbed in the small intestine. Four classes have been identified: physically inaccessible starch (RS1), native starch granules (RS2), retrograded starch (RS3), and chemically modified starch (RS4).
- Other synthetic carbohydrate compounds derived from cellulose (such as methyl cellulose and hydroxypropylmethyl cellulose). Unlike cellulose, they are soluble but they are hardly fermented by the microflora.
- Lignin is not a polysaccharide but it is chemically bound to hemicelluloses in plant cell walls.
- Other minor components associated with fibre, such as phytic acid (inositol hexaphosphate), tannins, cutins and phytosterols.

EFSA also mentioned the analytical methods, noting that several methods needed to be applied in tandem in order to capture all of the above fractions because none of the methods currently available are optimal for measuring the range of components now generally accepted as dietary fibre.

Traditionally, dietary fibre components have been classified according to their solubility into insoluble fibre (celluloses, lignins, some hemicelluloses) and soluble fibre (pectins, gums, mucilages). This difference determines their physicochemical properties and their nutritional effects. Soluble fibres form a gel-like network (alginates, carrageenan, pectins) or a viscous network (xanthan gum, some hemicelluloses) under certain physicochemical conditions, and in this way they bind water. Fibre from cereals is generally insoluble in water, whereas vegetables, fruit and nuts contain higher proportions of soluble fibre. Furthermore, most soluble fibres are fermented in the colon by bacteria. Insoluble fibre is only fermented to a limited extent in the colon. Although this classification is widely accepted, it may be misleading because some insoluble fibres are in fact fermented in the large bowel and solubility in water does not always predict physiological effects (Dikeman and Fahey 2006). Furthermore, some soluble fibres, such as the majority of FOS, hardly bind water.

3. Intake

Current recommendations for dietary fibre intake are related to energy intake, and thus depend on age and gender. The general recommendation for adequate intake (AI) is 14 g/1000 kcal (USDA 2005), half derived from cereal bran and the other half from fruits and vegetables (Nayak et al. 2000). AI is the recommended average daily intake based on observed or experimentally determined approximations or estimates of fibre intake by a group of apparently healthy people assumed to have an adequate intake. AI is used when the Recommended Dietary Allowance (RDA) cannot be determined. Using the energy guideline of 2000 kcal/d for women and 2600 kcal/d for men, the recommended daily dietary fibre intake is 28 g/d for adult women and 36 g/d for adult men. The same recommendation is applied in children over one year of age (Food and Nutrition Board 2002). Thus the recommended AI for children and adolescents is as follows: 1–3 years, 19 g/d; 4–8 years, 25 g/d; 9–13-year-old boys, 31 g/d; 9–13-year-old girls, 26 g/d; 14–18-year-old boys, 38 g/d; and 14–18-year-old girls, 26 g/d. However, in general, individual dietary fibre intake does not appear to reach even half the AI (Wu et al. 2003) and, furthermore, it has been decreasing over the past decade (Stevens et al. 2002).

Recommendations for increasing dietary fibre intake emphasise greater consumption of fibre-rich fruits, vegetables, legumes, cereals and whole-grain products. In addition, fibre supplements may be prescribed as an adjunct to the dietary treatment of certain illnesses. Because dietary fibre increases water retention in the colon, resulting in bulkier, softer stools, recommendations for water intake should be increased in parallel with increases in dietary fibre (Anderson et al. 2009).

Observations from the Women's Health Initiative (Howard et al. 2006) indicate that consumers are not as effective in modifying dietary habits as they try to be. Initiatives should not therefore focus exclusively on foods but they should also promote education both for consumers and for health professionals (Anderson et al. 2009).

With regard to this situation, the European Commission has regulated nutrition claims and the conditions applying to them concerning fibre (Regulation EC No. 1924/2006). The claim "source of fibre" is authorised when fibre levels exceed 3 g/100 g or 1.5 g/100 kcal. The claim "high fibre" is permitted if fibre levels exceed 6 g/100 g or 3 g/100 kcal. Furthermore, the claim "increased fibre" can be indicated if fibre levels are 30% higher than a similar food for which no claim is made. The Council Directive of 24 September 1990 (90/496/EEC), recently modified by Regulation (EC) No. 1137/2008, details the regulation concerning nutrition labelling for foodstuffs.

The Food and Drug Administration (FDA) has approved two health claims for dietary fibre. The first claim states that, along with a decreased consumption of fats (< 30% of calories), an increased consumption of dietary fibre from fruits, vegetables and whole grains may reduce some types of cancer (FDA 2008a). Increased consumption is defined as six or more one-ounce equivalents, with three ounces derived from whole grains. A one-ounce equivalent would be consistent with one slice of bread, ½ cup of oatmeal or rice, or five to seven crackers.

The second FDA claim supporting the health benefits of dietary fibre states that diets low in saturated fat (< 10% of calories) and cholesterol and high in fruits, vegetables and whole grains, have a decreased risk of leading to coronary heart disease (FDA 2008b). For most people, an increased consumption of dietary fibre is considered to be approximately 25 to 35 g/d, of which 6 g are soluble fibre.

4. Dietary fibre and health

4.1 Dietary fibre and cardiovascular health

Dietary fibre has been shown to enhance cardiac and circulatory health. Studies have been performed on the effect of fibre on certain illnesses, such as coronary heart disease (CHD), and on the major risks of those illnesses.

Streppel et al. (2008) indicated that for every 10 g of additional fibre added to the diet, the risk of mortality from CHD decreased by 17% to 35%. Looking at the type of fibre, whole-grain fibre may afford greatest protection (Anderson et al. 2009). Psyllium and oat β-glucan are the most widely used sources of soluble fibre and have been approved for health claims related to protection from CHD (FDA 1998).

Whole-grain fibre intake is also associated with a significant reduction in the prevalence of ischaemic stroke (Mozaffarian et al. 2003). Other types of fibre, such as fibre from fruit and vegetable, are also associated with a decrease in the risk of this disease (Johnsen et al. 2003) and have favourable effects on the progression of carotid artery atherosclerosis (Wu et al. 2003) and peripheral vascular disease (Merchant et al. 2003).

High levels of cholesterol and low-density lipoproteins (LDL) are major risk factors for coronary artery diseases. Several mechanisms have been proposed to explain the effect of dietary fibre on the blood lipid profile. The cholesterol-lowering effect of fibre is mediated partly by a decreased absorption of intestinal bile acid, leading to increased faecal bile acid loss and *de novo* synthesis in the liver (Anderson et al. 1984). It has been also suggested that dietary fibre increases the activity of the enzyme cholesterol-7-α-hydroxylase, the main rate-limiting enzyme in the hepatic conversion of cholesterol to bile acids (Roy et al. 2002), contributing to a greater depletion of hepatic cholesterol. Secondarily, this depletion has a stimulatory effect on endogenous cholesterol synthesis (Fernández 2001). In addition, Jones et al. (1993) described a reduction in hepatic lipogenesis stimulated by insulin.

It is thought that soluble fibre modifies the volume and viscosity of the intestinal contents, which will ultimately alter hepatic cholesterol and lipoprotein metabolism, also resulting in a lowering of plasma LDL-cholesterol concentration (Trautwein et al. 1999). Furthermore, it has been suggested that the fermentation of dietary fibre by the intestinal microflora could modify short-chain fatty acid formation, reducing acetate and increasing propionate synthesis. This in turn reduces the endogenous synthesis of cholesterol, fatty acids and very low density lipoproteins (Cheng and Lai 2000). And finally, fibre-rich foods such as grains, fruits and vegetables, usually contain additional compounds, including vitamins, minerals, phytochemicals, antioxidants and other micronutrients that will neutralise free radicals, counteracting their negative action on lipoprotein oxidation (Anderson et al. 2000).

Recent reviews are available on the effect of dietary fibre on cardiovascular health (Babio et al. 2010; Sánchez-Muniz 2012). Epidemiological studies have shown cardiovascular protection to be more strongly associated with insoluble fibre than soluble fibre (Rimm et al. 1996). However, insoluble fibre, such as that from wheat bran or cellulose, has not been reported to have any significant effect on blood cholesterol (Solà et al. 2007). This could suggest that the effects observed in epidemiological studies may be due not only to the fibre but also to the presence of other bioactive and antioxidant phytochemical substances in foodstuffs (Solà et al. 2007) or to the effect that fibre has on other risk factors such as blood pressure, body weight and postprandial blood glucose or insulin levels (Wu et al. 2003). Soluble fibre has a demonstrated cholesterol-lowering effect in patients at high risk of cardiovascular disease (Jiménez et al. 2008). However, the efficacy of soluble fibre in lowering serum lipid levels in a free-living population of healthy persons was not confirmed (Chen et al. 2006).

Increasing the consumption of dietary fibres such as oat fibre is associated with a moderate reduction in systolic and diastolic blood pressure (Davy et al. 2002). It has been suggested that the effect on LDL and high-density lipoprotein (HDL) concentrations affects the arterial endothelium and smooth muscle, modifying arterial contractile tone (Kim et al. 2000). Nonetheless, it has been speculated that fibre may influence cardiac index and total peripheral resistance through effects on the nervous systems or through modification of the concentrations of certain local or systemic factors (Berardi 2010). With regard to the role of the kidney in blood pressure control, dietary fibre may alter angiotensin-converting enzyme (ACE) activity. This enzyme contributes to the formation of angiotensin II, a powerful vasoconstrictor that induces the formation of the hormones noradrenaline, aldosterone and vasopressin (Berardi 2010). ACE is also involved in the conversion of bradykinin (a vasodilator and natriuretic and diuretic agent) into inactive degradation products. Furthermore, dietary fibre is usually associated with minerals and antioxidant compounds in food that may influence the production of regulators of vasomotor tone. Moreover, the blood-pressure lowering effects of dietary fibre may be associated with the retention of minerals, such as sodium, in their matrix (Bocanegra et al. 2009), as certain minerals have been related to blood pressure (González-Muñoz et al. 2010).

Other major risks factors for cardiovascular disease, such as diabetes, obesity and dyslipidaemia, are also less prevalent among individuals with higher levels of fibre consumption (Lairon et al. 2005).

4.2 Dietary fibre and diabetes

Epidemiological studies suggest that a higher intake of dietary fibre has a significant protective role against type 1 and type 2 diabetes (Anderson et al. 2009). This effect is associated with substantial improvements in postprandial blood glucose and insulin responses (Slavin et al. 1999).

Meyer et al. (2000) observed that women consuming an average of 26 g/d of dietary fibre had a 22% lower risk of developing diabetes when compared with women consuming only 13 g/d. This was supported by the findings of Schulze et al. (2004) in a group of men and women who presented a decrease in their risk of diabetes with the consumption of an additional 12 g/d of dietary fibre. Currently, Bantle et al. (2008) from the American Diabetes Association recommends that diabetic patients consume 14 g/1000 kcal/d of fibre to improve blood glucose control.

It appears that insoluble fibre and soluble fibre have different effects on the control of type 2 diabetes. Most research demonstrates a strong inverse relationship between insoluble fibre, such as that from whole grains, and the risk of type 2 diabetes, whereas soluble fibre from fruits or vegetables has not been shown to have any effect (Lattimer and Haub 2010).

The mechanisms of action of insoluble fibre are in part related to an increased rate of intestinal transit, which will decrease the absorption of nutrients such as simple carbohydrates. It has also been observed that an increased intake of cereal fibre accelerates the secretion of glucose-dependent insulinotropic polypeptide, a hormone that stimulates postprandial insulin release (Weickert et al. 2005). Furthermore, the fermentation of short-chain fatty acids reduced the postprandial glucose response (Ostman et al. 2002). And finally, insoluble fibre can result in reduced appetite and food intake (Samra and Anderson 2007). The inverse relationship between cereal grains and diabetes may also be attributed to an increased consumption of magnesium, as this element has been shown to decrease the incidence of type 2 diabetes (Meyer et al. 2000).

Metabolic syndrome, which is a cluster of abnormalities including insulin resistance, dyslipidaemia, visceral adiposity and hypertension, can be also ameliorated and perhaps reversed by a high intake of dietary fibre or whole grain foods (Anderson 2008). In general it has been observed that the use of psyllium or plantago ovata (Sierra et al. 2001), guar gum (Butt et al. 2007), pectin (Bantle et al. 2008), Konjac mannan (Vuksan et al. 2000) or arabinoxylan (García et al. 2007) can be associated with a better postprandial metabolic response. However, insoluble fibre has not been shown to affect carbohydrate metabolism. Although prospective studies have shown that dietary fibre protects the individual from diabetes, clinical trials are needed to corroborate the beneficial effects of fibre on the incidence of diabetes.

4.3 Dietary fibre and weight control

Excess weight is a major threat to human health because it increases the risk of many of the major causes of mortality, including heart disease, diabetes, hypertension, stroke, dyslipidaemia and some cancers (Malnick and Knobler 2006).

In epidemiological studies, high fibre and whole grain intake is associated with lower body weight and the prevention of weight gain compared to diets low in fibre and whole grains (Du et al. 2010). Koh-Banerjee et al. (2004) reported that for every 40 g/d increase in whole grain intake, weight gain decreased by 500 g.

Pereira and Ludwig (2001) proposed three physiological mechanisms through which dietary fibre regulates body weight: intrinsic, colonic and hormonal. The intrinsic effects of a high-fibre diet are related to the low energy content to this type of diet. The bulking and viscosity properties of dietary fibre are predominantly responsible for influencing satiation during a meal and satiety between meals (Burton-Freeman 2000). Furthermore, fibre-rich foods require more effort and/or time of mastication, which also leads to increased satiety. The colonic effects are related to the fermentation of short-chain fatty acids; this also increases satiation and decreases glucose and free fatty acids. The fall in glucose and free fatty acid levels reduces insulin secretion, thus reducing fat deposition and improving fat oxidation. The hormonal effects of orexigenic or anorexigenic hormones are related to increased intestinal intraluminal viscosity, particularly when using soluble fibre, which slows transit time in the small intestine, triggering the secretion of glucagon-like peptide-1 (Reimer and McBurney 1996), cholecystokinin, ghrelin (Weickert et al. 2006) and peptide YY (Reimer et al. 2010). These gut hormones induce satiety.

Soluble fibre and insoluble fibre do not act in the same way in weight control. Soluble fibre has been found to reduce weight gain when added to a low-fat diet but to increase it if added to a high-fat diet (Baer et al. 1997). Several mechanisms have been proposed to explain how soluble fibre could increase weight gain. Soluble fibre favours the growth of bacterial populations in the large intestine (Davidson and McDonald 1998), increasing the fermentation and utilization of short-chain fatty acids, and thus energy absorption. Furthermore, soluble fibre forms a viscous material which delays intestinal transit (Schneeman 1998) and may allow for more complete digestion and absorption. Insoluble fibre seems to have the opposite effect to that of soluble fibre. When insoluble fibre intake was increased in a high-fat diet, body weight decreased (Isken et al. 2010). Insoluble fibre probably causes an increased rate of transit through the gastrointestinal tract that would result in diminished food digestion and nutrient absorption.

Factors related to weight control such as appetite have also been studied. In a systematic review about the effect of fibre on satiety and food intake, Clark and Slavin (2013) observed different effects depending on the type of fibre, particle size, dose and the type and duration of methods to assess appetite. The different types of fibre also modify gut hormone secretion (Anderson 2008) and other mechanisms related to weight control.

In the case of childhood obesity, some evidence suggests that fibre intake may also play a role in its treatment and in its future prevention (Pashankar and Loening-Baucke 2005). It is clear that more studies are needed to clarify the effect of fibre on weight control.

4.4 Dietary fibre and constipation

Constipation can be defined as a condition in which the stools are abnormally hard and difficult to pass, whatever the frequency of bowel movements (Bisanz 2005). At present, around 15% of the worldwide population suffers from constipation (Peppas et al. 2008). High-fibre food is usually recommended to prevent and manage constipation in adults and children. However, the results of the studies performed have not been uniformly positive. An interesting review of this subject was done by Gelinas (2013).

The physiological effects of dietary fibre depend on the type of fibre (soluble or insoluble). Insoluble fibre has higher laxative potential than soluble fibre (AACC 2001). Furthermore, differences in the bulking potential of fibre-rich foods depend on the resistance of the fibres to bacterial degradation, particularly the ratio of fermentable to non-fermentable components. Bacteria, which represent 30% to 55% of dry faecal weight (Achour et al. 2007), absorb a considerable volume of water and increase stool softening (Mälkki 2001).

However, a high-fibre diet does not appear to be a lasting medical solution for treating constipation and other associated diseases (Tan and Seow-Choen 2007). Water binders would not be useful for people with slow transit or with a disorder of defecation (Voderholzer et al. 1997). Moreover, gas formation may worsen the problem in some cases because of abdominal pain and bloating (Levitt 2003).

In children, the medical community is undecided whether diet can prevent or alleviate constipation (Pijpers et al. 2009). Observational studies indicate that dietary fibre has the potential to prevent constipation, but results are conflicting and further research is thus needed to confirm this effect.

4.5 Dietary fibre and other gastrointestinal disorders

The consumption of high-fibre foods or fibre supplements is recommended for a variety of gut disorders such as gastro-oesophageal reflux disease, duodenal ulcers, inflammatory bowel disease, irritable bowel syndrome and diverticular disease.

Soluble fibre, such as guar gum, has a positive effect on the control of gastro-oesophageal reflux disease and duodenal ulcer (Smits 1974) as this type of fibre reduces gastric acid secretion.

Irritable bowel syndrome, a complex disorder with a variety of pathogenic factors, produces abdominal pain or discomfort, bloating and diarrhoea and/or constipation. Fibre consumption can affect those symptoms in different extent depending on the fibre type. While wheat bran often increases symptoms (Harju 1984), other fibre supplements such as methylcellulose (Smits 1974) and partially hydrolysed guar gum (Giannini et al. 2006) appear to alleviate them. Results with psyllium and other fibres are contradictory; whilst some studies show a possible benefit (Prior and Whorwell 1987), others point to a lack of evidence to support this effect (Bijkerk et al. 2004; Chouinard 2011).

Other diseases related to a deficiency of fibre, such as a diverticular disease, can be prevented or alleviated by a generous intake of dietary fibre (Frieri et al. 2006).

4.6 Dietary fibre and cancer

The protective effect of fibre against cancer was already being discussed 40 years ago (Burkitt 1973). However, it is difficult to analyse the positive effects of the fibre because high-fibre foods such as vegetables and fruits also contain other micronutrients that might themselves protect against cancer.

There is evidence of the beneficial effect of fibre against colorectal cancer (Ben et al. 2014). Dietary fibre would appear to absorb carcinogens which are thus excreted from the intestinal tract in the faeces, preventing an interaction of faecal mutagens with the intestinal epithelium. Furthermore, the development of health-promoting bacteria would produce anti-carcinogenic compounds and stimulate the immune system (Kaczmarczyk et al. 2012). It has been reported that insoluble fibre, including wheat bran, appears to be more protective than soluble fibre (Harris and Ferguson 1993). Dietary fibre intake has also been associated with a reduced risk of gastric cancer (Zhang et al. 2013) and oesophageal cancer (Tang et al. 2013).

A number of publications discuss the effect of fibre on breast and ovarian cancer (McEligot et al. 2009). A possible mechanism for the protective effect of fibre against breast cancer is that a high fibre intake results in increased faecal losses of oestrogens, which are associated with an increased risk of breast cancer (Roberton et al. 1991). However, the data on this relationship are unclear.

4.7 Dietary fibre and mineral and vitamin bioavailability

There are concerns that a high fibre intake may impair mineral absorption due to chelation with fibres. However, the inhibitory effects of fibre indicated by some investigators (Van Dokkum 1992) may be related to the presence of phytate in the fibre (Harrington et al. 2001). Phytate is a well-documented inhibitor of iron, zinc and calcium absorption, and the removal of phytate has been shown to improve the bioavailability of these elements. Furthermore it has been stated that the growth of health-promoting bacteria favoured by dietary fibre would facilitate the absorption of certain minerals, particularly calcium (Roberfroid 2007).

Some studies have demonstrated that high fibre intake can reduce vitamin E (Kahlon et al. 1986) and vitamin D (Dagnelie et al. 1991) levels. This finding is due to the reduction in bile acid reabsorption.

4.8 Dietary fibre and other health benefits

Other health benefits derived from the stimulation by dietary fibre of health-promoting bacteria in the colon have been proposed (Roberfroid 2007), including: protection against intestinal infection; lowering of intestinal pH due to the formation of acids after the assimilation of carbohydrates; a reduction in the number of potentially harmful bacteria; the production of vitamins and antioxidants; and stimulation of the immune response, cognition and memory (Kaczmarczyk et al. 2012).

5. Reasons to include fibre in bakery products

The reasons to include fibre in bakery products are very varied and they will determine the type and the quantity of fibre used. The most common reasons are the following:

5.1 Nutritional benefits

As described above, fibre intake has numerous nutritional benefits. Furthermore, the majority of studies demonstrate that fibre consumption by humans is lower than recommended. Deficient fibre intake is even more problematic in individuals with coeliac disease; several studies have demonstrated that people who follow a gluten-free diet consume less fibre than the rest of the population (Mariani et al. 1998; Wild et al. 2010). The inclusion of fibre in gluten-free products is thus an area of particular interest, despite the fact that a study on commercially available gluten-free breads (Hager et al. 2011a) showed that the average fibre content of gluten-free white breads is higher than that of standard breads.

One of the points that should be considered when talking about the nutritional benefits of fibre is the recommended ratios of soluble to insoluble fibre. To comply with the recommended ratio in a given product, it is usually necessary to use mixtures of fibres because most individual preparations will not achieve these proportions alone. It is also known that the nutritional properties of fibres depend on their structure, and this may be modified by the process of product elaboration. We must therefore ensure that the chosen fibre has the ideal features to fulfil the intended role in the final product. The β-glucans, or products rich in these substances, such as oat bran, are an example of this issue. β-glucans with a high molecular weight have better nutritional properties (such as reducing serum cholesterol and regulating blood glucose concentrations) than β-glucans with low molecular weight (Lazaridou and Biliaderis 2007). It is therefore appropriate to choose β-glucans with a high molecular weight as the ingredient. However, β-glucanases, present in certain cereal flours, can reduce the molecular weight of β-glucans, reducing therefore their nutritional advantages (Tiwari and Cummins 2009); this problem is exacerbated by the favourable conditions for the activity of these enzymes during some stages of processing, such as dough fermentation. In fact, Tiwari et al. (2013) observed a reduction of over 35% in β-glucan concentrations during the fermentation of breads with added oat and oat bran. Thus, if we do not wish to accept the possibility that the elaboration process may reduce the nutritional benefits of this ingredient, it is essential either to minimise the quantity of β-glucanases in the formula or to use a production process that does not enhance β-glucanase activity.

When fibre-rich ingredients are added instead of purified fibre, the other components of those ingredients can contribute to the nutritional advantages of the final product. Thus, cereal bran and some by-products from the fruit processing industry have high levels of antioxidant substances, minerals and vitamins. In breads enriched with bran, this may be considered useful to reduce the negative effect of phytates on mineral bioavailability. Fungal phytases (Sanz-Penella et al. 2008, 2012), phytase-producing bifidobacteria (Sanz-Penella et al. 2009) and the hydrothermal treatment of bran before its addition to the formula (Mosharraf et al. 2009) have been used successfully during bread-making. It is also possible to reduce the quantity of phytase and to increase mineral availability by adding sourdough or lactic acid to the formula (Larsson and Sandberg 1991).

5.2 Improved organoleptic characteristics

The incorporation of fibre can improve the organoleptic characteristics and the shelf-life of bakery products. The inclusion of 2% insoluble fibre to bread delays staling phenomena (Gomez et al. 2003), and the addition of small quantities of hydrocolloids improves bread volume and shelf-life by reducing crumb hardening (Rosell et al. 2001; Guarda et al. 2004). The delay in staling after the addition of fibre has been demonstrated by several authors in standard breads (Santos et al. 2008; Pla et al. 2013) and in pre-cooked breads (Ronda et al. 2014). The effect has been related to slower recrystallisation of amylopectin molecules. A special case is breads for individuals with coeliac disease; hydrocolloids are typically used as gluten substitutes in these breads (Gallagher et al. 2004; Lazaridou et al. 2007; Turabi et al. 2008; Sabanis and Tzia 2011). Hydrocolloids allow dough to retain the gas produced during fermentation and thus produce a spongier product more similar to wheat bread.

Without hydrocolloids, gluten-free breads would not increase in volume during fermentation, a sponge-like structure would not develop and the texture would be too hard. However, the levels of fibre necessary to achieve these effects are much lower than the levels needed to obtain high-fibre products, and it is not therefore possible to include labelling claims referring to their fibre content. Certain fibres, such as inulin, can modify Maillard reactions by accelerating crust browning during baking, and it has therefore been suggested that they could be used to reduce baking time (Poinot et al.

2010). However, it must be taken into account that, apart from crust browning, other phenomena take place during baking, such as loaf expansion, starch gelatinization, protein denaturalisation and a degree of dehydration, particularly in the superficial layers. It is also possible to introduce cereal bran in order to give more flavour or a specific texture to the final product.

In the case of gluten-free breads, in which hydrocolloids are usually added as gluten substitutes, the addition of certain soluble fibres such as inulin (Capriles and Areas 2013), polydextrose or nutriose (Martínez et al. 2014) can increase the specific volume and cell density of breads, decrease hardness, accelerate Maillard reactions in the crust and improve consumer acceptability. In general, the effects on volume, texture and cell density appear to be related to the effect of the fibre on dough rheology, as fibre decreases dough consistency.

One of the main problems of enriching bakery products with fibre is poorer consumer acceptability, as shown in most research studies. In general, the addition of fibre to bread dough results in decreased product acceptability (Frutos et al. 2008). This decrease is due partly to the effect of fibre on bread volume and texture, but also to the influence of the different fibres on the colour, flavour and aroma of the pieces. There are thus marked differences between one fibre and another. Angioloni and Collar (2011) stated that fibres with large particle size produce viscoelastic solutions to improve bread acceptability. Martin et al. (2013) demonstrated that the decrease in acceptability of fibre-rich baguettes depended on the production process, and characteristics such as taste, flavour and texture may therefore contribute to minimise the negative effect on acceptability of the addition of fibre to bakery products. In some cases, imitation of the original product may not be the most appropriate strategy, and the development of a new product with its own organoleptic characteristics and good acceptability among target consumers may be more effective. However, one of the aspects that has received least attention is the effect of fibre on the taste and flavour of the product. It is known that these are key issues in organoleptic assessment by consumers and in their purchasing decisions. In some fibre-enriched bakery products, considered as sources of fibre, it has a marked and almost always negative influence on flavour and taste, as it produces unusual flavours. In some cases, these effects can be concealed by the presence of other ingredients with a more pleasant taste (creams, toppings, fillings, etc.), but when this masking is not possible, fibre should not be added to the product. In fact, Sapirstein et al. (2012) demonstrated that the addition of wheat bran to bread modified taste, particularly in the crust, and there were even differences between types of bran (white or red wheat bran).

5.3 Calorie reduction

Calorie reduction is one of the main reasons for incorporating fibre into bakery products. Among the macronutrients of food, carbohydrates and proteins provide 4 Kcal/g and fats 9 Kcal/g, while water does not provide any calories. Until recently, legislation considered that fibre did not provide any calories, though most fibres do have a small caloric contribution. The substitution of carbohydrates, proteins or fat by fibre therefore represented a major reduction of calorie content. Fibre is now considered to provide 2 Kcal/g, and calorie reduction is therefore somewhat less, especially when substituting carbohydrates or proteins. In the case of bread, fibre is used mainly to substitute flour (mainly carbohydrate) and to a lesser extent proteins. But in these cases, the greatest reduction in calorie content occurs due to an increase in the volume of water in the formulation. Most types of fibre allow, and even need, a large amount of water in the formulation, and in most cases the final product also contains a large amount of water, depending on the properties of the fibre. By increasing the amount of water in the final product, the calorie content is significantly reduced. In these cases, it is necessary to choose fibres that allow the greatest increase in water content in the formulation, as the differences between fibres mainly affect this parameter and water retention during baking. It should be taken into account that larger amounts of water will facilitate mould development, and special hygienic measures, such as the addition of antimicrobial substances, should therefore be taken or the shelf-life of the product should be reduced. For products such as cakes or cookies, many authors state that it is possible to replace fat with fibre and that this can produce a significant reduction in calorie content. It is also possible to substitute sugars, such as oligosaccharides, with some types of fibre.

5.4 Use of by-products

The earliest research dealing with increasing fibre content in breads looked at the use of bran, a by-product of the cereal milling industry with a high mineral, vitamin, antioxidant and fibre content. Table 1 lists studies in which the addition of bran to bakery products has been investigated. Research using other cereal brans has also been performed. It is now known that aspects such as the cereal cultivar, particle size, and the treatments received before incorporation into the dough affect the suitability of a given fibre for inclusion into the baking process. Wheat, barley, rye and oat bran cannot be used in gluten-free products because they contain certain substances that are toxic to this group of individuals. One possibility is to use bran from other cereals such as maize or rice (Kadan and Phyllippy 2007), but whilst maize bran is too hard and the organoleptic characteristics are not well studied, rice bran must undergo stabilization treatment because of its high oil content. Studies on gluten-free breads have looked at the inclusion of defatted rice bran (Sharif and Butt 2006) or a heat-treated bran obtained to inactivate the lipoxidative enzymes (Soares et al. 2009). Another possibility is the addition of pseudocereal whole flours, which have high fibre content (Alvarez-Jubete et al. 2009, 2010).

   Much of the research into the fibre enrichment of bakery products is focused on the inclusion of high-fibre ingredients derived from different processing industries, including fruit (apple, pineapple, ...) and vegetable (potato skins, ...) processing, sugar production (cane and beet), and brewing or other forms of production of alcoholic drinks (see Table 2). In some cases, the ingredients are prepared simply by milling, but in other cases they receive more complex treatments in order to increase the fibre content or minimise possible unpleasant tastes or smells. When designed for use in the bakery industry, these ingredients must be of constant quality, with high levels

Table 1. Studies on the addition of bran to bakery products.

Product	Bran	Reference
Bread	Wheat bran and shorts	Larsson and Sandberg (1991); Rao and Rao (1991); Belisle et al. (1993); Czuchajowska and Pomeranz (1993); Sidhu et al. (1999); Al-Hooti et al. (2000); Al-Saqer et al. (2000); Salmenkallio-Marttila et al. (2001); Aamodt et al. (2004); Katina et al. (2006); Gandra et al. (2008); Sanz-Penella et al. (2008); Gul et al. (2009); Seyer and Gelinas (2009); Noort et al. (2010); Purhagen et al. (2012); Sanz-Penella et al. (2012); Sapirstein et al. (2012); Schmiele et al. (2012); Almeida et al. (2013b); Curti et al. (2013); Kaprelyants et al. (2013); Martin et al. (2013)
	Microparticulated wheat bran	Kim et al. (2013)
	Fermented wheat bran	Katina et al. (2012)
	Heat-treated wheat bran	Nelles et al. (1998); De Kock et al. (1999)
	Extruded wheat bran	Gomez et al. (2011)
	Defatted rice bran	Sharif and Butt (2006)
	Toasted rice bran	Sharma and Chauhan (2002); Soares et al. (2009)
	Extruded rice bran	Sharma and Chauhan (2002)
	Infrared-treated rice bran	Tuncel et al. (2014a,b)
	Corn bran	Sosulski and Wu (1988); Gul et al. (2009)
	Oat bran	D'Appolonia and Youngs (1978); Krishnan et al. (1987); Sosulski and Wu (1988); Dhinda et al. (2012); Purhagen et al. (2012); Tiwari et al. (2013)
	Barley bran	Chaudhary and Weber (1990)
	Rye bran	Purhagen et al. (2012)
Flat bread	Wheat bran	Basman and Koksel (1999, 2001); Shenoy and Prakash (2002); Majzoobi et al. (2013)
	Heat treated wheat bran	Mosharraf et al. (2009)
Bake-off bread and frozen doughs	Wheat bran	Almeida et al. (2013a); Ronda et al. (2014)
	Extruded rice bran	Quilez et al. (2013)
	Steam-treated rice bran	Quilez et al. (2013)
Gluten-free bread	Rice bran	Kadan and Phyllippy (2007); Phimolsiripol et al. (2012)
Cakes and muffins	Rice bran	Sloan and James (1988); Hudson et al. (1992); Lebesi and Tzia (2011)
	Oat bran	Hudson et al. (1992); Lee et al. (2004); Lebesi and Tzia (2011)
	Wheat bran	Brockmole and Zabik (1976); Springsteen et al. (1977); Shafer and Zabik (1978); Lebesi and Tzia (2011)
Cookies	Wheat bran	Nandeesh et al. (2011)
	Rice bran	Sharma and Chauhan (2002)

of fibre, and must not add any undesirable organoleptic characteristics to the final product. The addition of these ingredients can be of further benefit if they contain other compounds such as antioxidants and minerals.

Table 2. Studies on the addition of fibre to bread.

Product	Fibre	Reference
Bread	Inulin	Praznik et al. (2002); Wang et al. (2002); Rosell et al. (2006, 2010); Collar et al. (2007, 2009); Santos et al. (2008); Angioloni and Collar (2009, 2011); Poinot et al. (2010); Hager et al. (2011b); Salinas and Puppo (2014)
	Polydextrose	Angioloni and Collar (2009, 2011)
	β-glucans	Brennan and Cleary (2007); Skendi et al. (2010); Hager et al. (2011b)
	Barley fractions	Knuckles et al. (1997); Cavallero et al. (2002); Jacobs et al. (2008)
	Resistant starch	Yeo and Seib (2009); Sanz-Penella et al. (2010); Gomez et al. (2013); Almeida et al. (2013b)
	Pectins	Sivam et al. (2011)
	Locust bean guar	Wang et al. (2002); Angioloni and Collar (2009, 2011); Almeida et al. (2013b)
	Psyllium fibre	Park et al. (1997)
	Carrageenan	Belisle et al. (1993)
	Sugar beet fibre	Ozboy and Koksel (1999); Rosell et al. (2006, 2010); Collar et al. (2007); Filipovic et al. (2007); Santos et al. (2008); Simovic et al. (2010)
	Sugarcane bagasse	Sangnark and Noomhorm (2004)
	Wheat arabinoxylans	Bonnand-Ducasse et al. (2010)
	Legume hulls and fibres	Sosulski and Wu (1988); Wang et al. (2002); Johnson et al. (2003); Dalgetty and Baik (2006); Rosell et al. (2006, 2010); Collar et al. (2007); Santos et al. (2008)
	Potato fibre	Kaack et al. (2006)
	Cocoa fibre	Collar et al. (2009)
	Insoluble commercial fibres	Gomez et al. (2003)
	Brewers' spent grain	Prentice and D'Appolonia (1977); Hassona (1993); Stojceska and Ainsworth (2008)
	Fruit fibre	Masoodi and Chauhan (1998); Miller (2011); Salgado et al. (2011); Pla et al. (2013); Bchir et al. (2014)
	Seed spice residues	Chien and Potty (1996)
	Palm date flour and fibre	Dedelahaye et al. (1994); Borchani et al. (2011); Ahmed et al. (2013)
	Artichoke powder and fibre	Praznik et al. (2002); Frutos et al. (2008)
	Cellulose derivatives	Angioloni and Collar (2009, 2011)
Flat bread	Palm date seeds	Almana and Mahmoud (1994)
	Barley fractions	Izydorczyk et al. (2008)
	Coffee silverskin	Pourfarzad et al. (2013)
Bake-off bread and frozen doughs	Pectins	Rosell and Santos (2010); Skara et al. (2013)
	Resistant starch	Rosell and Santos (2010); Almeida et al. (2013a)
	Inulin and polydextrose	Filipovic et al. (2008); Polaki et al. (2010); Skara et al. (2013); Ronda et al. (2014)
	Locust bean and guar gums	Polaki et al. (2010); Almeida et al. (2013a); Skara et al. (2013)
	Cellulose derivatives	Polaki et al. (2010)
	Sugar beet fibre	Filipovic et al. (2008)

Table 2. contd....

Table 2. contd.

Product	Fibre	Reference
Scones (Quick bread)	Inulin and oligofructose	Roessle et al. (2011)
Rye bread	Grape by-product	Mildner-Szkudlarz et al. (2011)
Gluten-free bread	Cereal fibres	Sabanis et al. (2009a,b); Martinez et al. (2014)
	Psyllium fibre	Mariotti et al. (2009); Cappa et al. (2013)
	Sugar beet fibre	Cappa et al. (2013)
	Polydextrose	Martínez et al. (2014)
	Nutriose	Martínez et al. (2014)
	Potato fibre	Martínez et al. (2014)
	Pea fibre	Martínez et al. (2014)
	Inulin	Korus et al. (2006); Hager et al. (2011b); Capriles and Areas (2013); Ziobro et al. (2013)
	Resistant starch	Korus et al. (2009)
	β-glucans	Hager et al. (2011b); Perez-Quirce et al. (2014)

6. Selection criteria

When choosing the type of fibre to be added to a bakery product, we must consider not only the organoleptic and nutritional properties of the fibre, as commented above, but also the functional characteristics, legal aspects and price.

6.1 Functional characteristics

Raw materials rich in fibre differ in their functional properties, including water absorption capacity, thickening power, etc. These characteristics depend on the percentage and type of fibre, the presence of other components and particle size. These properties affect dough behaviour during kneading, handling and fermentation, dough expansion during baking and hardening of the final product during storage. In general, fibres that have minimal effects on the original properties of dough are preferred, but in some cases it can be advisable to use fibres with specific characteristics when particular nutritional or organoleptic attributes are sought. For example, fibre with a high water absorption capacity is useful when the aim is to produce a low calorie product. We must always be aware that the strategies applied to improve any production process will differ depending on the type of fibre used.

6.2 Legislation

When companies develop new products, they should always take into account the legislation of the countries where the products are to be produced and sold. Legislation can curb the use of certain ingredients. In the case of fibre-enriched products, labelling is one of the most important aspects to be considered. Several legislative systems regulate the use of different nutritional and health claims, such as "product rich in fibre", but those may change over time and vary from country to country. Mialon et al. (2002) showed that the perceived healthiness and nutritional value of breads and "English" muffins was increased by providing information on dietary fibre content, and perceived sensory intensities were also increased. It is generally known that the acceptability of fibre-enriched breads and cakes is increased when information on their fibre content is provided. Moriartey et al. (2010), in a study of β-glucan-enriched bread, demonstrated that such information not only increased the global acceptability of the product but also improved the assessment of appearance and flavour. This study also found that women and people who were used to eating whole grains were more receptive to this type of information. These results are consistent with the comments of Baixauli et al. (2008), who observed that consumers concerned about the nutritional attributes of foods were more sensitive to information on the fibre content of muffins. That study also found that the information was more effective when bran was added rather than resistant starch, as resistant starch was considered to be more "unnatural" than bran. The strategies to follow should therefore be based on the type of product and the potential consumers. On the other hand, in a study on fibre-enriched French baguettes, Ginon et al. (2009) observed that nutritional information about potential health benefits did not induce a significant change in willingness to pay. However, when bread was labelled as a "source of fibre", buying intention was slightly improved. Hellyer et al. (2012) also observed that consumers reacted positively to the inclusion of health benefit information in whole grain bread, but this reaction was not influenced by the specificity of the information. It is important to take into account that consumer reactions may be influenced by other factors such as age, social class and cultural level.

6.3 Price

Price is one of the aspects less widely analysed in research studies, despite being one of the most important for the food industry. Companies must be aware of the price of raw materials and processing costs to determine the possible price of a final product. The industrial development of fibre-enriched foods must therefore take into account the increased production costs caused both by the cost of the fibre or fibre-enriched ingredient and by possible changes that may need to be made to the process (longer processing, stronger flours, additives, etc.). It is also important price stability, as the price of some raw materials can be highly volatile worldwide, and to ensure a steady supply throughout the year and avoid problems of shortages.

7. Effects on processing

7.1 Kneading

Kneading is one of the most problematic aspects in the development of fibre-enriched products. In theory, the development of fibre-enriched products should include more water due to the increased water absorption capacity of the fibre. However, correct calculation of the amount of water to be added is complex. In general, the specifications to obtain a consistent product are based on assays of the water absorption capacity determined by centrifugation of a sample of fibre or of fibre plus flour; but these assays provide little information about the quantity of water required for kneading. The farinographic characteristics are more useful (Stauffer 1990), but it is always necessary to perform a bake test before making a final decision. It should also be noted that gluten or flours with a high protein content are added to many fibre-enriched breads and require a further increase in the water content of the formula. Study of the amount of water to be used in the formula should therefore be done on the final formulation. In general, the addition of fibre or bran leads to an increase in farinographic absorption (Park et al. 1997; Gomez et al. 2003, 2011; Rosell et al. 2006; Izydorczyk et al. 2008; Noort et al. 2010; Miller 2011; Schmiele et al. 2012; Bchir et al. 2014), but the intensity of this effect depends on the type of fibre. In addition, water absorption capacity of dough can be affected by differences in the structure or in the molecular weight of a specific type of fibre, for instance β-glucans of high molecular weight increase farinographic absorption more than those of low molecular weight (Skendi et al. 2010). Almeida et al. (2010) demonstrated that fibre with a high water absorption index, such as locust bean gum, noticeably increased farinographic absorption, while resistant starch hardly changed this parameter. This agrees with the studies performed by Rosell et al. (2001) and Guarda et al. (2004), who found that the addition of 0.5% of different hydrocolloids significantly increased farinographic absorption. The effect of inulin on water absorption was also smaller than the effect of other fibres (Wang et al. 2002; Rosell et al. 2006). In a study of the addition of different types of bran, Purhagen et al. (2012) observed that wheat and rye brans increased water absorption whereas oat bran, with a different chemical composition, had hardly any effect. However, oat bran increased development time and dough stability to a greater extent than the other types of bran. It is important to note that fibre blends may have synergistic or antagonistic effects (Rosell et al. 2006; Almeida et al. 2010).

Kneading time might be also modified by fibres. Stauffer (1990) stated that fibre-enriched dough showed anomalous behaviour because the fibre absorbed the water present in the dough very quickly; this would suggest that the dough needed more water. However, after further kneading the dough relaxed and began to form the elastic structure of typical bread. This situation can lead to two peaks of maximum consistency in the farinographic analysis, and only the second peak must be considered. In general, the addition of fibre increases development time during kneading (Park et al. 1997; Shenoy and Prakash 2002; Gomez et al. 2003; Noort et al. 2010; Skendi et al. 2010), although this effect depends on the type of fibre used and its percentage. For example, resistant starch hardly affects development or even reduces it (Almeida et al. 2010). These authors also noted that dough with a high proportion of locust bean gum and wheat bran had a low tolerance to excessive mixing, which is consistent with the findings of other authors with other types of fibre (Shenoy and Prakash 2002; Izydorczyk et al. 2008; Noort et al. 2010; Schmiele et al. 2012). In contrast, low doses of fibre increase dough tolerance, as observed by Gomez et al. (2003) and Bchir et al. (2014); although resistant starch has a much smaller effect than other fibres studied.

Correct calculation of the amount of water to be added is also very important in gluten-free breads. Although the kneading operation is not designed to develop the gluten network, it is important in dough rheology. In this case, the study of fundamental dough rheology is used rather than farinograph analysis. Again, considerable differences exist between fibres. For example, the addition of fibres such as β-glucans, with a high water holding capacity (water-binding), makes it necessary to increase the amount of water in the formulation in order to achieve a rheology similar to the control dough (Hager et al. 2011b; Perez-Quirce et al. 2014), the same happens with hydrocolloids (Lazaridou et al. 2007). On the other hand, the addition of fibres like inulin requires the amount of water to be reduced (Hager et al. 2011b).

7.2 Handling and fermentation

The addition of fibre to bread dough can significantly modify the texture and rheology of doughs. This effect has been demonstrated in many studies using conventional rheological measurements (Korus et al. 2009; Mariotti et al. 2009; Sabanis et al. 2009b; Bonnand-Ducasse et al. 2010; Angioloni and Collar 2011; Hager et al. 2011b; Sivam et al. 2011; Ahmed et al. 2013), dough texture, uniaxial extension tests (Collar et al. 2007; Angioloni and Collar 2009; Miller 2011; Schmiele et al. 2012; Mis and Dziki 2013) and biaxial extension tests (Wang et al. 2002; Gomez et al. 2003, 2011; Bchir et al. 2014). Properties such as dough stickiness, extensibility and tenacity are important for predicting the behaviour of doughs in operations such as forming, particularly in industrial processes. The incorporation of fibre usually increases dough viscosity and elasticity (Bonnand-Ducasse et al. 2010; Sivam et al. 2011). In general, dough tenacity increases and extensibility decreases, but this effect varies depending on the type of fibre studied (Wang et al. 2002; Gomez et al. 2003, 2011; Schmiele et al. 2012; Bchir et al. 2014). Some authors attribute the changes in dough tenacity and extensibility generated by the addition of fibre to the dilution of the gluten network, which is responsible for dough consistency and on which these parameters depend, at least in part. However, the high water absorption capacity of some fibres is also important as it leads to competition with the gluten. This situation explains the lack of uniformity in the results, and the differences observed between the fibres studied. Interactions have even been detected between different fibres (Collar et al. 2007). Obviously in the case of gluten-free breads the differences are due to the different water absorption capacity and thickening power of each fibre, and not to their interaction with the protein network, because this does not develop in the same way without gluten. Therefore, a detailed study must be conducted in each case, analysing the formulation and kneading conditions (hydration, mixing time, etc.), as these will also influence the rheological properties of the doughs. In fact, in some cases the differences observed are a consequence of not adapting the kneading conditions to the requirements of the fibre-enriched dough. For example, the addition of small percentages of hydrocolloids (0.5%) increases tenacity and decreases the extensibility of doughs analysed with the alveograph, without adjusting moisture, but they had the opposite effect when tested with the extensograph after moisture adjustment (Rosell et al. 2001). These differences are due in part to differences between the uniaxial extension (extensograph) and biaxial (alveograph) tests, but to a greater extent are due to changes in the preparation of the doughs.

In general, the addition of fibre does not affect gas production during the fermentation process, but it modifies the ability of the dough to retain the gas produced. Various authors agree that the height reached by the dough during fermentation is reduced by the addition of fibre (Wang et al. 2002; Sangnark and Noomhorm 2004) or by the addition of bran (Czuchajowska and Pomeranz 1993; Sanz-Penella et al. 2008). These authors attributed this effect to the disruption and/or dilution of the gluten network responsible for gas retention during fermentation. In these cases it may be interesting to reduce fermentation times to avoid dough breakdown. Factors such as the type of fibre or the percentage and particle size of bran also influence the magnitude of this phenomenon.

7.3 Product quality

The addition of fibre and bran to bread dough usually results in a fall in the volume of traditional breads (Frutos et al. 2008; Rosell and Santos 2010; Schmiele et al. 2012; Tiwari et al. 2013) unless hydrocolloids are added at proportions of up to 0.5%; this addition may actually increase loaf volume (Rosell et al. 2001; Guarda et al. 2004). The fall in volume is consistent with the lack of development during the fermentation process, and thus with the decreased gas retention capacity of these doughs. This decrease is therefore commonly attributed to dilution of the gluten network, as well as to interactions between the fibre and the protein network. In some cases, the high tenacity of fibre-enriched doughs (especially after the addition of hydrocolloids) also hinders dough expansion. However, this effect can be minimised by correcting dough moisture as discussed above. In the case of gluten-free breads, the addition of hydrocolloids, which permit gluten replacement, increases loaf volume, because gas retention during fermentation is more dependent on dough consistency, largely thanks to the presence of these fibres, than on the development of a protein network. But an excess of hydrocolloids may also be negative. It is thus necessary to optimise the formula, and the percentage of hydrocolloids added will differ according to the type of hydrocolloid chosen. The addition of fibre can also modify the pasting properties of flours because fibre competes with starch for the water necessary for gelatinization phenomena (Rosell et al. 2010). These changes may affect the volume and texture of the final products because the pasting properties and, specifically, the pasting temperature, influence the time at which expansion stops during baking due to the creation of a rigid structure. In turn, dough behaviour after baking and, specifically, retrogradation phenomena, also influence the final texture of the products obtained. As in other cases, it is not possible to talk about a general tendency as the different types and percentages of fibre influence these properties in different ways.

The addition of fibre also influences the moisture of the loaves, which is increased (Frutos et al. 2008; Miller 2011; Schmiele et al. 2012; Almeida et al. 2013a,b). This effect is due to the ability of the different fibres to retain water, though it must be kept in mind that there is often no direct relationship between the weight of the loaves and the water-holding capacity of the fibres measured at room temperature. The presence of fibres may also improve water retention during storage, although this effect is also influenced by the type of fibre used. Almeida et al. (2013a) observed that the addition of locust bean gum and wheat bran reduced moisture loss during the storage of pre-cooked breads, but the addition of resistant starch had a smaller effect, particularly during the initial days of storage. In the case of hydrocolloids, these effects are seen at doses lower than 0.5% (Guarda et al. 2004). The effects of the addition of fibre on loaf moisture and volume are usually observed as changes in the final texture of the bread, which typically becomes harder (Frutos et al. 2008; Rosell and Santos 2010). Changes in the texture of fibre-enriched breads may affect the crumbliness of bread during cutting and the resistance of loaves to fold (cutability), typically leading to increased crumbliness and decreased cutability, as demonstrated by Purhagen et al. (2012) in studies with bran-enriched breads.

8. Improvement of fibre-enriched products

In general, the addition of insoluble fibre or inulin must not exceed 10% to 15%, and studies on gums and hydrocolloids do not include percentages over 5% to 10%; this is partly due to the drastic changes that occur in dough rheology. The problems of incorporating fibre into conventional bread dough are largely related to gluten dilution, as mentioned above. To minimise these problems it is necessary not only to adapt the process conditions but also to increase the gluten network, either in quantity or quality, to obtain a reinforced structure that will retain the gas formed during fermentation. A number of authors have therefore proposed the addition of vital gluten at levels of around 5% (Rao and Rao 1991; Czuchajowska and Pomeranz 1993; Ozboy and Koksel 1999; Filipovic et al. 2007; Simovic et al. 2010). It was also found that the appropriate choice of flour improved the effect of the addition of fibre, with preference for the use of flour with a high protein content and good protein quality (Aamodt et al. 2004). The inclusion of substances that favour the creation of a strong gluten network, including oxidizing agents such as ascorbic acid (Rao and Rao 1991; Al-Saqer et al. 2000), emulsifiers such as SSL or DATEM (Rao and Rao 1991; Al-Saqer et al. 2000; Aamodt et al. 2004; Gomez et al. 2013), strengthening enzymes such as certain lipases and xylanases (Katina et al. 2006; Jacobs et al. 2008; Stojceska and Ainsworth 2008; Ghoshal et al. 2013) or glucose oxidase, and oxidants such as hexose oxidase (Gul et al. 2009), also improved the quality of enriched breads or, at least, reduced the fall in volume. Sanz-Penella et al. (2008) also proposed the addition of α-amylases to improve the fermentation process and to increase the final volume of breads with added bran.

The inclusion of hydrocolloids such as guar gum or pectins can also increase the volume of bran-enriched breads (Rao and Rao 1991) or inulin-enriched part-baked breads (Skara et al. 2013). We have already mentioned that hydrocolloids, thanks to their functional properties, may act as bread improvers, and an interesting strategy to increase the amount of fibre in bread-making has been to study the addition of mixtures of soluble and insoluble fibres (Belisle et al. 1993; Angioloni and Collar 2009; Polaki et al. 2010). These strategies enable the amount of fibre to be increased, but there is still a maximum percentage of fibre that should not be exceeded in order to avoid perceiving a clear deterioration in bread quality. This proportion is around 20%, though it varies greatly depending on the type of fibre and type of baking process used. Because of this, some authors have even proposed the use of up to 30%. The studies of these mixtures usually use specific experimental designs, such as surface response methodology. Furthermore, the choice of the most appropriate baking process can improve the final quality of the bread. Jacobs et al. (2008), in the production of breads with barley fibre-rich fractions, observed that the sponge and dough method achieved enriched breads with higher volumes than the direct method (straight dough) or short process. This is consistent with the observations of Rao and Rao (1991) and Katina et al. (2006), in their studies on the incorporation of wheat bran. It should also be kept in mind that changes in the formulation can affect the optimal conditions for kneading and fermentation, and these conditions must be recalculated in each case.

In some cases the addition of some fibres can be increased or the negative effects of fibre incorporation can be minimised by modifying the type of fibre. When adding wheat bran to traditional breads, the volume effects are smaller if particle size is increased; this may be due to a better interaction with the gluten or to the possibility that negative compounds are released by a greater reduction in particle size (De Kock et al. 1999; Noort et al. 2010; Sanz-Penella et al. 2012). However, the effect varies depending on the type of product manufactured and the size of particle added; in flat breads to which barley fibre-rich fractions were added, no differences were observed related to particle size (Izydorczyk et al. 2008) whereas, again with flat breads, when wheat bran was added, the breads with the finest wheat bran particle size were preferred by panellists (Majzoobi et al. 2013). These differences may be related to the fact that flat breads do not need to achieve a high volume during fermentation and the negative effect of particle size reduction on gas retention therefore had no noticeable effect on organoleptic quality. Differences have also been observed between breads depending on the bran layers used (external or internal layers) and on the milling procedure (Curti et al. 2013; Kaprelyants et al. 2013). These differences are related in some cases to a different chemical composition or variations in enzymatic activities, and in other cases to different particle size. The hydrothermal treatment of bran, such as extrusion, also improves the volume of bread when the improver is added (Mosharraf et al. 2009; Gomez et al. 2011). Other treatments, such as dry-heat treatment (De Kock et al. 1999), hydration or oxidation of the bran (Nelles et al. 1998) or bran prefermentative treatments (Salmenkallio-Marttila et al. 2001), have also been studied. These treatments either reduce enzyme activity (heat treatment) or minimise the presence of reducing substances. In the case of the addition of bran, only the appropriate choice of bran, depending on the wheat cultivar, may have any noticeable influence on results (Nelles et al. 1998; Al-Saqer et al. 2000). Specifically, Seyer and Gelinas (2009) found a high correlation between the specific volume of whole breads and the mechanical properties (low friability) of wheat bran. Katina et al. (2012) also proposed the modification of wheat bran by fermentation. Enzymatic reactions during fermentation modify the functional and nutritional properties of bran and may improve bread quality. Those authors observed that bran fermentation could increase bread volume and decrease bread hardness, probably due to the solubilisation of arabinoxylans.

The case of rice bran is of particular interest due to its high oil content and the short shelf-life resulting from rancidity. To minimise this risk, rice bran is usually subjected to a stabilization treatment such as extrusion, toasting, steam cooking, infrared treatment or defatting. The type of treatment used to stabilise rice bran will also affect the enriched breads. Quilez et al. (2013) demonstrated that extruded rice brans (high temperature treatment) produced better part-cooked breads than steam-cooked rice brans, as extruded rice brans were associated with greater dough development during fermentation, a higher specific volume and a better sensory evaluation, but acceptability still did not equal non-enriched breads.

In the elaboration of gluten-free breads, the correct selection of rice bran may improve the specific volume, texture and acceptability of breads, with preference for breads with a high content of soluble fibre (Phimolsiripol et al. 2012). In these breads, fibre selection may have a noticeable influence on bread quality. Martínez et al. (2014) observed that fibres that decreased dough consistency, such as some soluble fibres (polydextrose or nutriose), improved the specific volume of gluten-free breads and decreased hardness. The same authors observed that the size and shape of insoluble fibres also had a demonstrable effect on bread quality. Small, elongated fibres were preferred to other fibres as they produced a higher volume with lower hardness. These results are consistent with the observations made by Ziobro et al. (2013) in their study of the inclusion of different types of inulin in gluten-free breads. These authors observed that inulins with a low level of polymerisation—and thus with low thickening power—enabled breads with a higher volume and lower hardness to be obtained compared with inulins with a high level of polymerisation. In both the above studies, the cell density of the bread was also analysed, and was found to be finer and more uniform after the addition of polydextrose or nutriose compared with other insoluble fibres.

Keywords: Fibre, health benefits, nutritional benefits, improved organoleptic characteristics, by-products

References

AACC. 2001. The definition of dietary fibre. Cereal Foods World, 46: 112–126.

Aamodt, A., E.M. Magnus and E.M. Faergestad. 2004. Effect of protein quality, protein content, bran addition, DATEM, proving time, and their interaction on hearth bread. Cereal Chemistry, 81: 722–734.

Achour, L., S. Nancey, D. Moussata, I. Graber, B. Messing and B. Flourié. 2007. Faecal bacterial mass and energetic losses in healthy humans and patients with a short bowel syndrome. European Journal of Clinical Nutrition, 61: 233–238.

Ahmed, J., A.S. Almusallam, F. Al-Salman, M.H. Abdul Rahman and E. Al-Salem. 2013. Rheological properties of water insoluble date fiber incorporated wheat flour dough. LWT—Food Science and Technology, 51: 409–416.

Al-Hooti, S.N., J.S. Sidhu and J.M. Al-Saqer. 2000. Utility of CIE tristimulus system in measuring the objective crumb color of high-fiber toast bread formulation. Journal of Food Quality, 23: 103–116.

Almana, H.A. and R.M. Mahmoud. 1994. Palm date seeds as an alternative source of dietary fiber in saudi bread. Ecology of Food and Nutrition, 32: 261–270.

Almeida, E.L., Y.K. Chang and C.J. Steel. 2010. Effect of adding different dietary fiber sources on farinographic parameters of wheat flour. Cereal Chemistry, 87: 566–573.

Almeida, E.L., Y.K. Chang and C.J. Steel. 2013a. Dietary fibre sources in frozen part-baked bread: Influence on technological quality. LWT—Food Science and Technology, 53: 262–270.

Almeida, E.L., Y.K. Chang and C.J. Steel. 2013b. Dietary fibre sources in bread: Influence on technological quality. LWT—Food Science and Technology, 50: 545–553.

Al-Saqer, J.M., J.S. Sidhu and S.N. Al-Hooti. 2000. Instrumental texture and baking quality of high-fiber toast bread as affected by added wheat mill fractions. Journal of Food Processing and Preservation, 24: 1–16.

Alvarez-Jubete, L., E.K. Arendt and E. Gallagher. 2009. Nutritive value and chemical composition of pseudocereals as gluten-free ingredients. International Journal of Food Sciences and Nutrition, 60: 240–257.

Alvarez-Jubete, L., E.K. Arendt and E. Gallagher. 2010. Nutritive value of pseudocereals and their increasing use as functional gluten-free ingredients. Trends in Food Science & Technology, 21: 106–113.

Anderson, J.W. 2008. Dietary fiber and associated phytochemicals in prevention and reversal of diabetes. pp. 111–142. *In*: V.K. Pasupuleti and J.W. Anderson (eds.). Nutraceuticals, Glycemic health and type 2 diabetes. Blackwekk Publishing Professional, Ames, Iowa.

Anderson, J.W., P. Baird, R.H. Davis, S. Ferreri, M. Knudtson, A. Koraym, V. Waters and C.L. Williams. 2009. Health benefits of dietary fiber. Nutrition Reviews, 67: 188–205.

Anderson, J.W., T.J. Hanna, X. Peng and R.J. Kryscio. 2000. Whole grain foods and heart disease risk. Journal of the American College of Nutrition, 19: 291S–299S.

Anderson, J.W., L. Story, B. Seiling, W.J. Chen, M.S. Petro and J. Story. 1984. Hypocholesterolemic effects of oat-bran or bean intake for hypercholesterolemic men. The American Journal of Clinical Nutrition, 40: 1146–1155.

Angioloni, A. and C. Collar. 2009. Gel, dough and fibre enriched fresh breads: Relationships between quality features and staling kinetics. Journal of Food Engineering, 91: 526–532.

Angioloni, A. and C. Collar. 2011. Physicochemical and nutritional properties of reduced-caloric density high-fibre breads. LWT—Food Science and Technology, 44: 747–758.

Babio, N., R. Balanza, J. Basulto, M. Bulló and J. Salas-Salvadó. 2010. Dietary fibre: influence on body weight, glycemic control and plasma cholesterol profile. Nutrición Hospitalaria, 25: 327–340.

Baer, D.J., W.V. Rumpler, C.W. Miles and G.C. Fahey. 1997. Dietary fiber decreases the metabolizable energy content and nutrient digestibility of mixed diets fed to humans. Journal of Nutrition, 127: 579–586.

Baixauli, R., A. Salvador, G. Hough and S.M. Fiszman. 2008. How information about fibre (traditional and resistant starch) influences consumer acceptance of muffins. Food Quality and Preference, 19: 628–635.

Bantle, J.P., J. Wylie-Rosett, A.L. Albright, C.M. Apovian, N.G. Clark, M.J. Franz, B.J. Hoogwerf, A.H. Lichtenstein, E. Mayer-Davis, A.D. Mooradian and M.L. Wheeler. 2008. Nutrition recommendations and interventions for diabetes: a position statement of the American Diabetes Association. Diabetes Care, 31: S61–78.

Basman, A. and H. Koksel. 1999. Properties and composition of Turkish flat bread (Bazlama) supplemented with barley flour and wheat bran. Cereal Chemistry, 76: 506–511.

Basman, A. and H. Koksel. 2001. Effects of barley flour and wheat bran supplementation on the properties and composition of Turkish flat bread, yufka. European Food Research and Technology, 212: 198–202.

Bchir, B., H. Rabetafika, M. Paquot and C. Blecker. 2014. Effect of pear, apple and date fibres from cooked fruit by-products on dough performance and bread quality. Food and Bioprocess Technology, 7: 1114–1127.

Belisle, P.R., B.A. Rasco, K. Siffring, B. Bruinsma, R. Moss, P. Resmini and M.E. Camire. 1993. Baking properties and microstructure of yeast-raised breads containing wheat bran–carrageenan blends or laminates. Food Structure, 12: 489–496.

Ben, Q., Y. Sun, R. Chai, A. Qian, B. Xu and Y. Yuan. 2014. Dietary fiber intake reduces risk for colorectal adenoma: A meta-analysis. Gastroenterology, 146: 689–699.

Berardi, C. 2010. Regulación renal de la tension arterial. Eliminación de residuos nitrogenados. Insuficiencia renal. pp. 541–554. *In*: M.D. Dvorkin, D.P. Cardinali and R.H. Iermoli (eds.). Bases fisiológicas de la práctica médica. 14th Spanish edition. Panamericana, Buenos Aires.

Bijkerk, C.J., J.W.M. Muris, J.A. Knottnerus, A.W. Hoes and N.J. De Wit. 2004. Systematic review: the role of different types of fibre in the treatment of irritable syndrome. Alimentary Pharmacology and Therapeutics, 19: 245–251.

Bisanz, A.K. 2005. Bowel management in patients with cancer. pp. 313–345. *In*: J.A. Ajani, P.M. Lynch, N.A. Janjan and S.A. Curley (eds.). Gastrointestinal Cancer. Springer, New York.

Bocanegra, A., S. Bastida, J. Benedí, S. Ródenas and F.J. Sánchez-Muniz. 2009. Characteristics and nutritional and cardiovascular-health properties of seaweeds. Journal of Medicinal Food, 12: 236–258.

Bonnand-Ducasse, M., G. Della Valle, J. Lefebvre and L. Saulnier. 2010. Effect of wheat dietary fibres on bread dough development and rheological properties. Journal of Cereal Science, 52: 200–206.

Borchani, C., M. Masmoudi, S. Besbes, H. Attia, C. Deroanne and C. Blecker. 2011. Effect of date flesh fiber concentrate addition on dough performance and bread quality. Journal of Texture Studies, 42: 300–308.

Brennan, C.S. and L.J. Cleary. 2007. Utilisation Glucagel (R) in the beta-glucan enrichment of breads: A physicochemical and nutritional evaluation. Food Research International, 40: 291–296.

Brockmole, C.L. and M.E. Zabik. 1976. Wheat bran and middlings in white layer cakes. Journal of Food Science, 41: 357–360.

Burkitt, D.P. 1973. Some diseases characteristic of western civilisation. British Medical Journal, 1: 274–278.

Burton-Freeman, B. 2000. Dietary fiber and energy regulation. Journal of Nutrition, 130: 272S–275S.

Butt, M.S., N. Shahzadi, M.K. Sharif and M. Nasir. 2007. Guar gum: a miracle therapy for hypercholesterolemia, hyperglycemia and obesity. Critical Reviews in Food Science and Nutrition, 47: 389–96.

Cappa, C., M. Lucisano and M. Mariotti. 2013. Influence of Psyllium, sugar beet fibre and water on gluten-free dough properties and bread quality. Carbohydrate Polymers, 98: 1657–1666.

Capriles, V.D. and J.A.G. Areas. 2013. Effects of prebiotic inulin-type fructans on structure, quality, sensory acceptance and glycemic response of gluten-free breads. Food & Function, 4: 104–110.

Cavallero, A., S. Empilli, F. Brighenti and A.M. Stanca. 2002. High ($1\rightarrow3$, $1\rightarrow4$)-beta-glucan barley fractions in bread making and their effects on human glycemic response. Journal of Cereal Science, 36: 59-66.

Chaudhary, V.K. and F.E. Weber. 1990. Barley bran flour evaluated as dietary fiber ingredient in wheat bread. Cereal Foods World, 35: 560–562.

Chen, J., J. He, R.P. Wildman, K. Reynolds, R.H. Streiffer and P.K. Whelton. 2006. A randomized controlled trial of dietary fiber intake on serum lipids. European Journal of Clinical Nutrition, 60: 62–68.

Cheng, H.H. and M.H. Lai. 2000. Fermentation of resistant rice starch produces propionate reduced serum and hepatic cholesterol in rats. Journal of Nutrition, 130: 1991–1995.

Chien, L.Y. and V.H. Potty. 1996. Studies on use of de-aromatised spices as a source of dietary fibre and minerals in bread. Journal of Food Science and Technology-Mysore, 33: 285–290.

Chouinard, L.E. 2011. The role of psyllium fibre supplementation in treating irritable bowel syndrome. Canadian Journal of Dietetic Practice and Research, 72: e107–e114.

Clark, M.J. and J.L. Slavin. 2013. The Effect of Fiber on Satiety and Food Intake: A Systematic Review. Journal of the American College of Nutrition, 32: 200–211.

Collar, C., C.M. Rosell, B. Muguerza and L. Moulay. 2009. Breadmaking performance and keeping behavior of cocoa-soluble fiber-enriched wheat breads. Food Science and Technology International, 15: 79–87.

Collar, C., E. Santos and C.M. Rosell. 2007. Assessment of the rheological profile of fibre-enriched bread doughs by response surface methodology. Journal of Food Engineering, 78: 820–826.

Council Directive of 24 September 1990 (90/496/EEC) relative to nutrition labelling for foodstuffs.

Curti, E., E. Carini, G. Bonacini, G. Tribuzio and E. Vittadini. 2013. Effect of the addition of bran fractions on bread properties. Journal of Cereal Science, 57: 325–332.

Czuchajowska, Z. and Y. Pomeranz. 1993. Gas-formation and gas retention. II. Role of vital gluten during baking of bread from low-protein or fiber-enriched flour. Cereal Foods World, 38: 504–511.

D'Appolonia, B.L. and V.L. Youngs. 1978. Effect of bran and high-protein concentrate from oats on dough properties and bread quality. Cereal Chemistry, 55: 736–743.

Dagnelie, P.C., F.J. Vergote, W.A. van Staveren, H. van den Berg, P.G. Dingjan and J.G. Hautvast. 1991. High prevalence of rickets in infants on macrobiotic diets. American Journal of Clinical Nutrition, 51: 202–208.

Dalgetty, D.D. and B.K. Baik. 2006. Fortification of bread with hulls and cotyledon fibers isolated from peas, lentils, and chickpeas. Cereal Chemistry, 83: 269–274.

Davidson, M.H. and A. McDonald. 1998. Fiber: forms and functions. Nutrition Research, 18: 617–624.

Davy, B.M., C.L. Melby, S.D. Beske, R.C. Ho, L.R. Davrath and K.P. Davy. 2002. Oat consumption does not affect resting casual and ambulatory 24 h arterial blood pressure in men with high-normal blood pressure to stage I hypertension. Journal of Nutrition, 132: 394–398.

De Kock, S., J. Taylor and J.R.N. Taylor. 1999. Effect of heat treatment and particle size of different brans on loaf volume of brown bread. LWT—Food Science and Technology, 32: 349–356.

Dedelahaye, E.P., M. Cedres, A. Alvarado and A. Cioccia. 1994. Wheat bran substitution by defatted palm meal flour in fiber rich cookies and bread elaboration. Archivos Latinoamericanos de Nutricion, 44: 122–128.

Dhinda, F., A.J. Lakshmi, J. Prakash and I. Dasappa. 2012. Effect of ingredients on rheological, nutritional and quality characteristics of high protein, high fibre and low carbohydrate bread. Food and Bioprocess Technology, 5: 2998–3006.

Dikeman, C.L. and G.C.J. Fahey. 2006. Viscosity as related to dietary fiber: A review. Critical Reviews in Food Science and Nutrition, 46: 649–663.

Du, H., D.L. van der A, H.C. Boshuizen, N.G. Forouhi, N.J. Wareham, J. Halkjær, A. Tjønneland, K. Overvad, M.U. Jakobsen, H. Boeing, B. Buijsse, G. Masala, D. Palli, T.I.A. Sørensen, W.H.M. Saris and E.J.M. Feskens. 2010. Dietary fiber and subsequent changes in body weight and waist circumference in European men and women. American Journal of Clinical Nutrition, 91: 329–336.

FDA. 1998. US Department of Health and Human Services. Health claims: soluble fiber from certain foods and coronary heart disease—final rule. Federal Registration, 63: 8103–8121.

FDA. 2008a. Health claims: Fiber-containing grain products, fruits and vegetables and cancer. *In*: Code of Federal Regulations. Food and Drug Administration, Silver Spring, MD, USA, Volume 2.

FDA. 2008b. Health claims: fruits, vegetables, and grain products that contain fiber, particularly soluble fiber, and risk of coronary heart disease. *In*: Code of Federal Regulations. Food and Drug Administration, Silver Spring, MD, USA, Volume 2.

Fernández, M.L. 2001. Soluble fiber and nondigestible carbohydrate effects on plasma lipids and cardiovascular risk. Current Opinion in Lipidology, 12: 35–40.

Filipovic, J., S. Popov and N. Filipovic. 2008. The behavior of different fibers at bread dough freezing. Chemical Industry & Chemical Engineering Quarterly, 14: 257–259.

Filipovic, N., M. Djuric and J. Gyura. 2007. The effect of the type and quantity of sugar-beet fibers on bread characteristics. Journal of Food Engineering, 78: 1047–1053.

Food and Nutrition Board. 2002. Dietary reference intakes for energy, carbohydrates, fiber, fat, protein and amino acids. National Academy of Sciences, Washington, DC.

Frieri, G., M.T. Pimpo and C. Scarpignato. 2006. Management of clonic diverticular disease. Digestion, 73: S58–S66.

Frutos, M.J., L. Guilabert-Anton, A. Tomas-Bellido and J.A. Hernandez-Herrero. 2008. Effect of artichoke (*Cynara scolymus* L.) fiber on textural and sensory qualities of wheat bread. Food Science and Technology International, 14: 49–55.

Gallagher, E., T.R. Gormley and E.K. Arendt. 2004. Recent advances in the formulation of gluten free cereal based products. Trends in Food Science and Technology, 15: 143–152.

Gandra, K.M., M. Del Bianchi, V.P. Godoy, F.P. Collares Queiroz and C.J. Steel. 2008. Application of lipase and monoglyceride in fiber enriched pan bread. Ciencia e Tecnologia de Alimentos, 28: 182–192.

García, A.L., B. Otto, S.C. Reich, M.O. Weickert, J. Steiniger, A. Machowetz, N.N. Rudovich, M. Möhlig, N. Katz, M. Speth, F. Meuser, J. Doerfer, H.J. Zunft, A.H. Pfeiffer and C. Koebnick. 2007. Arabinoxylan consumption decreases postprandial serum glucose, serum insulin and plasma total ghrelin response in subjects with impaired glucose tolerance. European Journal of Clinical Nutrition, 61: 334–341.

Gelinas, P. 2013. Preventing constipation: a review of the laxative potential of food ingredients. International Journal of Food Science and Technology, 48: 445–467.

Ghoshal, G., U.S. Shivhare and U.C. Banerjee. 2013. Effect of xylanase on quality attributes of whole-wheat bread. Journal of Food Quality, 36: 172–180.

Giannini, E.G., C. Mansi, P. Dulbecco and V. Savarino. 2006. Role of partially hydrolysed guar gum in the treatment of irritable bowel syndrome. Nutrition, 22: 334–342.

Ginon, E., Y. Loheac, C. Martin, P. Combris and S. Issanchou. 2009. Effects of fibre information on consumer willingness to pay for French baguettes. Food Quality and Preference, 20: 343–352.

Gomez, A.V., D. Buchner, C.C. Tadini, M.C. Añon and M.C. Puppo. 2013. Emulsifiers: effects on quality of fibre-enriched wheat bread. Food and Bioprocess Technology, 6: 1228–1239.

Gomez, M., S. Jimenez, E. Ruiz and B. Oliete. 2011. Effect of extruded wheat bran on dough rheology and bread quality. LWT—Food Science and Technology, 10: 2231–2237.

Gomez, M., F. Ronda, C.A. Blanco, P.A. Caballero and A. Apesteguia. 2003. Effect of dietary fibre on dough rheology and bread quality. European Food Research and Technology, 216: 51–56.

González-Muñoz, M.J., F.J. Sánchez-Muniz, S. Ródenas, M.I. Sevillano, M.T. Larrea Marín and S. Bastida. 2010. Differences in metal and metalloid content in the hair of normo- and hypertensive postmenopausal women. Hypertension Research, 33: 219–224.

Gray, J. 2006. Dietary fibre: Definition, analysis, physiology and health. International Life Sciences Institute, Brussels.

Guarda, A., C.M. Rosell, C. Benedito and M.J. Galotto. 2004. Different hydrocolloids as bread improvers and antistaling agents. Food Hydrocolloids, 18: 241–247.

Gul, H., M.S. Ozer and H. Dizlek. 2009. Improvement of the wheat and corn bran bread quality by using glucose oxidase and hexose oxidase. Journal of Food Quality, 32: 209–223.

Hager, A.S., C. Axel and E.K. Arendt. 2011a. Status of carbohydrates and dietary fiber in gluten-free diets. Cereal Foods World, 56: 109–114.

Hager, A.S., L.A.M. Ryan, C. Schwab, M.G. Gaenzle, J.V. O'Doherty and E.K. Arendt. 2011b. Influence of the soluble fibres inulin and oat beta-glucan on quality of dough and bread. European Food Research and Technology, 232: 405–413.

Harju, E. 1984. Guar gum benefits duodenal ulcer patients by decreasing gastric acidity and rate of emptying of gastric contents 60 to 120 minutes postprandially. American Surgery, 50: 668–672.

Harrington, M.E., A. Flynn and K.D. Cashman. 2001. Effects of dietary fibre extracts on calcium absorption in the rat. Food Chemistry, 73: 263–269.

Harris, P.J. and L.R. Ferguson. 1993. Dietary fibre: its composition and role in protection against colorectal cancer. Mutation Research/Fundamental and Molecular Mechanisms of Mutagenesis, 290: 97–110.

Hassona, H.Z. 1993. High-fiber bread containing brewers spent grains and its effect on lipid-metabolism in rats. Nahrung-Food, 37: 576–582.

Hellyer, N.E., I. Fraser and J. Haddock-Fraser. 2012. Food choice, health information and functional ingredients: An experimental auction employing bread. Food Policy, 37: 232–245.

Howard, B.V., L. Van horn, J. Hsia, J.E. Manson, M.L. Stefanick, S. Wassetheil-Smoller, L.H. Lewis,Kuller, A.Z. LaCeroix, R.D. Langer, N.L. Lasser, C.E. Lewis, M.C. Limacher, K.L. Margolis, W.J. Mysiw, J.K. Ockene, L.M. Parker, M.G. Perri, L. Philips, R.L. Prentice, J. Robbins, J.E. Rossouw, G.E. Sarto, I.J. Schatz, L.G. Snetselaar, V.J. Stevens, L.F. Tinker, M. Trevisan, M.Z. Vitolins, G.L. Anderson, A.R. Assaf, T. Bassford, S.A.A. Beresford, H.R. Black, R.L. Brunner, R.G. Brzyski, B. Caan, R.T. Chlebowski, M. Gass, I. Granek, P. Greenland, J. Hays, D. Haber, G. Heiss, S.L. Hendrix, A. Hubbell, K.C. Johnson and J.M. Kotchen. 2006. Low-fat dietary pattern and risk of cardiovascular disease: the Women's Health Initiative randomized controlled dietary modification trial. The Journal of American Medical Association, 295: 655–666.

Hudson, C.A., M.M. Chiu and B.E. Knuckles. 1992. Development and characteristics of high-fiber muffins with oat bran, rice bran, or barley fiber fractions. Cereal Foods World, 37: 373–378.

Isken, F., S. Klaus, M. Osterhoff, A.F.H. Pfeiffer and M.O. Weickert. 2010. Effects of long-term soluble vs. insoluble dietary fiber intake on high-fat diet-induced obesity in C57BL/6J mice. The Journal of Nutritional Biochemistry, 21: 278–284.

Izydorczyk, M.S., T.L. Chornick, F.G. Paulley, N.M. Edwards and J.E. Dexter. 2008. Physicochemical properties of hull-less barley fibre-rich fractions varying in particle size and their potential as functional ingredients in two-layer flat bread. Food Chemistry, 108: 561–570.

Jacobs, M.S., M.S. Izydorczyk, K.R. Preston and J.E. Dexter. 2008. Evaluation of baking procedures for incorporation of barley roller milling fractions containing high levels of dietary fibre into bread. Journal of the Science of Food and Agriculture, 88: 558–568.

Jiménez, J.P., J. Serrano, M. Tabernero, S. Arranz, M.E. Díaz-Rubio, L. García-Diz, I. Goñi and F. Saura-Calixto. 2008. Effects of grape antioxidant dietary fiber in cardiovascular disease risk factors. Nutrition, 24: 646–653.

Johnsen, S.P., K. Overvad, C. Stripp, A. Tjonneland, S.E. Husted and H.T. Sorensen. 2003. Intake of fruit and vegetables and the risk of ischemic stroke in a cohort of Danish men and women. American Journal of Clinical Nutrition, 78: 57–64.

Johnson, S.K., P.L. McQuillan, J.H. Sin and M.J. Ball. 2003. Sensory acceptability of white bread with added Australian sweet lupin (*Lupinus angustifolius*) kernel fibre and its glycaemic and insulinaemic responses when eaten as a breakfast. Journal of the Science of Food and Agriculture, 83: 1366–1372.

Jones, P.J., C.A. Leitch and R.A. Pederson. 1993. Meal frequency effects on plasma hormone concentrations and cholesterol synthesis in humans. American Journal of Clinical Nutrition, 57: 868–874.

Kaack, K., L. Pedersen, H.N. Laerke and A. Meyer. 2006. New potato fibre for improvement of texture and colour of wheat bread. European Food Research and Technology, 224: 199–207.

Kaczmarczyk, M.M., M.J. Millier and G.G. Freund. 2012. The health benefits of dietary fiber: Beyond the usual suspects of type 2 diabetes mellitus, cardiovascular disease and colon cancer. Metabolism, 6: 1058–1066.

Kadan, R.S. and B.Q. Phillippy. 2007. Effects of yeast and bran on phytate degradation and minerals in rice bread. Journal of Food Science, 72: C208–C211.

Kahlon, T.S., F.I. Chow, J.L. Hoefer and A.A. Betshart. 1986. Bioavailability of vitamins A and E as influenced by wheat bran and bran particle size. Cereal Chemistry, 63: 490–493.

Kaprelyants, L., S. Fedosov and D. Zhygunov. 2013. Baking properties and biochemical composition of wheat flour with bran and shorts. Journal of the Science of Food and Agriculture, 93: 3611–3616.

Katina, K., R. Juvonen, A. Laitila, L. Flander, E. Nordlund, S. Kariluoto, V. Piironen and K. Poutanen. 2012. Fermented wheat bran as a functional ingredient in baking. Cereal Chemistry, 89: 126–134.

Katina, K., M. Salmenkallio-Marttila, R. Partanen, P. Forssell and K. Autio. 2006. Effects of sourdough and enzymes on staling of high-fibre wheat bread. LWT—Food Science and Technology, 39: 479–491.

Kim, B.K., A.R. Cho, Y.G. Chun and D.J. Park. 2013. Effect of microparticulated wheat bran on the physical properties of bread. International Journal of Food Sciences and Nutrition, 64: 122–129.

Kim, S.C., K.K. Seo, H.W. Kim and M.Y. Lee. 2000. The effects of isolated lipoproteins and triglyceride, combined oxidized low density lipoprotein (LDL) plus triglyceride, and combined oxidized LDL plus high density lipoprotein on the contractile and relaxation response of rabbit cavernous smooth muscle. International Journal of Andrology, 23: 26–29.

Knuckles, B.E., C.A. Hudson, M.M. Chiu and R.N. Sayre. 1997. Effect of beta-glucan barley fractions in high-fiber bread and pasta. Cereal Foods World, 42: 94–99.

Koh-Banerjee, P., M.V. Franz, L. Sampson, S.M. Liu, D.R. Jacobs, D. Spiegelman, W. Willett and E. Rimm. 2004. Changes in whole-grain, bran, and cereal fiber consumption in relation to 8-y weight gain among men. American Journal of Clinical Nutrition, 80: 1237–1245.

Korus, J., K. Grzelak, K. Achremowicz and R. Sabat. 2006. Influence of prebiotic additions on the quality of gluten-free bread and on the content of inulin and fructooligosaccharides. Food Science and Technology International, 6: 489–495.

Korus, J., M. Witczak, R. Ziobro and L. Juszczak. 2009. The impact of resistant starch on characteristics of gluten-free dough and bread. Food Hydrocolloids, 23: 988–995.

Krishnan, P.G., K.C. Chang and G. Brown. 1987. Effect of commercial oat bran on the characteristics and composition of bread. Cereal Chemistry, 64: 55–58.

Lairon, D., N. Arnault, S. Bertrais, R. Planells, E. Clero, S. Hercberg and M.C. Boutron-Ruault. 2005. Dietary fiber intake and risk factors for cardiovascular disease in French adults. American Journal of Clinical Nutrition, 82: 1185–1194.

Larsson, M. and A.S. Sandberg. 1991. Effect of incorporating wheat bran on the rheological characteristics and bread making quality of flour. Journal of Food Science and Technology-Mysore, 28: 92–97.

Lattimer, J.M. and M.D. Haub. 2010. Effects of dietary fiber and its components on metabolic health. Nutrients, 2: 1266–1289.

Lazaridou, A. and C.G. Biliaderis. 2007. Molecular aspects of cereal beta-glucan functionality: Physical properties, technological applications and physiological effects. Journal of Cereal Science, 46: 101–118.

Lazaridou, A., D. Duta, M. Papageorgiou, N. Belc and C. Biliaderis. 2007. Effects of hydrocolloids on dough rheology and bread quality parameters in gluten-free formulations. Journal of Food Engineering, 79: 1033–1047.

Lebesi, D.M. and C. Tzia. 2011. Effect of the addition of different dietary fiber and edible cereal bran sources on the baking and sensory characteristics of cupcakes. Food and Bioprocess Technology, 4: 710–722.

Lee, S., G.E. Inglett and C.J. Carriere. 2004. Effect of nutrim oat bran and flaxseed on rheological properties of cakes. Cereal Chemistry, 81: 637–642.

Levitt, M.D. 2003. Laxative preparation. WO Patent 03/000299.

Majzoobi, M., A. Farahnaky, Z. Nematolahi, M.M. Hashemi and M.J.T. Ardakani. 2013. Effect of different levels and particle sizes of wheat bran on the quality of flat bread. Journal of Agricultural Science and Technology, 15: 115–123.

Mälkki, Y. 2001. Physical properties of dietary fiber as keys to physiological functions. Cereal Foods World, 46: 196–199.

Malnick, S.D.H. and H. Knobler. 2006. The medical complications of obesity. Quarterly Journal of Medicine, 99: 565–579.

Mariani, P., M.G. Viti, M. Montuori, A. La Vecchia, E. Cipolletta, L. Calvani and M. Bonamico. 1998. The gluten-free diet: A nutritional risk factor for adolescents with celiac disease? Journal of Pediatric Gastroenterology and Nutrition, 27: 519–523.

Mariotti, M., M. Lucisano, M.A. Pagani and P.K.W. Ng. 2009. The role of corn starch, amaranth flour, pea isolate, and psyllium flour on the rheological properties and the ultrastructure of gluten-free doughs. Food Research International, 42: 963–975.

Martin, C., H. Chiron and S. Issanchou. 2013. Impact of dietary fiber enrichment on the sensory characteristics and acceptance of french baguettes. Journal of Food Quality, 36: 324–333.

Martínez, M.M., A. Diaz and M. Gómez. 2014. Effect of different microstructural features of soluble and insoluble fibres on gluten-free dough rheology and bread-making. Journal of Food Engineering, 142: 49–56.

Masoodi, F.A. and G.S. Chauhan. 1998. Use of apple pomace as a source of dietary fiber in wheat bread. Journal of Food Processing and Preservation, 22: 255–263.

McEligot, A.J., M. Mouttapa, A. Ziogas and H. Anton-Culver. 2009. Diet and predictors of dietary intakes in women with family history of breast and/or ovarian cancer. Cancer Epidemiology, 33: 419–423.

Merchant, A.T., F.B. Hu, D. Spiegelman, W.C. Willett, E.B. Rimm and A. Ascherio. 2003. Dietary fiber reduces peripheral arterial disease risk in men. Journal of Nutrition, 133: 3658–3663.

Meyer, K.A., L.H. Kushi, D.R. Jacobs, J. Slavin, T.A. Sellers and A.R. Folsom. 2000. Carbohydrates, dietary fiber, and incident type 2 diabetes in older women. American Journal of Clinical Nutrition, 71: 921–930.

Mialon, V.S., M.R. Clark, P.I. Leppard and D.N. Cox. 2002. The effect of dietary fibre information on consumer responses to breads and "English" muffins: a cross-cultural study. Food Quality and Preference, 13: 1–12.

Mildner-Szkudlarz, S., R. Zawirska-Wojtasiak, A. Szwengiel and M. Pacyński. 2011. Use of grape by-product as a source of dietary fibre and phenolic compounds in sourdough mixed rye bread. International Journal of Food Science and Technology, 46: 1485–1493.

Miller, R.A. 2011. Increased yield of bread containing citrus peel fiber. Cereal Chemistry, 88: 174–178.

Mis, A. and D. Dziki. 2013. Extensograph curve profile model used for characterising the impact of dietary fibre on wheat dough. Journal of Cereal Science, 57: 471–479.

Moriartey, S., F. Temelli and T. Vasanthan. 2010. Effect of health information on consumer acceptability of bread fortified with beta-glucan and effect of fortification on bread quality. Cereal Chemistry, 87: 428–433.

Mosharraf, L., M. Kadivar and M. Shahedi. 2009. Effect of hydrothermaled bran on physicochemical, rheological and microstructural characteristics of Sangak bread. Journal of Cereal Science, 49: 398–404.

Mozaffarian, D., S.K. Kumanyika, R.N. Lemaitre, J.L. Olson, G.L. Burke and D.S. Siscovick. 2003. Cereal, fruit and vegetable fibre intake and the risk of cardiovascular disease in elderly individuals. The Journal of American Medical Association, 289: 1659–1666.

Nandeesh, K., R. Jyotsna and G.V. Rao. 2011. Effect of differently treated wheat bran on rheology, microstructure and quality characteristics of soft dough biscuits. Journal of Food Processing and Preservation, 35: 179–200.

Nayak, S.K., P. Pattnaik and A.K. Mohanty. 2000. Dietary fiber: a low-calorie dairy adjunct. Indian Food Industry, 19: 268–271.

Nelles, E.M., P.G. Randall and J.R.N. Taylor. 1998. Improvement of brown bread quality by prehydration treatment and cultivar selection of bran. Cereal Chemistry, 75: 536–540.

Noort, M.W.J., D. van Haaster, Y. Hemery, H.A. Schols and R.J. Hamer. 2010. The effect of particle size of wheat bran fractions on bread quality—Evidence for fibre protein interactions. Journal of Cereal Science, 52: 59–64.

Ostman, E.M., H.G. Liljeberg Elmstahl and I.M. Bjorck. 2002. Barley bread containing lactic acid improves glucose tolerance at a subsequent meal in healthy men and women. Journal of Nutrition, 132: 1173–1175.

Ozboy, O. and H. Koksel. 1999. Utilization of sugar beet fiber in the production of "high fiber bread". Zuckerindustrie, 124: 712–715.

Park, H., P.A. Seib and O.K. Chung. 1997. Fortifying bread with a mixture of wheat fiber and psyllium husk fiber plus three antioxidants. Cereal Chemistry, 74: 207–211.

Pashankar, D.S. and V. Loening-Baucke. 2005. Increased prevalence of obesity in children with functional constipation evaluated in an academic medical center. Pediatrics, 116: e377–e380.

Peppas, G., V.G. Alexiou, E. Mourtzoukou and M.E. Falagas. 2008. Epidemiology of constipation in Europe and Oceania: a systematic review. BMC Gastroenterology, 8: 1–7.

Pereira, M.A. and D.S. Ludwig. 2001. Dietary fiber and bodyweight regulation. Observations and mechanisms. Pediatric Clinics of North America, 48: 969–980.

Perez-Quirce, S., C. Collar and F. Ronda. 2014. Significance of healthy viscous dietary fibres on the performance of gluten-free rice-based formulated breads. International Journal of Food Science and Technology, 49: 1375–1382.

Phimolsiripol, Y., A. Mukprasirt and R. Schoenlechner. 2012. Quality improvement of rice-based gluten-free bread using different dietary fibre fractions of rice bran. Journal of Cereal Science, 56: 389–395.

Pijpers, M.A., M.M. Tabbers, M.A. Benninga and M.Y. Berger. 2009. Currently recommended treatments of childhood constipation are not evidence based: a systematic literature review on the effect of laxative treatment and dietary measures. Archives of Disease in Childhood, 94: 117–131.

Pla, M.D., A.M. Rojas and L.N. Gerschenson. 2013. Effect of butternut (cucurbita moschata duchesne ex poiret) fibres on bread making, quality and staling. Food and Bioprocess Technology, 6: 828–838.

Poinot, P., G. Arvisenet, J. Grua-Priol, C. Fillonneau, A. Le-Bail and C. Prost. 2010. Influence of inulin on bread: Kinetics and physico-chemical indicators of the formation of volatile compounds during baking. Food Chemistry, 119: 1474–1484.

Polaki, A., P. Xasapis, C. Fasseas, S. Yanniotis and I. Mandala. 2010. Fiber and hydrocolloid content affect the microstructural and sensory characteristics of fresh and frozen stored bread. Journal of Food Engineering, 97: 1–7.

Pourfarzad, A., H. Mandavian-Mehr and N. Sedaghat. 2013. Coffee silverskin as a source of dietary fiber in bread-making: Optimization of chemical treatment using response surface methodology. LWT—Food Science and Technology, 50: 599–606.

Praznik, W., E. Cieslik and A. Filipiak-Florkiewicz. 2002. Soluble dietary fibres in Jerusalem artichoke powders: Composition and application in bread. Nahrung-Food, 46: 151–157.

Prentice, N. and B.L. D'Appolonia. 1977. High-fiber bread containing brewer's spent grain. Cereal Chemistry, 54: 1084–1095.

Prior, A. and P.J. Whorwell. 1987. Double blind study of ispaghula in irritable bowel syndrome. Gut, 28: 1510–1513.

Purhagen, J.K., M.E. Sjoo and A.C. Eliasson. 2012. Fibre-rich additives—the effect on staling and their function in free-standing and pan-baked bread. Journal of the Science of Food and Agriculture, 6: 1201–1213.

Quilez, J., M. Zator, J. Salas-Salvado and L. Alvarez. 2013. Different stabilization treatments of rice bran added to wheat flour determine different properties in partially baked wheat bread. Italian Journal of Food Science, 25: 222–228.

Rao, P.H. and H.M. Rao. 1991. Effect of incorporating wheat bran on the rheological characteristics and bread making quality of flour. Journal of Food Science and Technology-Mysore, 28: 92–97.

Regulation (EC) No 1137/2008 of the European Parliament and of the Council of 22 October 2008 adapting a number of instruments subject to the procedure laid down in Article 251 of Treaty to Council Decision 1999/468/EC, with regard to the regulatory procedure with scrutiny.

Regulation (EC) No. 1924/2006 of the European Parliament and of the Council of 20 December 2006 on nutrition and health claims made on foods (OJ L 404, 30.12.2006, p. 9).

Reimer, R.A. and M.I. McBurney. 1996. Dietary fiber modulates intestinal proglucagon messenger ribonucleic acid and postprandial secretion of glucagon-like peptide-1 and insulin in rats. Endocrinology, 137: 3948–3956.

Reimer, R.A., X. Pelletier, I.G. Carabin, M. Lyon, R. Gahler, J.A. Parnell and S. Wood. 2010. Increased plasma PYY levels following supplementation with the functional fiber PolyGlycopleX in healthy adults. European Journal of Clinical Nutrition, 64: 1186–1191.

Rimm, E.B., A. Ascherio, E. Giovannucci, D. Spiegelman, M.J. Stampfer and W.C. Willet. 1996. Vegetable, fruit and cereal fiber intake and risk of coronary heart disease among men. The Journal of the American Medical Association, 275: 447–451.

Roberfroid, M.B. 2007. Inulin-type fructans: functional food ingredients. Journal of Nutrition, 137: S2493–S2502.

Roberton, A.M., L.R. Ferguson, H.J. Hollands and P.J. Harris. 1991. Adsorption of a hydrophobic mutagen to dietary fibre preparations. Mutation Research, 262: 195–202.

Roessle, C., A. Ktenioudaki and E. Gallagher. 2011. Inulin and oligofructose as fat and sugar substitutes in quick breads (scones): a mixture design approach. European Food Research and Technology, 233: 167–181.

Ronda, F., J. Quilez, V. Pando and Y.H. Roos. 2014. Fermentation time and fiber effects on recrystallization of starch components and staling of bread from frozen part-baked bread. Journal of Food Engineering, 131: 116–123.

Rosell, C.M. and E. Santos. 2010. Impact of fibers on physical characteristics of fresh and staled bake off bread. Journal of Food Engineering, 98: 273–281.

Rosell, C.M., J.A. Rojas and C. Benedito de Barber. 2001. Influence of hydrocolloids on dough rheology and bread quality. Food Hydrocolloids, 15: 75–81.

Rosell, C.M., E. Santos and C. Collar. 2006. Mixing properties of fibre-enriched wheat bread doughs: A response surface methodology study. European Food Research and Technology, 223: 333–340.

Rosell, C.M., E. Santos and C. Collar. 2010. Physical characterization of fiber-enriched bread doughs by dual mixing and temperature constraint using the Mixolab®. European Food Research and Technology, 231: 535–544.

Roy, S., H.C. Freake and M.L. Fernandez. 2002. Gender and hormonal status affect the regulation of hepatic cholesterol 7 alpha-hydroxylase activity and mRNA abundance by dietary soluble fiber in the guinea pig. Atherosclerosis, 163: 29–37.

Sabanis, D. and C. Tzia. 2011. Effect of hydrocolloids on selected properties of gluten-free dough and bread. Food Science and Technology International, 17: 279–291.

Sabanis, D., D. Lebesi and C. Tzia. 2009a. Development of fibre-enriched gluten-free bread: a response surface methodology study. International Journal of Food Sciences and Nutrition, 60: 174–190.

Sabanis, D., D. Lebesi and C. Tzia. 2009b. Effect of dietary fibre enrichment on selected properties of gluten-free bread. LWT—Food Science and Technology, 42: 1380–1389.

Salgado, J.M., B.S. Rodrigues, C.M. Donado-Pestana, C.T.D. Dias and M.C. Morzelle. 2011 Cupuassu (*theobroma grandiflorum*) peel as potential source of dietary fiber and phytochemicals in whole-bread preparations. Plant Foods for Human Nutrition, 66: 384–390.

Salinas, M.V. and M.C. Puppo. 2014. Rheological properties of bread dough formulated with wheat flour-organic calcium salts-for-enriched inulin systems. Food and Bioprocess Technology, 7: 1618–1628.

Salmenkallio-Marttila, M., K. Katina and K. Autio. 2001. Effects of bran fermentation on quality and microstructure of high-fiber wheat bread. Cereal Chemistry, 78: 429–435.

Samra, R. and G.H. Anderson. 2007. Insoluble cereal fiber reduces appetite and short-term food intake and glycemic response to food consumed 75 min later by healthy men. American Journal of Clinical Nutrition, 86: 972–979.

Sánchez-Muniz, F.J. 2012. Dietary fibre and cardiovascular health. Nutrición Hospitalaria, 27: 31–45.

Sangnark, A. and A. Noomhorm. 2004. Effect of dietary fiber from sugarcane bagasse and sucrose ester on dough and bread properties. LWT—Food Science and Technology, 37: 697–704.

Santos, E., C.M. Rosell and C. Collar. 2008. Gelatinization and retrogradation kinetics of high-fiber wheat flour blends: a calorimetric approach. Cereal Chemistry, 85: 457–465.

Sanz-Penella, J.M., C. Collar and M. Haros. 2008. Effect of wheat bran and enzyme addition on dough functional performance and phytic acid levels in bread. Journal of Cereal Science, 48: 715–721.

Sanz-Penella, J.M., J.M. Laparra, Y. Sanz and M. Haros. 2012. Influence of added enzymes and bran particle size on bread quality and iron availability. Cereal Chemistry, 89: 223–229.

Sanz-Penella, J.M., J.A. Tamayo-Ramos, Y. Sanz and M. Haros. 2009. Phytate reduction in bran-enriched bread by phytase-producing bifidobacteria. Journal of Agricultural and Food Chemistry, 57: 10239–10244.

Sanz-Penella, J.M., M. Wronkowska, M. Soral-Smietana, C. Collar and M. Haros. 2010. Impact of the addition of resistant starch from modified pea starch on dough and bread performance. European Food Research and Technology, 231: 499–508.

Sapirstein, H.D., S. Siddhu and M. Aliani. 2012. Discrimination of volatiles of refined and whole wheat bread containing red and white wheat bran using an electronic nose. Journal of Food Science, 77: S399–S406.

Schmiele, M., L.Z. Jaekel, S.M.C. Patricio, C.J. Steel and Y.K. Chang. 2012. Rheological properties of wheat flour and quality characteristics of pan bread as modified by partial additions of wheat bran or whole grain wheat flour. International Journal of Food Science and Technology, 47: 2141–2150.

Schneeman, B.O. 1998. Dietary fiber and gastrointestinal function. Nutrition Research, 18: 625–632.

Schulze, M.B., S. Liu, E.B. Rimm, J.E. Manson, W.C. Willett and F.B. Hu. 2004. Glycemic index, glycemic load, and dietary fiber intake and incidence of type 2 diabetes in younger and middle-aged women. American Journal of Clinical Nutrition, 80: 348–356.

Seyer, M.E. and P. Gelinas. 2009. Bran characteristics and wheat performance in whole wheat bread. International Journal of Food Science and Technology, 44: 688–693.

Shafer, M.A.M. and M.E. Zabik. 1978. Dietary fiber sources for baked products—Comparison of wheat brans and other cereal brans in layer cakes. Journal of Food Science, 43: 375–379.

Sharif, K. and M.S. Butt. 2006. Preparation of fiber and mineral enriched pan bread by using defatted rice bran. International Journal of Food Properties, 9: 623–636.

Sharma, H.R. and G.S. Chauhan. 2002. Effects of stabilized rice bran—Fenugreek blends on the quality of breads and cookies. Journal of Food Science and Technology-Mysore, 39: 225–233.

Shenoy, A. and J. Prakash. 2002. Wheat bran (*Triticum aestivum*): Composition, functionality and incorporation in unleavened bread. Journal of Food Quality, 25: 197–211.

Sidhu, J.S., S.N. Al-Hooti and J.M. Al-Saqer. 1999. Effect of adding wheat bran and germ fractions on the chemical composition of high-fiber toast bread. Food Chemistry, 67: 365–371.

Sierra, M., J.J. García, N. Fernández, M.J. Díez, A.P. Calle and A.M. Sahagún. 2001. Effects of ispaghula husk and guar gum on postprandial glucose and insulin concentrations in healthy subjects. European Journal of Clinical Nutrition, 55: 235–243.

Simovic, D.S., N. Filipovic, Z. Seres, J. Gyura, A. Jokic and B. Pajin. 2010. Optimization of the formula of bread enriched with sugar beet fibres. Acta Alimentaria, 39: 488–497.

Sivam, A.S., D. Sun-Waterhouse, G.I.N. Waterhouse, S.Y. Quek and C.O. Perera. 2011. Physicochemical properties of bread dough and finished bread with added pectin fiber and phenolic antioxidants. Journal of Food Science, 76: H97–H107.

Skara, N., D. Novotni, N. Cukelj, B. Smerdel and D. Curic. 2013. Combined effects of inulin, pectin and guar gum on the quality and stability of partially baked frozen bread. Food Hydrocolloids, 30: 428–436.

Skendi, A., C.G. Biliaderis, M. Papageorgiou and M.S. Izydorczyk. 2010. Effects of two barley beta-glucan isolates on wheat flour dough and bread properties. Food Chemistry, 119: 1159–1167.

Slavin, J.L., M.C. Martini, D.R. Jr. Jacobs and L. Marquart. 1999. Plausible mechanisms for the protectiveness of whole grains. American Journal of Clinical Nutrition, 70: 459S–463S.

Sloan, S. and C. James. 1988. Extruded full-fat rice bran in muffins. LWT—Food Science and Technology, 21: 245–247.

Smits, B.J. 1974. The irritable bowel syndrome. Practitioner, 213: 37–46.

Soares, M.S., P.Z. Bassinello, M. Caliari, P.F.C. Gebin, T.D. Junqueira, V.A. Gomes and D.B.C.L. Lacerda. 2009. Quality of breads with toasted rice bran. Ciencia e Tecnologia de Alimentos, 29: 636–641.

Solà, R., G. Godàs, J. Ribalta, J.C. Vallvé, J. Girona, A. Anguera, M. Ostos, D. Recalde, J. Salazar, M. Caslake, F. Martín-Luján, J. Salas-Salvadó and L. Masana. 2007. Effects of soluble fiber (Plantago ovata husk) on plasma lipids, lipoproteins, and apolipoproteins in men with ischemic heart disease. American Journal of Clinical Nutrition, 85: 1157–1163.

Sosulski, F.W. and K.K. Wu. 1988. High-fiber breads containing field pea hulls, wheat, corn, and wild oat brans. Cereal Chemistry, 65: 186–191.

Springsteen, E., M.E. Zabik and M.A.M. Shafer. 1977. Note on layer cakes containing 30 to 70 percent wheat bran. Cereal Chemistry, 54: 193–198.

Stauffer, C.E. 1990. Functional additives for bakery foods. Van Nostrand Reinhold. New York (USA).

Stevens, J., K. Ahn, I. Juhaer, D. Houson, L. Steffan and D. Couper. 2002. Dietary fiber intake and glycemic index and incidence of diabetes in African-American and white adults: the ARIC study. Diabetes care, 25: 1715–1721.

Stojceska, V. and P. Ainsworth. 2008. The effect of different enzymes on the quality of high-fibre enriched brewer's spent grain breads. Food Chemistry, 110: 865–872.

Streppel, M.T., M.C. Ocke, H.C. Boshuizen, F.J. Kok and D. Kromhout. 2008. Dietary fiber intake in relation to coronary heart disease and all-cause mortality over 40 y: The Zutphen Study. American Journal of Clinical Nutrition, 88: 1119–1125.

Tan, K.Y. and F. Seow-Choen. 2007. Fiber and colorectal diseases: separating fact from fiction. World Journal of Gastroenterology, 13: 4161–4167.

Tang, L., F. Xu, T. Zhang, J. Lei, C.W. Binns and A.H. Lee. 2013. Dietary fibre intake associated with reduced risk of oesophageal cancer in Xinjiang, China. Cancer Epidemiology, 37: 893–896.

Thebaudin, J.Y., A.C. Legebvre, M. Hrrington and C.M. Bourgeois. 1997. Dietary fibres: nutritional and technological interest. Trends in Food Science and Technology, 8: 41–48.

Tiwari, U. and E. Cummins. 2009. Factors influencing beta-glucan levels and molecular weight in cereal-based products. Cereal Chemistry, 86: 290–301.

Tiwari, U., E. Cummins, N. Brunton, C. O'Donnell and E. Gallagher. 2013. A comparison of oat flour and oat bran-based bread formulations. British Food Journal, 115: 300–313.

Trautwein, E.A., A. Kunath-Rau and H.F. Erberdsobler. 1999. Increased fecal bile acid excretion and changes in the circulating bile acid pool are involved in the hypocholesterolemic and gallstone-preventive actions of psyllium in hamsters. Journal of Nutrition, 129: 896–902.

Tuncel, N.B., N. Yilmaz, H. Kocabiyik and A. Uygur. 2014a. The effect of infrared stabilized rice bran substitution on physicochemical and sensory properties of pan breads: Part I. Journal of Cereal Science, 59: 155–161.

Tuncel, N.B., N. Yilmaz, H. Kocabiyik and A. Uygur. 2014b. The effect of infrared stabilized rice bran substitution on B vitamins, minerals and phytic acid content of pan breads: Part II. Journal of Cereal Science, 59: 162–166.

Turabi, E., G. Sumnu and S. Sahin. 2008. Rheological properties and quality of rice cakes formulated with different gums and an emulsifier blend. Food Hydrocolloids, 22: 305–312.

USDA. 2005. Department of Agriculture, US Department of Health and Human Services. Dietary Guidelines for Americans USDA, Washington, DC.

Van Dokkum, W. 1992. Significance of iron bioavailability from iron recommendations. Biological Trace Element Research, 35: 1–11.

Voderholzer, W.A., W. Schatke, B.E. Mühldorfer, A.G. Klauser, B. Birkner and S.A. Müller-Lissner. 1997. Clinical response to dietary fiber treatment of chronic constipation. American Journal of Gastroenterology, 92: 95–98.

Vuksan, V., J.L. Sievenpiper, R. Owen, J.A. Swilley, P. Spadafora, K.L. Jenkins, E. Vidgen, F. Brighenti, R.G. Josse, L.A. Leiter, Z. Xu and R. Novokmet. 2000. Beneficial effects of viscous dietary fibre from Konjac-mannan in subjects with the insulin resistance syndrome: results of a controlled metabolic trial. Diabetes Care, 23: 9–14.

Wang, J.S., C.M. Rosell and C.B. de Barber. 2002. Effect of the addition of different fibres on wheat dough performance and bread quality. Food Chemistry, 79: 221–226.

Weickert, M.O., J. Spranger, J. Holst, B. Otto, C. Koebnick and M. Möhlig. 2006. Wheat-fibre-induced changes of postprandial peptide YY and ghrelin responses are not associated with acute alterations of satiety. British Journal of Nutrition, 96: 795–798.

Weickert, M.O., M. Mohlig, C. Koebnick, J.J. Holst, P. Namsolleck, M. Ristow, M. Osterhoff, H. Rochlitz, N. Rudovich, J. Spranger and A.F. Pfeiffer. 2005. Impact of cereal fibre on glucose-regulating factors. Diabetologia, 48: 2343–2353.

Wild, D., G.G. Robins, V.J. Burley and P.D. Howdle. 2010. Evidence of high sugar intake, and low fibre and mineral intake, in the gluten-free diet. Alimentary Pharmacology & Therapeutics, 32: 573–581.

Wu, H., K.M. Dwyer, Z. Fan, A. Shircore, J. Fan and J.H. Dwyer. 2003. Dietary atherosclerosis study. American Journal of Clinical Nutrition, 78: 1085–1091.

Yeo, L.L. and P.A. Seib. 2009. White pan bread and sugar-snap cookies containing wheat starch phosphate. A cross-linked resistant starch. Cereal Chemistry, 86: 210–220.

Zhang, Z., G. Xu, M. Ma, J. Yang and X. Liu. 2013. dietary fiber intake reduces risk for gastric cancer: a meta-analysis. Gastroenterology, 14: 113–120.

Ziobro, R., J. Korus, L. Juszczak and T. Witczak. 2013. Influence of inulin on physical characteristics and staling rate of gluten-free bread. Journal of Food Engineering, 116: 21–27.

15

Traditional Bread in Arab Countries...Key of Nutrition

Aly F. El Sheikha[1,2]

1. Introduction

Traditional foods constitute an essential aspect of people's cultural heritage, historical background and their environmental conditions. In addition, traditional foods represent an important component of people's diet and are very much related to their food habits and nutrition. During the last decades, the high rate of urbanization, labor migration and the increase in income have affected the life-styles of the population of the Arabic countries and resulted in an extensive increase in food import. This led to a high reduction in the consumption of traditional foods (Jönsson 2010).

It is hard to put a clear cut division between traditional and non-traditional foods, especially with the great change in the food situation in Arabic countries. Some traditional foods (e.g., bread) in Arabic countries have a high nutritive value and therefore can play an important role in providing essential nutrients. They can also supplement the main dishes and improve the nutritional composition of a meal (Musaiger 1993).

This chapter highlights the bread as one of the famous Arabic traditional foods and includes the methods of preparation and nutritive value. It is hoped that this chapter will be a useful publication for those interested in the field of nutrition and health.

[1] Minufiya University, Faculty of Agriculture, Department of Food Science and Technology, 32511 Shibin El Kom, Minufiya Government, Egypt.
[2] Al-Baha University, Faculty of Science, Department of Biology, P.O. Box 1988, Al-Baha, Saudi Arabia.
   Email: elsheikha_aly@yahoo.com

2. Bread in Arab countries......Means What For Them?

Arabs, the majority people in the Middle East, eat bread with every meal. In tradition and in daily life, bread is held to be a divine gift from God. The Egyptians call bread "Aysh" which means "life itself." In the Arab world, if a piece of bread falls on the floor, a person will pick it up and kiss it, then eat it. I used to see this happen at home when my mother dropped a piece of bread on the floor, not allowing it to be thrown away with the garbage. The Arabs claim that they cannot taste other foods without bread and the bread types they have to choose from are numerous and varied.[1]

2.1 In the past

The Spanish picked up this habit from the Arabs during their long stay in the Iberian Peninsula. In Spain, when a piece of bread falls on the floor, in the Arab fashion they will say: "Es pan de Dios" (in Arabic, 'aysh Allah means God's bread).[1]

Bread is pyramid builders' diet

The builders of the famous Giza pyramids in Egypt feasted on food from a massive catering-type operation, the remains of which scientists have discovered at a workers' town near the pyramids. The workers' town is located about 1,300 feet (400 meters) south of the Sphinx, and was used to house workers building the pyramid of pharaoh Menkaure, the third and last pyramid on the Giza plateau. The site is also known by its Arabic name, *Heit el-Ghurab*, and is sometimes called "the Lost City of the Pyramid Builders".[2]

How did the ancient Egyptians feed thousands of workers at Giza? and What kind of bread did the pyramid builders eat? We know from ancient texts that a staple diet of bread is one of the principal components of the diet for pyramid builders. The bakeries are the archaeological counterparts of the bakeries depicted in many scenes and limestone models from Old Kingdom (2575–2134 BC) tombs. The tomb scenes indicate that bread baking and beer brewing were part of the same production process, probably because lightly baked dough (in which the yeast was activated but not killed by the heat) was used for the beer mash. Froth from the beer may have gone back into the dough. Fragments of the large, bell-shaped bread pots like those we see in the tomb scenes litter the Lost City in the hundreds of thousands. Labeled bedja in the tomb scenes, the largest weigh up to 12 kilograms each (26.5 pounds) (Fig. 1). Evidence discovered from Elephantine Island in southern Egypt all the way to Palestine indicates that bread baking in bedja was a common and wide-spread practice for nearly 500 years.[3]

Low, stone walls surrounded the two bakeries, which were filled with homogenous black ash under a layer of mud brick tumble. Opposite the southern entrance to each

---

[1] http://www.backwoodshome.com/articles2/salloum135.html

[2] http://www.livescience.com/28961-ancient-giza-pyramid-builders-camp-unearthed.html

[3] http://www.aeraweb.org/lost-city-project/feeding-pyramid-workers/

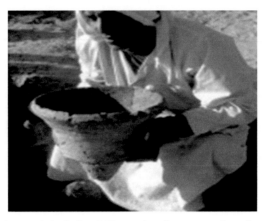

Figure 1. Large, crude ceramic bedja bread (Source: http://www.aeraweb.org/lost-city-project/feeding-pyramid-workers/).

bakery, large ceramic vats were embedded in the floor of the northwest corner. The ancient bakers had broken the bottoms of these vats, possibly by kneading the dough with their feet, but they continued using the vats by reinforcing them with pieces of limestone and granite. Marl clay floors were packed around the vats up to more than half their height, which would have made it difficult and tiring for the bakers to bend over their vats to do their work. It is possible that someone actually stood in the vats to mix the contents with their feet (Fig. 2).

All details concerned the historical backgrounds worldwide of bread were discussed before in Chapter 1 in this book (Aly F. El Sheikha).

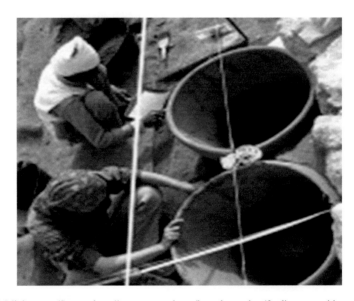

Figure 2. Mixing vats (Source: http://www.aeraweb.org/lost-city-project/feeding-pyramid-workers/).

2.2 In the present

People in Arab countries have always relied on bread as a low-cost source of sustenance. In Egypt, bread is known as aish, meaning "life". It is the inseparable companion of all dishes, even some desserts. The Fertile Crescent, stretching from the Egyptian Nile to the mouth of the Tigris and Euphrates, is where agriculture began, where wheat, lentils, chickpeas, sheep and goats and olives were first cultivated. Today, that same region is the largest importer of food in the world. The average per capita per day consumption of breads in different Arab Gulf and Mediterranean countries has been reported to be 355 g in Saudi Arabia (Al-Mohizea et al. 1995), 277 g in Kuwait (Eid and Bourisly 1986), 548, 444, 438 and 419 g in Libya, Egypt, Algeria and Morocco respectively (Pomeranz 1988).

Bread in the Arab spring

"Bread riots" have been occurring regularly since the mid-1980s, following policies brought to us by the World Bank and the International Monetary Fund. Among these were the reduction of agricultural subsidies and the encouragement of production of fruits and vegetables for export, at the expense of investing in local grain production. Export of value-added produce and the import of basic commodities such as wheat were monopolized by a small group of "entrepreneurs" protected by the security state who financially backed the ruling elite. The powerful countries provided encouragement and support. The US gave Egypt around $1.7 bn in 2010, exceeded only by the $2.4 bn it gave to Israel. Tunisia under President Ben Ali was viewed as the IMF model of "growth" and France offered to support him militarily through the uprising.

The first protests of the Arab spring in Tunisia in December 2010 were quickly dismissed as another bout of bread riots. Arab regimes responded by making adjustments to food prices and offering more subsidies. Increasing the subsidy slightly relieves the popular pressure but also increases the profit margins for importers and manufacturers. But this time round, truckloads of flour did not do the trick.[4]

Figure 3 is the best description of the new liberty in Arab spring as the Egyptian protesters said "We have tasted the bread of liberty and we want more of it".

3. In Arab world: bread between traditions and nutrition

Bread is highly regarded in the Arab world. If anybody notices a scrap of bread on the street, they would pick it up and put on the side where no one can step on it accidentally. Bread is an essential ingredient on the table in the Arabic cuisine. It is used on the side, in salads, or in certain dishes such as the "fatteh".

The traditional way of baking Middle Eastern bread is in highly heated brick ovens, with the loaves being slid into the ovens with wooden paddles (Fig. 4). Of course, the making of Middle Eastern bread in the modern countries of the Middle

---

[4] http://www.theguardian.com/lifeandstyle/2011/jul/17/bread-food-arab-spring

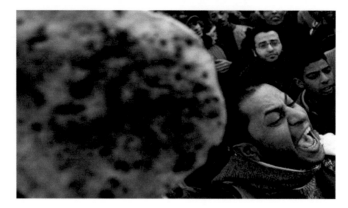

Figure 3. Egyptian protesters said "We have tasted the bread of liberty and we want more of it".

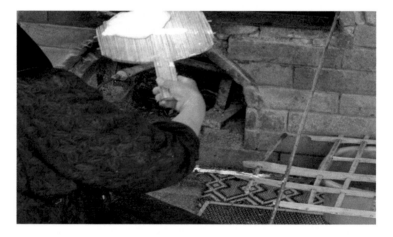

Figure 4. Woman slid the traditional Arab loaf into highly heated brick ovens with wooden paddle.

East and in North America is an automated process, from the flour to the piping hot bread. Today, in most cities and towns in the Middle East and in the major urban centers in both North and South America people usually buy pita bread commercially produced from Mediterranean and Middle Eastern bakeries and stores bypassing the work needed to make the bread. However, even though it takes time and energy to make your own homemade Middle Eastern breads, it can be one of your most exciting cooking experiences. The aroma coming from the kitchen, the delicious taste of bread fresh from the oven, and, above all, the pleasure you feel when you bake homemade bread are well worth the work involved. Just think of the mouth-watering aroma flowing out of the oven, especially from thyme-topped bread filling the room. It's an atmosphere one rarely forgets.[1]

3.1 Bread in Saudi Arabia

The people of Saudi Arabia are descended from tribes of nomadic sheep and goat herders and maintain many of the traditions of their past. Traditional foods like "fatir" (flat bread), and "arikah" (bread from the southwestern part of the country) are still eaten by Saudis today, although most Saudis have settled in towns and cities and no longer follow the nomadic lifestyle. Saudi Arabia is also home to Mecca, the origin and spiritual center of Islam. The culture, as well as the laws of Saudi Arabia, is founded on Islamic principles, including the dietary restrictions against eating pork or drinking alcohol.

In Saudi Arabia, cereals contribute 41 and 40 percent of the total available food energy and protein in the diet respectively. Wheat being the most commonly used for bread making, forms 64 percent of the total available cereals and per caput availability increased over 56 percent while other cereals like millet, sorghum, corn, etc. decreased by 64 percent during a period of one decade (Khan and Al-Kanhal 1998).

3.1.1 Saudi breads in traditional view

Millet Bread (Khoubez Al-Dokhn). Millet is a traditional cereal for a large sector of the inhabitants in the Northern and Southern regions of Saudi Arabia. Millet is used to prepare special bread (Khoubez Al-Dokhn). This bread is only prepared in the home.

The millet grains are ground in a stone mill. The flour mixed with salt and water kneaded by hand for 15–20 min. The prepared dough is set for 1 hr for fermentation. Pieces of about 300 g each one are separated, rounded and flattened with the palm of the hand. The leaves are baked in earthen oven at about 300°C for 15 min (Musaiger 1993).

Wheat Bread (Khoubez Samouli). Samouli bread is commonly consumed in Saudi Arabia. It is oblong in shape with varying sizes. It is usually consumed at breakfast or used for the preparation of sandwiches.

Samouli bread is prepared from a proportion of 1:2 of wheat flours of extraction rates 75 percent and 85 percent respectively. The flour is mixed with water, active dry yeast and salt for 15 min. The dough is allowed bulk fermentation for 30 min. The dough is then moulded and fermented in trays on which oil is spread. It is baked at 200–225°C for 20 min. The final product has a brown crust and a white crumb. The average weight of the small size loaf is 107 g (Musaiger 1993).

Khoubez Tannouri. Tannouri, or so called Iranian bread, is one of the most popular breads in Saudi Arabia. It is also commonly consumed in Bahrain, Qatar, Kuwait and the UAE. This bread has become one of the common breads consumed at breakfast and dinner.

It is prepared by dissolving yeast (0.12 g), salt (1.3 g) and sodium bicarbonate (0.3 g) in (55 g) water. The flour (100 g) is then added and mixed for 15 min. The dough obtained is cut into pieces, rounded, flattened and baked at 400–500°C in earthen oven for 30 to 60 sec.

3.1.2 Saudi breads in nutritional view

Tables 1 and 2 show the proximate composition, mineral and vitamin contents of various breads in Saudi Arabia. The contribution of calories from protein, fat and carbohydrates in various breads is given in Table 3.

Table 1. Proximate composition (wet basis) of Saudi breads.

Breads	g/100 g						Kcal/100 g
	Moisture	Protein (N X 5.7)	Fat	Available carbohydrates	Dietary fiber	Ash	Energy
Millet bread	43.3	8.1	1.9	40.2	5.7	2.4	202
Wheat breads							
Khoubez Samouli	32.1	9.2	1.4	54.8	2.7	1.1	267
Khoubez Tannouri	29.5	8.8	1.2	58.5	2.3	1.9	266
Tamees	29.4	8.7	2.3	56.3	2.3	1.4	281
Mafroud	26.4	9.4	0.9	60.6	2.1	0.6	288
Burr	31.9	9.1	0.4	52.9	4.8	1.0	252

Source: Adapted from Musaiger 1993; Al-Kanhal et al. 1999.

Table 2. Mineral and vitamin contents (wet basis) of Saudi breads.

Breads	mg/100 g								mg RE/100 g
	Ca	P	Na	K	Fe	Zn	Thiamin	Riboflavin	Vitamin A
Millet bread	23	250	102	198	7.8	1.0	0.02	0.13	122
Wheat breads									
Khoubez Samouli	38	320.8	304.3	101.4	2.5	0.9	0.07	0.04	ND*
Khoubez Tannouri	24.9	103.4	83.2	115.4	3.6	0.9	0.08	0.03	145
Tamees	3.5	86.4	794.6	0.7	1.8	ND	0.18	0.02	145
Mafroud	2.2	41.9	207.7	67.2	1.9	ND	0.01	0.04	45
Burr	3.3	173.4	393.6	224.2	2.9	ND	0.14	0.13	135

* ND = Not determined.
Source: Adapted from Musaiger 1993; Al-Kanhal et al. 1999.

Table 3. Food energy adequacy in Saudi breads.

Breads	Percent food energy (kcal)		
	Protein	Fat	Carbohydrates
Millet bread	15	8	77
Wheat breads			
Khoubez Samouli	13	5	82
Khoubez Tannouri	13	3	84
Tamees	12	7	81
Mafroud	13	3	84
Burr	14	2	84

Source: Adapted from Al-Kanhal et al. 1999.

3.2 Bread in Yemen

Yemen imports annually about 90 percent of its needs of wheat grains mainly for breadmaking and other bakery products. Milling of wheat grains take place in a local national milling plant situated in Aden (commercial capital of Rep. of Yemen) an international well known seaport as well as in another city which is considered the next seaport of Yemen (Al-Hoddidah) (Al-Mussali and Al-Gahri 2009).

3.2.1 Yemeni breads in traditional view

In Yemen alone there are more than 20 different kinds of bread, each made and baked differently. Bread has always been considered the staple food of choice in Yemen. Bread is consumed here at higher ratios than in other countries. It is reported that the amount of daily consumption ranged from 250–320 g per capita according to the imported quality of wheat (Al-Mussali 2004; Al-Mussali et al. 2007).

Bread is present at the table during all three main meals of the day as a main diet consumed either with fish, meat, mixed vegetables and legumes by the majority of Yemen people and present twice in few governorates, that use rice as a third meal, especially whose living in the coastal regions of the country. White wheat flour with about 90 percent is used for breadmaking of different kinds of bread in Yemen.

There are mainly five milling plants with a milling daily total capacity of about 7000 Mt of grains producing about 90 percent of their production white wheat flour with about 75 percent of extraction rate. There are several kinds of bread produced in Yemen. The most commonly consumed bread in Aden, Al-Hoddidah and other governorates throughout the country are pan bread, French type bread, flat bread, sliced bread (produced in bakeries) and the fifth one produced in public restaurants using earthen ovens for baking it which is named 'Mulwah' a flat unleavened bread with a diameter ranged 30–50 cm (Al-Mussali and Al-Gahri 2009).

Khoubez Yemeni. It is circular single layered bread and is made from wheat flour. This bread is prepared from wheat flour, salt, yeast and water. A proportion of 1:2 of flours of extraction rates 75 percent and 85 percent respectively are used. For preparation, the flour is first mixed with water. Other ingredients are then added, and mixed well for 15 min. The dough is then allowed to undergo bulk fermentation for 45 to 60 min. The dough is then cut into small pieces, rounded, flattened and baked at 450–550°C for 15 sec. The average weight of the final loaf is about 190 g (Musaiger 1993).

3.2.2 Yemeni breads in nutritional view

There is paucity of information on the nutritive composition of breads produced in Yemen. Therefore, our chapter put spotlight on the macronutrients and minerals available in the main popular breads commonly consumed all over the country, produced from wheat grains milled locally from the well-known national milling plants located in different main cities and their products distributed throughout Yemen.

The proximate composition and mineral contents of various breads in Yemen are given in Tables 4 and 5.

Table 4. Proximate composition of various Yemen breads.

Breads	Moisture	Protein	Fat	Ash	Carbohydrates	Energy
	(%)					(kcal/100 g)
Al-Mulwah bread	28.4	9.9	3.9	0.98	56.1	302
Khoubez Yemeni	31.6	10.1	0.3	0.80	56.8	270
Pan bread	32.4	11.2	1.8	0.79	53.6	276

Source: Adapted from Musaiger 1993; Al-Mussali and Al-Gahri 2009.

Table 5. Mineral contents of various Yemen breads.

Breads	Na	K	Mg	Mn	Cu	Fe	Zn
	mg/100 g						
Al-Mulwah bread	479.2	97.5	34.8	0.3	0.1	1.9	0.9
Khoubez Yemeni	112	ND*	ND	ND	ND	2.5	1.2
Pan bread	140.6	105.9	38.1	0.3	0.2	7.1	0.8

* ND = Not determined.
Source: Adapted from Musaiger 1993; Al-Mussali and Al-Gahri 2009.

3.3 Bread in Oman

Wheat and rice are the two staple foods in Oman (MNE 2006). Wheat is mainly consumed in the form of bread. Bread is a type of food which is made from cereal grains (mainly wheat) that have been ground into flour or meal, moistened with water, kneaded into dough, and then backed. The other ingredients which may be added to bread include milk, fat, eggs, salt and sugars (Samuel 2001).

3.3.1 Omani breads in traditional view

Bread has always been considered not only as the core component of diet of both rich and poor, but also for its versatile role in health and disease (Räsänen 2007). Together with various modern types of breads, some traditionally baked breads are also present in the local Omani markets.

In Oman, the breads are commonly consumed in a variety of ways and are served almost at all three meal times—breakfast, lunch and dinner—whereas the rice is mainly served at lunch time. Based on family purchases, Lebanese bread (Khubz Lebanani) is the most commonly consumed bread as compared to other types found in Oman. No exact quantification is however available on the consumption of these breads by Omani population (Ali et al. 2010).

Chapati. Unlike the chapati of the Indian-subcontinent, the chapati in the Gulf (e.g., Oman) mostly refers to unleavened bread made with oil. Chapati is generally produced and consumed fresh in home and restaurants. There are no bakeries preparing such bread. This bread is mainly prepared by Indian-subcontinent immigrants and commonly eaten with Indian dishes, which are popular in the Gulf.

Chapati is prepared by mixing 100 g of wheat flour with 55 g water and 0.7 g salt until a dough of firm consistency is formed. The dough is then cut into small pieces, rounded, flattened and grilled on a greased griddle over a stove at 183–205°C. The bread is turned over, after one side has been baked for 5 min. The final product is circular, one layered loaf, with an average weight of 82 g. Chapati is best eaten warm (Musaiger 1993).

3.3.2 Omani breads in nutritional view

The proximate composition of various breads in Sultanate of Oman is given in Table 6.

Table 6. Proximate composition of various Oman breads.

Breads	Moisture	Protein	Fat	Ash	Crude fiber	Energy
			(%)			(kcal/100 g)
Chapati	27.3	10.5	3.9	2.3	1.5	285
Rekhal	21.6	10.1	4.9	2.3	1.7	322
Goleh	51.4	4.3	6.6	1.9	1.2	214
Paratha	25.7	8.1	13.8	1.9	1.9	350

Source: Adapted from Musaiger 1993; Ali et al. 2010.

3.4 Bread in United Arab Emirates (UAE)

The daily consumption of bread is a deeply rooted tradition in many societies, including those in the UAE, as it is a main component of most meals. Some traditional bread is prepared at home daily. In addition, commercial breads are bought from local bakeries (Almousa et al. 2013).

3.4.1 UAE breads in traditional view

Khoubez Al-Rigag. Al-Rigag is traditional bread usually prepared at home by some families. People purchase it directly from home or from local market (which in turn depends on home preparation). Recently some modern bakeries began producing Al-Rigag but on a small scale, because its consumption remains limited to a few social occasions. Al-Rigag is especially eaten at the Muslim fasting month, Ramadan (Musaiger 1993).

Al-Rigag is thin, unleavened bread, the batter of which comprises flour (70 percent whole-meal flour with 30 percent white flour), salt and water, and is cooked on a hot metallic surface (Almousa et al. 2013). The flour is mixed with salt and water until a loose consistency elastic dough is formed. A handful of dough is then spread (in very thin layer) by hand on the top of an iron pan (Tawah). When the edges of the dough start drying, and lifting from the pan surface, the bread is removed by a knife and folded in half or in quarters. Sometimes an egg, some sugar and cardamom are added to the dough when it is on the pan. This sweet bread is commonly eaten with tea or at Sahoor (the meal before sunrise in Ramadan). Traditionally, dried palm leaves (khouse) are burnt to heat the pan. More recently, families are using modern gas burners (Musaiger 1993).

Chbab. Chbab is made by combining flour (50 percent white flour and 50 percent whole-meal flour), water, egg, sugar, vegetables oil and yeast. The batter is very thin due to the large amount of water used. It is baked by pouring the batter on a hot flat pan, and vegetable oil is added at the last stage of cooking to the top of the bread to brown the surface. This bread is well known because of its surface, which is full of air bubbles similar to the ones in pancakes (Almousa et al. 2013).

Khameer. It is prepared by mixing flour (100 percent white flour) with eggs, yeast, sugar, vegetable oil and ghee, and proving the dough in a warm place until the volume increases (yeast effect). Flat portions are formed; the surface covered with egg yolk and sesame, and it is baked on a flat pan (Almousa et al. 2013).

3.4.2 UAE breads in nutritional view

The nutrient compositions of traditional UAE breads are presented as a percentage of each composition in 100 g of the total bread weight (Table 7).

Table 7. Nutrient compositions of traditional UAE breads.

Breads	Moisture	Protein	Fat	Ash	Carbohydrates	Crude fiber	Energy
	(%)						(kcal/100 g)
Khoubez Al-Rigag	6.5	13.1	2.8	2.8	0.7	79.8	372
Chbab bread	39.2	1.8	8.4	2.5	0.5	47.6	273
Khameer bread	22.7	9.9	10.6	2.2	0.3	54.2	352

Source: Adapted from Musaiger 1993; Almousa et al. 2013.

3.5 Bread in Egypt

3.5.1 Egyptian breads in traditional view

A kind of rare tradition is also found in the Egyptian Coptic Church. Holy bread, called Qurban, is distributed after the service in the church. Qurban bread is round, decorated with a cross in the middle that is surrounded by twelve dots. The dots represent the twelve disciples of Jesus. It is very common for people visiting each other after mass to offer some and normally it can never be refused.[5]

In Upper Egypt, the traditionally baked bread is "Aysh Nashif" dry bread. These are huge, thin cracker-like round loaves that are easily stored for weeks in the dry climate of Upper Egypt. Once the dough has been made, it is rolled very thinly and then expertly placed on a long baton and placed in the oven. The technology is well-suited to the arid, and fuel wood-scarce area of Upper Egypt, for not only does the oven use the leavings of crops for fuel, but it also ably conserves the heat.

---

[5] http://www.touregypt.net/featurestories/copticchristians.htm

Bread-baking techniques were similar during British colonial times. Leeder (1918) described dry bread loaves as:

> *… Her great day is that of bread-making. All the women of a family are called to this task, for what with sifting the flour, mixing the leaven, and laboriously kneading the dough for the two to three hours which she thinks necessary, and then baking the many small loaves in her mud-oven, there is great activity.*
>
> *Such belief has the people in the medicinal virtues of helba [fenugreek seeds], of which I shall speak elsewhere, that she adds to her labor by pounding the seeds of this plant to mix in the bread.*
>
> *The native bread is a flat round cake, of a dusky color, very like a large stone: reminding us of Scripture again—"If a son shall ask bread … will ye give him a stone?" A piece of bread, with pickled turnip and a taste of salted curd, often makes a meal.*
>
> *I have sometimes seen the children eating this bread merely dipped in syrup, though vegetables are so cheap that it is rare not to be able to afford the relish of raw carrots, radishes, tomatoes, onions, and the tiny cucumber which is grown so abundantly in Egypt.*
>
> *In the hot weather every one eats the cucumber; indeed, without a dish of these cool and refreshing vegetables the people would often not eat at all.*
>
> *I have in other parts of the country eaten cakes with the whole seeds of sesame sprinkled thickly on the top…*

Figure 5 shows Coptic family eating bread with some onions or cucumbers, and water in an "Ulla" (clay bottle).

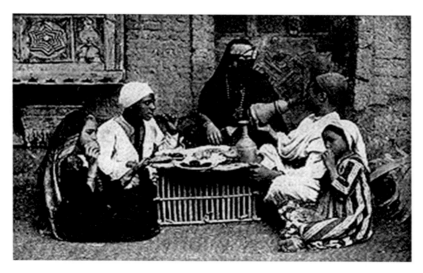

Figure 5. Bread, eaten by Coptic family with some onions or cucumbers, and water in an "Ulla" (clay bottle) (Source: Leeder 1918).

3.5.2 Egyptian breads in nutritional view

Fifty per cent of the calories consumed by Egyptians originate outside its borders. Egypt is the world's largest wheat importer, and no country in the region (except for Syria) produces more than a small fraction of the wheat it consumes. Should the global markets be unable to provide a country's need, or if there are not enough funds available to finance purchases and to offer price support, then the food of the poor will become inaccessible to them. Already, in Egypt, more than 40 percent of the population live below the poverty line and suffer from some form of malnutrition. Most of the poor in these countries have no access to social safety nets.[4]

Alian et al. (1997) determined the chemical content of balady (Egyptian bread) made of wholewheat flour and with flour of 72 percent extraction rate. They concluded in their results that balady bread contains moisture (33–34 percent), protein (11.8–11.9 percent), fat (2.53–2.55 percent), crude fiber (3.62–3.93 percent), ash (2.63–2.98 percent) and carbohydrate (78.91–78.98 percent). This is produced from wholewheat flour, but these nutrients obtained from white wheat flour of 72 percent extraction were in the range of 32–33 percent of moisture, 11.58–11.65 percent of protein, 1.4–1.6 percent of fat, 0.87–0.95 percent of crude fiber, 1.67–1.81 percent of ash and 84.1–84.2 percent of carbohydrates.

The micronutrients analyzed for the same study for balady bread ranged from 3.5–4.1 mg/100 g of Mn, 167–1751 mg/100 g of Mg, 2.20–3.04 mg/100 g of Zinc, 0.49–0.56mg/100 g of Cu, 30–321 mg/100 g of Ca and 310–3401 mg/100 g of phosphorus which were made from wholewheat flour, but the same nutrients were on the range of 2.25–2.51 mg/100 g of Mn, 126–1421 mg/100 g of Mg, 1.58–2.1 mg/100 g of Zinc, 0.42–0.421 mg/100 g of Cu, 21–221 mg/100 g of Ca and 190–2201 mg/100 g of phosphorus for the same balady bread made of white wheat flour of 72 percent extraction.

3.6 Other types of bread originated in the Arab world

3.6.1 Date bread (Khoubez Al-Tamer)

Khoubez al-tamer is commonly consumed in the Arabian Gulf countries. The date bread is baked in a special clay oven built in the ground and is often consumed with a traditional sweet (halwah), and Arabic coffee, during weddings, religious ceremonies, and other social occasions. Consumption of this kind of bread is on the decrease and few local bakeries still produce it.

Wheat flour, dates and/or date syrup (dibs), sugar, active dry yeast and water are the main ingredients used in the preparation of khoubez al-tamer. Sometimes sesame seeds are spread over the bread. For preparation, the sugar is dissolved in water, and then flour, dates and yeast are added. The ingredients are mixed well until dough of good consistency is formed. The dough is then cut into pieces, flattened and baked at 400°C in an earth clay oven until brown (Musaiger 1993).

This kind of bread is high in energy and minerals compared with other breads, due to the use of dates and date syrup (Table 8).

Table 8. Nutritional value of other types of bread originated to the Arab world.

I. Date bread (Khoubez Al-Tamer)							
Proximate composition (g/100 g edible portion)	Moisture	Protein	Fat	Ash	Carbohydrates	Crude fiber	Energy (kcal/100 g)
	22.4	8.8	1.9	1.2	0.5	65.2	307
Mineral composition (mg/100 g edible portion)	Ca		P	Na	Fe		Zn
	5.8		75	116	1.8		8.4
II. Sorghum bread (Khoubez Al-Thorah)							
Proximate composition (g/100 g edible portion, expressed on dry weight basis)	ND*	16.4	4.9	2.2	2.9	73.6	ND
Mineral composition (mg/100 g edible portion, expressed on dry weight basis)	Ca		P	Na	Fe		Zn
	27		187	174	4.2		2.5

* ND = Not determined.
Source: Musaiger 1993.

3.6.2 Sorghum bread (Khoubez Al-Thorah)

Sorghum is a basic ingredient in the preparation of several traditional foods which are commonly consumed in the southern part of the Arabian Peninsula. It is usually used for the preparation of flat thick bread (Khoubez Al-Thorah). This bread is prepared from two sorghum cultivars that are commonly grown in Saudi Arabia: white and reddish-white. This bread is only baked at home in an earthenware oven (Musaiger 1993).

Sorghum grains are ground in a stone mill and the flour obtained is passed through a 0.5 mm sieve. The flour is then mixed with salt and water. The mixture is kneaded by hand for 20 min until uniform dough is formed. Pieces (300 g each) of dough are scaled off, rounded and flattened with the palm of the hand into circular sheets (2–3 cm thick). The loaves are then baked in an earthenware oven at about 300°C for 15 min. The nutritional value of sorghum bread is given in Table 8.

Figure 6 illustrates some of the famous bread types originated in Arab world.

4. Conclusions

Bread is highly regarded in the Arab world. If anybody notices a scrap of bread on the street, they would pick it up and put on the side where no one can step on it accidentally. Bread is an essential ingredient on the table in the Arabic cuisine.

In conclusion, significant variability exists in traditions and nutritional views between various types of breads originated in Arab countries. This chapter highlights the bread as one of the famous Arabic traditional foods and includes the methods of preparation and nutritive value.

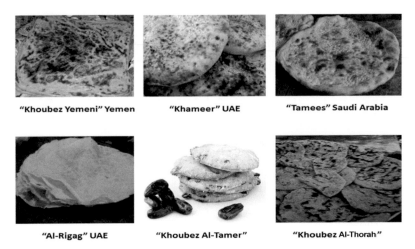

"Khoubez Yemeni" Yemen   "Khameer" UAE   "Tamees" Saudi Arabia

"Al-Rigag" UAE   "Khoubez Al-Tamer"   "Khoubez Al-Thorah"

Figure 6. Some of the famous bread types originated to Arab world.

5. Future perspectives

The rapid change in food habits in the Arabian countries has adversely affected the consumption of many traditional foods (of course bread is one of them). Consequently, traditional breads are gradually disappearing from the Arab tables.

The greatest challenge facing the Arab world is now how to transfer the awareness of the role of traditional breads in improving health and nutrition status of the Arab people. Many of traditional breads are healthy and nutritionally important in the diet and can make a significant contribution in meeting the nutritional requirements of the populations.

Nowadays, the Arabian countries have been making substantial efforts to increase their bread production and promote health and nutritional well-being of the community. Nevertheless, the traditional breads received little attention in nutrition programs, which is mainly due to the lack of information on the nutritive value of these indigenous breads.

Since the consumption of indigenous foods (including the breads) in the Arab world is decreasing at a very fast rate, it was found necessary to publish scientific documents which put the spotlight on traditional breads in this part of the world. It is hoped that this chapter will contribute in achieving of this aim and in the same time encourage the nutritionists, food technologists and social scientists to give this subject more attention in the future.

Keywords: Arab world, bread in Arab spring, Egypt, nutritional view, Oman, role of traditional bread, Saudi Arabia, traditional bread, traditional view, United Arab Emirates, Yemen

References

Ali, A., H.A.S. Al-Nassri, B. Al-Rasasi, M.S. Akhtar and B.S. Al-Belushi. 2010. Glycemic index and chemical composition of traditional Omani breads. International Journal of Food Properties, 13: 198–208.

Alian, A.M., A.R. Abdel-Latif and A.A. Yaseen. 1997. Production of balady and pan bread from whole wheat flour. Egyptian Journal of Food Science, 25: 213–230.

Al-Kanhal, M.A., I.S. Al-Mohizea, A.I. Al-Othaimeen and M.K. Khan. 1999. Nutritive value of various breads in Saudi Arabia. International Journal of Food Sciences and Nutrition, 50: 345–349.

Al-Mohizea, I.S., E.I. Mousa and M.A. Al-Kanahal. 1995. Bread consumption pattern in Riyadh area. Bulletin Faculty of Agriculture, 46: 417–428.

Almousa, A., M. Thomas, H. Siddieg, S. Varghese and S. Abusnana. 2013. The glycemic index of traditional types of bread in UAE. Journal of Nutrition & Food Sciences, 3: 1–6.

Al-Mussali, M.S. 2004. Evaluation of breadmaking industry in Yemen. 4th Scientific Symposium for bread day: Present and Future of Breadmaking in Yemen. Ministry of Trade & Industry/Agricultural Research & Extention Authority-16 July, Sanna. Yemen, 2004.

Al-Mussali, M.S. and M.A. Al-Gahri. 2009. Nutritive value of commonly consumed bread in Yemen. E-Journal of Chemistry, 6: 437–444.

Al-Mussali, M.S., F. Basunbel and H. Khamees. 2007. Bread from composite flour of wheat and millet. Yemeni Journal of Agricultural Research and Studies, 16: 5–18.

Eid, N. and N. Bourisly. 1986. Bread consumption in Kuwait. Nutrition Reports International, 33: 967–971.

Jönsson, H. 2010. Lecture: Bread as Culture; with a 66 slides PowerPoint presentation; Lund University.

Khan, M.A. and M.A. Al-Kanhal. 1998. Dietary energy and protein requirements for Saudi Arabia: A methodological approach. Eastern Mediterranean Health Journal, 4: 68–75.

Leeder, S.H. 1918. Modern Sons of the Pharaohs: A Study of the Manners and Customs of the Copts of Egypt. Hodder and Stoughton, London.

MNE. 2006. Ministry of National Economy. The draft survey of family income and expenditures; Ministry of National Economy: Muscat, Sultanate of Oman.

Musaiger, A.O. 1993. Traditional Foods in the Arabian Gulf Countries. Arabian Printing & Publishing House W.L.L., Manama.

Pomeranz, Y. 1988. Wheat Chemistry and Technology. American Association of Cereal Chemists (AACC), St. Paul, Minnesota.

Räsänen, L. 2007. Of all foods bread is the most noble: Carl von Linne (Carl Linneaus) on bread. Scandinavian Journal of Food Science and Nutrition, 51: 91–99.

Samuel, D. 2001. Brewing and baking. pp. 1–21. *In*: P.T. Nicholson and I. Shaw (eds.). Ancient Egyptian Materials and Technology. Cambridge University Press, Cambridge.

16

Nutritional and Nutraceutical Features of Regular and Protein Fortified Corn Tortillas

Sergio O. Serna-Saldivar

1. Introduction

Tortilla is ancestral unleavened bread obtained after lime-cooking or nixtamalization of corn (*Zea mays* L.) kernels, which are further ground into a cohesive dough or masa, which is subsequently formed into flat disks and baked into tortillas. Tortillas are still the single major food item consumed in Mexico and other Central America countries and greatly affect the nutritional status of the average population (Serna-Saldivar and Rooney 2003). In Mexico, the corn tortilla is still the single most widely consumed food with an average per capita consumption of 78.5 kg in 2012.

Hunger and malnutrition in developing countries are the most severe setbacks that face mankind. Protein-energy malnutrition (PEM), *Kwashiorkor*, *Marasmus* and other malnutrition problems inhibited growth and weakened human resources and in some way affected at least 850 million of 7.3 billion inhabitants of the world in year 2014 (FAO 2014). The most severe and widely spread forms of malnutrition are PEM followed by lack of micronutrients like vitamin A, iron and iodine. Malnutrition during the peri and postnatal periods causes an important loss in infant growth and development that affects other physiological stages during the life cycle. In addition, these people are more prone to infectious diseases and death at an early age. Poverty

Head and Professor, CIDPRO, Escuela de Ingeniería y Ciencias, Tecnologico de Monterrey. Av. Eugenio Garza Sada 2501 Sur CP 64849 Monterrey N.L., Mexico.
Email: sserna@itesm.mx

is the main underlying cause of malnutrition and its determinants. The grade and distribution of PEM and micronutrient deficiencies depend on issues such as the political and economic state, the level of education and sanitation, the season and climate conditions, domestic food production, cultural and religious food traditions, breast-feeding habits, prevalence of infectious illnesses, the existence of nutrition programs and the availability and quality of health and medical services (Muller and Krawinkel 2005).

Worldwide, PEM continues to be a major health burden in developing countries. The World Health Organization (WHO) estimates that about 60% of all deaths, occurring among children aged less than five years in developing countries, are attributed to malnutrition. PEM is also associated with comorbidities such as diarrheal diseases, and lower respiratory tract infections including tuberculosis, malaria and anaemia (Ubesie et al. 2012).

In developing countries, enrichment and fortification of staple foods, such as tortillas, are the most efficient ways to improve the nutritional status of the population and public health. It has been well documented that the nutritional quality of corn tortillas is upgraded by protein fortification especially with soybean proteins, utilizing quality protein corn (QPM) and enriching with selected minerals and vitamins (Amaya-Guerra et al. 2004, 2006; Bressani et al. 1974, 1979; Chavez and Chavez 2004; Serna-Saldivar and Amaya-Guerra 2008; Sproule et al. 1988; Stylianopoulos et al. 2001). The aim of this chapter is to review research related to the nutritional and nutraceutical properties of corn tortillas and the improvement of their nutritional value through protein fortification and enrichment with selected micronutrients.

2. The tortilla making process

Traditionally and commercially made tortillas are prepared after performing three major operations: lime-cooking, grinding and baking (Fig. 1). The modern lime-cooking processes use the same principles as the old traditional procedure first used by ancient Mesoamerican civilizations but the equipment and procedures have been mechanized to improve efficiency and manufacturing. Lime- cooking is considered the most important part of the process because it affects functionality, final tortilla features and nutritional value. Stone-grinding also plays a key role because it disrupts swollen starch granules of the nixtamal and distributes the hydrated starch and protein around the ungelatinized portions of the endosperm, forming masa with a given granulation (Serna-Saldivar 2010). Masa is transformed into tortillas after a baking step that forms the typical tortilla structure. In addition, baking inactivates all microorganisms and affects color and sensory properties of tortillas. Commonly, about 146 kg of table tortillas with 44–46% moisture are obtained from 100 kg of cleaned corn (Fig. 1, Serna-Saldivar 2010). Corn kernels are usually cooked with 2.5 to 3 parts water and 1% food grade.

Cooking time varies greatly from a few minutes to 1 hr depending on grain hardness and size. Processing wise, cooking is also affected by the interaction of temperature, time, lime-concentration, size of cooking vessel and frequency of agitation (Serna-Saldivar 2010; Serna-Saldivar et al. 1990). After lime-cooking, the nixtamal is

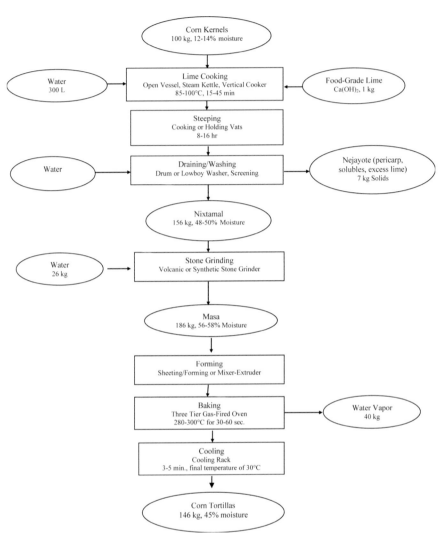

Figure 1. Flowchart and mass balance of the industrial processes for the manufacture of corn tortillas.

steeped for 8 to 16 hr in order to enhance the penetration of the lime-cooking solution. This step is critically important for production of fresh masa and is usually skipped for dry masa flour production. After steeping the nixtamal with approximately 48% moisture for fresh masa and 36% for dry masa flour operations is washed in order to remove excess lime and hydrolyzed pericarp tissue. Commonly, the clean nixtamal is ground using a system of two matching carved stones (volcanic or synthetic usually manufactured from aluminum oxide). The grinding operation consists of conveying the nixtamal through a center opening of one of the stones that conducts it into the grinding surfaces. The material is ground and kneaded while moving outwards. Water is frequently added during grinding to prevent excess heat generation, decrease masa temperature, and increase the moisture content in the masa. Masa particle size is the result of several interacting factors: (1) degree of *nixtamal* cooking; (2) carving design of the surface of the grinding stones; (3) pressure between stones; (4) amount of water added during milling; and (5) type of corn (Serna-Saldivar et al. 1990; Serna-Saldivar 2012).

Masa is formed into tortillas discs using a head that consists of two rotating smooth rolls that automatically presses the masa into a thin sheet of approximately 2 mm. The gap between the rolls determines product thickness and weight. The sheet of masa is continuously cut by an attachment located underneath the front roll. A set of cutting wires also helps in discharging the pieces of dough onto the conveying belt that feeds the oven. Different interchangeable cutter configurations are used for production of various products (Serna-Saldivar et al. 1990). In Mexico, most tortillas are formed with Celorio™ machines that consist of a mixer, extruder and former. The extrusion system forces the masa through a slot at the bottom of the unit. A gate cutter controls the discharge and regulates the shape and size of the masa product. The Celorio is exclusively used for table tortillas and requires a finely ground masa with higher moisture. The masa is usually hydrated to a larger extent (60% moisture). Tortillas extruded and formed with the Celorio unit generally puff during baking and retain their textural properties longer (Serna-Saldivar et al. 1990; Serna-Saldivar 2010). Regardless to the type of forming device, the formed masa pieces are baked into tortillas on a triple pass gas-fired oven (Fig. 1) at temperatures ranging from 280 to 302°C for 30 to 60 sec. Therefore, one side of the tortilla bakes twice as long as the other side. During baking about 10–12% moisture is lost from the masa. Baking causes starch gelatinization, protein denaturation, color development due to Maillard or browning reactions and the inactivation of microbial loads (Serna-Saldivar et al. 1990; Serna-Saldivar 2010). Tortillas are finally allowed to cool down to ambient temperature before packaging on cooling conveyors. Cooling is a key operation in terms of microbial shelf life and should be designed in order to minimize cross contamination.

2.1 Nutritional attributes of regular corn tortillas

The nutritional value of regular corn tortillas has been widely documented. The typical chemical composition of tortillas is depicted in Table 1. Tortillas are an important source of energy provided mostly by their high starch content, protein, dietary fiber, calcium and most B-vitamins.

Several significant chemical and nutritional changes occur when corn kernels are processed into tortillas. At equivalent moisture contents, tortillas contain less dietary fiber and fat than the original kernel. This is due to the loss of pericarp and germ tissues during nixtamalization. However, both products contain similar quantities of starch and protein. The raw kernels experience the loss of minerals associated to the pericarp and germ and gain relevant amounts of calcium due to the absorption of calcium hydroxide during lime-cooking (Bressani et al. 1958; Serna-Saldivar et al. 1987, 1988a; Serna-Saldivar and Amaya-Guerra 2008).

Table 1. Nutritional composition of corn tortillas (100 g serving).[a]

Nutrient	Table tortilla
Moisture, g	41.9
Total calories, kcal	238
Calories from fat, kcal	23
Digestible energy, kcal	224
Protein, g	6.5
Digestible protein, g	5.38
Fat, g	2.50
Saturated fat, g	0.33
Monounsaturated fat, g	0.65
Polyunsaturated fat, g	1.12
Total dietary fiber, g	7.4
Dietary insoluble fiber, g	6.3
Dietary soluble fiber, g	1.1
Starch, g	44.9
Resistant starch, g	0.84
Minerals, g	0.90
Calcium, mg	93
Phosphorus, mg	314
Magnesium, mg	70
Potassium, mg	205
Sodium, mg	13
Iron, mg	2.5
Zinc, mg	2.5
Copper, mg	0.07
Vitamins	
Thiamin or B_1, mg	0.11
Riboflavin or B_2, mg	0.07
Niacin or B_3, mg	1.50
Pyridoxin or B_6, mg	0.22
Folic acid, mcg	183

[a] From USDA (2014); Serna-Saldivar (2010).

2.1.1 Caloric density

Tortillas are considered an excellent source of calories due to their high content of starch and high energy digestibility (Tables 1 and 2, Serna-Saldivar et al. 1987, 1988a; Serna-Saldivar 2010; Sproule et al. 1988). The starch is in practical terms 100% absorbed and while being digested glucose is transported to blood more slowly; thus, favoring its value for diabetic people. The consumption of 100 g of tortillas (approximately three pieces) with 42% moisture supplies approximately 225 kcal of digestible energy (Table 1).

Table 2. Dry matter, energy and protein digestibilities of different types of corns lime cooked into nixtamal and baked into tortillas.

	Digestibility, %			Reference
	Dry matter	**Energy**	**Protein**	
Corn kernel	90.3	91.1	86.2	Serna-Saldivar et al. (1988a)
Nixtamal	92.9	93.8	79.3	
Tortilla	93.2	93.8	81.6	
Cooked corn kernel	91.5	91.6	85.4	Serna-Saldivar et al. (1987)
Nixtamal	92.0	92.6	84.6	
Regular corn kernel	91.4	92.9	86.1	Sproule et al. (1988)
Tortilla	94.3	94.3	83.8	
Tortilla chip	94.4	94.7	82.1	
QPM kernel	90.2	90.8	85.5	
QPM tortillas	93.6	94.0	80.9	
QPM chips	93.7	84.4	81.9	
Regular corn kernel	90.7	91.6	86.0	Serna-Saldivar et al. (1988b)
Regular tortilla	90.0	90.9	83.6	
Tortilla + 8% Defatted soybean meal	89.5	90.4	83.0	
Tortilla with 8% Soybean and 4% Sesame flours	89.6	91.0	83.1	

2.1.2 Protein

Corn tortillas contain approximately 6.5 and 5.4% total and digestible protein, respectively (Table 1). Significant changes to its protein fraction occur when corn is transformed into tortillas. Lime-cooking decreases slightly the rate of protein digestibility and the bioavailability of lysine, considered its most limiting essential amino acid (EAA) (Serna-Saldivar et al. 1987, 1988a). The protein digestibility of the tortilla is about 3 to 5% units lower (Table 2) compared to raw kernels (Serna-Saldivar et al. 1987, 1988a; Sproule et al. 1988). Research conducted with ileum-fistulated swine found 5% units lower lysine digestibility at terminal ileum in nixtamal compared to the same corn cooked without lime (Serna-Saldivar et al. 1987). The difference is attributed to the formation of lysinoalanine, lanthonine and ornithoalanine (Chu et al. 1976; De Groot et al. 1976).

The protein quality of the corn tortillas is considered marginal because of the low quantities of lysine and tryptophan to sustain regular growth in infants. These EAA are present in approximately half of the quantity required for optimum growth. Thus, the biological value (BV), net protein utilization (NPU), protein efficiency ratio (PER) and protein digestibility corrected amino acid score (PDCAAS) values are approximately one-half of those reported for animal products such as meat, fish, eggs and milk (Serna-Saldivar and Amaya-Guerra 2008).

2.1.3 Fiber

Dietary fiber in corn consists primarily of hemicellulose. Arabino-glucoronoxylans are the major hemicellulose components in the pericarp and β-glucans and xylans dominates in the endosperm cell walls. According to Martinez-Bustos et al. (2001) during the nixtamalization process fiber components from the germ, pericarp and tip cap are released increasing the contents of xylose, galactose and galacturonic acid.

Corn frees most of the pericarp and insoluble fiber after lime-cooking and steeping. The extents of cooking, steeping and degree of nixtamal washing affect the amount of pericarp lost in the nejayote (Serna-Saldivar et al. 1990). The xylans are susceptible to alkaline hydrolysis during processing (Ayala-Soto et al. 2014; Ghali et al. 1984; Nyman et al. 1984). Serna-Saldivar et al. (1987, 1988a) reported that corn tortillas contain on dry weight basis (dwb) 10.9% insoluble and 1.2% soluble dietary fiber. Bressani et al. (1990) determined insoluble and soluble dietary fiber in traditional processed tortillas and concluded that most of the losses occurred during lime-cooking. The raw corn contained on dwb 13.1 and 1.0% insoluble and soluble dietary fiber, respectively. Processing corn into masa lowered the insoluble fiber to 6.3% and increased soluble fiber to 1.75%. The concomitant effect of lime and the thermal treatment hydrolyzed insoluble fiber yielding soluble fiber components. Interestingly, baking the masa into tortillas augmented insoluble fiber to 6.9%. Recently, Ayala-Soto et al. (2014) studied the hydroxycinnamic and arabynoxylans profiles and antioxidant (AOX) capacity determined by the ORAC of the nejayote solids and concluded that these important nutraceuticals lost during lime-cooking and steeping negatively affects tortillas.

2.1.4 Minerals

Corn tortillas are an adequate source of phosphorus and calcium (Table 1). The first is intrinsically associated to the kernels whereas the second absorbed during lime-cooking. In an early research, Braham and Bressani (1966) found that rats absorbed more than 85% of the calcium present in tortillas. Interestingly, the supplementation of tortillas with lysine and other EAA from soybean (SB) flour enhanced calcium absorption. Serna-Saldivar et al. (1991, 1992a) demonstrated that the calcium in the tortilla is well absorbed, metabolized and deposited in the bones of rats fed diets of regular and QPM tortillas supplemented with beans. The calcium from these tortillas was better utilized than the calcium from regular counterparts. The same authors calculated that around 50% of the calcium ingested by the Mexican population comes from tortillas and related food items.

Tortillas are considered a poor source of iron, zinc and copper (Table 1) and their bioavailability is limited due to the presence of phytic acid. Tortillas are a poor source of iron because the raw grain has low quantities of this important mineral and part is lost during nixtamalization. A 100 g portion of tortillas provides about 2.5 mg iron (Table 1), about 15% of the recommended daily allowance (RDA).

According to the FAO (2014) the average iron consumption in the world is low especially among low socioeconomic groups and therefore the prevalence of anemia is still high particularly among childbearing women, and children. Iron deficiencies in these people are inversely related to bean and animal product consumption. In order to achieve a better iron status among tortilla consumers, the diets need to be fortified and/or supplemented with dietary iron and other known nutrients such as vitamin C and protein which improve iron absorption.

Mineral bioavailability in plant products is linked to phytic acid; specifically the concentration of phytic acid was inversely proportional to available iron. Urizar and Bressani (1997) showed a 3.7 to 34.6% decrease in phytic acid when corn was processed into 24 different types of nixtamal. The level of lime used for nixtamalization affects phytic acid concentration. Raw corn contained approximately 1% phytic acid whereas nixtamal cooked with 1.2% lime 25% lower phytic acid. They hypothesized the high calcium concentration provided by the lime saturated phytic acid thus allowing a better iron absorption and availability.

2.1.5 Vitamins

Tortillas contain significant amounts of most B-vitamins despite the losses experienced during lime-cooking. Losses of pericarp, germ and aleurone tissues during nixtamalization contribute to the decreased amounts of vitamins in tortillas. Tortillas are a poor source of lipid soluble vitamins (A, D, E, and K), and are devoid of water-soluble vitamins C and B_{12}. In an early study, Bressani et al. (1958) monitored changes in thiamine, riboflavin and niacin during tortilla processing of white and yellow corns. Approximately half of the thiamin losses were during lime-cooking and steeping. Figueroa-Cárdenas et al. (2001) evaluated the addition of vitamins, minerals and 4% defatted SB meal in tortillas produced from fresh masa or from dry masa flour (DMF). Thiamin, riboflavin, niacin and folic acid losses were about 36, 81, 29 and 46%, respectively. During nixtamal washing losses of thiamin, riboflavin and folic acid accounted for 18, 17 and 21%, respectively.

One documented advantage of lime-cooking is the release of bound niacin which makes it more bioavailable. That is the reason why Pellagra is virtually unknown in tortilla eating countries (Bressani 1990; Koetz and Neukom 1977; Wall and Carpenter 1988).

2.2 Nutraceutical properties of regular corn tortillas

Corn and its tortillas contain an array of nutraceuticals such as arabinoxylans, phenolics, carotenoids, polyunsaturated fatty acids, phospholipids, phytosterols and other minor nutrients such as policosanols and tocopherols (Serna-Saldivar 2010). These phytochemicals are mainly associated to the pericarp, germ and aleurone layer. Unfortunately, some of the phytochemicals are partially lost during the tortilla manufacturing process.

2.2.1 Dietary fiber

Dietary fiber is defined as the fraction of a given food which resist digestion by human gastrointestinal enzymes. The dietary fiber is mainly constituted of lignin, cellulose, hemicellulose and even starchy polymers, which comprises resistant starches (RS). The total dietary fiber is classed into insoluble or soluble. The first type has bulking action but may only be fermented to a limited extent in the large intestine. On the other hand, the soluble fiber has high affinity for water and upon hydration forms viscous masses and are commonly readily fermented in the colon. Current recommendations for dietary fiber intake for adults is 25 g. 100 g of tortillas provide between 6 and 9 g of total dietary fiber which represents about 25 to 35% of the RDA. The nixtamalization process is known to affect the removal of the pericarp and the dietary fiber content of masa and tortillas. The partial degradation of cell walls releases mainly the arabinoxylans, which act as tortilla texture improver.

2.2.2 Resistant starch

RS is considered as part of the dietary fiber because it also resists human enzymatic digestion and therefore do not provide digestible energy. Campas-Baypoli et al. (1999) documented changes of RS when corn was transformed into tortillas. As expected, the whole raw kernel had the lowest amounts of RS and when kernels were lime-cooked into nixtamal, ground into masa and baked into tortillas higher amounts of starch became resistant. The largest increment in RS was observed when masa pieces were baked. Most of the RS present in tortillas was classified as RS3 or retrograded. Similarly, Agama-Acevedo et al. (2005) analyzed the *in vitro* starch digestibility of commercial tortillas stored at refrigeration temperature for up to 72 h. RS3 represented more than 75% of the total RS. The RS increased slightly during storage. Likewise Rendón-Villalobos et al. (2002) determined RS values of nixtamal, masa and tortilla stored for 24 to 96 h. In general, a minor decrease in available starch content was observed with storage time. Tortilla contained slightly higher RS3 values (1.1–1.8%, dwb) compared to masa (0.7–0.9%). The same research group (Rendón-Villalobos et al. 2006) further evaluated tortillas stored for 7 or 14 d supplemented with commercial gums commonly used to improve texture. Interestingly, RS values increased with storage time and tortillas containing gums showed lower RS compared to the unsupplemented counterparts.

When RS reaches the large intestine it is readily fermented into the short chain fatty acids butyrate and propionate. These metabolites are the prime substrates for the energy metabolism in the colonocyte and act as growth factors to the healthy epithelium. In normal cells butyrate has been shown to induce proliferation at the crypt base, enhancing a healthy tissue turnover and maintenance. Raben et al. (1994) concluded that RS caused significant reductions in postprandial glycemia and insulinemia, and the sensation of satiety.

2.2.3 Phytochemicals

2.2.3.1 Phenolics

Lime-cooking and tortilla baking have a detrimental effect on phenolics due to their clear reduction especially after the thermal lime treatment. De la Parra et al. (2007) determined the concentration of phenolic compounds of five types of corns processed into masas, tortillas and fried tortilla chips. The observed range of total phenolic compounds in raw grains (244 to 320 mg gallic acid equivalents/100 g dwb), masa (125 to 198) and tortillas (137 to 207) strongly indicate a significant decline of these AOX. The amount of bound phenolics became approximately half after nixtamalization. Furthermore, they found that about 80% of the AOX capacity associated to raw kernels or their tortillas was due to bound moieties and that the different sorts of corns contained between 41 and 49.6 mol eq. of vitamin C/100 g. Interestingly, the AOX hydrophilic amount accounted for about 98% of the total AOX capacity.

Likewise, Mora-Rochin et al. (2010) investigated the effects of traditional nixtamalization and lime-cooking in a thermoplastic extruder on bound and free total phenolics of two Mexican pigmented (blue and red) and two commercial (white and yellow) whole corn flours processed first into DMF and then baked into tortillas. Tortillas prepared from extruded flours retained 88% of total phenolics compared to 62% in conventionally made tortillas. The AOX capacity of white, yellow, blue and red corns were 19.4, 19.1, 12.4 and 19.2 μmol eq. Trolox/100 g dwb, respectively. Interestingly, regular and extruded tortillas produced from these grains lost 36 and 15% of the total AOX capacity originally associated to uncooked kernels.

Guitérrez-Uribe et al. (2010) determined the phytochemical profile of different corn kernels which were optimally lime-cooked into nixtamal and their respective waste liquors commonly known as nejayote. White, yellow, white QPM, red, high-carotenoid and blue kernels, masas and nejayote solids were analyzed in terms of bound and free phenolics. Kernels, masas and nejayotes contained approximately 87, 82 and 91% of bound phenolics. Interestingly, total phenolics of nejayote solids were about twice as much compared to kernels and masas. Furthermore, the nejayote solids contained 40 and 8 times higher free and 191 and 61 times higher bound AOX capacities compared to raw kernels and masas, respectively. Thus, the nejayote solids, which are usually discarded and cause an environmental pollution problem, are a promising source of AOX which are effective to combat oxidative stress.

2.2.3.2 Ferulic acid

Ferulic acid is the most abundant hydroxycinnamic acid in all commercial cereals (Adom and Liu 2002; De la Parra et al. 2007; Serna-Saldivar 2010). It is generally found covalently bound to the cell wall by an ester bond. Approximately 75% is found in the aleurone layer and the pericarp while 15 and 10% to the germ and endosperm tissues, respectively. In corn and tortillas, ferulic moieties are found in free, conjugated and bound forms. Adom and Liu (2002) determined that corn contained 0.6, 7 and 93% of ferulic acid in free, soluble-conjugated and bound forms, respectively. Gutiérrez-Uribe et al. (2010) determined that levels of bound ferulic acid in blue corn were lower compared to other genotypes such as QPM or yellow. De la Parra et al. (2007) revealed a higher content of ferulic acid in varieties of blue corn when compared with yellow and white types whereas Mora-Rochin et al. (2010) assayed bound and free ferulic acids of different corns processed into tortillas by conventional nixtamalization or extrusion. The retention of total ferulic acid in regular tortillas was significantly lower compared to counterparts from extruded flours. Nonetheless, regular tortillas contained more free ferulic compared to counterparts produced from extruded flours indicating that harsher lime cooking schemes liberated more free moieties from cell walls. Rojas-García et al. (2012) determined free and bound ferulic acids associated to nejayote solids obtained after optimally lime-cooked blue, white, red, yellow, high-carotenoid and QPM types. Bound phenolics extracts contained higher ferulic compared to the free phenolics extracts. The bound phenolics extracts had higher induction of quinone reductase (QR) and particularly the normal yellow nejayote exerted the highest chemopreventive index tested in Hepa1c1c7 cells. In corn and tortillas, ferulic moieties are found in free, conjugated and bound forms. The different ferulic acid forms possess an ample range of therapeutic effects. They are considered potent AOX which prevent inflammation, cancer, low density lipoprotein (LDL)-oxidation (Asanoma et al. 1994; Huang et al. 1988; Kawabata et al. 2000) and neuron degeneration (Kanski et al. 2002).

2.2.3.3 Anthocyanins (ACN)

ACN are pigmented flavonoids existing in red, purple-pigmented and blue corn kernels. These flavonoids are set apart from others because they possess a net positive charge in acidic solutions. The main ACN are cyanidin and peonidin glycosides (Cortes et al. 2006; Del Pozo-Insfran 2006, 2007). Other important ACN are acylated mainly located in the endosperm's aleurone layer (Pedreschi and Cisneros-Zevallos 2007). The AOX effect of ACN is attributed specifically to the presence of hydroxyl groups in position 3' of the C ring and 3', 4', 5' of the B ring (Cone 2007). In general, the AOX of ACN aglycones is higher to that of glycosylated forms and decreases as the number of glycosidic residues increases in the molecule.

Cyanidin 3-glucoside is the most abundant ACN in blue and purple corns with concentrations varying from 15.4 to 110.2 mg/kg (Abdel Aal et al. 2006; Pedreschi and Cisneros-Zevallos 2007). Zaho et al. (2008) studied ACN rich extracts from a Chinese purple corn and found that contained 304.5 ± 16.32 mg eq. of cyanidin-3-O-glucoside/100 g dwb. The main ACN detected were cyanidin-3-(6'-malonylglucoside), cyanidin-3-O-glucoside-2-malonylglucoside, cyanidin-3-O-glucoside, peonidin-3-O-glucoside, peonidin-3-(6'-malonylglucoside), pelargonidin-3-(6''-malonylglucoside) and peonidin-3-(dimalonylglucoside). Pedreschi and Cisneros-Zevallos (2007) reported concentration values for most common ACN found in pigmented corns: 15.43 mg/kg for cyanidin-3-glucoside, 2.33 mg/kg for pelargonidin-3-glucoside, and 4.44 mg/kg for peonidin-3-glucoside.

Del Pozo-Insfran et al. (2006, 2007) processed a white and two blue corns into masa, tortillas and chips. ACN losses during the preparation of dough, tortillas and tortilla chips were 39, 53 and 78%, respectively. De la Parra et al. (2007), Salinas-Moreno et al. (2003) and Cortes et al. (2006) concluded that the lime-cooking and increasing concentrations of calcium hydroxide augmented ACN losses. Mora-Rochin et al. (2010) confirmed these results when regular blue tortillas were assayed. However, the production of tortillas from nixtamalized flours obtained via thermoplastic extrusion significantly reduced the losses of ACN and other AOX compounds.

Lopez-Martinez et al. (2011) assayed total phenolics and ACN contents, AOX activity and QR induction in the murine hepatoma (Hepa 1 c1c7 cell line) as a biological marker for phase II detoxification enzymes of white, blue, red and purple corns which were lime-cooked into masa and further baked into tortillas. As expected, the nixtamalization process reduced total phenolics, ACN and AOX activities and the ability for QR induction. Surprisingly, the blue variety and its corresponding masa and tortillas failed to induce QR.

Cumulative results of epidemiological, *in vitro* and *in vivo* studies suggest an inverse relationship between ACN consumption and the incidence of obesity, hyperglycemia and various degenerative diseases. These health benefits have been attributed to their strong AOX and antiradical activities (Fimognari et al. 2004; Tsuda et al. 2003). Moreover, the ACN stimulate the protective phase II enzyme system, glutathione peroxidase, glutathione reductase and glutathione S-transferase through the activation of the antioxidant response element (Shih et al. 2005; Wang and Stoner 2008), and inhibition of colorectal cancer in male rats F344 treated with 1,2-dimetilhydrazine and Pleckstrin Homology Domain Interacting Protein (PhIP). It was determined that the anti-mutagenic potency of the extracts was due primarily to the activity of glycosylated ACN, but the presence of acylated ACN also played an important role (Hagiwara et al. 2001; Pedreschi and Cisneros-Zevallos 2007).

2.2.3.4 Carotenoids and xantophylls

Other relevant groups of AOX are the carotenoids and xantophylls. Carotenoids are polyisoprenoids containing 40 carbons that impart the yellow color to the endosperm of cereals. Carotenoid hydrocarbons are known as carotenes and are the precursors of the oxygenated derivatives recognized as xantophylls. The absorption of these compounds is not regulated; therefore, their concentration in blood and peripheral tissues reflect ingestion. Carotenoids are minor constituents of corn and are only present in significant amounts in yellow genotypes. Blessin et al. (1963) determined that yellow corn contained most of its carotenoids in the corneous endosperm (74–86%) and soft (9–23%) endosperm portions. By far the predominant types are lutein (2–33 mg/kg) and zeaxanthin (0.6–27.4 mg/kg) followed by β-carotenes (0.1–5.4 mg/kg) (White and Weber 2003).

De la Parra et al. (2007) determined that the lime-cooking process significantly diminishes the lutein content in yellow, red and high-carotenoid corns. As expected, the high carotenoid and yellow genotypes contained the highest quantities of β-carotene. Processing of corn into tortillas and chips did not significantly affect lutein concentration, except in the yellow tortilla chips. Amounts of zeaxanthins were similar among masas, tortillas, and chips for white, red, blue and high-carotenoids corns whereas levels of zeaxanthin decreased in yellow corn after lime-cooking and tortilla baking. Recently, Gutiérrez-Uribe et al. (2014) studied the fate of lutein, zeaxanthin, cryptoxanthin, β-carotene and lipophilic AOX of yellow and white corn kernels processed into tortillas. As expected, lime-cooking significantly changed the extractability of carotenoids in masa and tortillas. No carotenoids were detected in the steepwater or nejayote. The lipophilic AOX activity increased 280 fold from kernel to masa but only 70% was retained in the baked tortillas. When masa was baked into tortillas, less than 10% of the carotenoids were retained due to the high temperatures employed during baking.

The main nutraceutical role of carotenoids is the molecular protection against free radicals. From the nutritional viewpoint, the most important metabolite is β-carotene because one molecule is converted in the human system into two molecules of retinol. The intake of β-carotenes and xanthophylls protects the skin against ultraviolet light and is associated with reduced risk of CVD, cancer and other chronic diseases. Lutein, zeaxanthin and cryptoxanthin prevent macular dystrophy or degeneration highly associated to blindness especially in geriatric patients and improves vision and functioning of the immune system (Fullmer and Shao 2001; Serna-Saldivar 2010).

2.2.3.5 Non-polar and polar lipids

Triglycerides and Fatty Acids. The majority of the corn oil is in the germ and is mainly constituted by triglycerides whereas the second major lipid class is phospholipids constituted by phosphatidyl choline, inositol, ethanolamine and serine. The corn kernels usually contain 3.5% oil whereas tortillas 2.5%. According to Saoussem (2013) the lipidic fraction contains between 5.2 and 8.7% of phospholipids. The corn oil is mainly formed by linoleic (> 40%) followed by palmitic acid. Linoleic is considered an essential fatty acid for humans and can be converted in the human system to linolenic and then to other important fatty acids and metabolites such as eicosapentaenoic (EPA), docosahexaenoic (DHA), eicosanoids and prostaglandins (Serna-Saldivar 2010). Among phospholipids, phosphatidyl choline is the chief component (37.5 to 68.1%) followed by phosphatidyls inositol (14.5 to 19.8%) and ethanolamine (10.3 to 13.9%). The fate of phospholipids throughout the different steps of corn tortilla processing is unknown. Nonetheless, since most of these polar lipids are present in the germ the quantities in the tortilla will depend on the germ losses incurred during nixtamalization. From the nutraceutical viewpoint, phosphatydyl choline and choline lower the risk of CVD and positively affect brain and mental development of both the fetus and infants and their chronic inadequacy may be related to Alzheimer's disease. Choline released from lecithin during metabolism is considered as one of the most important neurotransmissors and is commonly supplemented to newborns and geriatrics in order to maintain proper brain function (Canty 2001; Zeisel 1994). Phosphatidyl inositol and serine reduce blood triglycerides, fatty liver, bipolar disorders and neurodegenerative diseases. The deficiency of these phospholipids is also related to increased susceptibility to hepatic cancer (Majumder and Biswas 2006; Phillippy 2003). Inositol is essential for brain functioning and therefore is recommended for newborn babies and geriatrics. Furthermore, it helps in the synthesis of RNA and to transport lipids and cholesterol. As a result, inositol is considered hypocholesterolemic, cardioprotective and anticarcinogenic (Holub1982; Phillippy 2003; Vucenik and Shamsuddin 2006).

2.2.3.6 Phytosterols

Corn is considered an excellent source of phytosterols. The main sterol present is β-sitosterol followed by campesterol and stigmasterol (Chung and Ohm 2000). Little is known about the fate of phytosterols during nixtamalization. Since most of the phytosterols are associated to the germ and pericarp it is probable that significant amounts of these compounds are lost in the nejayote. Phytosterols are known to inhibit the absorption of cholesterol from the small intestine thus effectively lowering total blood cholesterol and LDL. A daily intake of only 1 to 3 g reduces cholesterol by 5 to 20% (White and Weber 2003; Serna-Saldivar 2010).

2.2.3.7 Tocopherols

Crude corn oil possesses significant amounts of tocol derivatives such as tocopherols and tocotrienols that are responsible for vitamin E activity. Among the structural parts of the corn kernel, tocol derivatives are most abundant in the germ (Chung and Ohm 2000; White and Weber 2003). The total tocols of corn ranges from 0.03 to 0.33% of the oil. The two major tocols are α-tocopherol and γ-tocopherol. These lipophilic compounds are considered to be the second most important mechanism of defense against free radicals and oxidative stress and prevent the oxidation of polyunsaturated fatty acids and LDL (Serna-Saldivar 2010). Vitamin E strengthens the immune system by lymphocytes-T (Bender 1992) and prevents chronic diseases (Serna-Saldivar 2010).

2.2.3.8 Policosanols

There are no scientific reports of the fate of policosanols during the tortilla making process. However, lime-cooking should reduce levels of policosanols significantly due to the partial removal of the pericarp during cooking, steeping and nixtamal washing. Harrabi et al. (2009) studied the total policosanol content of three different types of corn kernels and found that contents varied from 15.2 to 20.5 mg/kg dwb. Policosanols were mainly present in the corn pericarp (72.7–110.9 mg/kg) and germ (19.3–37.1 mg/kg). Corn pericarp policosanols were mainly triacontanol (33.63–46.29 mg/kg), dotriacontanol (22.31–39.46 mg/kg) and octacosanol (8.13–14.0 mg/kg). In contrast, the corn germ fraction contained mostly dotriacontanol (more than 50%) and was practically devoid of triacontanol. Policosanols exert various physiological activities such as lowering total blood and LDL cholesterol by approximately 20% and 25% respectively, while increasing HDL by 12%. There is also scientific evidence that policosanols provide additional beneficial effects on smooth muscle cell proliferation, reducing platelet aggregation and LDL peroxidation (Arruzazabala et al. 1994, 1996; Castano et al. 1996; Gouni-Berthold and Berthold 2002; Hargrove et al. 2004).

3. Strategies for the production of protein-fortified and enriched corn tortillas

Many efforts have been made to improve the nutritional value of tortillas by enrichment with vitamin/mineral premixes and/or protein fortification. Tortillas have been fortified with amaranth (*Amaranthus caudatus*), torula yeast (*Candida utilis*), quinoa (*Chenopodium quinoa*), flax (*Linum usitatissimum*), common beans

(*Phaseolus vulgaris*), chickpeas (*Cicer arietinum*) and different soybean (*Glycine max*) products. High protein quality tortillas can also be produced by the utilization of high-lysine genotypes or direct addition of lysine and tryptophan (Amaya-Guerra et al. 2004, 2006; Bressani 1990; Bressani et al. 1974, 1979; Del Valle and Perez-Villaseñor 1974; Figueroa-Cárdenas et al. 2001; Serna-Saldivar et al. 1988b; Sproule et al. 1988).

3.1 Enrichment with micronutrients

DMF are commonly enriched with selected minerals such as Fe and Zn and vitamins such as thiamin, riboflavin, niacin and folic acid and occasionally with other essential nutrients. The micronutrient premix is added during the last stage of the milling process with dosifiers commonly employed in the wheat milling industry. However, fresh masa processors do not enrich their products because of the difficulty to perform this task in small, low-technology plants. Dunn et al. (2007, 2008) proposed a commercial process for micronutrient fortification of tortillas prepared from fresh masa consisting of a dosification system that incorporates the micronutrient premix into the nixtamal feed stream as it passes into the milling stones. The dry dosification system proved to be readily adaptable yielded consistent fortification levels and gave sensory properties similar to unenriched tortillas. Additionally, the method was cost-effective, easy to implement, had minimal impact on the existing process, produced tortillas of comparable quality to currently unenriched counterparts, and resulted in an improvement in micronutrient content.

Independently of the enrichment program the aim is to provide key nutrients for people who depend on tortillas. DMF are usually enriched with 24–40 mg iron and 16–26 mg zinc/kg (Table 3). With this level of enrichment, corn tortillas (42% moisture content) will contain approximately 3.5 mg iron and 3.25 mg Zn/100 g serving. Iron is commonly added in the reduced form and zinc as an oxide. Iron is essential for the formation of hemoglobin and myoglobin and to prevent infectious diseases whereas zinc is required to sustain normal growth.

In terms of vitamins, DMF are commonly enriched with four important B-vitamins (Table 3) to reach the concentrations present in the raw kernel. With this level of enrichment corn tortillas (42% moisture content) will contain approximately 0.50 mg thiamin, 0.25 mg riboflavin, 3.65 mg niacin and 0.05 mg folic acid/100 g serving. The objectives of the enrichment programs are to lower the incidence of Beriberi, Pellagra, fetal malformations, such as neural tube defects, and low birth weight and promote a better cognitive development in preschool children. Recently, folic acid has gained attention because its supplementation lowers homocysteine, platelet aggregation and CVD especially in adults (Nygard et al. 1997; Serna-Saldivar and Amaya-Guerra 2008).

3.2 Protein quality of opaque-2 or QPM tortillas

The mutant genes that significantly increase the levels of lysine and tryptophan in opaque-2 corn later on transferred to the new QPM genotypes were first identified by Mertz et al. (1964) in the decade of the 1960s. Unfortunately, the improved protein quality of the opaque-2 grain was strongly linked with many undesirable agronomic

Table 3. Levels and types of micronutrients included in the Mexican dry masa flour enrichment program.

Nutrient	Level recommended (mg/kg)			Form	Daily requirement		Function
	Minimum	Optimum	Maximum		Infants	Adults	
Iron	24.0	30.0	40.0	Reduced iron	10 mg	15 mg	Prevents anemia, fatigue, dizziness and nervousness. Helps mental response and strengthens the immune system.
Zinc	16.0	20.0	26.0	Zinc oxide	10 mg	15 mg	Zn is essential to promote an adequate growth and cell replication. It promotes fertility and boosts the immune system. A pronounced deficiency results in loss of appetite, growth retardation, hypogonadism and dwarfism. Preschool children and pregnant women are the physiological stages more affected. Biochemically, Zn is essential and critical because important metalloenzymes require it.
Thiamin	4.0	5.0	8.0	Thiamin mononitrate	0.7 mg	1.4 mg	Deficiency is associated with abnormalities of carbohydrate metabolism. Clinical conditions associated with the prolonged intake of diets low in thiamin are called Beriberi whose primary symptoms involve the nervous and cardiovascular systems.
Riboflavin	2.4	3.0	5.0	Hydrochloridrate riboflavin	0.8 mg	1.6 mg	Riboflavin is essential to the functioning of vitamins B_6 and niacin.
Niacin	28.0	35.0	45.0	Nicotinamide	9 mg	18 mg	Niacin deficiency is associated with abnormalities of carbohydrate metabolism or efficiency of energy utilization. Clinical conditions associated with the prolonged intake of diets low in niacin are called Pellagra whose primary symptoms involve the nervous and cardiovascular systems.
Folic acid	0.4	0.5	0.8	Folic acid	50 µg	200 µg	Folic acid has gained attention because its deficiency has been associated with impaired cell division and fetal and placental malformations, mainly neural tube defects. In adults, folic acid lowers risk of CVD.

characteristics such as lower grain yield, poorer milling properties due to the soft endosperm and higher susceptibility of the kernels to insect and diseases. After years of continued effort, scientists from CIMMYT transformed the opaque-2 corn into new lines of QPM adapted to different agro-ecologies. QPM was the result of many years of recurrent selection where the high lysine potential of opaque-2 was combined with modifier genes that significantly improved the physical properties of the kernel and the agronomic performance of the crop. Today, QPM varieties and parental lines for hybrids are disseminated throughout the globe (Rooney and Serna-Saldivar 2003).

Animal trials and clinical studies have demonstrated the clear nutritional superiority of opaque-2 and QPM over regular corn. This is because QPM contains almost twice as much lysine and tryptophan which results in better nitrogen retention and growth. As a result these experimental subjects have growth rates of almost two times when compared with counterparts fed diets from regular corn. Opaque-2 or QPM tortillas have practically twice the PER value compared to regular counterparts (Amaya-Guerra et al. 2004, 2006; Bressani et al. 1968; Bressani 1992; Serna-Saldivar et al. 1992b; Sproule et al. 1988; Sullivan et al. 1989). As a result, recently QPM has regained value as a potential source for production of high quality and nutritious tortillas. This is because of the availability of new varieties and hybrids with good agronomic potential and functionality in the tortilla system (Melesio-Cuellar et al. 2008; Serna-Saldivar et al. 2008).

3.3 Protein fortification

Many protein supplements have been used to upgrade the protein quality of corn tortillas. Protein supplementation increases protein content, improves EAA scores and consequently protein utilization and growth. The nutritional value of tortillas can be upgraded by the addition of different types of soybean products, amaranth, fish meal, torula yeast, glandless cottonseed and by supplementation with lysine and tryptophan (Bressani and Marenco 1963; Bressani et al. 1968, 1974, 1979; Del Valle and Perez-Villaseñor 1974; Green et al. 1977; Figueroa Cárdenas et al. 2001; Sanchez-Marroquin et al. 1987; Serna-Saldivar et al. 1988b; Serna-Saldivar 1997). Bressani and Marenco (1963) determined that the addition of 3% fish meal, 5% meat flour, 5% whole egg flour, 5% casein, 8% skim milk powder, 8% SB protein, or 3% torula east improved significantly both quantity and quality of protein. The protein efficiency ratios of the fortified tortillas were at least twice as much compared to the regular counterparts. A highly significant correlation was found between PER and lysine content of the supplements indicating that this EAA is the limiting factor affecting protein quality. However, the processing attributes of the fortified masas and sensory or organoleptic properties of the resulting tortillas were not determined.

3.3.1 Fortification with essential amino acids

Lecuona-Villanueva et al. (2012) recently evaluated the texture of masa as well as the nutritional quality and acceptance of corn tortillas made either with DMF or by the traditional way both fortified with lysine and tryptophan or with a protein concentrate from *Phaseolus lunatus* added with these EAA (Uc-Cetz et al. 2003). Results showed that masa cohesion was significantly affected in the fortified tortillas made with DMF whereas adhesion was not affected by the different treatments. *In vitro* digestibility of proteins was improved by the fortification obtaining the highest values in tortillas made with DMF fortified with both the amino acids and the concentrate from *Phaseolus lunatus*. Sensory acceptance was greater for tortillas fortified with lysine and tryptophan alone. Presumably the protein quality of the fortified tortillas improved due to the higher amounts of lysine and tryptophan.

3.3.2 Fortification with Amaranth

Amaranth flour was composited with DMF or fresh masa commonly used to prepare tortillas. Fortified tortillas had similar organoleptic properties compared to unsupplemented counterparts. As expected, the protein content, PER and net protein rate improved in fortified tortillas (Sanchez-Marroquin et al. 1987).

3.3.3 Fortification with common beans

Mora-Aviles et al. (2007) fortified QPM tortillas with common beans in order to further improve their protein quality. In this study, amino acids and mineral changes that occur during nixtamalization and the chemical and nutritional characteristics of regular, commercial and QPM tortilla-bean combination were assessed. After nixtamalization, protein from QPM was reduced from 8.1% to 7.2%. Tryptophan was also reduced from 12.1 to 11.1 g/kg protein. When regular DMF was combined with beans the protein, tryptophan and lysine contents significantly increased. Both QPM and tortillas fortified with beans had an enhanced protein quality. Hernández-Salazar et al. (2006) determined *in vitro* starch digestibility and RS levels in tortillas fortified with beans and concluded that the inclusion of bean diminished starch digestibility and significantly increased RS values. This combination also reduced the glycemic index (Noriega et al. 2000).

3.3.4 Fortification with soybean products

Technological advances have made it possible to have SB protein available in various forms: as full fat meal, defatted flours, protein concentrates and isolates. These products differ in functional properties as well as in fat and protein content; however, EAA patterns on a protein basis are essentially the same. Nutritionally, these products have in common a highly digestible protein with ample amounts of lysine and an excellent EAA pattern (Bressani 1981). Furthermore, soybean products have made significant contributions to functionality of tortillas especially in terms of water absorption, tortilla yield and tortilla texture.

The different array of soybean products are the most promising sources for production of fortified corn tortillas because of their high availability, high protein, lysine and tryptophan contents, relatively low cost, and especially due to its proven complementary effect on corn proteins. Tortillas have been successfully fortified with full-fat soybean meal, defatted soybean flour, concentrates or isolates. The substitution levels recommended to double the PER and protein quality for these products is 8, 6, 5 and 4% respectively. At these levels of fortification the overall quality and characteristics of tortillas are not adversely changed (Chuck-Hernández et al. 2015; Serna-Saldivar et al. 1988b). Defatted soybean flour presents the advantage of better shelf stability although full-fat soybean flour produces a higher caloric density tortilla. The cheapest soybean sources are defatted soybean flour which contains less than 1% oil, 50% protein and 2.6% lysine and full-fat soybean that contain 17–20% oil, 36–38% protein and 2.2% lysine. Other advantage of these soybean sources is that they contain significant amounts of phytochemicals such as soluble and insoluble dietary fiber, phytosterols, isoflavones, flavonoids, soyasaponins and B-vitamins. Recently, Chuck-Hernández et al. (2015) assessed the functionality of five different defatted soybean proteins in tortillas manufactured in a pilot plant. The soybean proteins were added to increase the protein content of DMF between 20 to 25% (addition of about 6% defatted soybean flour or 4% soybean concentrate). The evaluated soybean ingredients depicted a pH between 6.6 and 6.8, protein of 42.4 to 67.1%, Urease Activity ranging 0.1 to 2.25, free amino nitrogen from 0.62 to 1.87 mg/g, reducing sugars from 5 to 88 mg/g, water absorption index (WAI) of 4.02 to 8.34, protein dispersability index (PDI) of 23 to 75% and fat absorption index (FAI) ranging from 2.5 to 3.1. EAA compositions of composited DMF showed twice the amount of lysine and tryptophan compared with the control treatment. Interestingly the sensory attributes of all soybean fortified tortillas were not different compared to control tortillas, but maximum texture force after five days of storage was higher for the low PDI defatted soybean flour and lower for a high PDI counterparts. Control and low PDI flours followed by the soybean concentrate were the best overall evaluated supplements according to the most relevant parameters for consumers and producers. These authors concluded that the best soybean proteins to be used in corn tortilla supplementation should preferably have reduced urease activity, water solubility and PDI.

3.3.5 Effect of tortilla fortification with soybean on growth and brain development of rats

The growth and brain development of laboratory rats fed typical indigenous tortilla based diets were determined throughout two generations (Stylianopoulos 1999; Stylianopoulos et al. 2001). The experiment compared three different types of tortillas: regular tortillas produced from DMF, tortillas obtained from fresh masa and tortillas produced from DMF fortified with 6% defatted soybean and enriched with vitamins B_1, B_2, niacin, and folic acid and the minerals iron and zinc. Female dams were mated 58 days post-weaning with males belonging to the same treatment with the aim of obtaining second-generation pups that were further subjected to regular lactation and 28-day post-weaned growth. Table 4 summarizes the main findings of this experiment. As expected, fresh masa or DMF tortillas contained lower amounts of lysine and tryptophan and inferior EAA scores compared to the soybean fortified tortillas. A highly significant difference in body weight after 28 days growth, daily gains and efficiency of food conversion was observed (Table 4). Growth rates expressed

Table 4. Effect of soybean-fortification and enrichment with selected micronutrients on the nutritional composition of tortilla-based Otomi diets and rat growth throughout two generations.[a]

	Tortilla from DMF	Tortilla from fresh masa	Tortilla fortified with defatted soybean meal	Control-casein
Chemical composition				
Moisture	6.26	6.72	7.19	9.85
Ash	1.71	2.22	1.96	4.09
Protein	8.94	9.24	10.56	10.06
Fat	2.80	2.85	3.90	5.23
Crude fiber	1.24	1.48	1.22	0.21
NFE[b]	85.31	84.21	82.36	80.41
Digestible energy[c]	377.2	372.6	378.0	369.6
Amino acid composition				
Leu	10.82	9.55	10.98	9.76
Ile	3.47	3.01	3.88	4.68
Lys	3.27	3.10	4.36	7.98
Met + Cys	3.47	2.92	3.69	2.98
Phe + Tyr	6.94	6.28	7.86	8.95
Thr	3.27	2.92	3.60	3.55
Trp	0.71	0.62	0.85	1.13
Val	4.69	3.98	4.92	6.37
EAA Score[d]	56.3	53.4	75.1	100
Mineral and vitamin composition				
Ca	122	168	137	465
Fe	10.2	9.4	16.6	21.6
Zn	6.4	5.0	9.0	16.2
Thiamin	0.95	1.33	2.82	1.73
Riboflavin	0.33	0.33	0.75	3.96
Niacin	5.17	7.01	14.87	10.07
Folic acid	9.2	10.0	29.0	74.5
First generation weanling rat growth for 28 d				
Initial weight, g	50.8	50.3	51.3	51.1
Final weight, g	78.9	81.4	15.8	112.4
Δ weight gain, g	28.13	31.13	54.50	61.25
Food consumption, g	259.0	261.7	276.0	298.3
Protein consumption, g	23.16	24.18	29.15	30.01
Δ Weight gain/ Protein consumption	1.46	1.59	2.05	2.34
Second generation weanling rat growth for 28 d				
Initial weight, g	14.2	18.3	14.3	35.4
Final weight, g	27.2	28.8	39.6	96.7
Δ weight gain, g	13.0	10.50	25.27	61.32
Food consumption, g	316	359.8	198.4	322.8
Protein consumption, g	25.44	29.28	18.22	31.60
Δ weight gain/ Protein consumption	0.51	0.36	1.73	2.03

[a] From Stylianopoulos (1999) and Stylianopoulos et al. (2001).

[b] NFE = Nitrogen free extract.

[c] Digestible energy = (% NFE × 4 kcal/g) + (% protein × 4 kcal/g) + (% ether extract × 9 kcal/g).

[d] EAA (Essential amino acid) score = Limiting EAA/ FAO/WHO requirement.

in terms of protein consumed by rats fed fresh masa and DMF tortillas were 1.59 and 1.46, respectively whereas counterparts fed soybean fortified tortilla and control diets had a higher growth performance (2.05 and 2.34). Growth of second-generation weanling pups fed DMF or fresh masa tortilla diets was 0.51 and 0.36 g gain/g protein consumed, respectively (Table 4). In contrast, counterparts fed soybean-fortified tortillas or control diets had significantly higher growth rates (1.73 and 2.03 g gain/g protein consumed, respectively). Therefore, weanling rats fed these diets gained from 3 to 4 times more weight than counterparts fed regular tortilla diets. This difference was higher than that documented in the first generation growth study demonstrating that prolonged malnutrition affected the second generation more severely. These findings agree with Gressens et al. (1997) who concluded that protein and energy malnutrition and deficiency of vitamins and minerals of mothers significantly retarded growth in second-generation individuals.

Interestingly, rats fed soybean fortified tortillas or the control-casein diets had 100% pregnancy rate while counterparts fed regular tortillas had less than 40% pregnancy rates (Table 4, Stylianopoulos 1999). The lower fertility was associated with the lower body weight produced by diets deficient in protein, vitamins and minerals. In addition, dams fed soybean-fortified tortillas and control-casein diets had 9 and 10 newborns, respectively, in contrast with fertile counterparts fed regular masa and DMF tortillas that delivered 4 and 7 pups, respectively (Table 4). At the end of lactation, females fed masa and DMF tortillas weaned only 4 and 7 pups, respectively. In contrast, a total of 32 and 45 rats were weaned by mothers fed fortified tortillas and casein-control diets, respectively.

Total content and concentration of brain DNA in first generation adult males and lactating females were similar for all diets. However, a significant change in these variables was observed in brains of second-generation subjects (Stylianopoulos 1999; Stylianopoulos et al. 2001). For animals fed soybean-fortified tortillas and control-casein diets, total DNA concentration and number of neurons were significantly higher than for counterparts fed regular tortillas. These results agree with Gressens et al. (1997), who concluded that severe protein malnutrition causes adverse effects on brain development and a reduction in cerebral DNA. The better EAA acid, protein quality and supplementation of key micronutrients of fortified tortillas enhanced DNA synthesis and the amount of cerebral DNA during intrauterine fetus development and lactation.

Amaya-Guerra et al. (2004) further researched the physiological and brain development of rats fed throughout two generations with an indigenous Otomi tortilla based diets described by Stylianopoulos (1999). The experiment compared casein control diet and five different types of tortillas: (1) a diet of tortillas obtained from fresh masa; (2) regular tortillas produced from enriched DMF containing vitamins B_1, B_2, niacin, folic acid and the microminerals iron and zinc; (3) tortillas produced from enriched DMF fortified with 6% defatted soybean meal; (4) tortillas produced from enriched QPM DMF; and (5) tortillas produced from enriched QPM flour fortified with 3% defatted soybean meal. Table 5 summarizes the main finding of this investigation. As expected, the growth of rats fed the soybean fortified DMF or QPM tortillas were significantly higher in both generations compared to counterparts fed the regular tortilla diets. The difference in growth rate among treatments was more evident in second-generation rats. Rats fed the soybean enriched DMF or QPM tortillas had the highest

Table 5. Effect of soybean fortification on digestibilities, nitrogen retention and growth of first and second-generation rats fed regular and quality protein corn tortillas.[a]

	Tortilla diets[b]					
	Fresh masa	Enriched DMF	Soybean fortified and enriched DMF	QPM DMF	Soybean fortified and enriched QPM DMF	Control -casein
Digestibilities						
Dry matter	90.14[a]	90.34[a]	88.24[a]	92.46[b]	89.63[a]	95.65[c]
Protein	85.70[a]	8565[a]	83.35[a]	86.94[b]	85.02[ab]	94.53[c]
Nitrogen retention and protein quality study						
Biological value, %	39.35[a]	55.64[b]	69.99[d]	64.23[c]	69.59[d]	72.21[e]
Net protein utilization Value, %	33.83[a]	47.75[b]	58.344[d]	55.89[c]	56.16[d]	68.27[e]
PDCAAS[b]	44.31[a]	50.19[b]	67.51[d]	62.94[c]	71.84[d]	94.53[e]
Fertility rate and reproduction						
% pregnancy rate	37.5[a]	77.7[b]	100[c]	100[c]	100[c]	100[c]
Pups/litter	3.4[a]	6.4[b]	9.0[c]	8.2[c]	9.3[c]	11.3[d]
Birth weight, g	4.2[a]	4.5[ab]	4.7[b]	4.5[ab]	4.9[b]	5.2[c]
Weanling weight, g	22.6[a]	29.8[b]	36.8[c]	34.8[c]	37.6[c]	42.1[d]
% survival, 21 days postpartum	26.4[a]	53.2[b]	74.6[c]	68.4[c]	77.4[c]	86.3[d]
First generation weanling rat growth study						
Δ weight [6] (g)	20.43[a]	39.78[b]	72.67[d]	64.38[c]	72.22[d]	87.67[e]
Food intake (g)	218.6[a]	298.6[b]	348.7[bc]	364.3[c]	321.5[bc]	332.3[bc]
Protein intake (g)	20.8[a]	28.1[b]	38.4[c]	35.0[c]	33.8[c]	36.2[c]
Δ weight/Protein intake	0.98[a]	1.41[b]	1.89[c]	1.84[c]	2.13[d]	2.42[e]
Second generation weanling rat growth study						
Δ weight (g)	15.48[a]	18.41[b]	47.54[cd]	44.14[c]	49.94[d]	81.33[e]
Food intake (g)	328.5[d]	307.6[c]	246.7[a]	268.9[b]	242.1[a]	323.0[d]
Protein intake (g)	31.3[c]	28.91[b]	27.14[ab]	25.82[a]	25.42[a]	35.21[d]
Δweight/Protein intake	0.49[a]	0.63[b]	1.75[c]	1.71[c]	1.96[d]	2.31[e]

[a] From Amaya-Guerra et al. (2004). Means with different letter(s) within row are statistically different ($P < 0.05$).

[b] Protein digestibility corrected amino acid score.

BV, NPU, and PDCAAS. The pregnancy rate, number of newborns/litter, litter weight, and newborn survival rate was also higher for rats fed soybean-fortified or QPM diets than their counterparts fed regular tortillas. Addition of 6% defatted soybean flour to the regular enriched dry masa flour or 3% to the enriched QPM DMF significantly improved nitrogen retention values and animal performance. Rats fed these soybean-fortified diets gained at least three times as much weight compared with counterparts fed regular tortillas produced from fresh masa. Therefore, the utilization of QPM flour saved half of the soybean flour without sacrificing nutritive value (Table 5).

Amaya Guerra et al. (2006) also investigated the brain development and memory performance of rats fed throughout two generations with the different tortilla-based diet described above. Results of this research are depicted in Tables 6 and 7. In both

Table 6. Effect of soybean fortification on brain and cerebellum weight, myelin, synapses density of neuron of first and second-generation rats fed regular and quality protein corn tortillas.[a]

Diet[b]	Brain weight mg	Cerebellum weight, mg	Myelin mg/g	Neuron syn-apses density, %	Protein/brain weight, mg/g	RNA/brain weight, mg/g	DNA/brain weight, mg/g	Protein/DNA	RNA/DNA
First generation (average age 158 days)									
FM	1024.3 ± 21.3[a]	174.4 ± 6.8[a]	86.6 ± 4.6[a]	26.4 ± 3.1[a]	96.76 ± 4.3[a]	3.66 ± 0.12[a]	6.96 ± 0.12[a]	13.90 ± 0.27[a]	0.55 ± 0.03[a]
REDMF	1130.9 ± 36.3[b]	205.8 ± 13.1[a]	124.2 ± 11.8[b]	29.8 ± 9.6[a]	96.72 ± 5.1[a]	4.05 ± 0.09[b]	6.82 ± 0.13[a]	14.18 ± 0.25[a]	0.59 ± 0.02[a]
FEDMF	1460.4 ± 36.8[d]	340.0 ± 6.3[c]	187.4 ± 4.6[c]	41.5 ± 3.4[b]	108.67 ± 5.4[b]	4.41 ± 0.18[c]	6.84 ± 0.22[a]	15.88 ± 0.37[b]	0.64 ± 0.02[b]
EQPM	1324.5 ± 42.3[c]	302.6 ± 7.2[b]	181.0 ± 7.2[a]	43.6 ± 1.6[b]	105.43 ± 3.2[b]	4.52 ± 0.15[c]	6.75 ± 0.22[a]	15.61 ± 0.46[b]	0.66 ± 0.03[b]
FEQPM	1503.4 ± 24.8[d]	354.2 ± 8.6[cd]	193.0 ± 6.3[a]	42.3 ± 2.6[b]	106.86 ± 4.4[b]	4.43 ± 0.17[c]	6.82 ± 0.17[a]	15.66 ± 0.39[b]	0.65 ± 0.03[b]
Control	1671.1 ± 29.6[e]	368.3 ± 5.0[d]	190.7 ± 5.3[a]	47.5 ± 2.2[c]	123.74 ± 7.3[c]	4.61 ± 0.11[c]	6.78 ± 0.12[a]	18.25 ± 0.20[c]	0.67 ± 0.02[b]
Second generation (average age 62 days)									
FM	394.6 ± 4.6[a]	61.2 ± 4.7[a]	68.8 ± 6.8[a]	32.5 ± 5.8[a]	86.76 ± 3.3[a]	3.86 ± 0.04[a]	5.79 ± 0.06[a]	14.98 ± 0.33[a]	0.66 ± 0.02[a]
REDMF	412.2 ± 8.3[b]	64.9 ± 5.2[a]	126.8 ± 3.9[b]	34.6 ± 3.7[a]	91.43 ± 2.6[a]	4.01 ± 0.04[b]	6.11 ± 0.08[b]	14.96 ± 0.29[a]	0.66 ± 0.03[a]
FEDMF	656.0 ± 21.6[d]	99.0 ± 2.6[c]	136.7 ± 3.4[c]	36.4 ± 5.2[a]	101.45 ± 2.1[b]	4.30 ± 0.06[c]	6.25 ± 0.04[c]	16.23 ± 0.22[b]	0.69 ± 0.02[a]
EQPM	578.6 ± 19.7[c]	91.7 ± 3.4[b]	128.6 ± 4.2[b]	36.5 ± 5.2[a]	99.64 ± 2.8[b]	4.23 ± 0.04[c]	6.28 ± 0.04[c]	15.86 ± 0.32[b]	0.67 ± 0.03[a]
FEQPM	694.3 ± 22.3[d]	99.3 ± 2.3[c]	131.3 ± 5.5[bc]	32.8 ± 5.9[a]	102.63 ± 3.4[b]	4.27 ± 0.06[c]	6.25 ± 0.04[c]	16.42 ± 0.4[b]	0.68 ± 0.03[a]
Control	803.4 ± 18.6[e]	104.3 ± 2.6[d]	142.6 ± 2.3[d]	38.6 ± 4.3[a]	109.61 ± 2.6[c]	4.31 ± 0.06[c]	6.36 ± 0.06[d]	17.23 ± 0.24[c]	0.68 ± 0.02[a]

[a] From Amaya-Guerra et al. (2006).

[b] FM = Tortilla-based diet from fresh masa; RDMF = Tortilla-based diet from regular dry masa flour; FEDMF = Tortilla-based diet from soybean fortified and enriched dry masa flour; QPM = Tortilla-based diet from quality protein corn; FEQPM = Tortilla-based diet from soybean fortified and enriched QPM dry masa flour; Control = Casein-based diet. Means ± SD with different letter(s) within column were statistically different (P < 0.05).

Table 7. Effect of soybean fortification on short term, long term and working memories and learning performance of first and second-generation rats fed regular and quality protein corn tortillas.[a]

Diet[b]	Short term memory		Long term memory	Working memory		Learning performance	
	Latency sec	Number of errors	Days to obtain a positive result	Latency sec	Number of errors	Latency sec	Number of errors
First generation (average age 64 days)							
FM	15.1 ± 2.3[a]	4.5 ± 0.23[c]	4.9 ± 0.32[b]	16.2 ± 0.53[a]	4.2 ± 0.21[a]	----[3]	----[3]
REDMF	14.3 ± 3.2[a]	4.3 ± 0.12[c]	5.3 ± 0.28[b]	16.7 ± 0.43[a]	5.7 ± 0.32[b]	32.1 ± 2.54[c]	18.4 ± 1.58[c]
FEDM	13.9 ± 1.2[a]	3.9 ± 0.23[b]	3.3 ± 0.52[a]	17.1 ± 0.32[a]	6.8 ± 0.22[c]	21.3 ± 1.24[a]	9.5 ± 1.46[a]
EQPM	14.4 ± 1.6[a]	3.7 ± 0.23[b]	3.1 ± 0.47[a]	16.4 ± 0.51[a]	5.8 ± 0.20[b]	26.4 ± 1.41[b]	12.6 ± 0.55[b]
FEQPM	13.6 ± 2.3[a]	3.6 ± 0.38[b]	3.9 ± 0.34[a]	16.8 ± 0.44[a]	7.9 ± 0.38[d]	21.4 ± 1.54[a]	11.4 ± 0.60[a]
Control	13.6 ± 1.6[a]	2.1 ± 0.42[a]	3.6 ± 0.11[a]	17.2 ± 0.51[a]	5.7 ± 0.34[b]	19.6 ± 1.12[a]	12.3 ± 0.32[ab]
Second generation (average age 62 days)							
FM	----[c]	----[c]	----[c]	----[c]	----[c]	----[c]	----[c]
REDMF	18.6 ± 2.1[b]	4.3 ± 0.2[b]	9.4 ± 2.3[b]	28.9 ± 0.6[c]	8.6 ± 0.4[c]	----[c]	----[c]
FEDMF	13.4 ± 2.0[a]	3.6 ± 0.2[a]	5.1 ± 1.6[a]	20.2 ± 1.2[a]	5.1 ± 0.4[a]	34.4 ± 2.0[b]	15.4 ± 1.80[b]
EQPM	13.8 ± 2.3[a]	4.1 ± 0.2[b]	6.2 ± 0.8[a]	23.6 ± 0.8[b]	7.6 ± 0.4[bc]	42.4 ± 2.4[c]	16.7 ± 1.62[b]
FEQPM	13.1 ± 1.6[a]	3.2 ± 0.2[a]	5.2 ± 1.1[a]	21.1 ± 1.2[a]	6.1 ± 0.4[b]	32.9 ± 2.6[b]	14.8 ± 2.78[b]
Control	12.7 ± 1.6[a]	2.9 ± 0.4[a]	4.1 ± 1.6[a]	18.9 ± 2.3[a]	6.8 ± 0.8[b]	19.3 ± 3.6[a]	8.4 ± 0.56[a]

[a] From Amaya Guerra et al. (2006). Means ± SD with different letter(s) within column were statistically different (P < 0.05).

[b] FM = Tortilla-based diet from fresh masa; RDMF = Tortilla-based diet from regular dry masa flour; FEDMF = Tortilla-based diet from soybean fortified and enriched dry masa flour; QPM = Tortilla-based diet from enriched dry masa flour from quality protein corn; FEQPM = Tortilla-based diet from soybean fortified and enriched QPM dry masa flour; Control = Casein-based diet.

[c] Rats could not complete the test.

generations, brain and cerebellum weights and myelin concentration were significantly higher in rats fed the soybean-fortified tortillas. There was no significant difference in brain DNA in first generation rats; however, second-generation rats fed QPM, soybean fortified-QPM and soybean-fortified DMF tortillas had higher brain DNA, neuron size and brain activity as estimated by the RNA/DNA ratio (Table 6). Short-term and long-term memory performance in the Morris maze significantly improved among rats fed the QPM and soybean-fortified tortillas. Second-generation rats fed these diets had a superior working memory and learning performance (Table 7).

3.3.6 Effect of dry masa flour soybean fortification and enrichment with selected micronutrients on humans

A long-term blind human study evaluated the effects of soybean fortification and enrichment with selected micronutrients of DMF in two neighboring rural Otomi communities located in the state of Querétaro, México: the community of Rincon (experimental group that received the fortified and enriched DMF) and the community of Yosphi (control group that received the regular DMF) (Chavez and Chavez 2004). Families having at least one child of 5 years or less were selected and given either the regular or the fortified/enriched DMF. A total of 125 families from the Rincon community and 145 families from the Yosphi community, respectively, participated in the study. These communities were chosen because of their high daily consumption of tortillas and represented a good model for all indigenous ethnic groups of Mexico. The total caloric or energy daily consumption was low (1714 kcal/capita for el Rincon and 1980 kcal/capita in Yosphi). Tortillas and related products provided between 76 and 80% of the total caloric intake. Families were provided the fortified or regular DMF in lots of 2.5 to 3.5 kg/d corresponding to 350 to 400 g/capita/d. Both sorts of DMF were well-accepted by the communities and there were not any significant differences in the organoleptic acceptability of these products. The average protein content in the soybean-fortified DMF ranged from 7.9 to 11.3% (dwb) whereas the available lysine was 242 ± 52 mg/100 g whereas values for regular DMF were $7.7 \pm 0.8\%$ and 139 ± 36 mg/100 g, respectively (Chavez and Chavez 2004).

The study stressed the monitoring of weight gains and height every other month for all infants and children. Also specialists performed clinical evaluations periodically. Infants and children receiving the soybean-fortified DMF grew 49% more than counterparts fed the regular DMF. The weight gains in the subjects fed the fortified/enriched blend were 92% of the expected for normal subjects, even considering that at the beginning of the study the community presented bouts of diarrhea, Chicken Pox and other infectious diseases. The control subjects suffered more diseases and in some instances weight losses when compared to those consuming the fortified diet. Therefore, subjects fed fortified tortillas had less incidence of moderate and severe malnutrition and had a higher proportion of individuals that fell into the category of normal subjects (Table 8). This two-year study clearly indicated that the intervention with soybean improved the nutritional status of all physiological stages (Chavez and Chavez 2004). At the beginning of the experiment some of the adult female members of the Rincon community were classified as malnourished (13.1% with < 17 kg/m^2)

Table 8. Effects of addition of defatted soybean and selected micronutrients to dry masa flours on a long-term blind intervention study performed with humans inhabiting in two neighbouring communities.[a]

	Regular dry masa flour provided at Yosphi	Soybean fortified and enriched dry masa flour provided at Rincon[b]
Protein in dry masa flour, %	7.6	10.5
Protein absorption, %	83.0	84.32
Nitrogen balance, g N/d	2.39	3.29
Preschool child growth, Δ weight/year	0.7	1.6
Malnutrition after 8 months intervention, %		
Slight	29.0	34.3
Moderate	29.0	14.1
Severe	9.0	6.1
Normal nourished after 8 months intervention, %	33.0	45.5
Adolescent change of BMI after 2 years intervention	19.9 to 21.8 (+1.9)	22 to 25 (+3)
Change of serum thiamine (B_1) after 1 year intervention, nmg/L	17.0 to 18.0 (+1)	12.0 to 34.3 (+22.3)
Change of serum riboflavin (B_2) after 1 year intervention, nmg/L	28.1 to 30.0 (+1.9)	35.0 to 74.0 (+39)
Incidence of diseases	25% less compared to Humans at Josphi	
Duration of disease	32% less compared to Humans at Josphi	
Average weight gain during pregnancy, kg	7.41 ± 1.7	8.5 ± 1.5
Average weight of newborns, kg	2.92 ± 0.64	3.13 ± 0.31
Newborns with birth weights below 2.5 kg, %	26.4	3.3
Bayley scale of infant development[c]	64.3 ± 4.2	73.8 ± 5.3

[a] From Chavez and M de Chavez (2004). Tortilla and related products provided between 76 and 80% of the total caloric intake.

[b] The dry masa flour was fortified with 6% defatted soybean flour, 4.2 to 5 mg/kg thiamine, 3 to 3.2 mg/kg riboflavin, 30.8 to 36 mg/kg niacin, 30 mg/kg iron and 10 mg/kg zinc. Folic acid was also added (300 μg/kg) to flours provided after the first half of the study.

[c] The Bayley scales of infant development is a standard test to assess the motor (fine and gross), language (receptive and expressive), and cognitive development of infants. Tests were applied to 1–3 year old infants.

or underweight (28.3% with 17 to 20 kg/m^2) according to the body mass index. In contrast no adult females in the control community were classified as malnourished while 23.2% were underweight. After only five months of supplementation, there were no malnourished subjects in the experimental community and after 10 months the percentage of underweight subjects was practically equal in both communities (around 21%). Clinical tests showed that subjects that consumed the fortified/enriched tortillas improved their hair, nails and skin conditions. Abnormal hair, nails and skin decreased from 82 to 33, 71 to 39 and 65 to 21% of the tested individuals, respectively (Chavez and Chavez 2004).

Blood serum analysis in children showed a significant increase in iron levels as measured by blood hemoglobin. Hemoglobin increased from 11.7 to 12.7 g/100 mL in preschool and from 12.6 to 14.2 g/100 mL in school-aged children. Children of the control community had a non-significant decrease in iron levels. The folic acid (2.7 to 5.2 ng/ml) and vitamin B_{12} (108.6 to 209.2 pg/ml) plasma values almost doubled after one year in subjects fed the fortified tortillas. Plasma levels of thiamin, riboflavin and pyridoxine stayed about the same for the subjects fed the control DMF products. Levels of serum thiamin tripled while riboflavin and pyridoxine doubled in subjects fed fortified tortillas. Interestingly, pregnant women belonging to the Rincon gave birth to newborns with significantly higher weights (210 gr higher compared to counterparts of Yoshpi) and only 3% of the babies had lower birth weights than 2.5 kg. The Rincon infants performed approximately 10 points better in the Bayley scales of infant development test which assesses the fine and gross motor capabilities, receptive and expressive language and cognitive development (Table 8, Chavez and Chavez 2004).

This long term human study practically reached the same conclusions of controlled animal studies in which growth, reproductive performance, brain development and memory performance were tested (Stylianopoulos et al. 2001; Amaya-Guerra et al. 2004, 2006). Undoubtedly, the best and most practical strategy to enhance nutrition and health of tortilla dependent subjects in marginal areas is by the low cost improvement of protein quality with soybean proteins and enrichment with selected vitamins and minerals.

4. Conclusion

In Latin America most of the corn is transformed into tortillas and related products via the nixtamalization process. The lime-cooking process significantly affects the nutritional and nutraceutical profiles of this important staple food. Resulting tortillas are considered an excellent source of energy due to their high starch content and bioavailable calcium and recently have also gained popularity because they are an excellent choice for gluten intolerant or celiac people. The tortilla lacks of good quality protein and adequate levels of key micronutrients such as iron, zinc and vitamins A, D, E and B_{12}. Furthermore, corn suffers during nixtamalization important losses of relevant phytochemicals that are known to prevent chronic diseases and cancer. Simple phenolics, anthocyanins, carotenes, xantophylls, phytosterols, arabinoxylans, essential trace minerals and B-vitamins leach into the steep water or nejayote or partially destroyed during the alkaline thermal process. From a practical viewpoint, the consumption of tortillas without the supplementation of high quality protein foods can lead to *Kwashiorkor* in infants. This is due to the lack of two essential amino acids: lysine and tryptophan. Thus, the supplementation of tortillas with legumes such as soybeans (*Glycine max*) or common beans (*Phaseouls vulgaris*) or animal products is the best alternative to alleviate protein malnutrition. Tortillas are also the ideal vehicle for the incorporation of micronutrients such as Fe, Zn, B-vitamins and vitamin A which are deficient in diets of people inhabiting in developing countries. These micronutrients plus an enhanced protein quality allows the proper physiological and cognitive development of babies during pregnancy and infants during the first critical years of their life cycle. Apparently, the best alternative to produce highly nutritious tortillas is with the fortification with any of the soybean proteins available in the market and the addition of selected micronutrients lacking in the diet of low socioeconomic groups. The addition of soybean and a micronutrient premix does not negatively affects organoleptic properties of tortillas and only increases the cost of the product less than 5%.

Abbreviations

ACN	:	anthocyanins
AOX	:	antioxidant capacity
BV	:	biological value
CVD	:	cardiovascular diseases
DMF	:	dry masa flour
dwb	:	dry weight basis
EAA	:	essential amino acids
FAI	:	fat adsorption index
FAO	:	Food Agriculture Organization
HMG-CoA	:	hydroxymethylglutarate coenzyme A
NPU	:	net protein utilization
ORAC	:	oxygen radical absorbance capacity
QPM	:	quality protein corn
QR	:	quinone reductase
LDL	:	low density lipoproteins
PDI	:	protein dispersability index
PDCAAS	:	protein digestibility corrected amino acid score
PEM	:	protein-energy malnutrition
PER	:	protein efficiency ratio
RDA	:	recommended daily allowance
RS	:	resistant starch
SB	:	soybean
WAI	:	water adsorption index
WHO	:	World Health Organization of the United Nations

Keywords: anthocyanidins, carotenoids, corn, dietary fiber, dry masa flour, enrichment, lime-cooking, fortification, nixtamalization, phenolic compounds, phospholipids, phytosterols, policosanols, protein quality, resistant starch, soybeans, tocopherols, tortillas

References

Abdel Aal, E.S., J.C. Young and I. Rabalski. 2006. Anthocyanin composition in black, blue, pink, purple, and red cereal grains. Journal of Agriculture and Food Chemistry, 54: 4696–4704.

Adom, K.K. and R.H. Liu. 2002. Antioxidant activity of grains. Journal of Agriculture and Food Chemistry, 50: 6182–6187.

Agama Acevedo, E., R. Rendón-Villalobos, J. Tovar, S.R. Trejo-Estrada and L.A. Bello-Pérez. 2005. Effect of storage time on *in vitro* digestion rate and resistant starch content of tortillas elaborated from commercial corn masas. Archivos Latinoamericanos de Nutrición, 55(1): 1–9.

Amaya-Guerra, C., M.G. Alanis-Guzman and S.O. Serna-Saldivar. 2004. Effects of soybean fortification on protein quality of tortilla based diet from regular and quality protein maize. Plant Foods and Human Nutrition, 59(2): 45–50.

Amaya-Guerra, C., S.O. Serna-Saldivar and M.G. Alanis-Guzman. 2006. Soybean fortification and enrichment of regular and quality protein maize tortillas affects brain development and maze performance of rats. British Journal of Nutrition, 96: 161–168.

Arruzazabala, M.L., D. Carbajal, R. Mas, V. Molina, S. Valdes and A. Laguna. 1994. Cholesterol lowering effects of polycosanol on rabbits. Biology Research, 27: 205–208.

Arruzazabala, M.L., S. Valdes, R. Mas, L. Fernandez and D. Carbajal. 1996. Effect of polycosanol successive dose increase on platelet aggregation in healthy volunteers. Pharmacological. Research, 34: 181–185.

Asanoma, M., K. Takahashi, M. Miyabe, K. Yamamoto, N. Yoshimi, H. Mori and Y. Kawazoe. 1994. Inhibitory effect of topical application of polymerized ferulic acid, a synthetic lignin, on tumor promotion in mouse skin two stage tumorigenesis. Carcinogenesis, 15(9): 2069–2071.

Ayala-Soto, F., S.O. Serna-Saldívar, S. García-Lara and E. Pérez-Carrillo. 2014. Sugar and hydroxycinnamic acids profiles and antioxidant capacity of arabinoxylans extracted from different maize fiber sources. Food Hydrocolloids, 35: 471–475.

Bender, D.A. 1992. Vitamin E: tocopherols and tocotrienols. Chapter 4. *In*: Nutritional Biochemistry of the Vitamins. Cambridge University Press; Cambridge, UK.

Blessin, C.W., J.D. Brecher and R.J. Dimler. 1963. Carotenoids of corn and sorghum. V. Distribution of xantophylls and carotenes in hand dissected and dry milled fractions of yellow dent corn. Cereal Chemistry, 40: 582–586.

Braham, J.E. and R. Bressani. 1966. Utilización del calcio del maíz tratado con cal. Nutrición Bromatología y Toxicología, 6: 14–19.

Bressani, R. 1981. The role of soybean in food systems. Journal of the American Oil Chemists Society, 58: 392–400.

Bressani, R. 1990. Chemistry, technology and nutritive value of maize tortillas. Food Reviews. International, 6(2): 225–264.

Bressani, R. 1992. Nutritional Value of High Lysine Maize in Humans. Chapter 12. *In*: E.T. Mertz (ed.). Quality Protein Maize. American Association of Cereal Chemists: St. Paul., MN.

Bressani, R., V. Benavides, E. Acevedo and M.A. Ortiz. 1990. Changes in selected nutrient contents and in protein quality of common and quality protein maize during rural tortilla preparation. Cereal Chemistry, 67: 515–518.

Bressani, R., J.E. Braham, L.G. Elias and M. Rubio. 1979. Further studies on the enrichment of lime treated corn with whole soybean. Journal of Food Science, 44: 1707–1710.

Bressani, R., L.G. Elias and R.A. Gomez-Brenes. 1968. Protein quality of opaque-2 corn: Evaluation in rats. Journal of Nutrition, 97: 173–180.

Bressani, R. and E. Marenco. 1963. The enrichment of lime treated corn flour with protein, lysine and tryptophan and vitamins. Journal of Agriculture and Food Chemistry, 11: 517–522.

Bressani, R., B. Murillo and L.G. Elias. 1974. Whole soybean as a means of increasing protein and calories in maize based diets. Journal of Food Science, 39: 507–580.

Bressani, R., R. Paz y Paz and N.S. Scrimshaw. 1958. Corn nutrient losses: Chemical changes in corn during preparation of tortillas. Journal of Agriculture and Food Chemistry, 6: 770–773.

Campas-Baypoli, O.N., E.C. Rosas-Burgos, P.I. Torres-Chávez, B. Ramírez-Wong and S.O. Serna-Saldivar. 1999. Physicochemical changes of starch during maize tortilla production. Starch/Starke, 51: 173–177.

Canty, D.J. 2001. Lecithin and Choline: New roles for old nutrients. Chapter 26. *In*: R.E.C. Wildman (ed.). Handbook of Nutraceuticals and Functional Foods. CRC Press: Boca Raton, FL.

Castano, G., L. Tula, M. Canetti, M. Morera, R. Mas, J. Illnait, L. Fernandez and J.C. Fernandez. 1996. Effects of policosanol in hypertensive patients with type II hypercholesterolemia. Current Therapy Research, 57: 691–699.

Chavez, A. and M. Chavez. 2004. La Tortilla de Alto Valor Nutritivo. McGraw Hill: Mexico, D.F.

Chu, N.T., P.L. Pellet and W.W. Nawar. 1976. Effect of alkali treatment on the formation of lysinoalanine in corn. Journal of Agriculture and Food Chemistry, 24: 1084–1085.

Chuck-Hernández, C., E. Perez-Carrillo, C. Soria-Hernández and S.O. Serna-Saldivar. 2015. A holistic assessment of maize tortillas enriched with five different soybean proteins. Cereal Chemistry (In Press).

Chung, O.K. and J.B. Ohm. 2000. Cereal Lipids. Chapter 14 (pp. 417–478). *In*: K. Kulp and J. Ponte (eds.). Handbook of Cereal Science & Technology, Second Edition, Marcel Dekker; New York.

Cone, K.C. 2007. Anthocyanin synthesis in maize aleurone tissue. Plant Cell Monograph, 8: 121–139.

Cortes, G.A., M.Y. Salinas, E. San Martín-Martinez and F. Martínez-Bustos. 2006. Stability of anthocyanins of blue maize (*Zea mays* L.) after nixtamalization of separated pericarp-germ tip cap and endosperm fractions. Journal of Cereal Science, 43: 57–62.

De Groot, A.P., P. Slump, N.J. Feron and L. Van Beek. 1976. Effects of alkali treated proteins: Feeding studies with free and protein bound lysinoalanine in rats and other animals. Journal of Nutrition, 106: 1527–1538.

De la Parra, C., S.O. Serna-Saldivar and R.H. Liu. 2007. Effect of processing on the phytochemical profiles and antioxidant activity of corn production of masa, tortillas and tortilla chips. Journal of Agriculture and Food Chemistry, 55: 4177–4183.

Del Pozo-Insfran, D., C. Brenes-Hernandez, S.O. Serna-Saldivar and S.T. Talcott. 2006. Polyphenolic and antioxidant content of white and blue corn (*Zea mays* L.) products. Food Research International, 39(6): 696–703.

Del Pozo-Insfran, D., S.O. Serna-Saldivar, C. Brenes-Hernandez and S. Talcott. 2007. Polyphenolics and antioxidant capacity of white and blue corns processed into tortillas and chips. Cereal Chemistry, 84: 162–168.

Del Valle, F.R. and J. Perez-Villaseñor. 1974. Enrichment of tortilla with soy protein by lime cooking of whole raw corn-soybean mixtures. Journal of Food Science, 39: 244–274.

Dunn, M., S.O. Serna-Saldivar, D. Sanchez and R.W. Griffin. 2008. Commercial evaluation of a continuous micronutrient fortification process for nixtamal tortillas. Cereal Chemistry, 85(6): 746–752.

Dunn, M., S.O. Serna-Saldivar and E.A. Turner. 2007. Industrial approaches to micronutrient fortification of traditional nixtamal tortillas. Cereal Foods World, 52(5): 240–248.

FAO. 2014. Statistical database. Rome, Italy. Electronic page http://apps.fao.org.

Figueroa-Cárdenas, J. de D., M.G. Acero Godinez, N.L. Vasco Mendez, A. Lozano Guzmán, L.M. Flores Acosta and J. Gonzalez Hernandez. 2001. Fortificación y evaluación de tortillas de nixtamal. Archivos Latinoamericanos de Nutrición, 51(3): 293–302.

Fimognari, C., F. Berti, M. Nüsse, G. Cantelli-Forti and P. Hrelia. 2004. Induction of apoptosis in two human leukemia cell lines as well as differentiation in human promyelocytic cells by cyanidin-3-O-glucopyranoside. Biochem. Pharm., 67: 2047–2056.

Fullmer, L.A. and A. Shao. 2001. The role of lutein in eye health and nutrition. Cereal Foods World, 46(9): 408.

Ghali, Y., O.H. El Sayed, R. Farag, N. Ibrahim and A. Bassiyouni. 1984. Effect of steeping on the structure of corn hull hemicellulose. Starch/Starke, 36: 23–26.

Gouni-Berthold, I. and H.K. Berthold. 2002. Policosanol: clinical pharmacology and therapeutic significance of a new lipid lowering agent. American Heart Journal, 143: 356–365.

Green, J.R., J.T. Lawhon, C.M. Cater and K.F. Mattil. 1977. Utilization of whole undeffatted glandless cottonseed kemels and soybeans to protein-fortify corn tortillas. Journal of Food Science, 42(3): 790–794.

Gressens, P., S.M. Muaku, L. Besse, E. Nsegbe, J. Gallego, B. Delpech, C. Gaultier, P. Evrard, J.M. Keteslegers and D. Maiter. 1997. Maternal protein restriction early in rat pregnancy alters brain development in the progeny. Developmental Brain Research, 103(1): 21–35.

Gutiérrez-Uribe, J.A., C. Rojas-García, S. García-Lara and S.O. Serna-Saldivar. 2010. Phytochemical analysis of wastewater (nejayote) obtained after lime-cooking of different types of maize kernels processed into masa for tortillas. Journal of Cereal Science, 52: 410–416.

Gutiérrez-Uribe, J.A., C. Rojas-García, S. García-Lara and S.O. Serna-Saldivar. 2014. Effects of lime-cooking on carotenoids present in masa and tortillas produced from different types of corns. Cereal Chemistry, 91(5): 508–512.

Hagiwara, A., K. Miyashita, T. Nakanishi, M. Sano, S. Tamano, T. Kadota, T. Koda, M. Nakamura, K. Imaida, N. Ito and T. Shirai. 2001. Pronounced inhibition by a natural anthocyanin, purple corn color, of 2-amino-1-methyl-6-phenylimidazo[4,5-b]pyridine (PhIP)-associated colorectal carcinogenesis in male F344 rats pretreated with 1,2-dimethylhydrazine. Cancer Letters, 171: 17–25.

Hargrove, J.L., P. Greenspan and D.K. Hartle. 2004. Nutritional significance and metabolism of very long chain fatty alcohols and acids from dietary waxes. Experimental Biology Medicine, 229: 215–226.

Harrabi, S., S. Boukhchina, P.M. Mayer and H. Kallel. 2009. Policosanol distribution and accumulation in developing corn kernels. Food Chemistry, 115: 918–923.

Hernández-Salazar, M., E. Agama-Acevedo, S.G. Sayago-Ayerdi, J. Tovar and L.A. Bello-Pérez. 2006. Chemical composition and starch digestibility of tortillas prepared with non-conventional commercial nixtamalized maize flours. International Journal of Food Sciences and Nutrition, 57: 143–150.

Holub, B.J. 1982. The nutritional significance, metabolism, and function of myo-inositol and phosphatidylinositol in health and disease. Advanced Nutrition Research, 4: 107–141.

Huang, M.T., R.C. Smart, C.Q. Wong and A.H. Conney. 1988. Inhibitory effect of curcumin, chlorogenic acid, caffeic acid and ferulic acid on tumor promotion in mouse skin by 12-o-tetradecanoylphorbol-13-acetate. Cancer Research, 48(21): 5941–5946.

Kanski, J., M. Aksenova, A. Stoyanova and D.A. Butterfield. 2002. Ferulic acid antioxidant protection against hydroxyl and peroxyl radical oxidation in synaptosomal and neuronal cell culture systems *in vitro*: structure-activity studies. The Journal of Nutritional Biochemistry, 13: 273–281.

Kawabata, K., T. Yamamoto, A. Hara, M. Shimizu, Y. Yamada, K. Matsunaga, T. Tanaka and H. Mori. 2000. Modifying effects of ferulic acid on azoxymethane induced colon carcinogenesis in F344 rats. Cancer Letters, 157(1): 15–21.

Koetz, R. and H. Neukom. 1977. Nature of bound nicotinic acid in cereals and its release by thermal and chemical treatment. p. 305. *In*: T. Hoyden and O. Kvale (eds.). Physical, chemical and biological changes in food caused by thermal processing. Applied Science Publishers: London, Great Britain.

Lecuona-Villanueva, A., D.A. Betancur-Ancona, L.A. Chel-Guerrero and A.F. Castellanos-Ruelas. 2012. Protein fortification of corn tortillas: effects on physicochemical characteristics, nutritional value and acceptance. Food and Nutrition Sciences, 3: 1658–1663.

Lopez-Martinez, L.X., K.L. Parkin and H.S. Garcia. 2011. Phase II-inducing, polyphenols content and antioxidant capacity of corn (*Zea mays* L.) from phenotypes of white, blue, red and purple corns processed into masa and tortillas. Plant Foods for Human Nutrition, 66: 41–47.

Martinez Bustos, F., H.E. Martinez Flores, E. Sanmartin Martinez, F. Sanchez Sinencio, Y.K. Chang, D. Barrera Arellano and E. Rios. 2001. Effects of the components of maize on the quality of masa and tortillas during the traditional nixtamalisation process. Journal of Science and Food Agriculture, 81: 1455–1462.

Majumder, A. and B. Biswas. 2006. Biology of Inositols and Phosphoinositides. Springer Science & Business Media: New York.

Melesio-Cuellar, J.L., R.E. Preciado-Ortiz, A.D. Terron-Ibarra, G. Vazquez-Carrillo, P. Herrera-Macias, C.A. Amaya-Guerra and S.O. Serna-Saldivar. 2008. Potencial productivo, propiedades físicas y valor nutrimental de híbridos de maíz de alta calidad proteínica sembrados en México. Agricultura Técnica de México, 34: 225–233.

Mertz, E.T., L.S. Bates and O.E. Nelson. 1964. Mutant gene that changes protein composition and increases lysine content of maize endosperm. Science, 145: 279–280.

Mora-Aviles, A., B. Lemus-Flores, R. Miranda-López, D. Hernández-López, J.L. Pons-Hernández, J.A. Acosta-Gallegos and S.H. Guzmán-Maldonado. 2007. Effects of common bean enrichment on nutritional quality of tortillas produced from nixtamalized regular and quality protein maize flours. Journal of the Science of Food and Agriculture, 87(5): 880–886.

Mora-Rochin, S., J.A. Gutierrez-Uribe, S.O. Serna-Saldivar, P. Sánchez-Peña, C. Reyes-Moreno and J. Milán-Carrillo. 2010. Phenolic content and antioxidant activity of tortillas produced from pigmented maize processed by conventional nixtamalization or extrusion cooking. Journal of Cereal Science, 52: 410–416.

Muller, O. and M. Krawinkel. 2005. Malnutrition and health in developing countries. CMAJ, 173 (3): 279–286.

Noriega, E., L. Rivera and E. Pedralta. 2000. Glycaemic and insulinaemic indices of Mexican foods high in complex carbohydrates. Diabetes, Nutrition & Metabolism, 13(1): 13–19.

Nygard, O., J.E. Nordrehaug, H. Refsum, P.M. Ueland, M. Farstad and S.E. Vollset. 1997. Plasma homocysteine levels and mortality in patients with coronary artery disease. New England Journal of. Medicine, 337: 230–236.

Nyman, M., M. Siljestrom, B. Pedersen, K.E. Bach Knudsen, N.G. Asp, C.G. Johansson and O. Eggum. 1984. Dietary fiber content and composition in six cereals at different extraction rates. Cereal Chemistry, 61: 14–19.

Pedreschi, R. and L. Cisneros-Zevallos. 2007. Phenolic profiles of Andean purple corn (*Zea mays* L.) Food Chemistry, 100: 956–963.

Phillippy, B. 2003. Inositol phosphates in foods. Advances in Food and Nutrition Research, 45: 1–60.

Raben, A., A. Tagliabue, N.J. Christensen, J. Madsen, J.J. Holst and A. Astrup. 1994. Resistant starch: the effect on postprandial glycemia, hormonal response, and satiety. American Journal of Clinical Nutrition, 60(4): 544–551.

Rendón-Villalobos, R., E. Agama-Acevedo, J.J. Islas-Hernández, J. Sánchez-Muñoz and L.A. Bello-Pérez. 2006. *In vitro* starch bioavailability of corn tortillas with hydrocolloids. Food Chemistry, 91(4): 631–636.

Rendon-Villalobos, R., L.A. Bello-Pérez, P. Osorio-Díaz, J. Tovar and O. Paredes-López. 2002. Effect of storage time on *in vitro* digestibility and resistant starch content of nixtamal, masa, and tortilla. Cereal Chemistry, 79(3): 340–344.

Rojas-García, C., S. García-Lara, S.O. Serna-Saldívar and J.A. Gutiérrez-Uribe. 2012. Chemopreventive effects of free and bound phenolics associated to steep waters (nejayote) obtained after nixtamalization of different maize types. Plant Foods for Human Nutrition, 67: 94–99.

Rooney, L.W. and S.O. Serna-Saldivar. 2003. Food Uses of Whole Corn and Dry Milled Fractions. Chapter 13 (pp. 495–535). *In*: P. White and L. Johnson (eds.). Corn Chemistry and Technology, Second Edition, American Association of Cereal Chemists: St. Paul, MN.

Salinas-Moreno, Y., M.H. Soto, F. Martínez-Bustos, R.P. Ortega and J.L. Arellano-Vásquez. 2003. Effect of alkaline cooking process on anthocyanins in pigmented maize grain. Agrociencia, 37: 617–628.

Sanchez-Marroquin, A., A. Feria-Morales, S. Maya and V. Ramos-Moreno. 1987. Processing, nutritional quality and sensory evaluation of amaranth enriched corn tortilla. Journal of Food Science, 52: 1611–1614.

Saoussem, H. 2013. Phospholipids. Chapter 6. *In*: L.M.L. Mollet and F. Toldra (eds.). Food Analysis by HPLC. CRC Press: Boca Raton, FL.

Serna-Saldivar, S.O. 1997. The Fortification and Enrichment of Corn Tortillas: An Industrial Approach. Chapter 3. *In*: Fortification of Corn Masa with Iron and/or Other Nutrients—A Literature and Industry Experience Review. SUSTAIN, US Agency for International Development: Washington, DC.

Serna-Saldivar, S.O. 2010. Cereal Grains: Properties, Processing and Nutritional Attributes. CRC Press (Taylor & Francis Group): Boca Raton, FL.

Serna-Saldivar, S.O. 2012. Cereal Grains: Laboratory Reference and Procedures Manual. CRC Press (Taylor & Francis Group). Boca Raton, FL, USA.

Serna-Saldivar, S.O. and C.A. Amaya-Guerra. 2008. El Papel de la Tortilla Nixtamalizada en la Nutrición y Alimentación. Chapter 3 (pp. 105–151). *In*: M. Rodriguez Garcia, S.O. SernaSaldivar and F. Sanchez Senecio (eds.). Nixtamalización del Maíz a la Tortilla: Aspectos Nutrimentales y Toxicológicos. Universidad de Querétaro, Series Ingeniería: Querétaro, Qro., México.

Serna-Saldivar, S.O. and L.W. Rooney. 2003. Tortillas. pp. 5808–5813. *In*: B. Caballero, L. Trugo and P. Finglas (eds.). Encyclopedia of Food Sciences and Nutrition. Second Edition. Academic Press: London, UK.

Serna-Saldivar, S.O., R. Canett, J. Vargas, M. Gonzales and S. Bedolla. 1988b. Effect of soybean and sesame addition on the nutritional value of maize/decorticated sorghum tortillas produced by extrusion cooking. Cereal Chemistry, 65: 44–48.

Serna-Saldivar, S.O., M.H. Gomez, A.R. Islas-Rubio, A.J. Bockholt and L.W. Rooney. 1992b. The Alkaline Processing Properties of Quality Protein Maize. Chapter 16. *In*: E.T. Mertz (ed.). Quality Protein Maize, American Association of Cereal Chemists: St. Paul, MN.

Serna-Saldivar, S.O., M.H. Gomez and L.W. Rooney. 1990. The chemistry, technology and nutritional value of alkaline-cooked corn products. Chapter 4. *In*: Y. Pomeranz (ed.). Advances in Cereal Sci. & Technology. Vol X., American Association of Cereal Chemists: St. Paul, MN.

Serna-Saldivar, S.O., P. Herrera-Macias, C.A. Amaya-Guerra, J.L. Melesio-Cuellar, R.E. Preciado-Ortiz, A.D. Terron-Ibarra and G. Vazquez-Carrillo. 2008. Evaluation of the lime-cooking and tortilla making properties of quality protein maize hybrids grown in Mexico. Plant Foods and Human Nutrition, 63(3): 119–125.

Serna-Saldivar, S.O., D.A. Knabe, L.W. Rooney and T.D. Tanksley. 1987. Effect of lime treatment on energy and protein digestibilities of maize and sorghum. Cereal Chemistry, 64: 247–252.

Serna-Saldivar, S.O., D.A. Knabe, L.W. Rooney, T.D. Jr. Tanksley and A.M. Sproule. 1988a. Nutritional value of sorghum and maize tortillas. Journal of Cereal Science, 7: 83–94.

Serna-Saldivar, S.O., L.W. Rooney and L.W. Greene. 1991. Effects of lime treatment on the bioavailability of calcium in diets of tortillas and beans: growth/metabolic studies. Cereal Chemistry, 68: 565–570.

Serna-Saldivar, S.O., L.W. Rooney and L.W. Greene. 1992a. Effects of lime treatment on the bioavailability of calcium in diets of tortillas and beans: Bone and plasma composition in rats. Cereal Chemistry, 69: 78–81.

Shih, P.H., C.T. Yeh and G.C. Yen. 2005. Effects of anthocyanidin on the inhibition of proliferation and induction of apoptosis in human gastric adenocarcinoma cells. Food and Chemical Toxicology, 55: 1557–1566.

Sproule, A.M., S.O. Serna-Saldivar, A.J. Bockholt, L.W. Rooney and D.A. Knabe. 1988. Nutritional evaluation of tortillas and tortilla chips from quality protein maize. Cereal Foods World, 33(2): 233–236.

Stylianopoulos, C. 1999. Efecto de la fortificación y del enriquecimiento de tortillas de maíz en el crecimiento fisiológico y cerebral de ratas durante dos generaciones. MSc Thesis. Tecnológico y de Monterrey: Monterrey, N.L., México.

Stylianopoulos, C., S.O. Serna-Saldívar and G. Arteaga MacKinney. 2001. Effects of fortification and enrichment of maize tortillas on growth and brain development of rats throughout two generations. Cereal Chemistry, 79(1): 85–91.

Sullivan, J.S., D.A. Knabe, A.J. Bockholt and E.J. Gregg. 1989. Nutritional value of quality protein maize and food corn for starter and growth pigs. Journal of Animal Science, 67: 1285–1292.

Tsuda, T., F. Horio, K. Uchida, H. Aoki and T. Osawa. 2003. Dietary cyanidin 3-O-β-D-glucoside-rich purple corn color prevents obesity and ameliorates hyperglycemia in mice. Journal of Nutrition, 133: 2125–2130.

Ubesie, A.C., N.S. Ibeziako, C.I. Ndiokwelu, C.M. Uzoka and C.A. Nwafor. 2012. Under-five Protein Energy Malnutrition Admitted at the University of In Nigeria Teaching Hospital, Enugu: a 10 year retrospective review. Nutrition Journal, 11: 43–50.

Uc-Cetz, H., V. Pérez-Flores, L. Chel-Guerrero and A. Betancur-Ancona. 2003. Production of corn tortillas added with a protein concentrate from *Phaseolus lunatus*. Food Technology, 38(1): 7–16.

Urizar, A.L. and R. Bressani. 1997. Efecto de la nixtamalizacion del maíz sobre el contenido de ácido fítico, calcio y hierro total y disponible. Archivos Latinoamericanos de Nutrición, 47(3): 217–223.

USDA. 2014. Nutrient Data Laboratory. Agricultural Research Service. Electronic page: http://www.nal.usda.gov/fnic/foodcomp.

Vucenik, I. and A.M. Shamsuddin. 2006. Protection against cancer by dietary IP6 and inositol. Nutrition Cancer, 55(2): 109–125.

Wall, J.W. and K.J. Carpenter. 1988. Variation in availability of niacin in grain products. Food Technology, 42(10): 198–204.

Wang, L.S. and G.D. Stoner. 2008. Anthocyanins and their role in cancer prevention. Cancer Letters, 269: 281–290.

White, P. and E.J. Weber. 2003. Lipids of the Kernel. Chapter 10 (pp. 355–395). *In*: P.J. White and L.A. Johnson (eds.). Corn Chemistry and Technology. Second Edition. American Association of Cereal Chemists: St. Paul, MN.

Zhao, X., M. Corrales, C. Zhang, X. Hu, Y. Ma and B. Tauscher. 2008. Composition and thermal stability of anthocyanins from chinese purple corn (*Zea mays* L.). Journal of Agriculture and Food Chemistry, 56(22): 10761–10766.

Zeisel, S. 1994. Choline and human nutrition. Annual Review of Nutrition, 14: 269–296.

17

The Influence of Bread Enriched with Bioactive Components on Body Weight Control, Carbohydrate Metabolism, and Lipid Profile

Joanna Bajerska[1,*] and *Sylwia Mildner-Szkudlarz*[2]

1. Introduction

Over the past several decades, the incidence of overweight and obesity has increased worldwide to epidemic proportions. Based on the latest available data, more than half (52%) of the adult population in the European Union are overweight or obese (WHO 2010). Obesity is a predisposing factor for the development of type-2 diabetes (T2D), hypertension, and cardiovascular disease (CVD). Weight loss reduces the risk of insulin resistance and atherosclerosis through favorable changes in blood pressure, blood lipids, and lipoprotein, as well as in insulin levels (Dattilo and Kris-Etherton 1992). However, the perception of the general public is that weight loss therapy, with its calorie-restricted diets, is difficult to implement, and the concomitant increase of physical activity level is difficult to achieve (Wing and Hill 2001). Therefore

[1] Poznań University of Life Sciences, Department of Human Nutrition and Hygiene, Wojska Polskiego 28, PL-60-637, Poznań, Poland.
 Email: joanna.bajerska@up.poznan.pl
[2] Poznań University of Life Sciences, Department of Food Science and Nutrition, Wojska Polskiego 28, PL-60-637, Poznań, Poland.
 Email: mildners@up.poznan.pl
* Corresponding author

developing effective strategies for body-weight management is a priority not only for researchers and the pharmaceutical and food industries, but most of all for the population that is currently overweight or obese. In line with the ancient Asian concept that "food and medicine are one"—a precept also widely accepted among the Western population—we can observe a trend towards identifying or producing food with functions that might help body-weight regulation and reduce the risk of (or delay the onset of) major diseases related to obesity. Such food products are referred to as "functional foods" which, besides their major functions of providing the necessary nutrients for humans, may also prevent nutrition-related diseases and improve the physical and mental well-being of consumers (Siró et al. 2008). In this area, food technologists may offer products that are aimed especially for obese people and which act to positively influence their energy metabolism while providing the physiological sensation of satiety (Serrano et al. 2012).

Worldwide, bread is one of the most widely consumed foodstuffs, with an average consumption ranging from 41 to 303 kg/year per capita (Rosell 2011). Therefore breads seem an ideal vehicle for delivering functionality to the consumer in an acceptable form (Aldrick 2007). It is, however, important to develop a functional bakery product which has both physiological effectiveness and consumer acceptance (Alldrick 2012). In late 2003, Unilever introduced an innovation in the bakery sector in the form of a white bread called Blue Band Goede Start, which was the first white bread containing the nutritional elements normally available in brown bread: fibers; vitamins B_1, PP and B_6; iron; zinc; and inulin (Siró et al. 2008).

Incorporation into the diet of functional bread enriched with bioactive ingredients that may reduce energy intake or its bioavailability, while increasing energy expenditure or otherwise reducing stored fat, seems to be a beneficial solution in weight loss and prevention of weight (re)gain. One ingredient that could be added to the white bread formula is dietary fiber. It is speculated that dietary fiber reduces nutrient absorption while increasing the rate of passage and stimulating production of gut hormones (Lattimer and Haub 2010).

It has also been indicated that food ingredients rich in protein and fiber can enhance satiety and reduce energy intake, acutely contributing to body-weight loss, while preventing and treating obesity related diseases (Belski 2011). Over the past two decades, polyphenols and methylxanthines have attracted the interest of the public and of the scientific community for their role in modulating obesity and associated disorders (Meydani and Hasan 2010) by stimulating thermogenesis and decreasing nutrient absorption (for example, fat) from the intestinal tract (Dulloo 2011). Furthermore, the addition of antioxidant dietary fiber (that is, fiber with associated antioxidant compounds) to the bread formula may help to increase the feeling of satiety from foods (Jiménez et al. 2008) or increase postprandial energy expenditure while reducing the respiratory quotient in humans (Dulloo 2011). It seems that the use of these metabolically active ingredients as additions to or replacement for the flour in bread may affect different processes of energy intake and expenditure, and may be the best strategy for tackling obesity, control and preventing the majority of nutrition-related diseases. However, prior to its market launch, the metabolic effects of the formulated functional breads should be clinically demonstrated. The impact of the consumption of bread enriched with bioactive food ingredients on satiety, glycemic index, energy or fat fecal extraction, weight loss, as well as on blood pressure, lipid profile, and glycaemia, has been reported in clinical and laboratory animal and human studies and presented in Tables 1 and 2.

2. Breads enriched with bioactive components

2.1 Bread enriched with dietary fiber

Dietary Fiber (DF) is those edible parts of plants (or analogous carbohydrate sources) that are resistant to digestion and absorption in the human intestine, and which undergo complete or partial fermentation in the large intestine, while promoting beneficial physiological effects including improvements in both the feeling of satiety and decreases in the transit time through the intestinal tract, as well as control of both blood glucose and cholesterol concentration (Madan and Narsaria 2013). Thus, DF intake reduces the risk of developing the following diseases: coronary heart disease, stroke, hypertension, diabetes, obesity, and certain gastrointestinal disorders (Anderson 2009). DF can be categorized as soluble or insoluble. The intake of soluble fibers may increase satiety and reduce the digestibility of nutrients. In addition, it may have the ability to bind bile acids and decrease the reabsorption of bile acids and cholesterol from the intestine (Lattimer and Haub 2010; Madan and Narsaria 2013). Soluble DF also undergoes fermentation to short-chain fatty acids in the colon, thus reducing the endogenous synthesis of cholesterol (Madan and Narsaria 2013). Insoluble fibers increase and soften the stool bulk, thereby shortening transit time through the intestinal tract (Lunde et al. 2011). Lunde et al. (2011) concluded that replacing some of the digestible carbohydrates in bread with 17% pea fiber (providing ~20 g of dietary fiber in a portion of bread) prolonged subjects' satiety over a longer period, while at the same time keeping postprandial blood glucose levels, significantly lower than following intake of the control bread (Table 1).

Recently, great attention has been paid to the health properties of flaxseed (FS) fiber. FS contain ~30% dietary fiber, of which one third is water-soluble and belongs to the group of heterogeneous polysaccharides (Kristensen et al. 2012). In a study conducted by Kristensen et al. (2008), it was found that the addition of whole FS to rye breads (6 g/100 g) significantly reduced the digestibility of fat and energy in humans (Table 1). Although in a later study by the same authors it was observed that rye bread enriched with FS dietary fiber (providing 5 g of dietary fibers from FS daily) significantly increased fecal fat excretion as compared to the control bread, much more extended effects were seen following consumption of a flaxseed drink. The authors explained that thermal process may decrease the ability of baked products to induce dietary fiber viscosity resulting from either reduced hydration of the dietary fiber or its reduced molecular weight in the baked products (Kristensen et al. 2012). The next explanation is that endogenous enzymes in the bread reduce the viscosity of FS fibers, thereby decreasing its clinical effectiveness as a functional ingredient (Kristensen et al. 2012). However, many of the animal and human studies with dietary fiber as a functional ingredient in bread have focused on improvements in glycemic control and preventing hypercholesterolemia (Beck et al. 2010). For example, in a

Table 1. Pooled results from human studies on the effect of different functionality on energy and lipid absorption, body weight, fat mass, lipids and carbohydrate profiles.

Functional bread	Functional ingredient	Experimental design	Duration	Addition levels	BW, BMI, WC, FM Functional bread vs. control bread	TC, HDL-C, TG, BG Functional bread vs. control bread	Satiety	Energy intake	References
Bread enriched with β-glucan	Fiber	46 patients with T2D and LDL-C greater than 3.37 mmol; 3-week randomized, double-blind study; bread enriched with β-glucan or control white bread.	3 weeks	3 g/day of β-glucan	BW: −0.64 kg, NS BMI: −0.26 kg/m², NS WC: −1.02 cm, NS	LDL-C: (−0.55 mmol/l); P < 0.01; TC: (−0.68 mmol/l); P < 0.01; HDL-C (−0.02 mmol/l) NS; TG: (−0.15 mmol/l) NS BG: (−0.65 mmol/l) NS; BI: (−7.0 µU/ml); P < 0.05; Homa-IR: (−3.41); P < 0.05; SBP: (−7.9 mmHg); NS; DBP: (−1.01 mmHg); NS	-	-	Liatis et al. 2009
Bread enriched with defatted flaxseed (DFS)	Fiber	16 subjects (8 T2D + 8 normal healthy); 200 g bread enriched with DFS + dietary regimen	8 weeks	Flour substituted with 10% DFS	BMI: after 2 months of dietary intervention, in both group BMI ↓ (P < 0.5)	BG: healthy: ↓3%; diabetic: ↓14% (P < 0.5); TC: healthy: ↓14% (P < 0.05); diabetic: ↓19% (P < 0.05); HDL-C: healthy: ↑9% (P < 0.01); diabetic: ↑8% (P < 0.01); LDL-C: healthy: ↓23% (P < 0.05); diabetic: ↓26% (P < 0.05); TG: healthy: ↓19% (P < 0.01); diabetic: ↓17% (P < 0.05); MDA: healthy: ↓25% (P < 0.01); diabetic: ↓16% (P < 0.05)	-	-	Mohamed et al. 2012

| Bread enriched with Flaxseed (FS) | Fiber | 11 healthy young men aged 24.6 ± 2.7 years; randomized crossover study with 300 g of one of four rye bread (RB) + basal diets | One week | (1) RB (control); (2) RB + 6.2 g sunflower seeds (SU)/100 g rye flour, (3) RB + 6.2 g whole flaxseed (FS) g/100 g rye flour; (4) Low extraction rate rye grain flour + 6.8 g SU and + 6.1 g FS/100 g flour | - | - | - | After RB + SU or RB + FL ↓apparent digestion of fat and energy. The effect on energy digestibility of FL was more pronounced than that of SU. | Kristensen et al. 2008 |
| Bread enriched with FS | Fiber | 17 young subjects (10 women and 7 men); three dietary intervention periods; double-blind randomized crossover design; three different diets | One week | (1) Low-fiber control diet (Control) (2) Diet + 3 flax drink per day = 5.2 g fibers/10 MJ (4) Diet + FS bread eaten 3 times per day = 5.2 g fibers/10 MJ | - | Flax drink vs. control ↓T-C by 12% and LDL-C by 15%, (P < 0.01), Flax bread vs. control ↓T-C by 7% and LDL-C by 9%, (P < 0.05) | - | Flax drink vs. control ↑ fecal fat extraction by 50% ↑ fecal energy excretion by 23%, (P < 0.05), Flax bread vs. control ↑ fecal fat excretion (P < 0.05). | Kristensen et al. 2012 |

Table 1. contd....

Table 1. contd.

Functional bread	Functional ingredient	Experimental design	Duration	Addition levels	BW, BMI, WC, FM Functional bread vs. control bread	TC, HDL–C, TG, BG Functional bread vs. control bread	Satiety	Energy intake	References
Bread enriched with pea fiber, rapeseed oil	Fiber and monosaturated fatty acid	10 women after overnight fast; three experiments; crossover design; ingestion of various types of bread, all providing 25g available carbohydrates (CHO)	One day	Bread 1: 61 g (4.6% fiber, 2.8% fat); Bread 2: 119 g (17% pea fiber, 1% rapeseed oil); Bread 3: 133 g (17% pea fiber, 9% rapeseed oil)	-	Intake of bread 2 and 3 (in amounts providing 25 g CHO) ↓ postprandial blood glucose (PPG), the incremental area under the glucose versus time curve (IAUC) (during 15 to 75 min), GP, ($P < .05$), vs. Bread 1	After ingestion bread 2 and 3 vs. bread 1 ↑ satiety ($P < 0.05$) from 60 min up to 120 min	-	Lunde et al. 2011
Bread enriched with LKF	Protein and fiber	16 subjects, randomized controlled crossover trial lupin bread (LB) vs. white bread (WB)	One day	Substituting 40% of the wheat flour with LKF	-	-	Breakfast: after LB ↑ satiety vs. WB	LB for breakfast ↓ energy intake (−488 kJ; 95% CI: −798, −178) for lunch vs. BW; LB for lunch ↓ within-meal energy intake (−1028kJ; 95% CI: −1338, −727) vs. WB	Lee et al. 2006

Bread enriched with LKF	Protein and fiber	20 subjects aged 20.1–44.8 years, BMI 18.4–24.8 kg/m², consumed two kinds of bread at breakfast: whole grain Bürgen bread (BB) and lupin bread (LB)	One day	Two slices of BB or LB (all 1300 kJ) with 10g margarine and 30 g strawberry jam for breakfast	–	–	After LB and BB ↑ satiety vs. WB LB produced ↓ smaller PG and PI responses vs. WB	–	Keogh et al. 2011
Bread enriched with LKF	Protein and fiber	88 overweight and obese subjects; parallel-design randomized controlled trial; LB and WB eaten ad libitum, 15%–20% of daily EI	16 weeks	Substituting 40% of the wheat flour with LKF	BW: −0.4 kg (−1.3, 0.6), NS FM: −0.5 kg (−1.1, 0.2), NS	TC: −0.08 mmol/l (−0.38, 0.22); NS TG: 0.09 mmol/l (−0.10, 0.21); NS BG: 0.10 mmol/l (−0.11, 0.30); NS		–	Hodgson et al. 2010
Bread enriched with green tea extract (GTE)	Catechins and caffeine	55 obese subjects; a single-blind, randomized, controlled design, subject received either rye bread enriched with GTE or plain rye bread	12 weeks	1.1% GTE: 280g for women, 360 g for men	BW: −0.97 kg (−2.2 to 0.3); NS FM: −0.67 kg (−1.5 to 0.2); NS WC: −1.22 (−2.4 to −0.02); p < 0.05	SBP: −4.6 (−9.06, −0.15); p < 0.05 DBP: −3.8 (−6.66, −0.89); p < 0.05 BG: −0.16 (−0.46, 0.15); NS HDL-C: 0.07 (−0.04, 0.18); NS TG: −0.23 (−0.54, 0.08); NS		–	Bajerska et al. (paper awaiting publication)

Table 1. contd....

Table 1. contd.

Functional bread	Functional ingredient	Experimental design	Duration	Addition levels	BW, BMI, WC, FM Functional bread vs. control bread	TC, HDL-C, TG, BG Functional bread vs. control bread	Satiety	Energy intake	References
Bread enriched with red or white beetroot	Betalains, dietary nitrate	Subjects ($n = 14$) were randomly assigned to one of three different bread products: white bread (WB), white bread enriched with white beetroot (WBT); and white bread enriched with red beetroot (RBT)	24-h	200 g WB (control) or 200g WBT or 200 g RBT	-	Bread enriched with 100 g RBT or WBT ↓ SBP and DBP over a period of 24 h. Total urinary NOx significantly ↑ after RBT, but did not reach significance for WBT vs. WB	-	-	Hobbs et al. 2012
Bread enriched with plant sterols (PS)	Plant sterols	Subjects ($n = 68$), double-blind, six-week, dietary intervention trial: habitual (1 week), baseline (1 week) Intervention trial: rye bread enriched with low dose (LD) of PS (2 weeks), rye bread enriched with high dose (HD) of PS	4 weeks	LD of plant sterols: 2 g/day HD of plant sterols: 4 g/day	-	Bread enriched with LD of plant sterols vs. control ↓ T-C: 5.1%, LDL-C: 8.1%, Apo/apoA1: 8.3%; T-C/HDL-C: 7.2%, Bread enriched with HD of plant sterols vs. control ↓ T-C: 6.5%, LDL-C: 10.4%, Apo/apoA1: 5.5% T-C/HDL-C: 3.7%	-	-	Söderholm et al. 2012

LKF: lupin kernel flour; LB: lupin bread; WB: wheat bread; BB: whole grain Bürgen Bread; EI: energy intake; BW: body weight; BMI: body mass index; WC: waist circumference; FM: fat mass; TC: total cholesterol; HDL-C: high-density cholesterol; LDL-C: low-density cholesterol; T2D: Type 2 diabetes; T-C: total cholesterol; TG: triglycerides; BG: blood glucose; PV: average postprandial blood glucose peak value; PG: postprandial glucose; NS: non-significant; SBP: systolic blood pressure; DBP: diastolic blood pressure; I: insulin; FS: flaxseed; DFS: defatted flaxseed; GTE: green tea extract; RB: rye bread.

Table 2. Pooled results from animal studies on the effect of different functionalities on energy and lipid absorption, body weight, fat mass, lipids and carbohydrate profiles.

Functional bread	Animals	Follow-up	Experimental diet	Active substances	Dose	Energy and lipid absorption	Reported effects on body weight, fat mass	Reported effects on lipid and carbohydrate profiles	References
Bread enriched GTE	$N = 24$, 8-week-old male Wistar rats	6 weeks	1. ND: normal caloric diet; 2. hypercaloric diet (H) + control rye bread (RB); 3. H+RB+0.8% green tea extract (GTE); 4. H+RB+1.1% GTE	Catechins, caffeine	0.8% GTE 1.1% GTE	Only RB + 1.1% GTE ↑ feces energy excretion vs. H+RB	RB + 0.8% GTE and 1.1% GTE nonsignificant impact on BW gain and VFC vs. HRB	RB + 0.8% GTE and 1.1% GTE nonsignificant impact on insulin and leptin concentration vs. H + RB	Bajerska et al. 2013
Bread enriched saffron extract (SE)	$N = 24$, streptozotocin (STZ)-induced Wistar rats	5 weeks	1. High fat diet (HF); 2. HF + rye bread (RB); 3. HF + RB enriched with saffron 0.12% (S) powder (RB+S); 4. HF + 0.08% S (HF + S)	Crocetin, safranal, picrocrocin, crocins	Bread enriched with 0.12% S 0.08% S to the HF diet	-	HF + S, HF + RB, and HF + RB + S nonsignificant impact on BW, VFC vs. HF	S, RB, and RB+S ↓ BG, TG and ↑ HOMA-% β and insulin concentration vs. HF	Bajerska et al. 2013
Bread enriched powdered grape by-products (PGP) or extract from grape by-products (EGP)	$N = 24$, 8-week-old male Wistar rats	6 weeks	1. Cholesterol/cholic acid diet (HF); 2. HF + control mixed rye bread (CB); 3. HF + bread enriched with powdered grape by-products (PGP); 4. HF + bread enriched with extract from grape by-products (EGP)	Fiber, polyphenols	6% PGP 1.4% EGP	PGP and EGP breads ↑fecal fat, ↓ apparent digestion of fat vs. HF and HF + CB	PGP and EGP breads nonsignificant impact on BW vs. HF and HF + CB PGP bread but not EGP-bread ↓ visceral fat content vs. HF and HF+CB	PGP and EGP breads ↓ TC (19–38%) and LDL-C (27–50%) ↓ AI and ↑ HDL-C (19–23%) vs. HF and HF+CB. PGP and EGP breads ↓ fasting blood glucose vs. HF and HF + CB	Mildner-Szkudlarz and Bajerska 2013

Table 2. contd....

Table 2. contd.

Functional bread	Animals	Follow-up	Experimental diet	Active substances	Dose	Energy and lipid absorption	Reported effects on body weight, fat mass	Reported effects on lipid and carbohydrate profiles	References
Bread enriched flaxseed (FS)	N = 30, hypercholesterolemic Wistar rats	4 weeks	1. CB: Control bread; 2. WFS: Bread contains whole flaxseeds; 3. DFS: Bread containing defatted flaxseeds	Fiber	10% FS, 15% DFS	-	WFS and DFS breads nonsignificant impact on BW gain vs. CB	WFS and DFS breads ↓ T-C, LDL-C, TG vs. CB WFS but not DFS bread ↑ HDL-C	Mohamed et al. 2005

GTE: green tea extract; SE: Saffron extract; PGP: powdered grape by-products; EGP: extract from grape by-products; FS: flaxseeds; TC: total cholesterol; HDL-C: high-density cholesterol; LDL-C: low-density cholesterol; TG: triglycerides; HF: high-fat diet; BW: body weight; VFC: visceral fat content; HOMA-% β: Homeostatic model assessment of β-cell function.

study conducted by Mohamed et al. (2005), it was indicated that the incorporation of either bread supplemented with ground FS or defatted FS (replacing 10% and 15% of wheat flour, respectively) into high-fat/hypercholesterolemic diet breads significantly decreased the total cholesterol (T-C), the low-density cholesterol (LDL-C), and the triglyceride (TG) levels, as compared to the control breads in hypercholesterolemic rats (Table 2). Only in the group of rats fed on the breads supplemented with ground FS a significant increase in high-density cholesterol (HDL-C) concentration was seen. The consumption of both functional breads did not influence food intake or prevent weight gain in the rats. In a later study by the same authors, a significant reduction in body mass index (BMI) in both healthy and diabetic patients was observed following two months' dietary intervention, involving 200 g of bread enriched with defatted FS daily (the flour in this bread was replaced with 10% ground defatted FS, Table 1). Although the authors concluded that the administration of bread enriched with defatted FS together with a dietary regimen for two months improved the glycaemia and lipid profile and decreased oxidative stress in both diabetic and normal healthy subjects, they did not present the precise amounts of dietary fibers responsible for this beneficial effects (Mohamed et al. 2012).

In the study of Liatis et al. (2009), the effects of consuming oat β-glucan-enriched bread on the lipid profile and on glucose control in patients with type-2 diabetes was investigated (Table 1). The consumption of this functional bread provided 3 g of oat β-glucan per day. It was found that consumption of this functional bread led to significant reductions (compared with the control wheat bread) in T-C, LDL-C, and in fasting plasma insulin, as well as in the Homeostasis Model of Assessment measurement of Insulin Resistance (HOMA-IR). Although it was not major outcome in the study, patients in both groups lost weight after three weeks (1.03 kg in the oat β-glucan group vs. 0.39 kg in the controls), with the weight reductions being statistical significant only in the oat β-glucan group. However, the intergroup differences in body weight (–0.64 kg) were not statistical significant. The authors of this study did not attempt to explain the causes of the observed body-weight loss, as no specific dietetic plan was given and physical activity and dietary intake were not recorded (Liatis et al. 2009). It seems, however, that the lack of significant difference in weight loss between experimental groups could be connected to both the amount of DF incorporated into the diet and the duration of its consumption. According to Serrano et al. (2012), the amount of fiber needed to produce a feeling of satiety in humans and to induce body-weight loss should be higher than 8 g per day, but the incorporation of this amount in technologically modified foods is difficult. Moreover, it has been suggested that viscous fiber may produce acute satiety feelings after chronic consumption for longer than nine months (Serrano et al. 2012). Finally, the reduction in the viscosity of the fibers during the breadmaking process may be responsible for the decrease in the clinical effectiveness of such fiber as a functional ingredient (Kristensen et al. 2012).

2.2 Bread enriched with ingredients that are rich in dietary fiber and protein

Data suggest that both high-protein and high-DF diets can enhance satiety and acutely reduce energy intake, and may contribute to body-weight loss in the longer term

(Bielski et al. 2011). It seems that a practical approach to increasing both the protein and fiber content of foods is to incorporate high-protein and high-fiber ingredients into commonly consumed high-carbohydrate foods, such as breads (Belski et al. 2012; Hodgson et al. 2010). Lupin kernel flour (LKF) could serve as one such ingredient: it is derived from the endosperm of lupin, and contains 40–45% protein, 25–30% fiber, and negligible sugar and starch (Hodgson et al. 2010). It has been shown that the incorporation of LKF into bread can increase protein and fiber and reduce the carbohydrate content with little change in product acceptability (Hodgson et al. 2010). In a study conducted by Lee et al. (2006) it was shown that bread enriched with this high-protein, high-fiber LKF (with 40% wheat flour replacement), eaten for breakfast and lunch, significantly increased intrameal and intermeal satiety and reduced energy intake, as compared to wheat bread (Lee et al. 2006, Table 1). A study using lupin bread and the whole grain "Bürgen bread" for breakfast showed that these breads had a significant impact on fullness responses, compared with the white bread. Both lupin bread and the whole grain Bürgen bread produced smaller postprandial glucose and insulin responses than did white bread (Keogh et al. 2011). It was indicated that, if consumption of lupin bread has similar effects on satiety and energy intake in the longer term, such effects could translate into weight loss. For this reason, Hodgson et al. (2010) decided to assess the effects of lupin bread eaten ad libitum on body-weight and the lipid and carbohydrate profiles during a 16-week trial. However, the diet containing lupin bread resulted in only moderate changes in body weight, body composition, fasting blood lipids, and glucose and insulin concentrations in overweight men and women with mildly elevated total cholesterol concentrations. This lack of effect on body weight and body composition may have several possible explanations. It seems that the amount of protein and fiber, as well as the type of fiber in the experimental diet, may be important. The increase in protein in the lupin group was relatively small in comparison with other intervention studies that have shown a beneficial effect on weight loss in the ad libitum and energy-restricted settings. Although the dietary fiber intake from the lupin-enriched bread group was high (12.5 g per day), it seems that the nature of the dietary fiber may be crucial. The dietary fiber present in lupin flour is primarily insoluble (~70%). About 10% is present as soluble fiber (~1.25 g per day) and a further 20% as oligosaccharides (Hodgson et al. 2010).

2.3 Bread enriched with antioxidant dietary fiber

The addition of antioxidant dietary fiber (i.e., fiber with associated antioxidant compounds) to food formulations may help to increase the feeling of satiety resulting from foods. The concept of antioxidant dietary fiber (ADF) was first proposed by Saura-Calixto in 1998, with the criteria that one gram of ADF should have a DPPH free-radical scavenging capacity equivalent to that of at least 50 mg vitamin E, and dietary fiber content greater than 50% dry matter from the natural constituents of the material. Phenolic compounds associated with soluble dietary fiber may present different structures, including soluble flavonoids and phenolic acids. For example, the main phenolic compounds associated with dietary fiber in wine are flavan-3-ols and benzoic acids (Saura-Calixto et al. 2007). There is increasing interest in applying fruit-processing wastes as functional food ingredients, since they are rich sources of dietary fiber, and most of the beneficial bioactive compounds remain in the byproducts (Balasundaram et al. 2006). ADF may be incorporated with flour for making high-dietary-fiber bakery goods, while the polyphenols in ADF could contribute as antioxidants for improving the color, aroma, and taste of the final product. Wine grape pomace (WGP)—the residual seed and skins from winemaking—contains high phenolic compounds and dietary fiber (Mildner-Szkudlarz and Bajerska 2013).

A study conducted by above authors has shown that sensory acceptable mixed rye bread enriched with either dried powdered skins of grape by-product (PGP) or freeze-dried extract from the skins of grape by-product (EGP), incorporated into a high-fat/hypercholesterolemic diet, resulted in lowered fat and protein digestion, as well as lowered T-C, LDL-C, lipid peroxidation, glucose and leptin levels in Wistar rats (Table 2). Both the experimental breads also prevented visceral fat accumulation and led to increases in HDL-C, as well as plasma ferric-reducing antioxidant power levels. It was indicated that polyphenols may induce a higher rate of secretion of satiety peptides such as GLP-1 possibly on account of their effects in the inhibition of glucose uptake by enterocytes (McCarty 2005). However, in the study conducted by these authors, neither the addition of PGP nor of EGP influenced food intake as compared with the control rats. The authors explained that reduced lipid absorption and increased fat excretion in rats' feces, such as was observed after feeding the rats with both fortified breads, could be due to the associated effect of fruit dietary fiber and phenolic compounds in terms in inhibiting the activity of pancreatic lipase. On the other hand, the authors stated that, since feeding with the control bread significantly lowered TC, LDL-C, and lipid peroxidation compared with the high-fat diet, it may be that not only grape by-products, but also another components in the bread, acted to improve the lipid metabolism of the rats. It was suggested that methionine, lignans, betaine, tocotrienols, Mg, and other bioactive rye components are associated with a decreased risk of diabetes and cardiovascular disease (Fardet 2012).

2.4 Bread enriched with herbal and other botanical agents

2.4.1 Green tea

Green tea has been used for centuries for its medicinal properties in preventing hypertension, arteriosclerosis, hyperglycemia, hypercholesterolemia, and obesity. Considering that obesity is becoming one of the most severe health threats (especially due to the development of diabetes, hypertension, and cardiovascular disease), there is increasing interest in studying the role of green tea in the prevention of obesity. The antiobesity properties of green tea components have been demonstrated in most *in vitro* and *in vivo* models of obesity. Decreased adipocyte differentiation, lipogenesis, lipid absorption, and increased β-oxidation are among the proposed mechanisms for the action of green tea (Wolfram 2006). The green tea extract (GTE) that is available on the market as a body-weight control aid is usually offered in an encapsulation formula. However, some nutritionists worry that such substances may mislead the public into believing that there are dietary magic bullets that can ensure health, regardless of what is eaten (Saper 2004). Therefore, it may be beneficial to enrich customarily food items (for example, bread) with GTE. In a study conducted by Bajerska et al. (2013) rye bread enriched with green tea extract: GTRB (at two doses, 0.8% and 1.1%) was incorporated into the rats' hypercaloric diet. It was found that only the consumption of rye bread enriched with 1.1% GTE increased energy excretion in the feces, as compared with the control rye bread. However, in this group of rats, no significant suppression of body-weight gain or visceral fat accumulation was found, and no changes leptin or insulin levels were detected (Bajerska et al. 2013, Table 2). The authors, in their later study, examined whether the incorporation of the GTRB into the diet could improve weight-loss maintenance and control abnormalities linked to metabolic syndrome (Table 1). Although GTRB consumption did not significantly influence the maintenance of weight after weight loss therapy, HDL-C, TG, or BG levels, it did result in significant differences between the treatment groups in diastolic and systolic blood pressure. Moreover the proportion of subjects fulfilling the criteria of the metabolic syndrome after weight maintenance phase was significantly lower in the study group than in the control group. With regard to lower effectiveness of weight loss maintenance after consumption of GTRB, Wang and Zhou (2004) considered that green tea components incorporated into rye bread might be less stable following the breadmaking process. While Schramm et al. (2003) have demonstrated the ability of carbohydrates, in the form of white bread and sucrose, to enhance epicatechin bioavailability in humans but, in general, evidence on the importance of food matrix on the stability of the green tea components is lacking.

2.4.2 Saffron extract

There is evidence that the bioactive ingredients of saffron (S), such as crocetin, safranal, picrocrocin, and crocins, may have antihyperglycemic and antihyperlipidemic effects. For example, Mohajeri et al. (2008) indicated that an ethanolic extract of saffron in a dose of 40 mg/kg body weight administered by the intraperitoneal route significantly decreases blood glucose level by 33.9% in diabetic rats, in comparison with normal healthy rats, six hours after administration. Moreover, Sheng et al. (2006) have indicated that crocin has lipid-lowering properties, and that it selectively inhibits the activity of pancreatic lipase as a competitive inhibitor.

In a study conducted by Bajerska et al. (2013) the most consumer-acceptable rye bread enriched with saffron powder (SP) was designed to verify its antidiabetic properties, and to compare these effects with those of rye bread and SP alone, matched to a similar dose of bioactive components used in the high-fat diet in streptozotocin-induced rats (Table 2). Although rye bread enriched with SP incorporated in high-fat diets leads to the regeneration of β-cell function, increases in insulin secretion, and decreases in glucose and triglyceride level, the authors concluded that these effects were not significantly higher than those seen in the case of SP or rye bread incorporated into the high-fat diet in diabetic rats separately (Bajerska et al. 2013). The explanation for this observation may be the thermal processing involved in breadmaking, which may lead to the degradation of the majority of the saffron bioactive components. Raina et al. (1996) indicated that, in the processing of saffron, drying temperatures lower than 30°C or higher than 60°C produced greater carotenoid degradation. Moreover, we postulate that the bioactive components of saffron powder may be less bioaccessible in the digestive tract when included in bread, most likely due to the strong interaction of this compound with the processed food components (proteins and starch). Therefore, the authors' proposals are that the optimal method for improving the stability and bioavailability of saffron's active components from food matrices should be employed (for example, microcapsulation).

2.4.3 White and red beetroot

It has been postulated that the cardioprotective effects seen with the consumption of green leafy vegetables and beetroot may be due to their high dietary nitrate and betalain content (Lundberg and Weitzberg 2005; Webb et al. 2008). Hobbs et al. (2012) assessed whether red or white beetroot-enriched bread can influence blood pressure (Table 1). These studies demonstrated significant hypotensive effects of the two kinds of beetroot-enriched breads, similar to that observed following consumption of beetroot juice. The authors of this study suggest that nitrate in the beetroot is a major contributor to the blood pressure reduction observed, whereas betalains had a minimal influence. It was observed also that food processing had minimal impact on physiological effects of beetroot on the blood pressure (Hobbs et al. 2012). Therefore, enriching bread with beetroot may be a useful way for the delivery of dietary nitrate and for increasing vegetable consumption, with minimal impact on dietary habits.

2.4.4 Plant sterols

Plant sterols (PSs) occur naturally in vegetable oils, nuts, seeds, and grains. Their chemical structure resembles that of cholesterol. PSs possess serum cholesterol-lowering properties equal to that of plant stanols, and in the food industry they are widely used as ingredients in functional foods, either in nonesterified (less lipophilic) or esterified (more lipophilic) form (Piironen et al. 2008). Soderholm et al. (2012) have explored the influence of consumption of rye bread enriched with low dose (2 g/d) or high dose (4 g/d) plant sterols on serum lipid risk factors, including the apolipoprotein B (ApoB)/apolipoprotein A-I (ApoA1) ratio in normocholesterolemic subjects (Table 1). The authors concluded that consumption of rye bread enriched with both doses of plant sterols beneficially modifies cardiovascular lipid risk factors in normocholesterolemic subjects compared to the controls. Moreover, these results indicate that rye bread, as a vehicle, is able to deliver and release plant sterols into the intestine; the marked reduction in LDL-C suggests no significant interaction between rye fiber and plant sterols (Söderholm et al. 2012).

3. Conclusion

Breads enriched with various phytochemicals, such as DF, ADF and SP, have shown in animal studies the ability to diminish the negative impact of a high-fat or high-cholesterol diet in hypercholesterolemic or diabetic rats by improving glycemic control and blood lipid profile. Feeding of bread enriched with GTE or ADF has the potential to, respectively, increase fecal energy extraction and prevent visceral fat accumulation in rats. However, it should be noted that in the animal studies presented here, experimental breads were added to the animal diets in amounts which were evidently on a higher level than would normally be consumed by a human. When bread enriched with functional ingredients was incorporated into human diets, a lack of beneficial effect was seen in terms of reduction in body weight and the maintenance of this weight loss. Nevertheless, in short-term human studies, the consumption of functional breads enriched with DF alone (pea fiber), or in combination with protein (from lupin), improved the feeling of satiety. In longer dietary intervention studies, incorporation into the diet of the functional breads including FS, β-glucan or PSs was effective for glycemic control and serum lipid improvement, and in case of GTE, red or white beetroot, and PSs for improvement of blood pressure.

However, developing functional bread, the influence of food matrix on physiological responses of the phytochemicals incorporated into bread formula should be considered. Moreover, the optimal method (for example encapsulation) to improve the stability and bioavailability of phytochemical active components from food matrices should be employed.

Keywords: Bioactive components, body composition, body weight, carbohydrate metabolism, functional foods, lipid profile, rye bread

References

Alldrick, A.J. The Bakery: A potential leader in functional food applications. http://www.ucd.ie/t4cms/ ffnet%20funct%20fds%20final%20e-publication%20jan%202011.pdf (accessed 4 Nov 2012).

Anderson, J.W., P. Baird, R.H.Jr. Davis, S. Ferreri, M. Knudtson, A. Koraym, V. Waters and C.L. Williams. 2009. Health benefits of dietary fiber. Nutr. Rev., 67: 188–205.

Bajerska, J., S. Mildner-Szkudlarz, T. Podgórski and E. Oszmałek-Pruszyńska. 2013. Saffron (*Crocus sativus* L.) powder as an ingredient of rye bread: an anti-diabetic evaluation. J. Med. Food, 16: 847–856.

Bajerska, J., S. Mildner-Szkudlarz and E. Pruszynska-Oszmałek. 2013. May rye bread enriched with green tea extract be useful in the prevention of obesity in rats? Acta. Alimentaria, 42: 69–78.

Balasundaram, N., K. Sundaram and S. Samman. 2006. Phenolic compounds in plants and agri-industrial by-products: Antioxidant activity, occurrence and potential uses. Food Chem., 99: 191–203.

Beck, E.J., L.C. Tapsell, M.J. Batterham, S.M. Tosh and X.F. Huang. 2010. Oat beta-glucan supplementation does not enhance the effectiveness of an energy-restricted diet in overweight women. Br. J. Nutr., 103: 1212–1222.

Belski, R., T.A. Mori, I.B. Puddey, S. Sipsas, R.J. Woodman, T.R. Ackland, L.J. Beilin, E.R. Dove, N.B. Carlyon, V. Jayaseena and J.M. Hodgson. 2011. Effects of lupin-enriched foods on body composition and cardiovascular disease risk factors: a 12-month randomized controlled weight loss trial. Int. J. Obes. (Lond, 35: 810–819.

Dattilo, A.M. and P.M. Kris-Etherton. 1992. Effects of weight reduction on blood lipids and lipoproteins: a meta-analysis. Am. J. Clin. Nutr., 56: 320–328.

Dulloo, A.G. 2011. The search for compounds that stimulate thermogenesis in obesity management: from pharmaceuticals to functional food ingredients. Obes. Rev., 12: 866–883.

Fardet, A. 2012. New hypotheses for the health-protective mechanisms of whole-grain cereals: what is beyond fibre? Nutr. Res. Rev., 23: 65–134.

Hobbs, D.A., N. Kaffa, T.W. George, L. Methven and J.A. Lovegrove. 2012. Blood pressure-lowering effects of beetroot juice and novel beetroot-enriched bread products in normotensive male subjects. Br. J. Nutr., 108: 2066–2074.

Hodgson, J.M., Y.P. Lee, I.B. Puddey, S. Sipsas, T.R. Ackland, L.J. Beilin, R. Belski and T.A. Mori. 2010. Effects of increasing dietary protein and fibre intake with lupin on body weight and composition and blood lipids in overweight men and women. Int. J. Obes. (Lond), 34: 1086–1094.

Jiménez, J.P., J. Serrano, M. Tabernero, S. Arranz, M.E. Díaz-Rubio, L. García-Diz, I. Goñi and F. Saura-Calixto. 2008. Effects of grape antioxidant dietary fiber in cardiovascular disease risk factors. Nutrition, 24: 646–53.

Keogh, J., F. Atkinson, B. Eisenhauer, A. Inamdar and J. Brand-Miller. 2011. Food intake, postprandial glucose, insulin and subjective satiety responses to three different bread-based test meals. Appetite, 57: 707–710.

Kristensen, M., T.W. Damgaard, A.D. Sørensen, A. Raben, T.S. Lindeløv, A.D. Thomsen, C. Bjergegaard, H. Sørensen, A. Astrup and I. Tetens. 2008. Whole flaxseeds but not sunflower seeds in rye bread reduce apparent digestibility of fat in healthy volunteers. Eur. J. Clin. Nutr., 62: 961–967.

Kristensen, M., M.G. Jensen, J. Aarestrup, K.E. Petersen, L. Søndergaard, M.S. Mikkelsen and A. Astrup. 2012. Flaxseed dietary fibers lower cholesterol and increase fecal fat excretion, but magnitude of effect depend on food type. Nutr. Metab. (Lond), 3;9:8. doi: 10.1186/1743-7075-9-8.

Lattimer, J.M. and M.D. Haub. 2010. Effects of dietary fiber and its components on metabolic health. Nutrients, 2: 1266–1289.

Lee, Y.P., T.A. Mori, S. Sipsas, A. Barden, I.B. Puddey, V. Burke, R.S. Hall and J.M. Hodgson. 2006. Lupin-enriched bread increases satiety and reduces energy intake acutely. Am. J. Clin. Nutr., 84: 975–980.

Liatis, S., P. Tsapogas, E. Chala, C. Dimosthenopoulos, K. Kyriakopoulos, E. Kapantais and N. Katsilambros. 2009. The consumption of bread enriched with betaglucan reduces LDL-cholesterol and improves insulin resistance in patients with type 2 diabetes. Diabetes Metab., 35: 115–120.

Lundberg, J.O. and E. Weitzberg. 2005. NO generation from nitrite and its role in vascular control. Arterioscler. Thromb. Vasc. Biol., 25: 915–922.

Lunde, M.S., V.T. Hjellset, G. Holmboe-Ottesen and A.T. Høstmark. 2011. Variations in postprandial blood glucose responses and satiety after intake of three types of bread. J. Nutr. Metab., 2011: 437587.

Madan, J. and A. Narsaria. 2013. Hypolipidemic dietary components. Curr. Res. Nutr. Food Sci., 1: 59–70.

McCarty, M.F. 2005. A chlorogenic acid-induced increase in GLP-1 production may mediate the impact of heavy coffee consumption on diabetes risk. Med Hypotheses, 64: 848–853.

Meydani, M. and S.T. Hasan. 2010. Dietary polyphenols and obesity. Nutrients, 2: 737–751.

Mildner-Szkudlarz, S. and J. Bajerska. 2013. Protective effect of grape by-product-fortified breads against cholesterol/cholic acid diet-induced hypercholesterolaemia in rats. J. Sci. Food Agric., 93: 3271–3278.

Mohajeri, D.B., B.A. Tabrizi, G. Mousavi and M. Mesgari. 2008. Anti-diabetic activity of Crocus sativus L. (Saffron) stigma ethanolic extract in alloxan-induced diabetic rats. Res. J. Biol. Sci., 3: 1102–1108.

Mohamed, D.A., S.Y. Al-Okbi, D.M. El-Hariri and I.I. Mousa. 2012. Potential health benefits of bread supplemented with defatted flaxseeds under dietary regimen in normal and type 2 diabetic subjects. Pol. J. Food Nutr. Sci., 62: 103–108.

Mohamed, D.A., D.M. El-Hariri and S.Y. Al-Okbi. 2005. Impact of feeding bread enriched with flaxseed on plasma profile of hyperlipidemic rats. Pol. J. Food Nutr. Sci., 55: 431–436.

Piironen, V., D.G. Lindsay, T.A. Miettinen, J. Toivo and A.M. Lampi. 2008. Plant sterols: biosynthesis, biological function and their importance to human nutrition. J. Sci. Food Agric., 80: 939–966.

Raina, B.L., S.G. Agarwal, A.K. Bhatia and G.S. Gaur. 1996. Changes in Pigments and Volatiles of Saffron (*Crocus sativus* L.) During Processing and Storage. J. Sci. Food Agric., 71: 27–32.

Rosell, C.M. 2011. The science of doughs and bread quality. pp. 3–14. *In*: V.R. Preedy, R.R. Watson, V.B. Patel (eds.). Flour and Breads and their Fortification in Health and Disease Prevention. Academic Press, Elsevier, London, Burlington, San Diego.

Saper, R.B., D.M. Eisenberg and R.S. Phillips. 2004. Common dietary supplements for weight loss. Am. Fam. Physician, 70: 1731–1738.

Saura-Calixto, F. 1998. Antioxidant dietary fiber product: A new concept and a potential food ingredient. J. Agric. Food Chem., 46: 4303–4306.

Saura-Calixto, F., J. Serrano and I. Goñi. 2007. Intake and bioaccessibility of total polyphenols in a whole diet. Food Chem., 101: 492–501.

Schramm, D.D., M. Karim, H.R. Schrader, R.R. Holt, N.J. Kirkpatrick, J.A. Polagruto, J.L. Ensunsa, H.H. Schmitz and C.L. Keen. 2003. Food effects on the absorption and pharmacokinetics of cocoa flavanols. Life Sciences, 73: 857–869.

Serrano, J.C.E., A. Cassanyé and M. Portero-Otin. 2012. Trends in functional food against obesity, scientific, health and social aspects of the food industry, Dr. Benjamin Valdez (ed.). ISBN: 978-953-307-916-5, InTech, Available from: http://www.intechopen.com/books/scientific-health-and-social-aspects-ofthe food-industry/trends-in-functional-food-against-obesity.

Sheng, L., Z. Qian, S. Zheng and L. Xi. 2006. Mechanism of hypolipidemic effect of crocin in rats: croc in inhibits pancreatic lipase. Eur. J. Pharmacol., 543: 116–122.

Siró, I., E. Kápolna, B. Kápolna and A. Lugasi. 2008. Functional food. Product development, marketing and consumer acceptance—a review. Appetite, 51: 456–467.

Söderholm, P.P., G. Alfthan, A.H. Koskela, H. Adlercreutz and M.J. Tikkanen. 2012. The effect of high-fiber rye bread enriched with nonesterified plant sterols on major serum lipids and apolipoproteins in normocholesterolemic individuals. Nutr. Metab. Cardiovasc. Dis., 22: 575–582.

Wang, R. and W. Zhou. 2004. Stability of tea catechins in the breadmaking process. J. Agric. Food Chem., 52: 8224–8229.

Webb, A.J., N. Patel, S. Loukogeorgakis, M. Okorie, Z. Aboud, S. Misra, R. Rashid, P. Miall, J. Deanfield, N. Benjamin, R. MacAllister, A.J. Hobbs and A. Ahluwalia. 2008. Acute blood pressure lowering, vasoprotective, and antiplatelet properties of dietary nitrate via bioconversion to nitrite. Hypertension, 51: 784–790.

Wing, R.R. and J.O. Hill. 2001. Successful weight loss maintenance. Annu. Rev. Nutr., 21: 323–341.

Wolfram, S., Y. Wang and F. Thielecke. 2006. Anti-obesity effects of green tea: from bedside to bench. Mol. Nutr. Food Res., 50: 176–187.

World Health Organization. Global Strategy on Diet, Physical Activity and Health 2010. http://www.who.int/dietphysicalactivity/publications/facts/obesity/en/.

18

Gluten-Free Bread: Health and Technological Aspects

Julita Reguła[1] and Zenon Kędzior[2],*

1. Health and nutritional aspect

Bread is a staple foodstuff in the diet of many societies and in many cultures it is the most frequently consumed cereal product supplying the organism with essential nutrients. Basic raw materials for the production of bread include bread flours made from wheat and rye grain containing a mixture of proteins (prolamins), referred to jointly as gluten, responsible for the appropriate structure and quality of dough (Blomfeldt et al. 2011). However, there is a certain group of individuals who as a result of consumption of prolamins, i.e., gliadin from wheat, secalin from rye, hordein from barley and avenin from oats, suffer from such conditions as coeliac disease (also referred to as morbus visceralis, coeliac sprue, gluten enteropathy), allergy, gluten ataxia and a newly identified condition, i.e., non-celiac gluten sensitivity (Volta et al. 2013). Gliadin is the prolamin with the greatest toxic effect in individuals allergic to gluten, with the other prolamins exhibiting medium toxicity. Patients suffering from celiac disease and having no gluten tolerance, irrespective of the type of the disease and the intensity of symptoms (diarrhoea, vomiting, malnutrition), have to completely eliminate products containing the above mentioned prolamins from their diet (Hamer 2005).

---

[1] Department of Human Nutrition and Hygiene, Poznan University of Life Sciences, Wojska Polskiego 31, 60-624 Poznań, Poland.
Email: jumar@up.poznan.pl

[2] Institute of Food Technology, Poznan University of Life Sciences, Wojska Polskiego 31, 60-624 Poznań, Poland.
Email: kedziorm@up.poznan.pl

* Corresponding author

The term gluten-free food refers to products, in which the total gluten content is max. 20 mg/kg product. Gluten-free diet excludes the consumption of products and foodstuffs produced from any species of wheat, i.e., common wheat (*T. aestivum* L.), spelt (*T. aestivum* ssp. *spelta*), einkorn wheat (*T. monococcum* L.), emmer wheat (*T. dicoccum* L.), durum wheat, rivet wheat and kamut, as well as rye, triticale, barley and oats (Fig. 1, Table 1). Otherwise, their consumption by individuals with gluten intolerance leads to damage in the small intestine mucosa and development of several gastrointestinal symptoms (flatulence, diarrhoea, stomachache) as well as non-intestinal symptoms (confusion, headache, joint and muscle pain, anxiety as well as depressibility). Gluten proteins, rich in glutamine, constitute a substrate for tissue transglutaminase, under the influence of which they undergo deamination. Thus formed peptides are strongly immunogenic for genetically predisposed individuals. This leads to the infiltration of endothelial lymphocytes, resulting in damage to intestinal villi in the small intestine mucosa. As a consequence disturbed digestion, absorption and peristalsis are observed along with clinical symptoms developing as a result of these disorders. Undernutrition and malnutrition appear, leading to numerous systemic complications (Kaganoff 2007). Individuals with dysfunctional intestinal villi present impaired absorption of proteins, fats as well as vitamins A, D, E, K and B, hypoelectrolytemia, disorders of disaccharide metabolism and calcium and phosphorus metabolism, secondary hyperparathyroidism, muscle weakness, osteoporosis, anaemia caused by iron deficiency, megaloblastic anaemia, habitual abortions, infertility and atrophic lesions within the oral cavity and the tongue (Grzymisławski et al. 2010).

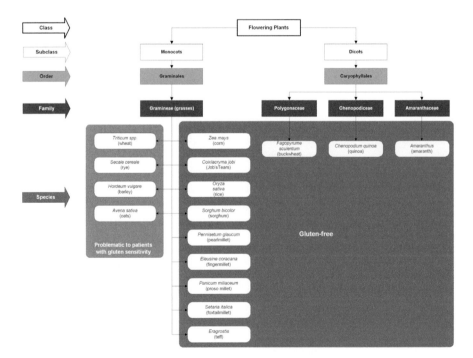

Figure 1. Taxonomy of the commonly used cereals and pseudocereals.

Table 1. Gluten-free and gluten-containing grain, seeds, flours and starches.

Gluten-free	Toxic (gluten-containing)
Adley (dehulled Job's Tears)	Grains:
Amaranth	Wheat, any species (common, durum, einkorn,
Arrowroot	emmer, rivet, Kamut, spelt, etc.) and products of
Bean (Garbanzo, Fava, Romano)	their processing
Buckwheat	Barley (products: groats, flakes, flour, malt,
Corn (maize)	extract, bran)
Flax	Oats (products: flakes, flour, bran)
Mesquite flour (milled dry pods of *Prosopis* genus)	Rye (products: flakes, flour, bran)
Millet, various species (e.g., proso millet, *Panicum*	Triticale
milliaceum, fonio, *Digitaria* genus, kodo, *Paspalum*	Common wheat and/or durum wheat products :
scrobiculatum, finger millet or ragi, *Eleusine*	Wheat flours (graham flour, wholegrain flour,
coracana)	matzo flour or matzah flour, chapatti flour, etc.)
Montina™ and other flours made from Indian	Semolina and pasta products
rice grass, *Achnatherum hymenoides* synonymes:	Grits and flakes
Oryzopsis hymenoides, Stipa hymenoides)	Couscous
Wild Indian rice (*Zizania* species)	Bulgur or burghul
Peas	
Quinoa	
Potato (flour, starch)	
Rice, all forms	
Sago	
Sesame	
Sorghum	
Soy (soya) flour	
Sunflower	
Tapioca	
Teff	

Source: Hozyasz and Słowik 2009.

It seems that at the exclusion of the allergen from the diet of patients with gluten intolerance the adoption of a gluten-free diet should limit disorders of mineral and vitamin metabolism in the organism. However, it has been observed that nutrient deficiencies occur in coeliac patients both treated and not treated with a gluten-free diet. Studies show tissue deficits of magnesium in approx. 20% patients following a gluten-free diet and in approx. 25% individuals with atrophy of small intestine mucosa. Probably magnesium deficiency in coeliac patients is caused by complex causes and depends not only on the atrophy of the small intestine mucosa, but also the consumption of insufficient amounts of magnesium (Rujner et al. 2004). Despite the application of gluten-free diet, metabolites of vitamin D_3 and calcitonin, the incidence rate of osteopenia and osteoporosis among children with celiac disease and reduced bone density is 60% (Szumera et al. 2004). In children with the diagnosed coeliac disease high deficiencies of Zn and Cu are also recorded, occurring as a result of frequent diarrhoeas and increased excretion in faeces (Altuntaş et al. 2000; Baeton et al. 2007). As a result of disturbed absorption 15% coeliac patients suffer from anaemia caused by iron deficiency (Fasano and Catassi 2001).

Nutrient deficiencies in coeliac patients should be supplemented with a properly balanced diet incorporating enriched gluten-free cereal products (Reguła and Śmidowicz 2014).

2. Nutritive value of gluten-free flours and produced bread

At present many types of gluten-free breads are commercially available, prepared most frequently from corn and potato flour and starch, and/or rice flour (Kawamura-Konishi et al. 2013; Matos et al. 2013; Onyango et al. 2011a). However, these raw materials in comparison to conventional cereals contain less vitamins B and minerals (Tables 3 and 4). Additives often used to improve processability and enhance nutritive value include buckwheat flour (Lin et al. 2009; Sakac et al. 2011; Mariotti et al. 2013) and soybean flour (Ribotta et al. 2004). Buckwheat flour contains 2-fold and soybean flour 6-fold greater amounts of protein than rice, corn or potato flour. Both buckwheat and soybean flour in comparison to other flours are very good sources of dietary fibre, minerals and vitamins B (Tables 2, 3 and 4). The greatest amounts of minerals are contained in soybean flour, while they are lowest in rice flour and starch and in potato starch. Neither rice nor potato starch contain any vitamins, while corn starch has much lower levels of vitamins than the other flours (Table 4). The greatest amounts of thiamin, riboflavin and folates are found in soybean flour, while buckwheat flour contains the highest levels of niacin and vitamin B_6.

A necessary condition for the preparation of gluten-free bread is to develop the product so as to eliminate the agent harmful for individuals allergic to gluten. A problem arises, connected with the fact that such an approach leads to reduced nutritive value of the final product. In the case of gluten-free bread the elimination of wheat, rye, barley and oat from the product leads to considerably reduced contents of protein, dietary fibre, vitamins B and minerals in the product (Tables 5 and 6) (Kunachowicz 2005; National Institute for Health and Welfare 2013; U.S. Department of Agriculture, Agricultural Research Service 2013). It is advisable to use buckwheat and soybean flours as well as flours and whole seeds of other edible plants and nuts in the production of gluten-free bread.

Table 2. Energy and basic nutrients (in 100 grams product) contained in flours and starches of cereal used in gluten-free bread.

Components	Buckwheat flour[1]	Millet flour	Rice			Corn		Soy Flour[3]	Potato	
			White	Brown	Starch	Flour[2]	Starch		Flour	Starch
Water (g)	11.1# 12.8*	10.7# 7.8*	11.9# 12.3*	11.9#	13.8*	10.9# 12.4*	11.2*	7.25# 6.8*	6.52#	15.0*
Energy (kcal)	335# 342*	373# 363*	366# 343*	363#	344*	361# 332*	348*	330# 424*	357#	337*
Protein (g)	12.6# 14,6*	10.7# 11.6*	5.95# 7.20*	7.23#	0.8*	6.93# 5.9*	0.2*	47.0# 45.0*	6.90#	0.60*
Total lipid (g)	3.10# 2.00*	4.25# 2.9*	1.42# 0.70*	2.78#	0.0*	3.86# 3.0*	0.0*	1.22# 23.5*	0.34#	0.1*
Carbohydrate (g)	70.6# 68.3*	73.0# 75.9*	80.1# 79.2*	76.5#	85.3*	76.8# 78.0*	88.5*	38.4# 20.1*	83.1#	83.9*
Fiber (g)	10.0# 1.90*	3.5# 3.2*	2.4# 2.3*	4.6#	0.0*	7.3# 7.6*	1.7*	17.5# 11.9*	5.9#	0.4*

Source: # U.S. Department of Agriculture, Agricultural Research Service 2013; * Kunachowicz et al. 1995.
[1] Buckwheat flour, whole-groat.
[2] Corn flour, whole-grain, yellow.
[3] Soy flour, defatted.

Table 3. Minerals (in 100 grams product) contained in flours and starches of cereal used in gluten-free bread.

Components	Buckwheat flour	Millet flour	Rice			Corn		Soya Flour	Potato	
			White	Brown	Starch	Flour	Starch		Flour	Starch
Calcium (mg)	41# 40*	14# 13*	10# 10*	11#	5.0*	7.0# 7.0*	11*	241# 269*	65#	39*
Iron (mg)	4.06# 4.00*	3.94# 4.3*	0.35# 1.10*	1.98#	0.4*	2.38# 3.0*	0.2*	9.24# 9.1*	1.38#	0.6*
Magnesium (mg)	251# 219*	119# 213*	35# 36*	112#	6.0*	93# 40*	3.0*	290# 300*	65#	8.0*
Phosphorus (mg)	337# 441*	285# 397*	98# 90*	337#	66*	272# 127*	14*	674# 753*	168#	59*
Potassium (mg)	577# 521*	224# 340*	76# 117*	289#	55*	315# 193*	7.0*	2384# 2307*	1001#	14*
Sodium (mg)	11# 1.0*	4.0# 1.0*	0.0# 3.0*	8.0#	3.0*	5.0# 2.0*	2.0*	20# 1.0*	55#	5.0*
Zinc (mg)	3.12# 3.75*	2.63# 3.66*	0.80# 0.80*	2.45#	0.66*	1.73# 0.84*	0.07*	2.46# 4.55*	0.54#	0.06*
Copper (mg)	0.60*	0.78*	0.20*	-	0.08*	0.10*	0.00*	1.53*	-	0.01*
Manganese (mg)	1.89*	1.61*	0.60*	-	0.50*	0.35*	0.00*	3.48*	-	0.17*

Source: # U.S. Department of Agriculture, Agricultural Research Service 2013; * Kunachowicz et al. 1995.
Buckwheat flour, whole-groat
Corn flour, whole-grain, yellow
Soy flour, defatted

Table 4. Vitamins (in 100 grams product) contained in flours and starches of cereal used in gluten-free bread.

Components	Buckwheat flour	Millet flour	Rice			Corn		Soya Flour	Potato	
			White	Brown	Starch	Flour	Starch		Flour	Starch
Thiamin (mg)	0.417# 0.196*	0.412# 0.196*	0.138# 0.080*	0.443#	0.00*	0.246# 0.371*	0.02*	0.698# 0.121*	0.228#	0.00*
Riboflavin (mg)	0.190# 0.117*	0.073# 0.117*	0.021# 0.030*	0.080#	0.00*	0.080# 0.100*	0.013*	0.253# 0.265*	0.051#	0.00*
Niacin (mg)	6.150# 5.63*	7.164# 5.63*	4.092# 1.90*	10.02#	0.00*	2.223# 1.32*	2.21*	2.612# 1.84*	5.611#	0.00*
Vitamin B$_6$ (mg)	0.582#	0.372#	0.436#	0.736#	-	0.370#	-	0.574#	0.769#	-
Folate (µg)	54#	42#	4.0#	16#	-	25#	-	305#	25#	-
Vitamin E (alpha-tocopherol) (mg)	0.32# 0.10*	0.11# 0.10*	0.11# 0.00*	1.20#	0.00*	0.42# 0.30*	0.00*	0.12# 0.60*	0.25#	0.00*

Source: # U.S. Department of Agriculture, Agricultural Research Service 2013; * Kunachowicz et al. 1995.
Buckwheat flour, whole-groat
Corn flour, whole-grain, yellow
Soy flour, defatted

Table 5. Comparison of basic composition (in 100 grams product) of chosen grades of gluten-free and wheat-rye traditional bread.

Components	Bread, naturally gluten-free^	Buckwheat bread*	Gluten-free bread, low protein*	Gluten-free bread, with milk*	Wheat-rye, commercially bread*	Wheat bread#
Water (g)	-	42.1	45.6	42.6	34.8	34.5
Energy (kcal)	236	217	205	224	248	270
Protein (g)	2.9	3.0	0.4	1.6	6.1	10.4
Total lipid (g)	4.4	3.0	1.3	3.0	1.3	3.44
Carbohydrate (g)	43.3	49.4	51.7	51.4	56.3	49.5
Fiber (g)	4.9	5.0	1.0	3.7	4.2	4.2

Source: * Kunachowicz et al. 2005; ^ National Institute for Health and Welfare 2013; # U.S. Department of Agriculture, Agricultural Research Service 2013.

Table 6. Comparison of vitamins and minerals (in 100 grams product) of chosen grades of gluten-free and wheat-rye traditional bread.

Components	Bread, naturally gluten-free^	Buckwheat bread*	Gluten-free bread, low protein*	Gluten-free bread, with milk*	Wheat-rye, commercially bread*	Wheat bread#
Calcium (mg)	8	14	11	49	17	138
Iron (mg)	0.5	2.9	0.4	0.5	1.2	3.52
Magnesium (mg)	12	40	4	8	29	46
Phosphorus (mg)	43.1	86	38	69	98	153
Potassium (mg)	55	106	18	55	148	182
Sodium (mg)	389	598	162	157	391	519
Zinc (mg)	0.5	0.88	0.15	0.24	1.17	1.18
Copper (mg)	-	0.20	0.01	0.01	0.13	-
Manganese (mg)	-	0.31	0.04	0.04	0.84	-
Thiamin (mg)	0.02	0.074	0.069	0.059	0.149	0.471
Riboflavin (mg)	0.06	0.066	0.061	0.082	0.080	0.270
Niacin (mg)	1.2	3.45	0.38	0.43	1.05	5.93
Vitamin B$_6$ (mg)	-	-	-	-	0.10	0.107
Folate (μg)	30.4	-	-	-	27.6	99
Vitamin E (alpha-tocopherol) (mg)	0.60	0.90	0.60	0.60	0.47	0.19

Source: * Kunachowicz et al. 2005; ^ National Institute for Health and Welfare 2013; # U.S. Department of Agriculture, Agricultural Research Service 2013.

3. Raw materials enriching gluten-free breads with nutrients

In order to improve its nutritive value bread is enriched with various additional raw materials such as flour from amaranth, buckwheat, millet, quinoa, soybeans or sorghum, seeds and fibre preparations as well as egg whites or egg powder (Gallagher et al. 2003; Gambuś 2005; Pruska-Kędzior et al. 2008; Mariotti et al. 2009) (Table 7). It has also been attempted to enrich gluten-free bread with milk powder, whey, buttermilk and calcium alone (Krupa-Kozak et al. 2009). Addition of these raw materials enriches bread with quality protein, increases the nutritive value of cereal proteins and thus enhances their utilisation as a result of greater contents of certain exogenous amino acids, primarily lysine, and increases contents of vitamins B and calcium.

Raw materials frequently proposed in the production of gluten-free bread include pseudocereals such as amaranth and quinoa, as well as the oldest cereal originally found in Ethiopia, i.e., teff. Alvarez-Jubete et al. (2009a, 2010) are of an opinion that the replacement of potato starch with flours from amaranth, quinoa and teff greatly increases contents of important nutrients such as protein, fiber, calcium, iron and vitamin E in the final product. The resultant breads also have a significantly higher content of polyphenol compounds and their *in vitro* antioxidant activity is also increased.

Table 7. Energy and nutritive value (in 100 grams product) in chosen raw materials used for supplement gluten-free bread.

Components	Amaranthus seeds#	Teff#	Quinoa#	Flax*	Pumpkin seeds*	Poppy seed*
Water (g)	11.3	8.82	13.3	6.0	6.8	601
Energy (kcal)	371	367	368	500	556	478
Protein (g)	13.6	13.3	14.12	24.5	24.5	20.1
Total lipid (g)	7.02	2.38	6.07	31	45.8	42.9
Carbohydrate (g)	65.2	73.13	64.2	35	18	24.7
Fiber (g)	6.7	8.0	7.0	3.9	5.3	20.5
Calcium (mg)	159	180	47	195	43	1266
Iron (mg)	7.61	7.63	4.57	17.1	15	8.1
Magnesium (mg)	248	184	197	291	540	458
Phosphorus (mg)	557	429	457	722	1170	1022
Potassium (mg)	508	427	563	762	810	963
Sodium (mg)	4.0	12.0	5.0	79.0	18.0	6.0
Zinc (mg)	2.87	3.63	3.10	7.80	7.5	3.34
Copper (mg)	-	-	-	0.40	1.57	0.42
Manganese (mg)	-	-	-	1.20	1.0	3.71
Thiamin (mg)	0.116	0.390	0.360	0.17	0.21	0.073
Riboflavin (mg)	0.200	0.270	0.318	0.16	0.32	0.120
Niacin (mg)	0.923	3.363	1.520	1.4	1.70	0.81
Vitamin B$_6$ (mg)	0.591	0.482	0.487	0.04	0.10	0.44
Folate (µg)	82	-	184	0.0	60	58
Vitamin E (alpha-tocopherol) (mg)	1.19	-	2.44	0.17	26	1.80

Source: # U.S. Department of Agriculture, Agricultural Research Service 2013; * Kunachowicz et al. 2005.

3.1 Amaranth

Amaranth belongs to the family *Amaranthaceae*. Primarily *Amaranthus cruentus*, *Amaranthus hypochondriacus* and *Amaranthus caudatus* are grown for food. The nutritive value of amaranth depends on the species, cultivar and cultivation practices. This cereal contains large amounts of protein and fat. Amaranth proteins consist of about 40% albumins, 20% globulins, 25–30% glutelins and 2–3% prolamins (Schoenlechner et al. 2008). Protein, accounting for 13 to 21% d.m., is rich in exogenous amino acids, particularly lysine constituting approx. 6% all amino acids, and tryptophan (approx. 1%) (Table 8) (Zheleznov et al. 1997; Venskutonis and Kraujalis 2013; U.S. Department of Agriculture, Agricultural Research Service 2013). Due to the advantageous amino acid composition and good digestibility of approx. 74%, amaranth protein has high nutritive value.

Table 8. Exogenous amino acids content of quinoa, teff and amaranthus.

Amino acid	Quinoa* (g/100 g protein)	Teff# (g/16 g N)	Amaranthus spp.^ (g/100 g protein)
Isoleucine	3.3–7.4	3.7	2.7–4.1
Leucine	5.8–7.5	8.5	4.2–6.3
Lysine	4.6–6.1	3.7	5.1–6.1
Phenylalanine + Tyrosin	6.2–7.5	9.5	6.0–8.5
Methyonine + Cystine	4.5–4.8	4.1	4.1–4.9
Threonine	2.5–3.8	4.5	3.3–4.0
Tryphtophan	1.1–1.2	1.3	0.8–1.82
Valine	4.0–6.0	5.5	3.9-4.7

Source: * Vega-Gálvez et al. 2010; #Ketema 1997; ^Grobelnik et al. 2009.

Amaranth seeds contain from 5.2 to 13% fat (Bressani et al. 1987; Budin et al. 1996; U.S. Department of Agriculture, Agricultural Research Service 2013) (Table 7), while according to Kraujalis and Venskutonis (2013) it is as much as 16.7%. According to He et al. (2002), unsaturated fatty acids are the primary fat components of amaranth seeds. Oil from 11 genotypes of four grain amaranth species contains palmitic (19.1% to 23.4%), oleic (18.7% to 38.9%), and linoleic acids (36.7% to 55.9%). Important components of the lipid fraction in amaranth include tocopherols, tocotrienols as well as squalene, which content in amaranth oil depending on the cultivar is estimated at 2% to 7% (He et al. 2002; Berganza et al. 2003; Ratusz and Wirkowska 2006). The predominant tocopherols in amaranth are α- and β-tocopherols. Amaranth oil is also a source of unique phytosterols, such as spinasterol, δ-7-stigmasterol and δ-7-ergosterol (Kaźmierczak et al. 2011). Among the above mentioned phytosterols the greatest content in amaranth is recorded for spinasterol, amounting to 46 to 54% total sterols.

The average carbohydrate content in amaranth seeds is 65%, with starch being the main component. In general, amaranth seeds contain 65% to 75% starch, 4% to 5% dietary fibers, 2 to 3 times higher content of sucrose in comparison to wheat grain, as well as nonstarch polysaccharide components (Burisová et al. 2001).

Amaranth seeds are also distinguished in terms of their high content of minerals, particularly readily available iron, magnesium and calcium (Alvarez-Jubete et al. 2010). Thanks to the considerable contents of iron, exceeding its levels in legumes, spinach and meat, amaranth products are valuable supplements to the diet of individuals with symptoms of anemia. Amaranth seeds also contain numerous microelements, mainly manganese, nickel, chromium, zinc, copper, selenium, iodine and cobalt. In terms of their vitamin contents amaranth seeds do not differ much from wheat, barley or rye and contain folic and pantothenic acids, niacin and vitamins B.

Amaranth seeds are a raw material frequently used to enrich gluten-free bread. According to Alvarez-Jubete et al. (2009), bread produced from 50% *A. caudatus* grain and 50% rice flour contained 3.4 times higher content of fat, 28% higher dietary fiber, and two times higher content of Mg as compared with the wheat control.

3.2 Quinoa

Quinoa (*Chenopodium quinoa* Willd.) is a plant grown in Argentina, Bolivia, Chile, Colombia, Ecuador and Peru for at least five thousand years. Quinoa seeds contain large amounts of proteins with a balanced amino acid composition (Table 7). The content of essential amino acids in quinoa is higher than in common cereals. The protein fraction is characterised by high levels of lysine as well as methionine and cysteine (Table 8) (Vega-Gálvez et al. 2010). Advantages of quinoa seeds also include high contents of fat, dietary fiber and minerals (Bhargava 2006). Quinoa fat is rich in essential unsaturated fatty acids and contains high concentrations of natural antioxidants such as α-tocopherol and γ-tocopherol (Ng et al. 2007). Ahamed et al. (1998) and Kozioł (1992) reported that quinoa fat has a high content of oleic acid (24–28%) and linoleic acid (39–52%).

Carbohydrate content in quinoa is similar to that in rice, amaranth seed and barley. Total dietary fiber of quinoa is comparable to that in cereals and the soluble fiber content is reported between 1.3% and 6.1% (Abugoch James 2009).

In comparison to cereals (rice, barley and wheat) quinoa contains more riboflavin (B_2), α-tocopherol (vitamin E) and carotene (Kozioł 1992; Repo-Carrasco et al. 2003). Moreover, quinoa seeds are good sources of calcium, magnesium, phosphorus, manganese, copper, zinc, potassium and iron. Konishi et al. (2004) when using scanning electron microscopy with energy dispersive X-ray observed that minerals such as P, K and Mg were located in the embryo, while Ca and P in the pericarp were associated with pectic compounds of the cell wall.

Apart from the above mentioned nutrients, quinoa also contains phenolic acids, flavonoids and saponins. Flavonoid content in quinoa seeds is high (on average 58 mg/100 g dry matter). Quercitin and kaempherol are primary flavonoids in quinoa (Repo–Carrasco–Valencia et al. 2010).

3.3 Teff

Teff [*Eragrostis tef* (Zucc.) Trotter], a plant botanically classified as *Eragrostis abyssinica, Poa cerealis* Salisb. and *Cynodon abyssinicus* Jacq. Raspail, in literature on human nutrition and medicine is referred to as teff grass and Abyssinian/Williams lovegrass. It is a cereal plant species from the *Poaceae* family, growing in the wild in north-eastern Africa. Teff grain contains 9.4–13.3% protein, 73.0% carbohydrates, 1.98–8% dietary fiber, 2.0–3.1% fat and 2.7–3.0% minerals (Bultosa and Taylor 2004). Proteins in teff grain include glutelins, albumins, prolamins and globulins found at 44.5%, 36.6%, 11.8% and 6.7%, respectively (Hozyasz and Słowik 2009). Teff is characterized by high contents of methionine, cysteine and—in comparison to other cereals—high contents of lysine (Table 8) (Tatham et al. 1996). Starch accounts for the greatest proportion of the carbohydrate fraction. This raw material also contains high amounts of minerals and vitamins. Apart from high contents of calcium, iron and zinc, this cereal contains folic acid and antioxidants in amounts exceeding those in wheat, barley or sorghum. Due to the high contents of dietary fiber and minerals teff constitutes a valuable component of gluten-free bread mixes.

4. Other raw materials

An excellent additive considerably enhancing the nutritive value of gluten-free bread is provided by seeds of oil flax cultivars, containing over 20% protein of high digestibility ranging from 85 to 90% and over 30% fat, containing predominantly unsaturated fatty acids, particularly α-linolenic acid. When replacing starch in bread with ground yellow seeds of flax cv. *Hungarian Gold* added at 12.5%, Gambuś (2005) in her study recorded an increase in protein contents by 77%, a 6-fold increase in the soluble dietary fiber as well as macro- and microelements, particularly Zn by 38%, K by 74%, Ca by 76%, P by 86%, Cu by 127%, Mg by 286% and Mn by 350% in relation to their original contents in conventional bread. Potential for modification and enrichment of bread with nutrients makes it possible to balance the nutrient profile of the product and to compensate for losses of nutrients caused by processing, particularly in gluten-free breads (Gambuś 2005).

Raw materials rich in minerals (Zn, Mg, Fe, Cu) and vitamins, capable of enriching the nutritive value of gluten-free bread in the opinion of Markiewicz et al. (2006) and Reguła and Siwulski (2007) include dried fruits, nuts, almonds, sunflower seeds, pumpkin, dried oyster mushroom and shiitake. In turn, Skibniewska et al. (2002) and Suliburska et al. (2009) claimed that fermented legume seeds are good sources of Fe, Cu, Zn and vitamins B. Fermentation of cereal products and legume seeds significantly increases bioavailability of minerals thanks to an increase in phytase activity and reduction of phytic acid content.

5. Concluding remarks

Recommended introduction of additives to the product as a good source of nutrients, protein, vitamins and minerals requires precise determination of bioavailability of these compounds. Enriched products typically contain greater amounts of nutrients. However, there is a limited body of information concerning the nutritive value of such food. Suliburska et al. (2011) presented an opinion that products enriched with, e.g., Ca and Fe are better sources of potentially available Ca and Fe than products not enriched with these nutrients. Obtaining a cereal product naturally enriched with nutrients of good bioavailability may be their good source in the nutrition of individuals with deficiencies of many nutrients, primarily patients with absorption and metabolism disorders.

6. Technological aspects of gluten-free bread formulation and production

Baking value of a cereal flour depends on the physicochemical properties of its main macromolecular components, i.e., the complex of gluten proteins, starch, and non-starch polysaccharides. Intrinsic polar lipids also affect the flour baking quality. Flour is mixed with water until forming a viscoelastic dough capable to retain gas bubbles released during fermentation over the time of the dough raising and oven baking. Viscoelastic properties and surface active behavior of wheat dough depend largely on physicochemical properties of two groups of gluten proteins, i.e., prolamins (gliadins) and glutenins, according to classical Osborne classification.

In dry, mature wheat grain and in wheat flour gluten proteins occur as storage proteins in the form of small particles of the size < 17 μm known in cereal science under the name of "wedge protein". Gluten proteins are present also in fine protein films called "adhering protein" covering individual starch granules. Upon dough mixing, gluten proteins hydrate, polymerize (aggregate) and form extensive, continue three-dimensional viscoelastic networks of gluten films enlacing individual starch granules. Covalent bonds (disulfide bridges), ionic, hydrogen and hydrophobic bonds, and van der Waals forces are involved in developing and stabilization of the gluten structure. The system of continuous gluten films network occluding dispersed hydrated starch granules and gas bubbles is interpenetrated by a dough aqueous phase, called also the "dough liquor". The aqueous phase is composed of solubilized in water macromolecules, like some proteins (albumins and globulins) and non-starch polysaccharides, and small molecules, including salts and surface-active polar lipids (Sahi 1994).

Physical resistance of wheat dough to the deformation resulting from viscoelastic properties of the gluten network combined with the capability of gas bubbles retention and stabilization due to interfacial properties of proteins, polysaccharides, and polar lipids governs the dough behavior during mixing, proofing, dividing and shaping, and thermal setting upon baking.

After removal of starch and soluble components of wheat dough in water in the process called gluten washing out, a viscoelastic artefact of aggregated gluten protein films called "gluten" or "vital gluten" is formed. It is possible to isolate vital gluten from barley dough and, after special preparation of rye flour (removal of non-starch polysaccharides) also from rye dough (Cunningham et al. 1955). These observations caused creation in the past a misleading term "gluten-free" cereals as the synonym of a food not yielding "vital gluten" and "harmless in celiac disease" or "safe in celiac disease", ignoring an association between occurring of the disease and the presence of celiac-inducing prolamins regardless of their capability of forming a gluten. The best illustration of this misunderstanding is naming maize a gluten-free cereal despite its capability of gluten forming when a maize meal (corn meal) is subjected to the process of starch production and a by-product, the corn meal gluten, an isolate of maize zein, is produced (Shukla and Cheryan 2001).

In a rye dough, gluten proteins are unable to fully develop the continuous three-dimensional gluten films structure mainly due to interfering action of non-starch polysaccharides, arabinoxylans (pentosans). Therefore, in rye dough viscosity plays more important role in its overall viscoelasticity than in wheat dough. Capability of gas retention in the dough is lower than in wheat dough and rye bread crumb shows smaller pores with thicker pores' walls compared to wheat bread crumb.

Alcoholic fermentation conducted by yeast provides CO_2 causing dough raising. The surface of the interface gas bubbles—wheat dough increases from ~8 m^2/100 g at the stage of dough mixing to ~42 m^2/100 at the end of proofing and reaches as much as ~65 m^2/100 g in the bread crumb (Van Vliet et al. 1992). Other benefit of dough fermentation is the formation of flavor precursors.

Specificity of physicochemical properties of rye flour proteins and arabinoxylans causes that rye and mixed wheat-rye dough reach optimal capability of gas retention and viscoelastic properties at lower pH than wheat dough. Therefore, these types of dough have to be submitted to acidifying by means of lactic fermentation conducted by the lactic acid bacteria (LAB) in the technological process of sourdough production. Sourdough technology improves bread structure, taste, flavor and digestibility not only in rye and mixed wheat-rye bread but also in wheat bread (Katina et al. 2005).

All types of bread stale upon storage due to complex process of retrogradation occurring in gelatinized starch. Bread staling is relatively quick in wheat white bread and much slower in rye bread, mixed rye-wheat bread and in any whole-grain bread due to increased content of non-starch polysaccharides.

7. Gluten-free bread technology

7.1 General remarks

Generally, two types of gluten-free bread recipes exist: formulations based on a mixture of various plant flours or mixture of starches and plant flours containing proteins of above 2%, and special gluten-free bread for phenylketonuria suffering subjects, of low protein content (> 1%) based on starch mixtures.

Absence of the structure forming gluten proteins causes that various hydrocolloids have to be used to form necessary water holding capability, cohesiveness, viscoelasticity and capability of gas retention of the gluten-free dough to assure obtaining of well raised bread, comparable in its porosity to traditional wheat bread. Lipids, like oils or shortenings, and emulsifiers are applied also to improve rheological and surface active properties of a gluten-free dough. Some recipes contain enzymes, mainly amylases but also proteases, transglutaminase or others, added to improve dough structure and fermentation process (Houben et al. 2012).

7.2 Starch

Starch is a main chemical component and nutrient in bread. Starch is introduced into gluten-free mixtures as a commercial native starch like maize (corn), potato, wheat or cassava/tapioca starch, or occurs as a principal component of the plant flours utilized in the recipes. Modified starches are used as hydrocolloids improving the dough structure.

Hydrated starch granules form in the dough a dispersed, solid elastic phase weakly associated with proteins matrix mainly by means of hydrogen bonds. In dough structure, these granules are often treated as an inert filler enlaced with protein films and a molecular dispersion of soluble polysaccharides (Tolstoguzov 1997; Tolstoguzov 2003). During dough fermentation, starch is a substrate to amylases and becomes a source of glucose for yeast and lactic acid bacteria providing CO_2 for raising dough. Dextrins formed during partial enzymatic hydrolysis of amylose and amylopectin influence rheological properties of dough, bread crumb texture and the staling process. In oven baking, starch undergoes to pasting (gelatinization) and forms a continuous gel interlaced with denatured proteins skeleton forming a bi-continuous spongy gel system transformed by the end of baking into a solid foam of open pores, i.e., bread crumb. It is strongly possible, that in starch gel a mixture of amylopectin and amylose preserve more or less shape of starch granules embedded in a thin continuous film of amylose (Keetels et al. 1996). During bread storage, the starch retrogradation phenomenon occurs, i.e., partial starch recrystallization takes place causing bread staling (Fadda et al. 2014).

There are a number of starch physicochemical properties important in bread making. The starch granules size distribution and degree of the granules mechanical damaging affect their hydration upon dough mixing and their accessibility to amylolytic enzymes. Proportions of amylose and amylopectin in starch granules, molecular weight distribution in amylose and amylopectin, degree of amylopectin branching, and degree of crystallinity of native starch granules influence the thermal properties, i.e., extent of starch swelling in water with increasing temperature, pasting temperature and time, viscosity of the hot paste and viscoelasticity of the starch gel. Last but not least, physicochemical properties of amylose and amylopectin influence strongly the process of retrogradation.

Starches of various botanical origin differ significantly in their physicochemical properties. Starch granules are relatively dense (1.34–1.65 g/cm³), insoluble, and swell only slightly in cold water (for example, undamaged wheat starch absorbs 0.44 g H_2O/g). Average apparent density of maize and potato starch granules is close to 1.637 and 1.617 g/cm³, respectively (French 1984). The density of wheat starch ranges from 1.55 to 1.59 g/cm³, and for rice appeared to be of 1.57 ± 0.23 g/cm³ (Ahmad et al. 2012). Starch granules differ in size and shape among plants. For example, maize starch has an average diameter of about 15 μm (5–25 μm). Wheat starch appears to have a bi-modal size distribution of 25–40 and 5–10 μm, potato starch shows an average size of 40 μm (10–70 μm), and rice starch has an average size of 5 μm (3–5 μm) (Shelton and Lee 2000). Amylose content in starch usually varies around 25% and covers a range of 18–30% in common wheat, 22.4–32.5% in normal maize, 5.0–28.4 in normal rice and 20.1–31.0% in potato (Singh et al. 2003).

Swelling power of starch increases tremendously with temperature reaching at 95°C as much as 22 g H_2O/g in maize, 23–30 g/g in rice and 11–59 g/g in potato. Wheat starch shows swelling power 18.3–26.6 g/g in 100°C (Singh et al. 2003). Significant differences in starch gelatinization, retrogradation and pasting properties occur depending on the starch botanical origin (Table 9). Comparison of retrogradation degree characterizing starches applied in the gluten-free formulations and wheat starch can help understanding particular susceptibility of the gluten-free bread to staling.

Table 9. Gelatinization, pasting and paste properties of starches from different botanical origins.

Starch origin	Gelatinization[a]			Retrogradation[b]	Pasting and pasta properties[c]			
	To (°C)	Range (°C)	Enthalpy (ΔH, J/g)	(%)	Pasting temperature (°C)	Viscosity (cP)		
						Peak	Hot paste	Final
Normal maize[d]	64.1 ± 0.2	10.8	12.3 ± 0.0	47.6	82.0	1824	1140	2028
Waxy maize[d]	64.2 ± 0.2	10.4	15.4 ± 0.0	47.0	69.5	2460	1008	1200
Normal rice[d]	70.3 ± 0.2	9.9	13.2 ± 0.6	40.5	79.9	1356	1152	1920
Waxy rice[d]	56.9 ± 0.3	13.4	15.4 ± 0.2	5.0	64 1	2460	1008	1200
Wheat[d]	57.1 ± 03	9.1	10.7 ± 0.2	33.7	88.6	1248	900	1848
Cattail millet[d]	67.1 ± 0.0	8.5	14.4 ± 0.3	53.8	74.2	2412	960	2496
Sorghum[e]	70.0 ± 2.1	7.6	11.7 ± 1.3	33.8	78.4	3420	1980	3516
Amaranth[f,g]	64.8 ± 0.4	16.3	8.2 ± 0.2	< 45[h]	75.7	820	620	710
Buckwheat[i]	61.2 ± 0.4	12.4	9.0 ± 0.8	52[j]	68.8	4589	2171	3986
Quinoa[k]	55.0± 0.6	12.0	8.8 ± 0.2	4.1	62.7	3932	3151	3978
Cassava[a]	64.3 ± 0.1	10.1	14.7 + 0.7	25.3	67.6	2076	732	1284
Potato[a]	58.2 ± 0.1	9.5	15.8 + 1.2	43.4	63.5	8424	1980	2772

[a] Starch gelatinization parameters were obtained by a differential scanning calorimetry. Range of gelatinization is the difference between conclusion temperature and onset temperatures.

[b] % retrogradation is the percentage of the enthalpy of the first run (i.e., native samples) and the second run (i.e., samples stored at 4°C for 7 days).

[c] As determined by a Rapid ViscoAnalyzer, using 8% (w/w, dry substance basis) starch in water (28 g of total weight). Source data given by [d]Jane et al. 1999, reported in RVU have been recalculated to centipoise using conversion rate 1 RVU = 12 cP.

[d] According to Jane et al. (1999). [e]mean values calculated according to the results reported by Singh et al. 2011, [f]Resio and Suarez 2001, [g]Choi et al. 2004, [h] 45% after 21 days (Baker and Rayas-Duarte 1998), [i]Li et al. 2014, [j]Estimated according to Lian et al. (2014); DSC analysis results. [k]Steffolani et al. (2013).

7.3 Proteins

7.3.1 General remarks

Main proteins of plant flours are the seed (grain) storage proteins. In cereals, monocotyledonous plants (synonym: monocots), dominating fractions of storage proteins are prolamins (gliadins) and glutelins. In pseudocereals, belonging to dicotyledonous plants (dicots), main storage proteins are globulins, and particularly 11S and 7S globulins. In some dicots used in gluten-free bread a storage albumin 2S can influence functional properties of the flour.

Cereal flours applied in gluten-free bread recipes contain gluten proteins similarly like wheat but these proteins show different aggregation behavior and gas bubbles retention capability due to its physicochemical characteristics and differences in polysaccharides contents and properties. Due to it, dough obtained with the use of these flours is much more sensible to deformation than wheat dough, it has lower gas retention capability and gives a lower loaf specific volume.

Storage globulins contained in pseudocereal flours have much poorer capability of structure formation in a dough than prolamins of "gluten free" cereals because of its compact, globular shape, more hydrophobic properties and absence of intermolecular covalent bonds, like disulphide bonds. Therefore, forces involved in structure stabilization in so concentrated hydrated systems as gluten-free dough are related to ionic interactions and hydrogen bondings. Some attempts were done to take advantage of intermolecular isopeptide ε-(γ-Glu)-Lys bonds formed by transglutaminase between pseudocereal or legume storage globulins molecules and/or cereal prolamins of rice flour to imitate in the gluten-free dough the structuring function of SS bonds in wheat dough (Moore et al. 2006; Marco et al. 2007; Marco and Rosell 2008a). However, particular caution should be kept using transglutaminase in gluten-free formulations because of risk of deamidation a glutamine in the sequence QPFPQPQLPYPQPQ widely occurring in gliadins leading to formation of the sequence QPFPQPELPYPQPQ being an active epitope, thought to be involved in the autoimmune response in coeliac suffers (Gerrard and Sutton 2005).

Protein classification according to its solubility into water soluble albumins, salt soluble globulins, prolamins soluble in water-alcohol mixtures and alkali soluble glutelins proposed by Osborne (Osborne 1924) still remains a useful first insight into understanding protein physicochemical properties. As it is shown in Table 10, in most cereals total contents of albumins and globulins range between 10 and 20% of total protein, and total contents of prolamins and glutelins reach the range of 60 to 80% of total protein. There are some exceptions like oats containing up to 60% of globulins and as little as ~20% of gluten proteins, and rice, containing mainly gluten proteins, particularly glutelins. In pseudocereals, albumin and globulin constitute up to 60–70% of total protein and prolamin and glutelin contents ranges from 15 and 40% of total protein.

In 1984 Shewry et al. proposed a new classification of gluten proteins dividing them into Prolamins I and Prolamins II (Fig. 2), according to their molecular weight, sulfur amino acids content and capability of polymerization (aggregation) *via* covalent bonds, i.e., disulphide bridges formed between two cysteine residues.

7.3.2 Wheat gluten proteins and bread making

In wheat dough, gliadins, high molecular weight (HMW) glutenin subunits (GS) and low molecular weight glutenin subunits (LMW-GS) are important factors in determining dough properties and final product quality. It is likely that HMW-GS are

Table 10. Protein content and protein fractional composition according to Osborne classification in flours of cereals and pseudocereals.

Cereal/ pseudocereal	Protein content	Albumins	Globulins	Prolamins	Glutelins
	(% of d.m.)	% of total protein	% of total protein	% of total protein	% of total protein
Wheat[a]	10–16	10–15	5–10	40–50 (69)	30–40
Rye[b]	9–14	15–35	5–10 (15–30)	20–45	30–40
Barley[c]	10–16	3–4	10–20	35–45	35–45
Oat[d]	8–20	5–10	50–60	7–16	5
Maize[e]	7–13	2–10	9–20	39–55	30–45
Rice[f]	8–10	2–5	2–8	1–5	80–90
Sorghum[g]	9–13	6–9	7–10	60–70	30–40
Millet[h]	14–18	13–23	9–5	40–47	20–28
Teff[i]	10–12	10–13	10–13	38–42	20–25
Buckwheat[j]	10–12	44–56	44–56	3–5	14–19
Amaranth[k]	13–18	8–21	19–59	2–19	6–44
Quinoa[l]	8–22	13–14	51–60	0.5–7	3–6

[a] Eliasson and Larsson (1993); Lasztity (1995); Shewry (2009), [b] Eliasson and Larsson (1993); Lasztity (1995); Lorenz (2000), [c] Shukla and Bushuk (1975); Eliasson and Larsson (1993); Lasztity (1995); Hockett (2000), [d] Shukla and Bushuk (1975); Eliasson and Larsson (1993); Lasztity (1995); McMullen (2000), [e] Shukla and Cheryan (2001), [f] Shukla and Bushuk (1975); Eliasson and Larsson (1993); Lasztity (1995), [g] Shewry 2002; de Mesa-Stonestreet et al. 2010, [h] Okoh et al. (1985); Lasztity (1995); McDonough et al. (2000), [i] Adebowale et al. 2011, [j] Range of values found by Radovic et al. (1996), Mickowska et al. (2013), [k] Range of values found by Bressani and Garcia-Vela (1990), Shewry (2002), Thanapornpoonpong et al. (2008), Mickowska et al. (2013), [l] Thanapornpoonpong et al. (2008), Jancurova et al. (2009), Bhargava and Srivastava (2013).

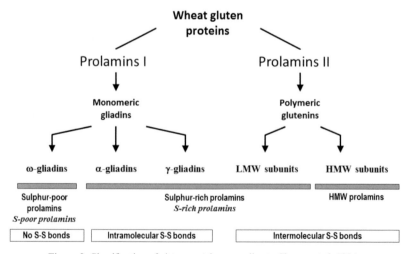

Figure 2. Classification of gluten proteins according to Shewry et al. 1984.

more important for dough strength, while gliadins and LMW-GS are more involved in dough extensibility (Bekes et al. 2006; Rasheed et al. 2014). Basing on wide collection of published results, it is possible to suggest that for dough strength, the interaction among glutenin fractions can be ranked as HMW-HMW > HMW-LMW > LMW-LMW, while for gluten extensibility, HMW-LMW > LMW-LMW > HMW-HMW (Bekes et al. 2006; Rasheed et al. 2014).

In quantitative terms, the relative proportion of gluten protein fractions, i.e., glutenins and gliadins, and their sub-fractions (particularly HMW-GS) are important determinants of bread-making quality. There is still a discussion concerning the role of the various protein classes on bread-making parameters such as dough properties, loaf volume, and crumb characteristics (Rasheed et al. 2014).

Diversity of proteins occurring in the gluten-free formulations causes that according to our current knowledge it is impossible to present such an overall classification of the protein impact on gluten-free dough functional properties.

7.3.3 Proteins of gluten-free cereals

7.3.3.1 Rice

In rice (*Oryza sativa* L.) seed and flour globulin is the most abundant storage protein. The prolamins are a smaller component of the storage proteins in rice; they are present in quantities of order of 5% of total protein. Prolamin and glutelin (a globulin-like protein) are deposited into separate protein bodies in rice seed. The rice prolamins are approximately 10,000 to 16,000 in M_r and are highly variable within and between different rice cultivars. The net charge of the rice prolamins varies also significantly. In Japanese rice cultivars five to nine prolamins of isoelectric points ranging from 5.6 to 8.3 were identified. The rice prolamins have a number of characteristics that are different from the prolamins of most other cereals (Muench et al. 1999).

Rice glutelin is only soluble in dilute acid or alkaline solutions, but it is considered a member of the 11S salt-soluble globulin family based on amino acid sequences homology and similarities in its biosynthesis. During biosynthetic process, the rice glutelin precursor of M_r 55,000–57,000 is proteolytically processed in protein bodies into acidic (α) and basic (β) polypeptides, which are covalently linked to each other by an interchain disulfide bond. The acidic subunits have M_r 28,500–30,800 with isoelectric point ranging from pH 6.5 to 7.5, while the basic subunits have M_r between 20,600 and 21,600 with pI between 9.4 to 10.3. At this storage site, the typical 11S globulin is assembled into a hexamer like in legume seeds, but more than half of rice glutelin polymerizes by disulfide bonding and hydrophobic interactions to form very large macromolecular complexes. The formation of higher-order structures may be one of the reasons why functional properties are lacking for rice glutelin (Takaiwa et al. 1999).

Rice glutelin can be classified into A and B types. The B type glutelin has fewer free cysteine residue that is not involved in interchain disulfide bonds, and may be able to self-assemble into an oligomer, similar to soybean glycinin which possesses superior food processing properties (Takaiwa et al. 1999; Katsube-Tanaka et al. 2004).

7.3.3.2 Maize, sorghum and Coix

In whole maize (*Zea mays* L.) grain, zein occurs as a heterogeneous mixture of disulfide-linked aggregates of average M_r 44,000. The zeins can be separated by

SDS-PAGE under reducing conditions into four groups, called α-, β-, γ- and δ-zeins varying in their apparent M_r from about 10,000 to 27,000 and characterized by their high hydrophobicity. Among these four groups, α-zeins are the most abundant and comprise 75–85% of total zeins (Lasztity 1995; Shukla and Cheryan 2001; Cabra et al. 2005).

The structure of maize glutelin has not been studied as intensively as that of zein. It is generally accepted that glutelin is a macromolecule composed of different polypeptide subunits linked together by disulfide bonds. Based on solubility the subunits may be classified into the three following groups: water-soluble and alcohol-soluble polypeptides, alcohol-soluble polypeptides, and alkali-soluble subunits. The classification of maize glutelin subunits still causes the difficulties. More detailed knowledge of the maize endosperm proteins is still needed to find an internationally agreed and more accurate classification (Lasztity 1995; Shukla and Cheryan 2001).

Studies on sorghum (*Sorghum bicolor* (L.) Moench) and Job's tears (*Coix lacryma-jobi* L.) prolamins called kafirins and coixins, respectively, revealed their close similarity to maize prolamins. Homologues of α-, β- and γ-zeins are also present in sorghum and *Coix*. However, the prolamins in these three species differ in their solubility properties indicating differences in sequence and structure which could affect their functional properties and utilization (Leite et al. 1999; Shewry 2002).

7.3.3.3 Millets

About 40% of the total proteins of pearl millet (*Pennisetum glaucum*) can be extracted in aqueous alcohol as prolamins called pennisetins. The amino acid compositions of these prolamins are similar to those of maize and sorghum prolamins. SDS-PAGE under reducing conditions shows a major band of M_r about 22,000 with minor bands of M_r about 20,000 and 10,000. However, analysis of total seed proteins by two-dimensional non-reducing/reducing SDS-PAGE showed that a high proportion of the prolamins is present as dimers of M_r 45,000–47,000. Comparison with the sequence of an α-zein fraction showed a lower level of homology than between zeins and kafirins (Leite et al. 1999; Shewry 2002).

Foxtail millet (*Setaria italica* (L.) Beauv.) prolamins (called setarins) account for over half of the total grain protein and comprise major bands of M_r between about 17,000 and 22,000 and a minor band of M_r about 12,000. However, the subunits are mainly present in oligomers and polymers which can be separated by gel filtration chromatography into two major size fractions: above 100,000 and 40,000–100,000 of M_r. The amino acid composition of these three fractions are similar to those of α-zeins. The most soluble fractions, α- and β-setarins, contain methionine-rich polypeptides of M_r 7,900 and 9,100, respectively (Leite et al. 1999; Shewry 2002; Mickowska et al. 2013).

Prolamins are the major protein group in teff (*Eragrostis tef* (Zucc.) Trotter.) grain and flour. The aqueous alcohol-soluble protein accounts for ~40% of total protein and it was rich in glutamine and leucine. The SDS-PAGE under non-reducing and reducing conditions revealed teff monomeric prolamins of M_r 20,300 and 22,800. Polymeric polypeptides of M_r approx. 36,100, 50,200, 66,200 and 90,000, respectively found under non-reducing conditions were absent under reducing conditions, indicating that these polypeptides are linked with disulphide bonds. There are several significant differences between teff and sorghum prolamins. Teff prolamins are more hydrophilic, less polymerized and have lower thermal stability. These differences probably make them more functional in bread making compared to sorghum prolamins (Leite et al. 1999; Adebowale et al. 2011).

Some species belonging to the genus *Digitaria* are important local crops in Africa, like white and black fonio: white fonio, synonyms—acha, hungry rice (*Digitaria exilis* (Kippist) Stapf) and black fonio, synonym—iburura (*Digitaria iburua*). In the past, grain of finger-grass, synonym crabgrass (*Digitaria sanguinalis* (L.) Scop.), were consumed in Europe and North America. In common terminology, various *Digitara* species are treated as a kind of millet. Like in other cereals, major component of *Digitaria* grains are carbohydrates accounting for more than 80% of grain, and their protein contents range from 6 to 11% d.m. (Irving and Jideani 1997; Carcea and Salvatorelli 1999; Jideani 1999).

Protein fractional composition of cultivated *Digitaria* species grain has been little studied. It was found in *Digitaria exilis* wholegrain flour, that the glutelin fraction represented about 60% of total protein and there remained significant insoluble protein residue. It is suggested that hydrophobic as well as covalent disulphide interactions are responsible for the relative insolubility of acha proteins in conventional solvents. SDS-PAGE analysis of wholegrain *Digitaria exilis* flour revealed that a major component of M_r 25,200 forms a basic structural component of the storage proteins (Jideani et al. 1994; Carcea and Salvatorelli 1999).

A high methionine contents have been found in the *Digitaria* prolamin and glutelin fractions accounting for about 5% (g aa/g protein) and about 2–7% protein, respectively. The glutelin fraction also had a high lysine content (> 5%) (Delumen et al. 1993; Carcea and Salvatorelli 1999).

7.3.4 Proteins of pseudocereals

7.3.4.1 Buckwheat

Buckwheat (*Fagopyrum esculentum* Moench) seeds and flour contain about 13.5% protein on a dry matter basis. Nearly 40% of total protein appears to be storage globulins, of which 13S and 8S globulins have been reported to account for about 33 and 6.5% of the total seed proteins, respectively. The 2S albumins account for about 25% of the total salt-soluble proteins. These albumins are a single chain proteins of M_r 8000–16,000. Some of the buckwheat albumins appeared heterodimeric comprising subunits of M_r about 7000–8000 and 4000–5000. Amino acid analysis showed a high content of methionine (9.21 mol%) but low amount of cysteine (0.7 mol%) (Segura-Nieto et al. 1999; Shewry 2002).

The buckwheat major storage globulin has a slightly higher sedimentation coefficient (13S) than classical 11S globulins occurring in legumes (11–12S). Nevertheless, this globulin has a typical legumin structure with its M_r of about 280,000 and the presence of six subunits each comprising large acidic (M_r 32,000–43,000) and small basic (M_r 20,000–23,000) chains. These chains are linked by disulphide bonds. Homology of the buckwheat 13S legumin basic subunit with the sequences of the soybean glycinins and pea legumins has been demonstrated (Radovic et al. 1996; Segura-Nieto et al. 1999; Shewry 2002).

Buckwheat globulins 8S have an M_r of about 57,000–58,000. Although physicochemical characteristics of these globulins are close to vicilin-like 7–8S globulins homology between these groups remains to be confirmed (Radovic et al. 1996; Shewry 2002; Milisavljevic et al. 2004).

7.3.4.2 Amaranth

There are three major species of amaranth cultivated for grain, *Amaranthus hypochondriacus*, *A. cruentus* and *A. caudatus*. Of these species, *A. hypochondriacus* has been most studied. All amaranth species have high seed protein contents, from about 13 to 18% dry weight. Albumins and globulins are the major seed and flour proteins in all three species, accounting for 40 to 80% of the total seed proteins. Similarly, the ratio of albumins to globulins observed for amaranth species ranges from about 4:1 to 1:5 (Segura-Nieto et al. 1999; Shewry 2002).

The 13S globulins (amaranthins) corresponding to 11S legume-type globulins are a major amaranth globulin group accounting for about 77–81% of the total fraction. According to gel filtration chromatography, their M_r range from 273,000 to 381,000. Under reducing conditions the 13S amaranthins dissociate into polypeptides of M_r 30,000–37,000 and 18,000–27,000, which were presumed to correspond to the acidic and basic subunits, respectively. The amaranth 8S globulins (conamaranthin) have a M_r of 50,000–75,000 and are not affected by reduction, which is consistent with their identification as subunits of 7S vicilin-type globulins. Conamaranthin has isoelectric point of pH 5.2–5.8 (Marcone and Yada 1998; Marcone 1999; Shewry 2002).

7.3.4.3 Quinoa

Quinoa (*Chenopodium quinoa* Willd.), and more recently kaniwa (syn. Kañiwa) (*Chenopodium pallidicaule* Aellen), the American relatives of a European famine plant goosefoot (*Chenopodium album* L.), are considered as potentially valuable gluten-free pseudocereals. Both quinoa and kaniwa have been reported to contain about 14–16% protein (Shewry 2002; Repo-Carrasco et al. 2003; Rosell et al. 2009; Repo-Carrasco 2011; Diaz et al. 2013; Steffolani et al. 2013).

Extracts of quinoa seed proteins can be fractionated into 11S globulins (chenopodin) and 2S albumins fractions, although the range of proportions of these fractions do not appear to have been determined. SDS-PAGE of the purified 2S albumins showed a group of bands of M_r about 8000–9000. These are thought to correspond to the large subunits of albumin heterodimers, with the small subunits not being resolved. Amino acid analysis of the fraction showed high cysteine (15.6 mol%) but less than 1 mol% methionine. Chenopodin has a typical 11S globulin structure, with a native M_r of about 320,000. It comprises six subunits, each consisting of acidic (M_r 32,000–39,000) and basic (M_r 22,000–23,000) chains associated by inter-chain disulphide bonds (Brinegar and Goundan 1993; Brinegar et al. 1996; Shewry 2002).

Protein fractional composition of kaniwa should be very close to those of quinoa although the proportions of 2S albumins to 11S and 7S globulins in kaniwa do not appear to have been determined.

7.4 Cereal flours

The cereal most frequently used at commercial scale as one of the principal components in gluten-free formulations is rice flour. Other cereal used in GF technology or recommended to be used is maize, mainly as starch (corn starch, maize starch) but also as a flour. Depending on rice flour particle size distribution and dough hydration pure rice bread specific volume varies from 1.8 to 5.7 cm³/g (Hager and Arendt 2013; de la Hera et al. 2014). Maize flour used as a significant component of a GF mixture (40 to 100% of the GF mixture) lowers rheological properties of the gluten-free dough and sensory-textural properties of the GF bread (Pruska-Kędzior et al. 2008; Renzetti et al. 2008; Renzetti and Arendt 2009). In some formulations it was proposed to use reduced quantities of maize flour (Gambus et al. 2007; Mezaize et al. 2009; Mezaize et al. 2010; Wolska et al. 2010), of order of 7 to 14% of GF mixture. Maize flour was used as the main component of GF recipes to produce special types of GF bread like the Portuguese *broa* (Brites et al. 2010), or flat sour maize bread (Edema and Sanni 2008). The specific bread volume at the presence of maize flours varies from ca. 2.6 cm³/g at 40% addition of maize flour to the gluten-free formulation (Pruska-Kędzior et al. 2008) to as low as 1.4 cm³/g at 100% maize flour recipe (Renzetti et al. 2008; Renzetti and Arendt 2009). It was found that depending on particle size distribution in maize flour and/or semolina specific loaf volume of pure maize bread has varied from 1.7 to 4.3 cm³/g (de la Hera et al. 2013).

Sorghum is a vital food crop in many regions of Africa and Asia but it still remains underutilized as a food in Europe and North America (Taylor et al. 2006). Traditionally, a flat bread used to be manufactured from sorghum flour, leavened like Ethiopian *injera* or puffed like chapatti or roti made in India (Murty and Kumar 1995). Sorghum flour has been appeared a valuable component of GF leavened bread (Schober et al. 2005; Schober et al. 2007; Schwab et al. 2008; Onyango et al. 2011a; Onyango et al. 2011b). Renzetti et al. (2008) noted specific bread volume of pure sorghum formulations ranging around 1.5–1.6 cm³/g. When enzymes like glucose oxidase, protease or transglutaminase have been added to the formulations, specific volume of sorghum bread increased to ca. 1.8 cm³/g (Renzetti et al. 2008; Renzetti and Arendt 2009). Schober et al. (2007) observed for optimized gluten-free bread containing 70% of sorghum flour the specific volume of order of 2.3–2.7 cm³/g.

Various millets are commonly used in Asia and Africa for flat bread manufacturing (Murty and Kumar 1995). Millet flours are considered as components of GF mixtures for leavened or leavened flat gluten-free bread manufacturing. European common millet (synonym—proso millet, *Panicum miliaceum* L.) flour was proposed to produce a sourdough for GF bread baking (Wolska et al. 2010). Nutritional and technological potential of various millets for baking gluten-free bread and cakes has been studied for such millet species as: pearl millet (synonym: cattail millet), finger millet (ragi) (*Eleusine coracana* (L.) Gaertn.), foxtail millet, Indian barnyard millet (*Echinochloa frumentacea* Link), and Japanese millet (*Echinochloa crus-galli* (L.) Beauv), kodo millet (*Paspalum scrobiculatum* L.), and fonio: white, and black (Kumari and Thayumanavan 1998; Taylor et al. 2006; Bernardi et al. 2010; Kamara et al. 2010; Jideani and Jideani 2011; Omary et al. 2012; Mickowska et al. 2013). Recently, special attention has been paid to application of the Ethiopian millet teff (*Eragrostis tef* (Zucc.) Trotter.) in gluten-free bread manufacturing (Moroni et al. 2010; Adebowale et al. 2011; Moroni et al. 2011; Hager and Arendt 2013; Wolter et al. 2013). Typical specific bread volume of pure leavened teff bread ranged from 1.7 to 1.8 cm^3/g (Renzetti et al. 2008; Renzetti and Arendt 2009).

7.5 Pseudocereal flours

Buckwheat, amaranth and quinoa flours have been the most frequently studied pseudocereals in gluten-free formulations. Water holding capacity of pseudocereal flours is higher than those of wheat flour (0.84 g H$_2$O/g) and equal or higher than of rye flour (1.13 g/g), and ranges from 1.13 g/g for buckwheat to 1.57 g/g for quinoa flour, while for amaranth and teff it was found of ~1.4 g/g (Collar and Angioloni 2014). Foam capacity of pseudocereal flours is lower than those of rye (26 ml) and wheat flour (14 ml) and ranges from 3 (buckwheat and quinoa) to 5 (teff) and 9 ml (amaranth). However, foam stability measured after 60 min is higher than in wheat (36%) and ranges from 33% (amaranth, no statistical difference as compared to wheat) to 60 (teff), and 100% (buckwheat and quinoa) while for rye flour it was 81% (Collar and Angioloni 2014).

In model wheat-rye bread (1:1 wheat and rye flour), a 5% additions of amaranth, buckwheat, quinoa or teff flour did not lower significantly the bread specific volume ranging around 3.1 cm^3/g (Collar and Angioloni 2014). However, 10% additives of binary mixtures of these pseudocereal flours mixed at the ratio 1:1, 15% additives of the ternary mixtures (pseudocereal flours at the ratio 1:1:1), and/or 20% quaternary mixtures (1:1:1:1) caused lowering bread specific volume to the level of 2.5–2.7 cm^3/g. It seemed that amaranth and teff flours affected bread specific volume stronger than buckwheat and quinoa (Collar and Angioloni 2014).

In true gluten-free formulations, pseudocereal flours are used in quantities ranging from 5% to 100%. In the gluten-free French-type bread based on rice flour (50% of the mix) and various starches, the specific loaf volume reached 2.5 cm^3/g and was a half lower than the specific volume of typical wheat French bread (5.3 cm^3/g). Replacing 5% of the gluten-free mix mass (in starch fraction) with buckwheat flour caused increasing the specific volume to 3.6 cm^3/g (Mezaize et al. 2009).

In breads containing 40–50% buckwheat flour in the gluten-free mix the specific loaf volume varied from 1.6 to 3.6 cm^3/g, depending on the mix composition and hydrocolloids used in the formulation (Pruska-Kędzior et al. 2008; Alvarez-Jubete et al. 2009b; Mariotti et al. 2013). In pure buckwheat bread the specific loaf volume was as low as 1.4 cm^3/g (Costantini et al. 2014).

In gluten-free formulations based on rice flour mixed with amaranth or quinoa flours at the ratio 1:1 the specific loaf volume was 1.3 and 1.4 cm^3/g, respectively (Alvarez-Jubete et al. 2009b).

7.6 Legume flours and protein isolates

Legume flours and legume protein isolates are used to enrich gluten-free recipes with protein. Soybean, pea, chickpea and lupin have been proposed as the components of the gluten-free mixes (Marco et al. 2007; Marco and Rosell 2008b; Mariotti et al. 2009; Sabanis and Tzia 2009; Minarro et al. 2012; Ziobro et al. 2013b).

Marco and Rosell (2008b) studied the effect of a 1 to 25% addition of pea or soybean protein isolates (protein contents > 90%) to rice flour on the physicochemical properties of rice dough.

Protein isolates induced a significant increase in the water absorption of the composite rice flour-protein isolate blends. However, significant lowering of overall viscoelasticity of the dough was observed comparing to control rice dough (a decrease of the storage G' and loss G'' moduli). Protein isolates also modified the mechanical and surface related textural properties.

Ziobro et al. studied the effect of the 8% replacement of starch with pea, lupine or soybean protein on viscoelastic properties of the dough and crumb specific volume in a starch-based recipe containing a 3.24% addition of pectin and guar gum (1:1) (Ziobro et al. 2013b). The partial replacement of starch with the proteins increased the overall viscoelastic properties of the dough comparing to the control. Soy protein reduced specific bread volume (2.6 and 2.2 cm^3/g for control and soy protein formulations, respectively), while the lupine protein addition increased significantly the bread volume (3.6 cm^3/g). Bread containing pea protein was the most acceptable among the analyzed samples. A decrease in crumb hardness and a drop in enthalpy of retrograded amylopectin observed after the addition of the protein preparations clearly indicate that such additions could effectively retard staling of starch based bread (Ziobro et al. 2013b).

7.7 Hydrocolloids

Hydrocolloids used as the structure forming components of gluten-free formulations are introduced as a single component or a mixture of two or more components. The most frequently used polysaccharides are: pectin, guar gum, carboxymethyl cellulose (CMC), hydroxymethylpropyl cellulose (HPMC), carrageenans, xanthan gum, locust bean gum and carob flour (both obtained from *Ceratonia siliqua* L., carob tree, St. John's-bread, or locust bean), inulin and modified starches. The level of the addition ranges from 0.5 to 5%. The choice of a single or a mixed hydrocolloids addition, proportions of the hydrocolloids in the complex systems and the level of their addition to a gluten-free formulation depend on the composition of a gluten-free mix, its initial rheological and interfacial properties, the effect on specific bread volume, expected lowering of the staling process, and are individually optimized (Rosell et al. 2001; Guarda et al. 2004; Gambus et al. 2007; Lazaridou et al. 2007; Anton and Artfield 2008; Kohajdová and Karovičová 2009; Witczak et al. 2010; Rosell et al. 2011; Houben et al. 2012; Witczak et al. 2012; Ziobro et al. 2013a; Ziobro et al. 2013b).

For example, the effect of hydrocolloids on dough rheology and bread quality parameters in gluten-free formulations based on rice flour and maize starch was studied by Lazaridou et al. (2007). The hydrocolloids added at 1% and 2% w/w (rice flour basis) were pectin, CMC, agarose, xanthan and oat β-glucan. The effect of hydrocolloids on the elasticity and resistance to deformation of dough, as determined by oscillatory and creep measurements, followed the order of xanthan > CMC > pectin > agarose > β-glucan (Lazaridou et al. 2007).

7.8 Lipids

Vegetable oil, shortenings or margarine are used as a factor plasticizing the dough and improving stabilization of the gas bubbles in the dough. Sunflower, rapeseed and olive oils are the most frequently used in the gluten-free bread formulations but shortenings and margarine are also applied. The level of fat additions varies from 2 to 12%, depending on formulation. The stabilization of the gas bubbles in bread dough is often enhanced by the addition of various emulsifiers (Houben et al. 2012).

8. Concluding remarks

It is difficult to present in a single chapter the abundance of potential gluten-free raw materials. Apart from the presented raw materials of plant origin also milk and dairy products, whole egg, egg white and yolk have been used to improve nutritional value of gluten-free bread and other baked goods (Schober et al. 2005; Moore et al. 2006; Marco and Rosell 2008a; Mezaize et al. 2009). Effects of whole or ground seeds rich in minerals, antioxidants, dietary fiber, and valuable oils on nutritional value and sensory properties of gluten-free bread are studied (Pruska-Kędzior et al. 2008; Mariotti et al. 2009; Houben et al. 2012; Costantini et al. 2014). It is expected also that enzymatic processes occurring in sourdough technology could enable controlled hydrolysis of the celiac-inducing epitopes of wheat, rye and barley prolamins opening a perspective of safe introduction of these raw materials to the gluten-free baked goods (Gobbetti et al. 2007).

Keywords: Bread, gluten-free, nutritive value, dough, protein, prolamins, glutenins, hydrocolloids, polysaccharides, rheology, viscoelasticity, surface-active properties, gas retention, fermentation, staling

References

Abugoch James, L.E. 2009. Chapter 1. Quinoa (*Chenopodium quinoa* Willd.): Composition, chemistry, nutritional, and functional properties. Advances in Food and Nutrition Research, 58: 1–31.

Adebowale, A.R.A., M.N. Emmambux, M. Beukes and J.R.N. Taylor. 2011. Fractionation and characterization of teff proteins. Journal of Cereal Science, 54(3): 380–386.

Ahamed, N.T., R.S. Singhal, P.R. Kulkarni and P. Mohinder. 1998. A lesser-known grain, *Chenopodium quinoa*: review of the chemical composition of its edible parts. Food Nutr. Bull., 19: 61–70.

Ahmad, M.Z., S. Akhter, M. Anwar, M. Rahman, M.A. Siddiqui and F.J. Ahmad. 2012. Compactibility and compressibility studies of assam bora rice starch. Powder Technology, 224(0): 281–286.

Altuntaş, B., B. Filik, A. Ensari, P. Zorlu and T. Teziç. 2000. Can zinc deficiency be used as a marker for the diagnosis of celiac disease in Turkish children with short stature? Pediatr. Int., 42: 682–4.

Alvarez-Jubete, L., E.K. Arendt and E. Gallagher. 2009a. Nutritive value and chemical composition of pseudocereals as gluten-free ingredients. Intl. J. Food Sci. Nutr., 60: 240–57.

Alvarez-Jubete, L., E.K. Arendt and E. Gallagher. 2010. Nutritive value of pseudocereals and their increasing use as functional gluten-free ingredients. Trends in Food Science & Technology, 21: 106–113.

Alvarez-Jubete, L., M. Auty, E.K. Arendt and E. Gallagher. 2009b. Baking properties and microstructure of pseudocereal flours in gluten-free bread formulations. European Food Research and Technology, 230(3): 437–445.

Anton, A.A. and S.D. Artfield. 2008. Hydrocolloids in gluten-free breads: A review. International Journal of Food Sciences and Nutrition, 59(1): 11–23.

Baeton, S.H., D.G. Kelly and J.A. Murray. 2007. Nutritional deficiencies in celiac disease. Gastroenterol Clin. North Am., 36: 93–108.

Baker, L.A. and P. Rayas-Duarte. 1998. Retrogradation of amaranth starch at different storage temperatures and the effects of salt and sugars. Cereal Chemistry, 75(3): 308–314.

Bekes, F., S. Kemeny and M. Morell. 2006. An integrated approach to predicting end-product quality of wheat. European Journal of Agronomy, 25(2): 155–162.

Berganza, B.E., A.W. Moran, G.M. Rodríguez, N.M. Coto, M. Santamaría and R. Bressani. 2003. Effect of variety and location on the total fat, fatty acids and squalene content of amaranth. Plant Food Hum. Nutr., 58: 1–6.

Bernardi, C., H. Sánchez, M. Freyre and C. Osella. 2010. Gluten-free bread formulated with prosopis ruscifolia (vinal) seed and corn flours. International Journal of Food Sciences and Nutrition, 61(3): 245–255.

Bhargava, A. and S. Srivastava. 2013. Quinoa: Botany, production and uses. CABI.

Bhargava, A., S. Sudhir and O. Deepak. 2006. *Chenopodium quinoa*—An Indian perspective. Industrial Crops and Products, 23: 73–87.

Blomfeldt, T.O., R. Kuktaite, E. Johansson and M.S. Hedenqvist. 2011. Mechanical properties and network structure of wheat gluten foams. Biomacromolecules, 12: 1702–1715.

Bressani, R. and L.A. Garcia-Vela. 1990. Protein fractions in amaranth grain and their chemical characterization. Journal of Agricultural and Food Chemistry, 38(5): 1205–1209.

Bressani, R., J.M. González, J. Zúñiga, M. Breuner and L.G. Elías. 1987. Yield, selected chemical composition and nutritive value of 14 selections of amaranth grain representing four species. J. Sci. Food Agric., 38: 347–56.

Brinegar, C. and S. Goundan. 1993. Isolation and characterization of chenopodin, the 11s seed storage protein of quinoa (*Chenopodium-quinoa*). Journal of Agricultural and Food Chemistry, 41(2): 182–185.

Brinegar, C., B. Sine and L. Nwokocha. 1996. High-cysteine 25 seed storage proteins from quinoa (*Chenopodium quinoa*). Journal of Agricultural and Food Chemistry, 44(7): 1621–1623.

Brites, C., M.J. Trigo, C. Santos, C. Collar and C.M. Rosell. 2010. Maize-based gluten-free bread: Influence of processing parameters on sensory and instrumental quality. Food and Bioprocess Technology, 3(5): 707–715.

Budin, J.T., W.M. Breene and D.H. Putnam. 1996. Some compositional properties of seeds and oils of eight *Amaranthus* species. J. Am. Oil Chem. Soc., 73: 475–81.

Bultosa, G. and J.R.N. Taylor. 2004. Tef. pp. 253–262. *In:* Encyclopedia of Grain Science, C. Wrigley, H. Corke, C. Walker Amsterdam.

Burisová, A., B. Tomášková, V. Sasinková and A. Ebringerová. 2001. Isolation and characterization of the non-starch polysaccharides of amaranth seeds. Chem. Pap., 55: 254–260.

Cabra, V., R. Arreguin, A. Galvez, M. Quirasco, R. Vazquez-Duhalt and A. Farres. 2005. Characterization of a 19 kda alpha-zein of high purity. Journal of Agricultural and Food Chemistry, 53(3): 725–729.

Carcea, M. and S. Salvatorelli. 1999. Extraction and characterisation of fonio (*Digitaria exilis* Stapf) proteins. pp. 51–58. *In:* P. Colonna and S. Guilbert (eds.). Biopolymer science: Food and non food applications, Inst. Natl. Recherche Agronomique, Paris.

Choi, H., W. Kim and M. Shin. 2004. Properties of korean amaranth starch compared to waxy millet and waxy sorghum starches. Starch-Starke, 56(10): 469–477.

Collar, C. and A. Angioloni. 2014. Pseudocereals and teff in complex breadmaking matrices: Impact on lipid dynamics. Journal of Cereal Science, 59(2): 145–154.

Costantini, L., L. Luksic, R. Molinari, I. Kreft, G. Bonafaccia, L. Manzi and N. Merendino. 2014. Development of gluten-free bread using tartary buckwheat and chia flour rich in flavonoids and omega-3 fatty acids as ingredients. Food Chemistry, 165: 232–240.

Cunningham, D.K., W.F. Geddes and J.A. Anderson. 1955. Preparation and chemical characteristics of the cohesive proteins of wheat, rye, barley and oats. Cereal Chemistry, 32(2): 91.

De La Hera, E., C.M. Rosell and M. Gomez. 2014. Effect of water content and flour particle size on gluten-free bread quality and digestibility. Food Chemistry, 151(0): 526–531.

De La Hera, E., M. Talegon, P. Caballero and M. Gomez. 2013. Influence of maize flour particle size on gluten-free breadmaking. Journal of the Science of Food and Agriculture, 93(4): 924–932.

De Mesa-Stonestreet, N.J., S. Alavi and S.R. Bean. 2010. Sorghum proteins: The concentration, isolation, modification, and food applications of kafirins. Journal of Food Science, 75(5): R90–R104.

Delumen, B.O., S. Thompson and W.J. Odegard. 1993. Sulfur amino acid-rich proteins in acha (*Digitaria-exilis*), a promising underutilized african cereal. Journal of Agricultural and Food Chemistry, 41(7): 1045–1047.

Diaz, J.M.R., S. Kirjoranta, S. Tenitz, P.A. Penttila, R. Serimaa, A.M. Lampi and K. Jouppila. 2013. Use of amaranth, quinoa and kaniwa in extruded corn-based snacks. Journal of Cereal Science, 58(1): 59–67.

Edema, M.O. and A.I. Sanni. 2008. Functional properties of selected starter cultures for sour maize bread. Food Microbiology, 25(4): 616–625.

Eliasson, A.C. and K. Larsson. 1993. Cereals in breadmaking: A molecular colloidal approach. Taylor & Francis.

Fadda, C., A.M. Sanguinetti, A. Del Caro, C. Collar and A. Piga. 2014. Bread staling: Updating the view. Comprehensive Reviews in Food Science and Food Safety, 13(4): 473–492.

Fasano, A. and C. Catassi. 2001. Current approaches to diagnosis and treatment of celiac disease: an evolving spectrum. Gastroenterol., 120: 636–651.

French, D. 1984.Organization of starch granules. pp. 183–248. *In*: R.L. Whistler, J.N. Bemiller and E.F. Paschall (eds.). Starch: Chemistry and technology, Academic Press.

Gallagher, E., A. Kunkel, T.R. Gormley and E.K. Arendt. 2003. The effect of dairy and rice powder addition on loaf and crumb characteristics, and on shelf life (intermediate and long-term) of gluten-free breads stored in a modified atmosphere. European Food Research and Technology, 218(1): 44–48.

Gambuś, H. 2005. Linseed (*Linum usitatissimum* L.) as a source of nutrients in gluten-free bread. Żywność. Nauka. Technologia. Jakość, 45(4): Supl. 61–74.

Gambuś, H., M. Sikora and R. Ziobro. 2007. The effect of composition of hydrocolloids on properties of gluten-free bread. Acta Scientiarum Polonorum Technologia Alimentaria, 6(3): 61–74.

Gerrard, J.A. and K.H. Sutton. 2005. Addition of transglutaminase to cereal products may generate the epitope responsible for coeliac disease. Trends in Food Science and Technology, 16(11): 510–512.

Gobbetti, M., C. Giuseppe Rizzello, R. Di Cagno and M. De Angelis. 2007. Sourdough lactobacilli and celiac disease. Food Microbiology, 24(2): 187–196.

Grobelnik, M.S., M. Turinek, M. Jakop, M. Bavec and F. Bavec. 2009. Nutrition value and use of grain amaranth: potential future application in bread making. Agricultura., 6: 43–53.

Grzymisławski, M., H. Stankowiak-Kulpa and M. Włochal. 2010. Coeliac disease—diagnostic and therapeutic standards. Forum Zaburzeń Metabolicznych, 1(1): 12–21.

Guarda, A., C.M. Rosell, C. Benedito and M.J. Galotto. 2004. Different hydrocolloids as bread improvers and antistaling agents. Food Hydrocolloids, 18(2): 241–247.

Hager, A.S. and E.K. Arendt. 2013. Influence of hydroxypropylmethylcellulose (HPMC), xanthan gum and their combination on loaf specific volume, crumb hardness and crumb grain characteristics of gluten-free breads based on rice, maize, teff and buckwheat. Food Hydrocolloids, 32(1): 195–203.

Hamer, R.J. 2005. Coeliac Disease: background and biochemical aspects. Biotechnol. Adv., 23(6): 401–408.

He, H.P., Y.Z. Cai, M. Sun and H. Corke. 2002. Extraction and purification of squalene from *Amaranthus* grain. J. Agric. Food Chem., 50: 368–72.

Hockett, E.A. 2000. Barley. *In*: K. Kulp (ed.). Handbook of cereal science and technology, second edition, revised and expanded, CRC Press, Taylor & Francis, pp. 81–126.

Houben, A., A. Hochstotter and T. Becker. 2012. Possibilities to increase the quality in gluten-free bread production: An overview. European Food Research and Technology, 235(2): 195–208.

Hozyasz, K.K. and M. Słowik. 2009. Teff—a valuable gluten-free cereal. Przegląd Gastroenterologiczny, 4 (5): 238–244.

Irving, D.W. and I.A. Jideani. 1997. Microstructure and composition of *Digitaria exilis* Stapf (acha): A potential crop. Cereal Chemistry, 74(3): 224–228.

Jancurova, M., L. Minarovicova and A. Dandar. 2009. Quinoa—a review. Czech Journal of Food Sciences, 27(2): 71–79.

Jane, J., Y.Y. Chen, L.F. Lee, A.E. Mcpherson, K.S. Wong, M. Radosavljevic and T. Kasemsuwan. 1999. Effects of amylopectin branch chain length and amylose content on the gelatinization and pasting properties of starch. Cereal Chemistry, 76(5): 629–637.

Jideani, I.A. 1999. Traditional and possible technological uses of *Digitaria exilis* (acha) and *Digitaria iburua* (iburu): A review. Plant Foods for Human Nutrition, 54(4): 363–374.

Jideani, I.A. and V.A. Jideani. 2011. Developments on the cereal grains *Digitaria exilis* (acha) and *Digitaria iburua* (iburu). Journal of Food Science and Technology, Mysore, 48(3): 251–259.

Jideani, I.A., R.K. Owusu and H.G. Muller. 1994. Proteins of acha (*Digitaria-exilis* Stapf)—solubility fractionation, gel-filtration, and electrophoresis of protein-fractions. Food Chemistry, 51(1): 51–59.

Kaganoff, M.F. 2007. Celiac disease: pathogenesis of a model immunogenetic disease. Clin. Invest., 117: 41–49.

Kamara, M.T., I. Amadou, F. Tarawalie and H.M. Zhou. 2010. Effect of enzymatic hydrolysis on the functional properties of foxtail millet (*Setaria italica* L.) proteins. International Journal of Food Science and Technology, 45(6): 1175–1183.

Katina, K., E. Arendt, K.H. Liukkonen, K. Autio, L. Flander and K. Poutanen. 2005. Potential of sourdough for healthier cereal products. Trends in Food Science and Technology, 16(1-3): 104–112.

Katsube-Tanaka, T., J.B.A. Duldulao, Y. Kimura, S. Iida, T. Yamaguchi, J. Nakano and S. Utsumi. 2004. The two subfamilies of rice glutelin differ in both primary and higher-order structures. Biochimica et Biophysica Acta (BBA)—Proteins and Proteomics, 1699(1–2): 95–102.

Kawamura-Konishi, Y., K. Shoda, H. Koga and Y. Honda. 2013. Improvement in gluten-free rice bread quality by protease treatment. Journal of Cereal Science, 58(1): 45–50.

Kaźmierczak, A., I. Bolesławska and J. Przysławski. 2011. Amaranth—its use in the prevention and treatment of certain civilization-related diseases. Nowiny Lekarskie, 80(3): 192–198.

Keetels, C., T. Vanvliet and P. Walstra. 1996. Gelation and retrogradation of concentrated starch systems .1. Gelation. Food Hydrocolloids, 10(3): 343–353.

Ketema, S. 1997. Tef (*Eragrostsis tef*) Series: Promoting the Conservation and Use of Underutilized and Neglected Crops. Institute of Plant Genetics and Crop Plant Research, Getersleben/International Plant Genetic Resources Institute, Rome.

Kohajdová, Z. and J. Karovičová. 2009. Application of hydrocolloids as baking improvers. Chemical Papers, 63(1): 26–38.

Konishi, Y., S. Hirano, H. Tsuboi and M. Wada. 2004. Distribution of minerals in quinoa (*Chenopodium quinoa* Willd.) seeds. Biosci. Biotechnol. Biochem., 68: 231–234.

Kozioł, M. 1992. Chemical composition and nutritional evaluation of Quinoa (*Chenopodium quinoa* Willd.). J. Food Comp. Anal., 5: 35–68.

Kraujalis, P. and P.R. Venskutonis. 2013. Optimisation of supercritical carbon dioxide extraction of amaranth seeds by response surface methodology and characterization of extracts isolated from different plant cultivars. J. Supercrit. Fluid, 73: 80–6.

Krupa-Kozak, U., M. Wronkowska, M. Soral-Śmietana, A. Troszyńska and J. Sadowska. 2009. The improvement of sensory quality and texture properties of gluten-free bread fortified with Ca. Czech Journal of Food Sciences, 27 (Spec. Iss.).

Kumari, S.K. and B. Thayumanavan. 1998. Characterization of starches of proso, foxtail, barnyard, kodo, and little millets. Plant Foods for Human Nutrition, 53(1): 47–56.

Kunachowicz, H., I. Nadolna, W. Kłys, K. Iwanow and B. Kruszewska. 1995. Gluten-free products composition and nutritive value. National Food and Nutrition Institute, Warsaw.

Kunachowicz, H., I. Nadolna, B. Przygoda and K. Iwanow. 2005. Tables of the nutritive value of food products and dishes. National Food and Nutrition Institute, Warsaw.

Lasztity, R. 1995. The chemistry of cereal proteins, second edition. Taylor & Francis, Boca Raton.

Lazaridou, A., D. Duta, M. Papageorgiou, N. Belc and C.G. Biliaderis. 2007. Effects of hydrocolloids on dough rheology and bread quality parameters in gluten-free formulations. Journal of Food Engineering, 79(3): 1033–1047.

Leite, A., G.C. Neto, A.L. Vettore, J.A. Yunes and P. Arruda. 1999. The prolamins of sorghum, coix and millets. pp. 141–157. *In*: P.R. Shewry and R. Casey (eds.). Seed proteins, Springer Netherlands.

Li, W.H., F. Cao, J. Fan, S.H. Ouyang, Q.G. Luo, J.M. Zheng and G.Q. Zhang. 2014. Physically modified common buckwheat starch and their physicochemical and structural properties. Food Hydrocolloids, 40: 237–244.

Lian, X.J., C.J. Wang, K.S. Zhang and L. Li. 2014. The retrogradation properties of glutinous rice and buckwheat starches as observed with FT-IR, C-13 NMR and DSC. International Journal of Biological Macromolecules, 64: 288–293.

Lin, L.Y., H.M. Liu, Y.W. Yu, S.D. Lin and J.L. Mau. 2009. Quality and antioxidant property of buckwheat enhanced wheat bread. Food Chemistry, 112(4): 987–991.

Lorenz, K. 2000. Rye. *In*: K. Kulp (ed.). Handbook of cereal science and technology, second edition, revised and expanded, CRC Press, Taylor & Francis, pp. 223–256.

Marco, C. and C.M. Rosell. 2008a. Effect of different protein isolates and transglutaminase on rice flour properties. Journal of Food Engineering, 84(1): 132–139.

Marco, C. and C.M. Rosell. 2008b. Functional and rheological properties of protein enriched gluten free composite flours. Journal of Food Engineering, 88(1): 94–103.

Marco, C., G. Pérez, P. Ribotta and C.M. Rosell. 2007. Effect of microbial transglutaminase on the protein fractions of rice, pea and their blends. Journal of the Science of Food and Agriculture, 87(14): 2576–2582.

Marcone, M. F. 1999. Evidence confirming the existence of a 7S globulin-like storage protein in *Amaranthus hypochondriacus* seed. Food Chemistry, 65(4): 533–542.

Marcone, M.F. and R.Y. Yada. 1998. Structural analysis of globulins isolated from genetically different amaranthus hybrid lines. Food Chemistry, 61(3): 319–326.

Mariotti, M., M. Lucisano, M. Ambrogina Pagani and P.K.W. Ng. 2009. The role of corn starch, amaranth flour, pea isolate, and *Psyllium* flour on the rheological properties and the ultrastructure of gluten-free doughs. Food Research International, 42(8): 963–975.

Mariotti, M., M.A. Pagani and M. Lucisano. 2013. The role of buckwheat and HPMC on the breadmaking properties of some commercial gluten-free bread mixtures. Food Hydrocolloids, 30(1): 393–400.

Markiewicz, K., H. Nowak-Polakowska, E. Markiewicz, R. Zadernowski, J.E. Bojarska and R.E. Łojko. 2006. Contents of selected macro- and microminerals and toxic elements in walnuts. Bromatologia i Chemia Toksykologiczna, 39(3): 237–241.

Matos, M.E. and C.M. Rosell. 2013. Quality indicators of rice-based gluten-free bread-like products: Relationships between dough rheology and quality characteristics. Food and Bioprocess Technology, 6(9): 2331–2341.

McDonough, C.M., L.W. Rooney and S.O. Serna-Saldivar. 2000. The millets. *In*: K. Kulp (ed.). Handbook of cereal science and technology, second edition, revised and expanded, CRC Press, Taylor & Francis, pp. 177–202.

McMullen, M.S. 2000. Oats. *In*: K. Kulp (ed.). Handbook of cereal science and technology, second edition, revised and expanded, CRC Press, Taylor & Francis, pp. 127–148.

Mezaize, S., S. Chevallier, A. Le Bail and M. De Lamballerie. 2009. Optimization of gluten-free formulations for French-style breads. Journal of Food Science, 74(3): 140–146.

Mezaize, S., S. Chevallier, A. Le-Bail and M. De Lamballerie. 2010. Gluten-free frozen dough influence of freezing on dough theological properties and bread quality. Food Research International, 43(8): 2186–2192.

Mickowska, B., P. Socha, D. Urminska and E. Cieslik. 2013. Immunodetection, electrophoresis and amino acid composition of alcohol soluble proteins extracted from grains of selected varieties of pseudocereals, legumes, oat, maize and rice. Cereal Research Communications, 41(1): 160–169.

Milisavljevic, M.D., G.S. Timotijevic, S.R. Radovic, J.M. Brkljacic, M.M. Konstantinovic and V.R. Maksimovic. 2004. Vicilin-like storage globulin from buckwheat (*Fagopyrum esculentum* Moench) seeds. Journal of Agricultural and Food Chemistry, 52(16): 5258–5262.

Minarro, B., E. Albanell, N. Aguilar, B. Guamis and M. Capellas. 2012. Effect of legume flours on baking characteristics of gluten-free bread. Journal of Cereal Science, 56(2): 476–481.

Moore, M.M., M. Heinbockel, P. Dockery, H.M. Ulmer and E.K. Arendt. 2006. Network formation in gluten-free bread with application of transglutaminase. Cereal Chemistry, 83(1): 28–36.

Moroni, A.V., E.K. Arendt and F. Dal Bello. 2011. Biodiversity of lactic acid bacteria and yeasts in spontaneously-fermented buckwheat and teff sourdoughs. Food Microbiology, 28(3): 497–502.

Moroni, A.V., E.K. Arendt, J.P. Morrissey and F. Dal Bello. 2010. Development of buckwheat and teff sourdoughs with the use of commercial starters. International Journal of Food Microbiology, 142(1-2): 142–148.

Muench, D.G., M. Ogawa and T.W. Okita. 1999. The prolamins of rice. pp. 93–108. *In*: P.R. Shewry and R. Casey (eds.). Seed proteins, Springer Netherlands.

Murty, D.S. and K.A. Kumar. 1995. Traditional uses of sorghum and millets. pp. 185–221. *In*: D.A.V. Dendy (ed.). Sorghum and millets: Chemistry and technology, American Association of Cereal Chemists, St. Paul, MN, USA.

National Institute for Health and Welfare, Nutrition Unit. 2013. Fineli. Finnish food composition database. Release 16. Helsinki. http://www.fineli.fi.

Ng, S.C., A. Anderson, J. Coker and M. Ondrus. 2007. Characterization of lipid oxidation products in quinoa (*Chenopodium quinoa*). Food Chem., 101: 185–192.

Omary, M.B., C. Fong, J. Rothschild and P. Finney. 2012. Effects of germination on the nutritional profile of gluten-free cereals and pseudocereals: A review. Cereal Chemistry, 89(1): 1–14.

Onyango, C., C. Mutungi, G. Unbehend and M.G. Lindhauer. 2011a. Modification of gluten-free sorghum batter and bread using maize, potato, cassava or rice starch. LWT—Food Science and Technology, 44(3): 681–686.

Onyango, C., C. Mutungi, G. Unbehend and M.G. Lindhauer. 2011b. Rheological and textural properties of sorghum-based formulations modified with variable amounts of native or pregelatinised cassava starch. LWT—Food Science and Technology, 44(3): 687–693.

Osborne, T.B. 1924. The vegetable proteins. Longmans Green and Co., London.

Pruska-Kędzior, A., Z. Kędzior, M. Gorący, K. Pietrowska, A. Przybylska and K. Spychalska. 2008. Comparison of rheological, fermentative and baking properties of gluten-free dough formulations. European Food Research and Technology, 227(5): 1523–1536.

Radovic, S.R., V.R. Maksimovic and E.I. Varkonjigasic. 1996. Characterization of buckwheat seed storage proteins. Journal of Agricultural and Food Chemistry, 44(4): 972–974.

Rasheed, A., X.C. Xia, Y.M. Yan, R. Appels, T. Mahmood and Z.H. He. 2014. Wheat seed storage proteins: Advances in molecular genetics, diversity and breeding applications. Journal of Cereal Science, 60(1): 11–24.

Ratusz, K. and M. Wirkowska. 2006. Characterization of seeds and lipids of amaranthus. Oilseed Crops, 27: 243–250.

Reguła, J. and M. Siwulski. 2007. Dried shiitake (*Lentinulla edodes*) and oyster (*Pleurotus ostreatus*) mushrooms as a good source of nutrient. Acta Sci. Pol., Technol. Aliment, 6(4): 135–142.

Reguła, J. and A. Śmidowicz. 2014. Share of dietary supplements in nutrition of coeliac disease patients. Acta. Sci.Pol., Technol. Aliment, 13(3): 301–307.

Renzetti, S. and E.K. Arendt. 2009. Effects of oxidase and protease treatments on the breadmaking functionality of a range of gluten-free flours. European Food Research and Technology, 229(2): 307–317.

Renzetti, S., F. Dal Bello and E.K. Arendt. 2008. Microstructure, fundamental rheology and baking characteristics of batters and breads from different gluten-free flours treated with a microbial transglutaminase. Journal of Cereal Science, 48(1): 33–45.

Repo-Carrasco, R. 2011. Andean indigenous food crops: Nutritional value and bioactive compounds. *In*: Department of Biochemistry and Food Chemistry, Vol. Ph.D., 188, Turku: University of Turku.

Repo-Carrasco, R., C. Espinoza and S.E. Jacobsen. 2003. Nutritional value and use of the andean crops quinoa (*Chenopodium quinoa*) and kaniwa (*Chenopodium pallidicaule*). Food Reviews International, 19(1-2): 179–189.

Repo–Carrasco–Valencia, R., J.K. Hellström, J. Pihlava and P.H. Mattila. 2010. Flavonoids and other phenolic compounds in Andean indigenous grains: Quinoa (*Chenopodium quinoa*), kañiwa (*Chenopodium pallidicaule*) and kiwicha (*Amaranthus caudatus*). Food Chemistry, 120: 128–133.

Resio, A.C. and C. Suarez. 2001. Gelatinization kinetics of amaranth starch. International Journal of Food Science and Technology, 36(4): 441–448.

Ribotta, P.D., S.F. Ausar, M.H. Morcillo, G.T. Perez, D.M. Beltramo and A.E. Leon. 2004. Production of gluten-free bread using soy bean flour. Journal of the Science of Food and Agriculture, 84: 1969–1974.

Rosell, C.M., G. Cortez and R. Repo–Carrasco. 2009. Breadmaking use of Andean crops quinoa, kañiwa, kiwicha, and tarwi. Cereal Chemistry, 86(4): 386–392.

Rosell, C.M., J.A. Rojas and C. Benedito De Barber. 2001. Influence of hydrocolloids on dough rheology and bread quality. Food Hydrocolloids, 15(1): 75–81.

Rosell, C.M., W. Yokoyama and C. Shoemaker. 2011. Rheology of different hydrocolloids-rice starch blends. Effect of successive heating-cooling cycles. Carbohydrate Polymers, 84(1): 373–382.

Rujner, J., J. Socha, M. Syczewska, A. Wojtasik, A. Kunachowicz and A. Stolarczyk. 2004. Magnesium status in children and adolescents with coeliac disease without malabsorption symptoms. Clinical Nutrition, 23(5): 1074–1079.

Sabanis, D. and C. Tzia. 2009. Effect of rice, corn and soy flour addition on characteristics of bread produced from different wheat cultivars. Food and Bioprocess Technology, 2(1): 68–79.

Sahi, S.S. 1994. Interfacial properties of the aqueous phases of wheat-flour doughs. Journal of Cereal Science, 20(2): 119–127.

Sakac, M., A. Torbica, I. Sedej and M. Hadnadev. 2011. Influence of breadmaking on antioxidant capacity of gluten free breads based on rice and buckwheat flours. Food Research International, 44(9): 2806–2813.

Schober, T.J., S.R. Bean and D.L. Boyle. 2007. Gluten-free sorghum bread improved by sourdough fermentation: Biochemical, rheological, and microstructural background. Journal of Agricultural and Food Chemistry, 55(13): 5137–5146.

Schober, T.J., M. Messerschmidt, S.R. Bean, S.H. Park and E.K. Arendt. 2005. Gluten-free bread from sorghum: Quality differences among hybrids. Cereal Chemistry, 82(4): 394–404.

Schoenlechner, R., S. Siebenhandl and E. Berghofer. 2008. Pseudocereals. Chapter 7 (pp. 149–190). *In:* E.K. Arendt and F.D. Bello (eds.). Gluten-free Cereal Products and Beverages. Academic Press.

Schwab, C., M. Mastrangelo, A. Corsetti and M. Gänzle. 2008. Formation of oligosaccharides and polysaccharides by *Lactobacillus reuteri* LTH5448 and *Weissella cibaria* 10M in sorghum sourdoughs. Cereal Chemistry, 85(5): 679–684.

Segura-Nieto, M., P.R. Shewry and O. Paredes-Lopez. 1999. Globulins of the pseudocereals: Amaranth, quinoa, and buckwheat. pp. 453–475. *In:* P.R. Shewry and R. Casey (eds.). Seed proteins, Springer Netherlands.

Shelton, R.D. and W.J. Lee. 2000. Cereal carbohydrates. pp. 385–416. *In:* K. Kulp (ed.). Handbook of Cereal Science and Technology, Second Edition, Revised and Expanded, Taylor & Francis, Boca Raton.

Shewry, P.R. 2002. The major seed storage proteins of spelt wheat sorghum, millets and pseudocereals. pp. 1–24. *In:* P.S. Belton and J.R.N. Taylor (eds.). Pseudocereals and less common cereals: Grain properties and utilization potential. Springer.

Shewry, P.R., B.J. Miflin and D.D. Kasarda. 1984. The structural and evolutionary relationships of the prolamin storage proteins of barley, rye and wheat. Philosophical Transactions of the Royal Society of London Series B-Biological Sciences, 304(1120): 297–308.

Shewry, P.R. 2009. Wheat. Journal of Experimental Botany, 60(6): 1537–1553.

Shukla, T.P. and W. Bushuk. 1975. Cereal proteins: Chemistry and food applications. CRC Critical Reviews in Food Science and Nutrition, 6(1): 1–75.

Shukla, R. and M. Cheryan. 2001. Zein: The industrial protein from corn. Industrial Crops and Products, 13(3): 171–192.

Singh, H., Y.H. Chang, N.S. Sodhi and N. Singh. 2011. Influence of prior acid treatment on physicochemical and structural properties of acetylated sorghum starch. Starch-Starke, 63(5): 291–301.

Singh, N., J. Singh, L. Kaur, N.S. Sodhi and B.S. Gill. 2003. Morphological, thermal and rheological properties of starches from different botanical sources. Food Chemistry, 81(2): 219–231.

Skibniewska, K., W. Kozirok, L. Fornal and K. Markiewicz. 2002. *In vivo* availability of minerals from oat products. Journal of Science of Food and Agriculture, 82: 1676–1681.

Steffolani, M.E., A.E. Leon and G.T. Perez. 2013. Study of the physicochemical and functional characterization of quinoa and kaniwa starches. Starch-Starke, 65(11-12): 976–983.

Suliburska, J., Z. Krejpcio and N. Kolaczyk. 2011. Evaluation of the content and the potential bioavailability of iron from fortified with iron and non-fortified food products. Acta Sci. Pol., Technol. Aliment, 10(2): 233–243.

Suliburska, J., Z. Krejpcio, E. Lampart-Szczapa and R.W. Wójciak. 2009. Effect of fermentation and extrusion on the release of selected minerals from lupine grain preparations. Acta Sci. Pol., Technol. Aliment, 8(3): 87–96.

Szumera, M., G. Sikorska-Wiśniewska, B. Gumkowska-Kamińska, P. Landowski and M. Korzon. 2004. Does a gluten-free diet and therapy influence a bone mineralisation in children with celiac disease? Pediatria Współczesna. Gastroenterologia, Hepatologia i Żywienie Dziecka, 6(3): 289–293.

Takaiwa, F., M. Ogawa and T.W. Okita. 1999. Rice glutelins. pp. 401–425. *In:* P.R. Shewry and R. Casey (eds.). Seed proteins, Springer Netherlands.

Tatham, A.S., R.J. Fido, C.M. Moore, D.D. Kasarda, D.D. Kuzmicky, J.N. Keen and P.R. Shewry. 1996. Characterisation of the major prolamins of tef (*Eragrostis tef*) and finger millet (*Eleusine coracana*). J. Cereal Sci., 24: 65–71.

Taylor, J.R.N., T.J. Schober and S.R. Bean. 2006. Novel food and non-food uses for sorghum and millets. Journal of Cereal Science, 44(3): 252–271.

Thanapornpoonpong, S.N., S. Vearasilp, E. Pawelzik and S. Gorinstein. 2008. Influence of various nitrogen applications on protein and amino acid profiles of amaranth and quinoa. Journal of Agricultural and Food Chemistry, 56(23): 11464–11470.

Tolstoguzov, V. 1997. Thermodynamic aspects of dough formation and functionality. Food Hydrocolloids, 11(2): 181–193.

Tolstoguzov, V. 2003. Thermodynamic considerations of starch functionality in foods. Carbohydrate Polymers, 51(1): 99–111.

U.S. Department of Agriculture, Agricultural Research Service. 2013. USDA National Nutrient Database for Standard Reference, Release 26. Nutrient Data Laboratory Home Page, http://www.ars.usda.gov/ba/bhnrc/ndl.

Van Vliet, T., A.M. Janssen, A.H. Bloksma and P. Walstra. 1992. Strain hardening of dough as a requirement for gas retention. Journal of Texture Studies, 23(4): 439–460.

Vega-Gálvez, A., M. Miranda, J. Vergara, E. Uribe, L. Puente and E.A. Martínez. 2010. Nutrition facts and functional potential of quinoa (*Chenopodium quinoa* Willd.), an ancient Andean grain: a review. J. Sci. Food Agric., 90: 2723–2726.

Venskutonis, P.R. and P. Kraujalis. 2013. Nutritional components of Amaranth seeds and vegetables: A Review on Composition, Properties, Comprehensive Reviews in Food Science and Food Safety, 12(4): 381–412.

Volta, U., G. Caio, F. Tovoli and R. De Gorgio. 2013. Non celiac gluten sensitivity: question still be answered despite increasing awereness. Cellular and Molecular Immunology, 10: 383–392.

Witczak, M., L. Juszczak, R. Ziobro and J. Korus. 2012. Influence of modified starches on properties of gluten-free dough and bread. Part I: Rheological and thermal properties of gluten-free dough. Food Hydrocolloids, 28(2): 353–360.

Witczak, M., J. Korus, R. Ziobro and L. Juszczak. 2010. The effects of maltodextrins on gluten-free dough and quality of bread. Journal of Food Engineering, 96(2): 258–265.

Wolska, P., A. Ceglinska and A. Dubicka. 2010. Production of bread using sourdoughs from gluten-free cereals. Zywnosc-Nauka Technologia Jakosc, 17(5): 104–111.

Wolter, A., A.S. Hager, E. Zannini and E.K. Arendt. 2013. *In vitro* starch digestibility and predicted glycaemic indexes of buckwheat, oat, quinoa, sorghum, teff and commercial gluten-free bread. Journal of Cereal Science, 58(3): 431–436.

Zheleznov, A.V., L.P. Solonenko and N.B. Zheleznova. 1997. Seed proteins of the wild and the cultivated *Amaranthus* species. Euphytica, 97(2): 177–182.

Ziobro, R., J. Korus, L. Juszczak and T. Witczak. 2013a. Influence of inulin on physical characteristics and staling rate of gluten-free bread. Journal of Food Engineering, 116(1): 21–27.

Ziobro, R., T. Witczak, L. Juszczak and J. Korus. 2013b. Supplementation of gluten-free bread with non-gluten proteins. Effect on dough rheological properties and bread characteristic. Food Hydrocolloids, 32(2): 213–220.

Index